D0820340

Chemical Carcinogens

Chemical Carcinogens

CHARLES E. SEARLE, Editor
Department of Cancer Studies
The Medical School
The University of Birmingham
Birmingham B15 2TJ England

ACS Monograph **173**

AMERICAN CHEMICAL SOCIETY

WASHINGTON, D. C.   1976

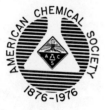

Library of Congress CIP Data

Chemical carcinogens.
  (ACS monograph; 173)
    Includes bibliographical references and index.
  1. Carcinogens. 2. Carcinogenesis.
  I. Searle, Charles E., 1922-   . II. Series: American
Chemical Society. ACS monograph; 173.
RC268.6.C48   .616.9'94'071   76-26515
ISBN 0-8412-0226-5   ACMOAG 173 1–788(1976)

Fourth Printing (corrected) 1978

GENERAL INTRODUCTION

American Chemical Society's Series of Chemical Monographs

By arrangement with the interallied Conference of Pure and Applied Chemistry, which met in London and Brussels in July 1919, the American Chemical Society undertook the production and publication of Scientific and Technologic Monographs on chemical subjects. At the same time it was agreed that the National Research Council, in cooperation with the American Chemical Society and the American Physical Society, should undertake the production and publication of Critical Tables of Chemical and Physical Constants. The American Chemical Society and the National Research Council mutually agreed to care for these two fields of chemical progress.

The Council of the American Chemical Society, acting through its Committee on National Policy, appointed editors and associates (the present list of whom appears at the close of this sketch) to select authors of competent authority in their respective fields and to consider critically the manuscripts submitted. Since 1944 the Scientific and Technologic Monographs have been combined in the Series. The first Monograph appeared in 1921, and up to 1972, 168 treatises have enriched the Series.

These Monographs are intended to serve two principal purposes: first to make available to chemists a thorough treatment of a selected area in form usable by persons working in more or less unrelated fields to the end that they may correlate their own work with a larger area of physical science; secondly, to stimulate further research in the specific field treated. To implement this purpose the authors of Monographs give extended references to the literature.

American Chemical Society
F. Marshall Beringer
Editor of Monographs

EDITORIAL BOARD

Contents

Preface

"HOW NEAR ARE WE to finding a cure for cancer?" is a question which workers in any field of cancer research are frequently asked. This perhaps illustrates several common misconceptions—that cancer is a single disease; that a single cancer cure will, once found, be capable of curing every new case of cancer; and that cancer research is only concerned with the search for this cure.

The term "cancer" covers, in fact, a wide range of disease entities affecting every organ of the body; some commonly, others only rarely. However, the cells constituting the cancers share in differing degrees the common characteristic of being unresponsive to the delicate controls that govern the healthy cells of the body—controls which ensure, for example, that the rapid cell proliferation which occurs in a wound ceases when the healing process is complete. In a malignant tumor the rate of cell growth exceeds the rate of cell death, and invasion and destruction of adjoining healthy tissue occurs. Surgical removal of such a tumor is, sadly, often only palliative since small fragments are commonly shed and dispersed to other parts of the body where some of them then give rise to secondary deposits (metastases).

The various forms of cancer differ greatly in the ease with which they can be successfully treated by the three main established techniques—surgery, radiotherapy, and chemotherapy. Cancer of the skin, common in white races exposed to powerful sunlight or resulting from occupational exposure to some oils and tars, can be treated with a high rate of success because the site is accessible and early diagnosis is possible. Two other forms which are now treatable with considerable success are choriocarcinoma, which affects a small proportion of women after childbirth, and Burkitt lymphoma, a disease afflicting particularly children in certain tropical areas. Both these conditions may respond rapidly and apparently permanently to treatment with drugs such as methotrexate or cyclophosphamide. It must be admitted, however, that these are somewhat special cases; choriocarcinoma is a tumor derived from fetal tissue and not from the mother while the Burkitt lymphoma is at present the cancer with the strongest evidence for being caused by a virus. The virus concerned, Epstein–Barr (EB) virus, has a worldwide distribution. Although it is normally responsible only for infectious mononucleosis (glandular fever), is can apparently also cause Burkitt lymphoma in a proportion of people whose immune system has been severely disturbed by malarial infection.

Other cancers differ greatly in their responsiveness to drug therapy. Those relatively sensitive include Hodgkin's disease, lymphosarcoma, and tumors of the ovary and testis while intestinal, breast, head and neck tumors, and melanoma are less responsive. Because of the widely held pessimistic views of the outcome of cancer treatment, however, it is worth mentioning that the International Union Against Cancer (UICC) quotes five-year survival rates of better than 50% for a considerable range of cancers detected at an early stage and still better than 25% for all stages. It is a tragedy of our time that tumors of the lungs and bronchi, among the most difficult to treat successfully, are now not only so common as to constitute an epidemic in many "Western" countries, particularly in Britain, but also are believed beyond reasonable doubt to be almost entirely caused by tobacco smoking and, hence, preventable. The incidence of this disease is still rising (British doctors, who smoke less than formerly, represent one group in which it is falling), and its prevention is now a social and behavioral problem rather than a medical one. Very recently, there has been growing interest in the evidence that tobacco smoking causes physical harm not only in smokers themselves but also in those (sometimes called "passive smokers") obliged to inhale the tobacco fumes.

Whatever future improvements are made in treating cancer by drugs, radiation, surgery, and/or immunological procedures, at present it seems improbable that a single mode of treatment ("the cure for cancer") will be found applicable to each and every variety of the disease. Much more likely is a continued stepwise progression in which some forms of cancer become amenable to improved procedures earlier than others. This is the process we have already seen with, for example, skin cancer and choriocarcinoma and are probably beginning to see with some forms of leukemia.

However, if such a universal cure were to become available this week, it would still be immeasurably better to prevent cancer from arising in the first instance wherever it is possible. That successful treatment of so much established cancer remains beyond our present capability makes prevention that much more vital.

Cancer Causation and Prevention

Not too long ago, the idea that a significant amount of human cancer might be preventable was barely considered. Sir Richard Doll quoted a professor of surgery who remarked that it was not only a waste of time but also faintly immoral to try to prevent cancer! However, epidemiological studies have revealed such enormous differences in the incidence of cancer between different localities that it has become difficult, if not impossible, to escape the conclusion that a major proportion of human cancer is of environmental origin.

That certain types of cancer are much commoner in some localities than in others has long been evident from comparisons of death rates (mortality). However, some cancers are much more easily diagnosed and treated than others, and therefore, building up a reliable global picture of the actual occurrence of the different types of cancer requires the collection of data on all diagnosed cases of cancer (morbidity) irrespective of their subsequent treatment and survival. For this purpose there now exists a large and growing number of cancer registries throughout the world furnishing data which are collated by the UICC.

In some countries registration of each case is compulsory while in others it depends on the voluntary cooperation of the clinicians responsible for the diagnosis. Where confidentiality prevents the inclusion of the patient's name, reliable morbidity studies are not at present possible.

In 1966 it was possible for the UICC to publish a volume, "Cancer Incidence in Five Continents," based on data from 32 registries. For the second volume, published in 1970, the number of collaborating registries had risen to 44, and it is now nearly double that number. The largest part of the 1970 volume consists of tables which list, for each registry area and for each of some 40 sites of cancer, computer-calculated incidence rates per 100,000 population for each five-year age group and also for all ages. Since there are differences in age distribution between the populations and also differences in the way in which the incidence of different cancers varies with age these incidence rates are then standardized in several ways to enable valid comparisons to be made between different registry areas. A selection of incidence data, age-standardized to a world population, is presented in Table I. The data, which are from 12 registry areas and for 8 important cancer sites, show how completely the cancer pattern in one locality can differ from that in another.

It will be seen that some registries cover entire countries (e.g., Denmark, Puerto Rico) and others well-defined parts of countries (the Birmingham region of the United Kingdom, Bombay in India, etc.). Some registries (e.g., California, Hawaii) present separate data for the different ethnic groups within their boundaries, making possible some particularly valuable studies of populations which now live remote from their countries of origin. For example, the table shows that the black population of one area of California develops more esophageal and prostate cancer but less rectal and breast cancer than the white population of the same area. Very significantly, however, the overall cancer patterns of the black population here and in Puerto Rico differ greatly from that found in the Ibadan area of Nigeria. Similarly, the incidence of cancer in the Japanese population of Hawaii differs not only from that in other inhabitants of Hawaii but also greatly from that in Japan itself. Though it is a slow process, the cancer patterns of migrant populations tend to shift towards those characteristic of the new environment. In the case of the Hawaii Japanese, this is towards more colorectal, breast, and prostate cancer but with a marked fall from the exceptionally high rate of stomach cancer which occurs in Japan.

By field surveys in areas much smaller than those covered by the usual statistics, even more striking differences in cancer incidence can be brought to light. There are numerous localized areas in the Transkei of South Africa, in East Africa and in areas bordering the Caspian Sea where the incidence of esophageal cancer is higher than anywhere in the world while within a few miles live other communities in which the disease is virtually unknown. In the Transkei the intensity of esophageal cancer is apparently of quite recent origin, and a correlation has been noted with mineral impoverishment of the soil and resultant poor crops, although various other dietary factors also come under suspicion as possible causative factors.

Table I. Average Annual Cancer Incidence Rates/100,000

Site and Incidence of Primary Tumors

Geographical Area	Years	Esoph-agus	Stomach	Colon
U.S., California,				
Alameda County: white	1960–64	4.1	15.3	24.0
black	1960–64	10.2	24.4	14.1
Puerto Rico	1964–66	17.5	28.6	4.9
Nigeria, Ibadan	1960–65	0.8	8.0	1.2
U.S., Hawaii:				
Filipino	1960–64	2.2	9.7	12.6
Caucasian	1960–64	5.7	16.9	19.3
Hawaiian	1960–64	14.3	45.9	20.2
Chinese	1960–64	7.6	9.5	35.9
Japanese	1960–64	6.8	47.6	20.7
Japan, Miyagi prefecture	1962–64	14.5	95.3	4.1
Canada, Quebec	1963–66	3.4	15.7	15.6
U.K., Birmingham region	1963–66	4.7	25.2	15.3
Denmark	1958–62	3.3	27.5	15.5
Germany, Democratic Republic	1964–66	2.8	36.8	8.2
Poland, Katowice district	1965–66	3.8	30.6	4.7
Yugoslavia, Slovenia	1961–65	6.4	46.1	5.7
India, Bombay	1964–66	13.0	10.0	4.1

[a] Source of data: R. Doll, C. Muir, J. Waterhouse (Eds.), "Cancer Incidence in Five Continents," Vol. II, Springer-Verlag for the International Union Against Cancer, 1970.

If it is accepted that the great geographical differences in cancer incidence are evidence for the environmental origin of much human cancer, we are led to the view that we should be able to identify some of the important factors responsible and hopefully to effect significant reductions in the human burden of cancer. This is a goal for which the extensive knowledge of chemical carcinogenesis already acquired is of paramount importance.

How much cancer in man is in fact caused by exposure to chemical substances? It is unfortunately still not possible to give even an approximate answer to this important question, although some authorities suggest that the proportion of chemically induced cancers could be as high as 90%. To a considerable extent the answer depends on the outcome of much current research into a possible viral etiology for a range of human cancers, particularly leukemias and cancer of the breast, cervix, and nasopharynx, in addition to the Burkitt lymphoma mentioned earlier. Certainly, viruses can induce cancer in many animal species, and we have no reason to suppose man is exempt.

On the other hand, exposure to chemical materials is known to cause a range of occupational cancers, mainly of the skin, bladder, lungs, and nasal sinuses while chemical carcinogens and co-carcinogens in tobacco smoke seem likely to be the chief causes of non-occupational respiratory cancer.

Site and Incidence of Primary Tumors

Rectum	Bronchus and Trachea	Urinary Bladder	Prostate	Breast[b]	All Sites
15.5	47.8	17.9	38.0	62.4	254.1
4.9	43.8	10.9	65.3	38.6	251.1
3.7	13.6	7.6	17.2	20.9	205.0
0.5	1.2	2.9	9.7	13.7	76.7
12.4	17.1	1.5	17.6	19.5	131.0
12.6	43.8	19.3	43.4	62.9	265.1
6.8	70.3	9.9	30.0	52.3	313.6
15.8	27.2	9.4	9.8	44.3	207.0
11.7	26.3	9.0	13.9	23.0	207.6
4.8	15.6	4.7	3.2	11.0	196.0
10.7	28.7	12.1	21.1	48.7	209.3
15.8	73.3	11.5	18.4	51.1	254.5
17.2	31.4	12.4	19.5	44.9	221.1
9.5	48.8	6.5	12.6	28.6	211.7
5.9	29.4	4.6	4.6	17.0	136.3
8.2	38.5	5.3	13.1	22.8	204.1
4.3	13.3	2.3	6.5	20.4	139.5

[b] In females only; all others in males only.

Moreover, our knowledge of chemical carcinogenesis in animals enables us to theorize, if not to prove, that many other human cancers could have chemical causes. This view has become more plausible since the recognition relatively recently of the versatile and potent nitroso carcinogens, some of which can be formed adventiously in the environment, and of the remarkable variety of strongly carcinogenic compounds which occur naturally in some fungi and higher plants.

As used here, the term "carcinogen" refers simply to an agent, exposure to which results in the eventual appearance of cancer which would not have occurred in the absence of such exposure. This makes no implication about its mode of action, in particular whether chemical carcinogens are capable of initiating malignant change by direct action or only by some indirect mechanism involving, for example, activation of latent oncogenic viruses, derepression of genes, or interference with normal immunologic defenses against malignancy.

Having referred briefly to viral carcinogenesis, reference should also be made here to physical carcinogenesis and to certain intrinsic factors influencing the appearance of cancer. It is well known that cancer can be induced in man by radiation in various ways. X-rays caused skin cancer and leukemia in early x-ray workers, ingestion of radium resulted in bone cancer in luminous dial painters, radiation from the atomic bombs released over Japan caused leukemia and later solid tumors in some survivors while skin cancer is a common malignancy in white races living in areas of intense sunlight. The carcinogenic action of ionizing radiation is, of course, a major reason why stringent safety precautions are necessary in occupations involving use of x-rays or radioactive materials.

The development of connective tissue tumors in rodents at the site of implanted plastic or metal films is also sometimes regarded as a form of physical carcinogenesis. This effect, which has an obvious bearing on the safety of implanted materials in surgical practice, depends on the dimensions of the film and on whether it is intact or perforated much more than on its chemical nature. Though these topics are outside the scope of this volume, chemical and physical carcinogenesis may become more closely linked in the future as we gain a greater understanding of the primary events occurring in malignant change.

Certain genetic abnormalities are associated with an increased risk of cancer. Thus, individuals with Down's syndrome (mongolism) in which an additional number 21 chromosome is present in each cell, have an enhanced risk of contracting leukemia. Sufferers from xeroderma pigmentosum, in which DNA repair mechanisms are defective, have a high risk of skin cancer, the actual direct cause being the ultraviolet component of sun light. Reduced competence of the body's immune system, whether arising from other rare genetic conditions or from treatment with immunosuppressive drugs, is also associated with increased risk of certain cancers. Immunosuppression is also an effect of a number of chemical carcinogens, a factor of possible significance in chemical carcinogenesis.

There is some evidence that first degree relatives of breast cancer patients may have an above average risk of the same cancer only, but such associations could arise from common exposure to environmental factors and, as far as the commoner cancers are concerned, there is no evidence that an overall susceptibility is inherited. Nevertheless, the individual's genetic makeup must still be of considerable importance in determining the outcome of exposure to environmental carcinogenic influences, except perhaps in those instances where exposure is so great that genetic factors become unimportant. It now seems increasingly likely that cancer, in the large majority of cases, results from the operation of a multiplicity of factors.

Recognition and Modification of Carcinogenic Activity

Our first leads to some major classes of chemical carcinogens came from the recognition of their effects on man—polynuclear aromatic carcinogens through occupational skin cancer, aromatic amines through occupational bladder cancer, and N-nitroso carcinogens less directly as a result of liver injury in a few exposed workers. The great majority of individual carcinogens are recognized, however, because they have induced cancer in experimental animals. Animals have generally been the small, easily bred, relatively cheap laboratory rats and mice. Even with these, life span tests still take two to three years to complete. Many other species, such as hamsters, rabbits, and newts, have also been used, but for obvious reasons utilization of animals such as dogs, pigs, or primates, has been much more restricted.

Many carcinogens are very potent, and identifying activity in these is relatively simple since a high proportion of treated animals will develop tumors within a few months. Carcinogens, however, differ enormously in their potency, and the difficulties of establishing carcinogenic activity increase as the potency of the substance decreases. To recognize weak carcinogens many more experimental and control animals are needed, the tests become more prolonged and increasingly expensive, and difficulties can still arise through inability to distinguish tumors induced by the test substance from a background of so-called spontaneous tumors. Nevertheless, it may still be very important to know whether or not a compound has even weak carcinogenicity if problems of human exposure are involved. Cyclamates, DDT, 8-hydroxyquinoline, and chloroform are just a few examples that come to mind.

Many instances are known of marked species differences in response to chemical carcinogens. Perhaps the most striking is that of the aromatic amines which are bladder carcinogens for man but affect other organs in most experimental animals. The potent agent of this class 2-fluorenylacetamide (2-acetamidofluorene) is actually inactive in the guinea pig, which metabolizes it without the vital step of N-hydroxylation which in other species leads to carcinogenesis. In mice especially, even different inbred strains differ greatly in their responses to carcinogens of various types and in their incidence of spontaneous tumors.

However, the resistance of the guinea pig to some carcinogens is rather a special case, and it has to be assumed that a substance shown to be carcinogenic in test animals is potentially a carcinogen for man also. The problem then arises of estimating the degree of hazard to man of exposure to a carcinogen at relative dose levels generally much smaller than those needed to give meaningful results in animal tests. What is the cancer risk to man, for instance, from the small traces of nitrosamines which sensitive analytical techniques find in various foods? Obviously, we must take all practicable steps to reduce human exposure to carcinogens to the minimum possible, but we probably will have to accept that complete elimination of all measurable carcinogens in the environment is an unrealistic and perhaps pointless objective.

For practical as well as humane reasons we would like to be able to recognize carcinogens reliably without carrying out prolonged animal experiments. Many *in vitro* tests have been devised, and in recent years much work has been done on carcinogenesis *in vitro*, in which cultured cells are "transformed" by carcinogen treatment into cells with more characteristics of malignant behavior. Before long, combined *in vivo/in vitro* tests may overcome some, but probably not all, disadvantages of such systems. Rapid *in vitro* screening tests of great current interest use mutant forms of bacteria, which are exposed to test chemicals alone or in the presence of enzymic metabolizing systems. Reversion to forms which can grow and form colonies in the absence of nutrients originally required is evidence for mutagenicity of the test chemical or a metabolite, a property which increasingly appears to correlate with carcinogenicity. Very recently these tests have become a focus of publicity and some controversy with the independent discovery by American and British workers that a high proportion of proprietary hair dyes are strongly mutagenic in the bacterial systems at a time when there is negligible information available on the carcinogenicity of the dyes or their constituents in animal systems. Even when carcinogenicity is firmly established by laboratory experiments there remain, of course, the problems already referred to of extrapolating these results to man, emphasizing the great importance of carrying out epidemiological studies directly on man wherever practicable.

In practice, exposure to a carcinogen is not simple, but subject to modification by a variety of influences which may act to increase or decrease the net carcinogenic effect. A pitfall in testing a carcinogen or a potential antitumor drug is that tumor development and growth may be inhibited by a general toxic action or by simple restriction of food intake, and many experiments have shown that administration of various chemicals can inhibit the action of carcinogens. Conversely, it has long been known that the effects of minimal amounts of carcinogens may be greatly magnified by the action of other substances (co-carcinogens) which may not themselves by carcinogenic. This is a phenomenon investigated particularly as a facet of skin carcinogenesis, and the effects of skin carcinogens in, for example, industrial mineral oils are thought to be considerably influenced by other substances present in the complex mixtures to which workers are exposed. It is also easier to understand the induction of human lung cancer (Chapter 7) if the effects of small amounts of polynuclear aromatic or other carcinogens are magnified by the co-carcinogens which are known also to be present in tobacco smoke (Chapter 2).

One field that is particularly complex concerns hormonal influences on chemical and viral carcinogenesis and on tumor growth. A prerequisite of significant enlightenment here may be a much better understanding of hormonal actions in the healthy organism.

Separate reviews are presented in this book on carcinogenicity testing, co-carcinogenesis, and hormonal influences on cancer, in Chapters 1, 2, and 3 respectively. It is appropriate here to draw attention to a quantitative aspect of carcinogenesis. It is an interesting and important point that, in a number of cases studied in detail, the response to a carcinogen is a function of the total carcinogen dose (d) and of the duration of exposure (t) raised to a power in the approximate range 2 to 6. It thus follows that long exposure to a carcinogen may be much more effective than exposure to the same amount over a shorter period. The significance of the exponent n in the equation $(dt^n = \text{constant})$ in relation to the primary events in the initiation of carcinogenesis is discussed in Chapter 4.

Alkylating Agents

Compounds of this type react directly, or nearly so, with nucleophilic centers in various biological macromolecules, resulting in vesicant and other toxic actions and, in a considerable number of known cases, in mutagenic and carcinogenic activities. Elucidation of their biological action is of fundamental importance to an understanding of the action of carcinogens of other types, and a major part of Chapter 4 is therefore devoted to a review of this field.

This is followed by a survey of the large range of alkylating agents that have been tested for mutagenic and carcinogenic activities. Many compounds of this varied class have important industrial uses and some of these, such as β-propiolactone and 1,3-propane sultone, are known from animal experiments to possess a considerable degree of carcinogenic activity. In man, some cases of lung cancer have been attributed to occupational exposure to mustard gas, some chlorinated ethers, and possibly methyl sulfate. However, as there is still relatively little known about the carcinogenic effects of these agents in man, this aspect of the subject is included with the main review.

Vinyl chloride, the raw material of a major part of the plastics industry, has recently come under intensive scrutiny as the cause of the normally very rare angiosarcoma of the liver in some exposed workmen. Though as an alkyl halide it bears a formal relationship to some alkylating carcinogens, it probably has an entirely different biological action (*see* Chapters 4, 7).

Occupational Skin Cancer and Polycyclic Aromatic Hydrocarbons

Almost invariably, the history of chemical carcinogenesis is taken as starting just two centuries ago when the London surgeon Percivall Pott recognized that cancer of the scrotum in chimney sweeps was an occupational disease which resulted from prolonged contact of the skin with soot. Remarkably for that time, this was followed only three years later by rules requiring Danish chimney sweeps to bath daily, an early health measure that has been said to have done more to prevent human cancer than the efforts of many research workers.

Soot is, of course, an extremely complex mixture of chemical substances. Among these are many polycyclic aromatic compounds possessing various degrees of carcinogenic activity (Chapter 5), and similar compounds to which man has been exposed have been held responsible for skin cancer in other occupations such as shale oil distillation, mule spinning in the cotton industry, and, still a significant hazard at the present time, in workmen in contact with cutting oils in engineering industries. The long-continued hazards of exposure to such materials and the possible return of shale oil to a position of importance in some areas fully justify the inclusion of the separate treatment of these materials as occupational cancer hazards given in Chapter 6.

It is less certain that the association of respiratory cancer with tobacco smoke and air pollution is caused by inhalation of carcinogens of this type, but with no firm evidence incriminating other classes of carcinogen, it seems most logical for respiratory carcinogenesis by smoking and other environmental factors to be considered in the following Chapter 7.

The first pure compounds recognized as chemical carcinogens some 45 years ago were the polycyclic aromatic hydrocarbons benzo[*a*]pyrene (formerly 3,4-benzopyrene) and dibenz[*a,h*]anthracene (1,2,5,6-dibenzanthracene). With several related compounds, these have ever since held a central place in cancer research and have been the source of endless speculation as to their importance as causes of human cancer other than those already mentioned. It has proved much more difficult than with more recently discovered carcinogens to elucidate their mode of action, in particular whether they are active in the body *per se* or only after metabolism to an ultimate carcinogen. It is fortunate that the review of the chemistry and biology of these important carcinogens (Chapter 5) has been written at a time when our knowledge of their metabolism has been advancing rapidly, although important questions still remain unanswered.

Occupational Bladder Cancer and Aromatic Amines

Another observation of an occupational cancer hazard led to recognition of the aromatic amine carcinogens such as 2-(or beta-)naphthylamine, 4-biphenylamine (4-aminobiphenyl), and benzidine (4,4′-diaminobiphenyl) (Chapter 8). Tumors are induced by these carcinogens in man predominantly in the urinary bladder, and, although Rehn's original observations were made in the German dyestuffs industry in the 1890's, occupational bladder cancer later became a serious problem in the chemical, rubber, and cable industries in a number of countries (Chapter 9) and necessitated legislation to protect workers.

Laboratory usage of these carcinogens, such as analytical procedures using benzidine and other carcinogens, also poses problems of personnel protection as described in Chapter 10. Hazards of this type arise in a range of occupations from analysts in hospital and other laboratories to students in colleges and even in schools and, although on a smaller scale than in manufacturing industries, cause particular concern where exposure of young persons with a long life expectancy is involved.

As with the polycyclic aromatic carcinogens, intense effort has gone into elucidating the action of the carcinogenic aromatic amines. Recognition of N-hydroxylation as the key step in conversion of the ingested amine to the active metabolite eventually led to rapid progress, and the close parallels now apparent between the biological actions of carcinogenic aromatic amines, nitro compounds, and azo dyes now make it possible to treat this major group of carcinogens in a unified way that would not have been possible a few years ago (Chapter 8).

N-Nitroso Carcinogens and Related Compounds

One of the major landmarks in the history of chemical carcinogenesis was the recognition in 1956 that N-nitrosodimethylamine (dimethylnitrosamine) is a strong carcinogen. The compound was under investigation because a number of men who had been using it as a solvent in their work had suffered from its severe toxic action on the liver. This discovery led to important developments in various directions. It was soon found that, in the range of open chain and cyclic nitrosamines tested in the following years, strong carcinogenicity is the rule rather than the exception. Further, the compounds show marked predilections for tumor induction in specific organs (organotropic action), and in a number of organs it became possible to induce tumors for the first time using carcinogens administered systemically rather than by direct application. The specific induction of tumors of the esophagus by certain dialkylnitrosamines administered intravenously is an unexpected and particularly good example of this and of an experimental discovery in this field with implications for cancer causation in man.

The closely related nitrosamide carcinogens, particularly N-ethyl-N-nitrosourea, have attracted great attention on account of their remarkable efficiency in inducing tumors of the brain and other parts of the nervous system in some species and by the special sensitivity of the nervous system to such agents in the periods shortly before and after birth. These discoveries may reasonably be compared with the thalidomide tragedy in the way in which they have focused attention on the vulnerability of the fetus to injury by agents reaching it through the maternal circulation. Ethylnitrosourea is, in fact, also teratogenic earlier in pregnancy, although it should not be assumed that these actions necessarily go together. Cancer induction in this way (transplacental carcinogenesis) may be considerably important in man, particularly with respect to cancer in childhood. Carcinogens of the nitrosourea type have not, however, been incriminated, and there is at present only one well authenticated example of human transplacental carcinogenesis in which the normal rarity of the disease facilitated its recognition. This is the occurrence of vaginal cancer in some 14–22-year old girls whose mothers had been treated with large doses of the synthetic hormone diethylstilbestrol during pregnancy (Chapters 3, 13).

The technical and patent literature contains proposed uses for nitroamines, both carcinogenic and inactive, in a variety of fields such as plastics, rubber, lubricants, pesticides, and chemical manufacture, and there seems no doubt that many such uses would represent considerable carcinogenic hazards to personnel. It is surely amazing that a review published as recently as 1971, which acknowledges the toxic and carcinogenic properties of nitrosamines, should not only refer to their uses in industrial processes but also describe the application of N-nitrosodimethylamine to food crops at 56–112 kg/hectare to counter nematode infection. There seems to be little available information on the extent to which nitrosamines are in fact used commercially, but in any event patenting or publication of such proposed uses has presumably been preceded by developmental work with associated health hazards unrecognized at the time by those involved.

At the present time, however, the main interest in nitroso carcinogen hazards is concerned not with their deliberate use but with their inadvertent formation from the ready interaction of amino compounds and nitrite. The much quoted incident which pinpointed this problem in 1961–62 was the poisoning of Norwegian sheep fed on nitrite-preserved fishmeal, which was subsequently found to contain highly toxic amounts of dialkylnitrosamines. Not surprisingly, much work has since been carried out to investigate the possibilities of nitrosamine contamination of food for human consumption.

Nitrosamines can also be formed by amine–nitrite interaction inside the body—another aspect of this field that is now receiving considerable attention. Some of the amines shown to generate nitroso derivatives in this way are normal food constituents derived from protein breakdown, while others are chemicals administered as drugs, for example, the vermifuge piperazine and the appetite suppressant phenmetrazine. Contrary to the widely held view, nitrosation of tertiary amines can also occur with elimination of one of the original substituent groups. This greatly extends the range of substances which have to be considered as potential nitroso carcinogen precursors. For some tertiary amines rather drastic conditions are necessary to obtain a significant degree of nitrosation *in vitro*, but *in vivo* reactions may possibly be facilitated by bacterial action as is known to occur with secondary amines. Concurrent administration to rats of nitrite and the analgesic aminopyrine, containing a dimethylamino group on the pyrazolone ring but no secondary nitrogen atom, has resulted in severe liver damage and death, the pathological effects being apparently identical with those caused by administering N-nitrosodimethyl-amine itself. Is this test now one that should be routinely carried out on all drugs in which nitrosamine formation is a possibility or can such drugs and nitrite be reliably kept apart?

Perhaps this monograph should have had a separate section devoted to the many facets of the nitrosamine hazard problem. In the event, however, such hazards are considered in the main review of these and related carcinogens in Chapter 11, but some aspects particularly relevant to foods are also discussed later with other carcinogens in foods (Chapter 14).

Naturally Occurring Carcinogens

The organic carcinogens so far mentioned are generally regarded as being made by man, sometimes intentionally as with industrial chemicals, sometimes inadvertently as with the polycyclic aromatic compounds formed by the action of heat on organic materials during incomplete combustion. There is in addition a range of carcinogens of quite different types found in the plant world. Apart from their great intrinsic interest these may also, in a number of cases, be of considerable importance as causes of human cancer.

The main growth of this field has taken place since 1960 when many young poultry in Britain died after being fed groundnut meal contaminated with *Aspergillus flavus*. This fungus produces as metabolites a group of compounds named aflatoxins, one of which, aflatoxin B_1, is currently the most potent chemical carcinogen known. The possible hazards for man of consuming similarly contaminated foods are obvious, and there is some epidemiological evidence from Africa linking the incidence of primary liver cancer with the aflatoxin content of the food.

Carcinogenic alkaloids based on the pyrrolizidine nucleus occur in plants of the *Senecio* and other species. These are also possible causes of human cancer, again particularly in Africa where they may be consumed for medicinal purposes or in times of food shortage. Cycasin is a potent toxic and carcinogenic agent present in Cycads, although in areas where these are used for food, methods of first removing the toxins are practiced.

Bracken fern produces an agent which causes acute poisoning or bladder tumors in cattle, depending on the amounts ingested. In experimental animals intestinal tumors also result from bracken feeding. The toxin could be one cause of human cancer in countries where bracken is eaten, possibly also where milk from cattle on bracken-infested pastureland is consumed. Moreover, if some recent observations are substantiated, bracken may have provided the first recognized case of cancer being induced in higher animals by the synergistic action of a chemical carcinogen and a virus. Bladder cancer caused by bracken is generally only seen in old cattle, but in Scotland two-year old cattle have recently been found with malignant esophageal tumors closely associated with virally induced papillomas, and the time of appearance of the tumors strongly suggests that bracken consumption is the additional factor which precipitates malignancy. A quite unexpected and potentially important finding during recent bracken research has been the discovery of carcinogenic and mutagenic activity in shikimic acid, an intermediate on the normal metabolic pathway to aromatic amino acids in plants.

Different aspects of these significant and intriguing natural carcinogens are described in several chapters of this book. Cycasin is a glycoside of methylazoxymethanol, an azomethane derivative with a biological action closely resembling that of N-nitrosodimethylamine. Cycasin and some related natural carcinogens are therefore described chiefly in Chapter 11, immediately after the nitroso and related carcinogens. This is followed (Chapter 12) by accounts of aflatoxins, pyrrolizidine alkaloids, and several other groups of natural carcinogens. The rationale of treating these compounds together is based purely on their occurrence in the plant world. Structurally the types differ greatly from each other and from carcinogens of other classes, and they are also generally more complex than the carcinogens described in other sections of this book. The chemical identity of the bracken carcinogen remains elusive, and Chapter 13 is an account of this fascinating but frustrating field by the leading worker who has been involved from its inception. The co-carcinogenic phorbol esters from croton oil were also described earlier in Chapter 2. Hazards arising from the presence of some of these materials in foods are referred to also in Chapter 14.

A relatively recent but important aspect of disease prevention may appropriately be referred to here, though it is not included in this monograph. In a series of lectures and papers (*see*, for example, *J. Amer. Med. Ass.* (1974) **229**, 1068) Burkitt and his colleagues discussed the range of degenerative diseases which afflict almost exclusively those living in advanced technological societies and which may reasonably be attributed in large measure to dietary factors. They consider that the significant factor is the almost complete lack of undigestible fiber in the diet of the advanced countries. Tests in many subjects in different localities have shown that a typical native African high fiber diet results in the daily passage of feces weighing some 400 g and with a total intestinal "transit time" of under $1\frac{1}{2}$ days. Comparable measurements for English volunteers resulted in little more than 100 g with transit times of 3–$3\frac{1}{2}$ days.

As a result of his studies in a hitherto unpopular field of research, Burkitt believes that this greatly retarded passage with its associated changes in bacteria, chemical composition, and pressure of the intestinal contents, is the major factor directly and indirectly responsible for a variety of ills such as appendicitis, diverticulosis of the colon, coronary heart disease, and (of more direct relevance here) cancer of the colon and rectum.

Other workers have demonstrated the great differences in the types of intestinal bacteria and content of steroids between countries with high and low incidence of these cancers, and there is an apparent direct correlation between the incidence of colon cancer in different countries and intestinal levels of deoxycholic acid. If confirmed, this would indicate a connection between a major form of cancer and an abnormal degree of exposure to an entirely natural substance of animal origin, which in tests many years ago gave evidence of being weakly carcinogenic. The possible metabolism of steroids in the intestine to compounds of the polycyclic aromatic hydrocarbon type is, however, another possibility under consideration.

Other writers have placed greater emphasis on other characteristics in the Western way of life as causes of disease, such as excessive consumption of protein, saturated fats, and refined sugar or insufficient vitamin C and physical activity. Extension of work in these areas, in which cooperation of human volunteers on controlled diets is practicable and particularly valuable, should make it possible to evaluate the significance of these various factors in our diet. This might then show the way not only to prevent some important forms of cancer but to effect great improvements in health generally. It certainly seems sensible, as Burkitt has urged, to examine the broad picture of environment in relation to disease, rather than to focus attention too closely on single environmental factors or on single disease entities.

Inorganic Carcinogenic Materials

A range of occupations in mineral mining and refining have been found to possess associated risks of cancer development, particularly in the lungs and nasal sinuses. Much of our knowledge in this field has come directly from investigations of the human situation rather than from laboratory experimentation. Many metals and their compounds have been tested for carcinogenicity in experimental animals, sometimes being administered by inhalation but often by routes such as subcutaneous or intramuscular injection. Such routes bear little relationship to the conditions of human exposure, but may still be of great value in extending our understanding of the mechanisms of tumor induction. The metal of outstanding carcinogenicity both for man and in animal experiments has been nickel. Connective tissue tumors arise in the vicinity of deposited sparingly soluble materials like nickel sulfide and oxide, soluble compounds showing toxic but not carcinogenic effects. Metallic salts administered in the diet have generally proved to be noncarcinogenic. It is particularly regretted that no account of these important aspects of chemical carcinogenesis could be included in this monograph.

A special case of an inorganic carcinogen is the fibrous mineral asbestos, mined in a number of forms and used in an extremely wide range of applications. Unfortunately, inhalation of its dust gives rise to asbestosis and cancer of the lung and, after a longer latent period, to mesothelioma of the pleura and peritoneum. Mesothelioma is for all practical purposes a tumor exclusively associated with asbestos exposure and, although rare, is becoming commoner. As with plastic film carcinogenesis, the shape and dimensions of the fibers seem to be more important than their chemical nature, and it has recently been found that glass fibers can also cause tumors if sufficiently fine. Chapter 15 reviews the asbestos cancer problem.

The practical problems of preventing occupational cancer are very different in the mineral sphere. At least until the recent recognition of vinyl chloride as an occupational carcinogen, it has been possible to find alternatives to dangerous industrial substances such as 2-naphthylamine without undue disruption of manufacture or to avoid introduction of substances such as 2-fluorenylacetamide into the environment. Technological societies depend so heavily on materials such as asbestos, nickel, and chromium, however, that prevention of their associated diseases must be largely a matter of ensuring high standards of occupational hygiene so as to avoid ingestion of dusts and fumes by personnel.

Mechanisms of Carcinogenesis

The important classes of chemical carcinogen recognized relatively early, the polycyclic aromatic hydrocarbons and aromatic amines, differ greatly in their chemical nature, and as the range of known carcinogens grew to include further widely differing types, such as the nitrosamines, aflatoxins, and asbestos, it became increasingly difficult to believe that they could share any underlying common mechanism of action.

This trend has been reversed in recent years, in large measure because essential steps in the metabolism of the aromatic amines have been elucidated. It now appears that most or all carcinogens are either potent electrophilic reactants or are converted by metabolic changes to such reactants. This may be a reflection of the fact that most active sites in biological macromolecules are nucleophilic centers, but it nevertheless appears to bring considerable order into a confused situation. An account of this coordinating view of chemical carcinogenesis has been written by its principal proponents in the concluding Chapter 16.

Dealing primarily with the metabolism of ingested cancer-inducing chemicals (referred to as "precarcinogens" by some authors and "procarcinogens" by others) to proximate and ultimate carcinogens, Chapter 16 may be regarded as complementary with the earlier part of the account of alkylating agents (Chapter 4) which reviews the way in which such agents, once formed, interact with biological macromolecules. DNA is commonly regarded as the most important target as far as mutagenesis is concerned and probably for carcinogenesis also. However, we have still not arrived at an understanding of the significant action of an ultimate carcinogen at the molecular level, of the relationships between carcinogenic and mutagenic activity, or of the fundamental distinguishing features of cancer cells which result in such profound changes of behavior in the body.

Some Practical Aspects of Chemical Carcinogens

Chemical carcinogenesis poses so many intriguing problems that its study would no doubt attract many research workers even if it had no direct relevance to present-day life. The accounts of the different aspects of chemical carcinogenesis which follow will, I hope, not only provide a valuable source of information but also convey something of the subject's fascination to readers in many other disciplines.

Of course, there are in fact severely practical reasons for the great effort that goes into identifying carcinogens and finding out how they act. Basically, we want to know just which chemical agents are hazardous to life and health so that we can avoid them or at least reduce their hazards to the minimum possible. Moreover, we now want to be able to identify carcinogenic hazards in advance, rather than belatedly after their effects on man have become apparent.

There is a further reason, the contribution that a deeper understanding of carcinogenesis could make to the treatment of cancer. This may not be an essential prerequisite to curing cancer—by breaking a chain of infection in London, John Snow stopped an epidemic of cholera long before the cholera "germ" was identified, and we think we know how most lung cancer can be avoided without understanding the biological action of tobacco smoke. Nevertheless, we believe that if we knew more about how carcinogens act we would also know more about the nature of cancer and might have access to new and more rational approaches to cancer treatment.

As far as preventing cancer by avoidance of exposure to chemical carcinogens is concerned, it seems self-evident that chemists, more than members of any other profession, need to be aware of at least the essentials of the subject. Chemical carcinogenesis has long ceased to be a topic relevant only to a few selected industries handling tar products, dyestuffs intermediates, or certain minerals. This is clearly shown by the many uses which have been proposed for nitroso carcinogens, the possible contamination of foods with nitrosamines or naturally occurring carcinogens, the possible formation of carcinogens in the body by nitrosation of a variety of amines and amides, the carcinogenic action of various drugs and plant constituents, the carcinogenic hazards of a number of laboratory procedures, and the printing in a teachers' journal of suggested experiments with benzidine for schoolchildren.

As far as I am aware, however, it is still exceptional for a chemist to learn anything about carcinogens during his training, although this is a deficiency that could easily be rectified with minimal incursion into college teaching schedules. If it is necessary for a student to learn the preparation, structure, and reactions of, say, benzidine, he should surely also learn that it has caused bladder cancer in industrial and possibly in laboratory workers. The textbook of organic chemistry which I used as a student was unusual in describing the carcinogenic polycyclic aromatic hydrocarbons in some detail, but updating this account many years later consisted mainly in inserting Kekulé double bonds in the former plain hexagons, perpetuating the now dangerous illusion that chemical carcinogenesis is only concerned with substances of a type unlikely to be encountered in industrial or laboratory practice. Nevertheless, if some instruction regarding carcinogens is at last included in a chemist's training, it will probably be more sensible for it to be placed in the broad context of occupational and environmental safety rather than isolated from those important areas.

The tremendous volume of published research on chemical carcinogens is distributed through a great range of journals, predominantly biological or medical in nature if not directly dedicated to cancer research. Despite the present-day relevance of carcinogenesis to chemists in many spheres of activity and their increasing appreciation of this, it is not easy for a chemist who requires information about a particular substance to find it. The position is, however, improving.

The International Agency for Research on Cancer was established in Lyon, France, in 1965 by the World Health Assembly and is concerned particularly with cancer epidemiology and environmental aspects of carcinogenesis. It has recently started to issue the valuable IARC Monographs on the Evaluation of the Carcinogenic Risk of Chemicals to Man. At the time of writing, the seven monographs issued since 1972 review the carcinogenicity of a considerable range of chemicals such as aromatic amines, nitroso compounds, organochlorine pesticides, sex hormones, antithyroid substances, nitrofurans, and metals and derivatives. Additional publications cover the important specific areas of nitrosamine analysis and transplacental carcinogenesis.

The series "Chemical Induction of Cancer" (J. C. Arcos and M. F. Argus, Academic) so far comprises an introductory volume (1968) and two volumes (1974) which cover conjugated aromatic systems of the polycyclic hydrocarbon, amine, nitro compound, and azo dye types. Also, 1974 saw the publication of a two-part multi-author volume "Chemical Carcinogenesis" (editors: P. O. P. Ts'o and J. A. DiPaolo, Marcel Dekker) which was based on a symposium held in 1972 at the Johns Hopkins Hospital in Baltimore. Now over 13 years since the publication of D. B. Clayson's classic "Chemical Carcinogenesis" (J. & A. Churchill, 1962), these references will undoubtedly perform a very valuable service in making information on chemical carcinogenesis more readily available.

A comprehensive but uncritical source of information widely used in cancer research laboratories is the series "Survey of Compounds Which Have Been Tested for Carcinogenic Activity," published by the U.S. Department of Health, Education, and Welfare. The first volume (1951) covered literature up to 1947, and the coverage of the six volumes issued to date extends to 1971. For a chemist seeking recent information on specific compounds, however, the best course will generally be to consult "Chemical Abstracts."

Nevertheless, I have felt for some time that a need existed for a single book which described our present knowledge of the chemistry, biology, and hazards of the known range of carcinogens in such a way as to be of value and interest to chemists in many fields of work, as well as to its more obvious readership of medical and scientific workers directly involved in cancer research. I hope this monograph will do much to satisfy this requirement, and I am very grateful to the American Chemical Society for having asked me to undertake what proved to be the protracted and frequently nerve-racking, but also rewarding and highly educational task of organizing this volume. My particular thanks are due here to F. Marshall Beringer, former Editor of the Monograph Series, and to Robert F. Gould, Head of the Books Department.

As originally planned, the coverage of this monograph would have been somewhat more comprehensive than eventually proved possible. For various reasons, sections on cancer epidemiology and on the cancer hazards associated with some drugs and pesticides could not be included, though reference will be found to these where appropriate elsewhere. The most serious omission—a review of occupational and experimental carcinogenesis by inorganic materials —has already been referred to. It is hoped that the value of the chapters which follow will enable these deficiences to be overlooked.

One common cause of confusion in the literature of chemical carcinogens has caused many problems during the preparation of the book. This concerns their chemical nomenclature which has undergone many changes, especially in the major fields of polycyclic aromatic compounds, aromatic amines, and N-nitroso compounds. The environmental polycyclic hydrocarbon carcinogen now correctly known as benzo[a]pyrene still frequently appears as 3,4-benzo-pyrene (with or without the 'o') and has also been named 1,2-benzopyrene. Similarly the former 9,10-dimethylbenz-1,2-anthracene is now 7,12-dimethyl-benz[a]anthracene. These changes are clarified at the beginning of Chapter 5. Alternative forms in the aromatic amine field include 4-(or p-)aminobiphenyl (or -diphenyl) for 4-biphenylamine, and in case of the carcinogen which has contributed so much to the elucidation of metabolic changes in this group, 2-acetylamino- or 2-acetamido-fluorene for 2-fluorenylacetamide. Also, carcino-gens of the type (alkyl)$_2$NN:O, correctly N-nitrosodialkylamines as used here, are widely known as dialkylnitrosamines, with sometimes additional variations in the order of alkyl substituents. The generic name "nitrosamines" has been retained in this book, however. Considerable effort has gone into attempting to use correct nomenclature uniformly in this volume, with clear indications of alternative forms, but it is probably unduly optimistic to hope that this has been completely successful.

It is a very sad duty to have to record here the death on October 2, 1974, of Dr. John Jull, a few weeks after he had completed his chapter. He had devoted his working life to cancer research, first in Leeds, England, and since 1962 at the University of British Columbia, Vancouver, where he was associate professor of physiology. Though he had worked for some time on the carcinogenic aromatic amines, he developed a keen interest in the importance of hormones in cancer. As his review "Endocrine Aspects of Carcinogenesis" (Chapter 3) makes clear, he became an outstanding authority in this field, and in February 1974 was vice-chairman of the Working Group on Sex Hormones which drew up Volume 6 of the IARC Monograph Series referred to above. His premature death has caused shock and sadness to a wide circle of friends and colleagues.

In conclusion, I express my warm thanks to all the contributors to this book for their most friendly cooperation, very hard work, and patience. I also wish to express my indebtedness to David Clayson for helpful discussion in the early planning stage, to my colleagues David Harnden and June Marchant for their valuable advice and encouragement, and to my family for their forbearance.

C. E. SEARLE

University of Birmingham
Birmingham, England
May 1975

1

Bioassays and Tests for Chemical Carcinogens

John H. Weisburger, Naylor Dana Institute for Disease Prevention, American Health Foundation, Valhalla, N. Y. 10595

CANCER IS A GENERIC TERM covering a variety of neoplastic diseases character-ized by uncontrolled, but not necessarily fast, tumor growth. It is estimated that 70–90% of cancer in man and animals is the result of environmental causes (1, 2). If factors causing such cancers in the environment were known and identified, it would be possible to design measures either to eliminate the carcinogenic risk altogether or at least to minimize its impact. Thus, in this sense, research on carcinogenic risks and efforts to reduce their action is an optimal application of preventive medicine. Success along those lines has been achieved in the past. For example, one of the first historic developments in this field was the discovery by a British surgeon, Sir Percival Pott, that chim-ney sweeps exhibited cancer of the scrotum as a result of their profession (*see* Chapter 6 and Ref. *3*). Hygienic measures taken to remove soot from cloth-ing and body prevented the onset of this type of cancer. Another example concerns the development of nasopharyngeal cancers by employees in factories where nickel was refined by a certain, now-obsolete technology (*4*). While the old process was in operation, staff in the factory developed this cancer whereas employees working there after technological alterations had been made were not at risk. Furthermore, in the synthetic dye industry, ex-posure to certain aromatic amines and related chemicals such as 2-naphthyl-amine induced cancer in the urinary bladder in a significant proportion of those contaminated (*5, 6*). As production of these dangerous chemicals ceased or as the systems used in synthesizing these chemicals were improved by remote control, sealed operation, the cancer risk was minimized or indeed abolished.

The examples cited are all cases of occupational cancers. However, the incidence of various types of cancer suggests that occupational cancers repre-sent only a small portion of the total cancer incidence in the world (*2, 7, 8, 9, 10*). In order to definitively solve "the cancer problem," it will be necessary to address the important question of the etiology of the various key types of

1

cancer affecting millions of people, such as gastric cancer in Japan and certain parts of Europe, liver cancer in Africa, or colorectal, breast, and prostate cancer in the Western world, particularly the Anglo-Saxon countries.

The best way of eliminating each type of cancer is to define precisely the nature of the carcinogenic chemical or mixture of chemicals which may operate in the environment and induce cancer. Occupational health statistics and epidemiology may give clues to suspicious agents which may be responsible for cancer in man. In order to obtain specific information, it is necessary to show that a suspected chemical can indeed reproduce the disease in an animal model or at least that it can induce cancer in such a model even though not necessarily at the same site as in man.

For this purpose, bioassay systems specifically designed to detect carcinogenic chemicals are required. Such systems are even more potentially useful in avoiding the spread of a carcinogenic risk caused by a new synthetic chemical which may cause cancer in man. Thus, the screening for carcinogenic activity of agents to be used in the environment for various technological or social reasons is designed to avoid a possible catastrophic cancer epidemic. For example, it is most fortunate that the chemical N-2-fluorenylacetamide was discovered to be a powerful carcinogen prior to the possible use of the parent 2-fluorenamine as an insecticide (11). Indeed, in 1938 before DDT was known and when insect pests were controlled with difficulty, 2-fluorenamine was a potent and promising insecticide. If this chemical had been used widely in the environment as a pesticide, it is quite probable that cancer would have assumed epidemic proportions in populations exposed by whatever route. Hence, one of the key aims of carcinogen bioassay is to assess the carcinogenic risk in chemicals early in the technological development stages. This is sound economic practice, for it seems wasteful and indeed imprudent to conduct carcinogen bioassays on an interesting chemical to be introduced into commerce late in the production stages. If it should be found to have adverse effects at that time, all the previous work leading to possible marketing would have been futile.

Thus, evaluation of the carcinogenic potential of environmental chemicals needs to concern itself with two types of agents, synthetic chemicals which may enter or currently are in the human environment and naturally occurring chemicals which may be responsible for existing human cancer.

Bioassay systems should present a sensitive, reliable, and specific tool for the detection of possible carcinogenicity in chemicals. They should be economical, fast, and foolproof. They should, if possible, mimic the human situation. Current practices in this field, while refined to some extent in modern times, are basically not much different from the pioneering procedures of years ago. Often they are not fast, are expensive, and sometimes even misleading when applied to the detection of weak carcinogenic entities. A great deal of effort is being exerted now to improve this particular technology. Such developments are soundly based on remarkable new advances in the basic understanding of the carcinogenic process.

Table I.   Direct-Acting Carcinogens

Alkylating agents—nitrogens or sulfur mustards, sulfonic esters and sultones, ethylene imines and imides, strained or α,β-unsaturated lactones, epoxides, peroxides, chloroalkyl ethers
Inorganic chemicals[a]—Be, Cd, Mn, Ni, Co, Pb, Cr, Ti
Some triphenylmethane dyes[a]

[a] Mechanism of action is unclear, and classification as direct-acting carcinogen is subject to revision as more data accumulate.

Before discussing the various procedures used to detect chemical carcinogens in animal models, certain underlying fundamental principles will be mentioned to give some insight into the complexities of the overall problem.

Nature of Chemical Carcinogens

Current views recognize the existence of three types of chemical carcinogens: primary or ultimate carcinogens, secondary or procarcinogens, and cocarcinogens, promoting agents, or factors.

Primary or Ultimate Carcinogens. A chemical of this type is a chemically and biologically reactive entity by virtue of its specific structure. Such a chemical can interact specifically with certain elements of tissues, cells, and cellular component macromolecules to yield modified macromolecules in cells which are typical of the neoplastic state. Examples of such chemical carcinogens are alkylating agents of various types. In general, current views indicate that a chemical which can be considered to be an electrophilic reagent and possibly also chemicals which can assume free radical character belong to this class (Table I).

Secondary Agents or Procarcinogens. The majority of carcinogenic chemicals with a great diversity of structures belong to this class (Table II). Characteristically they are often chemically, biochemically, and biologically inert. There are specific, spontaneous, or biochemically (*i.e.* host-mediated and -controlled) activation reactions which convert procarcinogens to the corresponding reactive ultimate carcinogens.

Some procarcinogens are often chemically or spontaneously converted to ultimate carcinogens by hydrolytic reactions. Obviously, such events can occur under a variety of circumstances in virtually all species. Thus, these chemicals often exhibit a broad spectrum of activity in many species and target organs.

Table II.   Procarcinogens—Agents Requiring Biochemical Activation

Polynuclear aromatic and heterocyclic hydrocarbons	Cycasin, safrole, ethionine
Aromatic and heterocyclic amines and azo dyes	Acetamide, thioamides
	Chlorinated hydrocarbons
Nitroaryl- and furan derivatives	Aflatoxin, mycotoxins
Nitrosamines, -amides, -ureas, -carbamates	Pyrrolizidine alkaloids
Alkyltriazenes, dialkylhydrazines	Bracken fern
	Carbamates (urethan)

Procarcinogens which require host-controlled biochemical activation, on the other hand, may exhibit a much more specific, and indeed sometimes restricted, type of activity since their activation depends on the presence of some specific enzyme system (*12–18*). Thus, it is clear how the same chemical which is carcinogenic in some systems can show no carcinogenic effect at all in a given species or tissue or under certain conditions if the required enzyme system is absent. Likewise, shifts in target organs or various other modifiers are understandable in terms of the presence and quantity of the appropriate enzyme systems (*19, 20*). Such enzymes can be present either in mammalian cells, the most common situation, but can also be of bacterial origin, as that derived from the microflora in the intestinal tract (*21, 22, 23*). Under some conditions chronic bacterial or parasitic infection in some organs like the urinary or gall bladder may also lead to release of a carcinogen which would not arise in a non-infected organ (*14, 24, 25*).

Promoting Agents or Co-carcinogens. These chemicals are not carcinogenic by themselves but serve to potentiate, sometimes quite dramatically, the effect of either a primary or a procarcinogen. Complex carcinogenic mixtures such as cigarette smoke and coal tars are believed to contain large amounts of co-carcinogens and relatively minor quantities of primary or procarcinogens (*26, 27, 28*).

In this connection, it seems appropriate to mention that cancer found in man and animals is, in many instances, probably the result of the simultaneous or sequential action of mixtures of agents. This point will need to be considered when investigating the precise nature of agents responsible for cancer in man. Up to now many bioassays and safety assessments have been conducted on single agents. While such studies have led to the discovery of a number of different chemical carcinogens (*29*) future studies must delineate the carcinogenic risk of specific and rationally selected mixtures which may affect man.

The best known co-carcinogen is that contained in an extract of croton resin. It promotes skin tumor formation in mice after an application of a carcinogenic polycyclic aromatic hydrocarbon such as 3-methylcholanthrene (*30, 31, 32*). After substantial efforts the chemical nature of the active principles in croton oil were identified as certain phorbol esters. These now form useful tools to investigate the nature of the carcinogenic process.

Carcinogenic Process

Overt cancer in man and animals caused by environmental chemicals or conditions is thought to be the end result of a complex series of individual reactions, subject to and controlled by a number of modifying factors.

1. Biochemical activation of a procarcinogen to the ultimate carcinogen, a reaction which competes with biochemical detoxification and elimination reactions

2. Interaction of such direct-acting or biochemically produced ultimate carcinogens with specific cellular and molecular receptors, mainly DNA, a

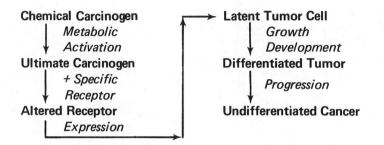

Figure 1. *Sequence of complex events during chemical carcino-genesis*

series of reactions subject to certain, as yet ill-defined, stereochemical conditions and competitive inhibitors. The altered DNA is subject to repair and restoration by repair enzyme systems, currently under extensive investigation.

3. Duplication of the abnormal receptor which subsequently may be immune to the operation of repair systems

4. Multiplication of the cells containing the abnormal receptor as early or latent tumor cells

5. Further growth to form a well differentiated tumor

6. Conversion of this tumor, by as yet unknown mechanisms called progression, to an independent undifferentiated cancer (Figures 1–4).

Many of these specific steps are controlled and modified by numerous endogenous and exogenous factors. Thus, species, strain, sex, and age differences are accounted for in part by the alteration of these elements in certain of these steps. In addition, immunologic and related factors may enhance or diminish the extent and rate of the carcinogenic process. Among the exogenous elements, nutritional and hormonal factors are involved heavily. Furthermore, there are many interactions between all of these elements as well as between synthetic and also naturally occurring chemicals which can

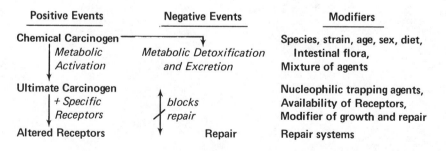

Figure 2. *First steps of chemical carcinogenesis, involving activation of procarcinogen and reaction of resulting ultimate or primary carcinogen with specific cellular receptors, including DNA. These reactions are controlled and modified by numerous factors, some of which are noted. See Refs. 13, 15, 17, 20, 36, 62, 85, 101 for detailed treatment.*

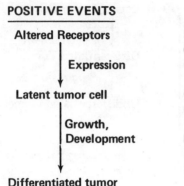

Figure 3. *Later steps in carcinogenic process involving elements affecting the development and growth of carcinogen-modified cells and constituents*

augment or decrease the overall effectiveness of one carcinogen in leading to cancer.

These basic elements can be used to reduce the impact of carcinogens in the human environment. On the other hand, and in the context of the current article, this background of information can be exploited to enhance the sensitivity of bioassay systems to detect chemical carcinogens.

Test Systems

A number of recent reviews have dealt with this subject (*33, 34, 35*). The ultimate goal of carcinogen test systems is to provide data permitting an evaluation of carcinogenic risk to man. It is quite obvious that man cannot

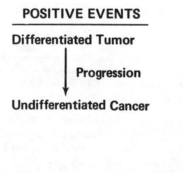

Figure 4. *Last steps in carcinogenic process leading to malignancy, including spread by metastasis. Much more fundamental information is required to understand fully these steps. It is these terminal steps which often are responsible for the fatal outcome if not controlled by the modifiers listed.*

be used for such studies, even though a few of the pioneers did make attempts along those lines. Thus, animal models are necessarily involved in assessing carcinogenic potency of chemicals.

The question can be asked whether the data obtained in such systems actually do reflect a carcinogenic risk to man. As noted above, some chemicals or mixtures, now numbering about 30, have been demonstrated unambiguously to have induced cancer in man (*14, 36*). Every one of these chemicals which have led to cancer in man are also carcinogenic in one or more animal models. It would seem, therefore, that the reverse would likely be true—that is, a chemical reliably carcinogenic in an animal model would also affect man (*37*).

A qualification can and should be introduced at this time. Man is not a homogeneous unique sample. In fact, man is highly heterogenous, lives under different environmental conditions and under varied dietary and other exposures, and thus necessarily would have widely varying response patterns to a given carcinogenic challenge. For example, it is universally admitted now, after many years of controversy, that heavy cigarette smoking does lead to lung cancer. However, even with equal numbers of cigarettes smoked per day, the response of different individuals varies a great deal. The smoking method, the inhalation depth, the nutritional status of the individual, the biochemical activation and detoxification systems, the ciliary and mucous clearance systems, and defense mechanisms all play a role in defining the overall outcome in this carcinogenic situation (*26*). Other examples with other carcinogens or carcinogenic situations could be cited. The fact is that, given a chemical carcinogen definitely active in one or more animal models, it can be stated that certain individuals of *Homo sapiens* would be at risk.

In addition to these practical considerations, the specific cellular and molecular systems in man are not now considered to be that different from the equivalent cellular and molecular systems in animals. Since these systems determine how a given exogenous chemical interacts, it is theoretically sound and logical to conclude that humans exposed to chemical carcinogens would not react much differently from the animal models, except as regards quantitative aspects and tissues affected (*37*).

Early workers used larger animals such as rabbits and sometimes dogs. The mouse was introduced in the assay of chemical carcinogens by the school of Kennaway, which was trying to determine the active carcinogenic principle in coal tar (*3*). Because it is now known that the overall carcinogenic process is in some way related to the lifespan of a given species, model bioassay systems have turned away, except for specialized studies, from longer lived animals such as dogs, cats, rabbits, or even primates and have concentrated on small rodents such as various strains of mice, rats, or hamsters which have an average lifespan, under good conditions, of two to three years.

Purity of Chemicals to be Tested

Cancer in man has rarely been caused by pure chemicals, with the exception of neoplasia resulting from drugs (*38, 39*). Since impurities in a chemical may modify, *i.e.*, enhance or diminish, toxicity and carcinogenicity, it is necessary to have detailed information on the nature of the chemical. Where the environmental chemical is a technical product, it may be useful to test both the technical product with its contaminants, which need to be known, and also the pure main ingredient. Data must be available on the stability of the chemical under the conditions of administration to animals or insertion into other bioassay systems.

Selection of Animals

A comprehensive bioassay in animals is best performed on more than one species. Indeed, examples are known where even powerful carcinogens which affect man are not active in all strains of all species. For example, 2-naphthylamine, for reasons that are not yet clear, fails to cause cancer in most strains of rats (*14, 29*). On the other hand, the mold product aflatoxin B_1, suspected as a cause of liver cancer in man, does not elicit a neoplastic response in the liver of mice under the customary bioassay conditions, although administration to newborn mice has produced a carcinogenic effect (*40*).

There are numerous strains of inbred and non-inbred rats, mice, and hamsters (*35, 41, 42, 43*). Controlling elements in the selection of a specific strain should be the ease of maintenance of the animals, their relative sensitivity to various test chemicals, freedom from nonneoplastic disease, and the occurrence of spontaneous cancer in as low an incidence as possible, as late as possible.

The rats most often used for carcinogen bioassay are the Wistar and Sprague–Dawley strains in the United States, the Donryu strain in Japan, and various types of Wistar-derived rats in Europe. However, some of these breeds exhibit a high incidence of spontaneous cancer, especially in endocrine-responsive organs, when kept for their full lifespan. They have, however, potential for specialized assay system. For example, the Sprague–Dawley strain female rats are excellent for the Huggins breast cancer assay (*44, 45*). Currently, many bioassay programs have standardized their systems on the highly inbred rat of the Fischer strain (*46*) and the non-inbred Osborne–Mendel strain. The latter is selected for its sensitivity to certain chlorinated hydrocarbons (*47*).

A greater variety of mouse strains is available for carcinogen testing. The non-inbred Swiss breeds are widely used for a variety of tests and are quite suitable, provided adequate control groups are used. Inbred strains such as AKR, which exhibit spontaneous leukemia and lymphoma early in life, or the C3H, which develop high yields of mammary lesions when milk agent is present, are not very useful. Strain A mice are excellent because of their tendency to give lung tumors in a short time with many carcinogens, but they cannot be used for long tests because of an elevated yield of spontaneous lung tumors (*48*). Strains such as Balb/C and hybrid strains such as the widely used model, C57BL X C3H F_1, exhibit adequate sensitivity, a relatively low spontaneous disease rate, and good longevity (*49*).

In addition to sensitivity to pulmonary tumor formation, several strains of mice readily develop liver tumors. This response has been criticized as not always reflecting a true carcinogenic risk to man, even though a number of human carcinogens do yield mainly liver tumors in mice (50).

Non-inbred hamsters have found favor, largely because of extensive tests by Shubik and Saffiotti (51). They are particularly suited for lung carcinogenesis studies because they are fairly resistant to infectious lung diseases which are so frequent in rats and even mice.

Recently a number of strains of inbred hamsters were developed mainly by Homburger (42). Their responsiveness to a variety of chemical carcinogens remains to be determined. When 3-methylcholanthrene is given orally, some such strains have responded with several types of cancer like those in the colon, which are of current interest as a model system (23, 52).

The quality of the animals is an important factor in the satisfactory conduct of carcinogen bioassays. Procurement of animals from unreliable sources can be a costly mistake if such animals jeopardize the collection of valid data, either through premature loss or through disease processes which may, in turn, affect their response. The cost of acquiring animals is only a minor item, compared to the overall expense of conducting carcinogen bioassay. Only the best quality will do (35).

Along these same lines, animals must be housed and maintained under optimal conditions. Intercurrent infection may affect the response (53). There should be no crowding of animals in cages or of cages in a given size animal room. Temperature and humidity need to be closely controlled. Soiled bedding and cages should be changed frequently. The water supply should be clean and the bottles, if used, sanitized and sterilized at each refilling. Water can be chlorinated to maintain sterility, or the pH can be adjusted carefully to about two. Automatic water supplies need to be monitored to insure a continuing supply of clean, fresh water.

There are a number of available commercial diets. Consideration has been given in recent years to formulating a standard diet for carcinogen bioassay which is uniform not only in composition, as are the commercial chows, but also in ingredients. A few laboratories use the formulation of semi-synthetic diets. Others have used vitamin-fortified commercial diets which can be autoclaved and are so used. Here again, the cost of the diet constitutes but a small part of the overall cost of the bioassays. No effort should be spared to acquire the best diet to insure long-term survival under optimal nutritional conditions. All animals, including concurrent controls, require maintenance under identical dietary and environmental conditions. The "spontaneous" tumor rate was found to depend on type and availability of diet, as shown by Ross and Bras (54).

Animals which have recently been weaned, typically at six to seven weeks of age, are usually used for bioassays and to evaluate the toxicity of test chemicals and mixtures. Older animals, especially after puberty, are often less responsive, and thus require a longer experimental period. In some instances, six- to seven-week-old animals have significantly greater tolerance to toxic chemicals than right at weaning. Hence, this may be an optimal age with respect to maximizing the sensitivity of the system and allowing the expression of carcinogenic potential, if present.

After tumors were successfully induced in newborn animals by viruses, this type of experimentation was used more in tests with chemicals (55, 56). With many types of chemicals tested, mice of various strains and hamsters appeared to be quite responsive when treated from birth; with rats this result was not so common. However, there have been few accurate comparative studies. The field of transplacental carcinogenesis has seen renewed interest, especially in the light of human findings with diethylstilbestrol (57, 58).

A modification of the bioassay system is currently being considered which involves continuing administration of test chemicals over two generations. The F_1 offspring are the key groups maintained for long-term observation. This refinement certainly appears to merit further examination with regard to sensitivity to several classes of carcinogens, particularly weak agents and/or lower dosages. Also, humans may be exposed to certain chemicals under similar long-term conditions, so that a rational and reasonable defense of such protocols can be made.

Administration of Test Chemicals

There are several possible ways to administer test chemicals. The mode selected depends in part on the ultimate application and dosages of the chemical in the human environment. Food additives or drugs given orally are best tested by feeding, but cosmetics would be applied to the skin, etc. On the other hand, if the question is asked whether a given chemical with a specific structure is endowed with carcinogenic potential, the route of administration is somewhat less important. However, great care must be taken to interpret any data wisely and rationally. This is meant to imply that with certain administration routes, such as subcutaneous injection or bladder implantation, tumors are produced not necessarily because the chemical itself is truly carcinogenic, but because the physicochemical nature of the chemical or solid, exhibiting a long residence time at the point of application or insertion, has produced a tissue reaction resulting in cancer (5, 14, 24, 25, 59–63). Thus, cancer at the site of subcutaneous injection or chemical in a pellet implated in the urinary bladder may or may not represent a true carcinogenic response and signify that the chemical structure is responsible for the effect obtained. Conclusions drawn must necessarily be based on a complete understanding of the mechanism involved.

Oral Intake. Chemicals can be mixed in food, administered in drinking water, or given by gavage or stomach tube. This mode is practiced often and appears to be quite reliable in detecting carcinogenic potential. Because chemicals can be mixed with the diet in almost any amount, artifacts may be obtained when a certain percentage of the diet is an inert chemical, nutritionally speaking. Also, deposits of the chemical or metabolites in certain tissues from intake of excessive amounts may lead to adverse effects in organs such as the kidneys and urinary bladder which would be avoided with lower, yet still meaningful, rational dosages. Unless crystalluria or similar effects can also be predicted to arise following intake of such a chemical by man, the animal data cannot be used to forecast a carcinogenic hazard to man and are thus irrelevant. Unless a chemical is a food itself or an important component thereof, it should not account for more than 5% of the diet. In fact, probably a top level of 2–3% would suffice properly to detect and evaluate even a weak carcinogen. Similar considerations hold where oral intake is secured through administration in the drinking water or by intubation.

The use of gavage or intragastric intubation offers the advantage of quantitative administration of a given dose. This operation can be performed repeatedly. If the animals are started on a regimen at weaning, they adapt readily and tolerate the daily handling. It is important to realize that administration by tube delivers the entire dose all at once. When the test chemical is dissolved in drinking water or incorporated in the diet, the chemical is delivered and absorbed over a period of time. Thus, with certain chemicals, somewhat different tolerated dosages or effects might result by these two different techniques of oral administration because of distinct peak tissue levels.

Another point which favors and often necessitates intragastric intubation, is the case of a chemical with an unacceptable taste. Animals might not consume this material when offered in diet or drinking water.

Cutaneous Application. The skin of mice or rabbits generally responds better than that of other species to carcinogenic challenges. Mouse skin has been a standard tool to detect and quantitate the carcinogenic potential of coal or tobacco tars. Except for liquid chemicals, a solvent, such as acetone, toluene, or some purified mineral, or edible oils, is usually necessary. Benzene is less desirable since it is metabolized to toxic phenol. Because of solubility problems lower amounts of chemical can be administered by the cutaneous route than by the oral route. It is generally true that tumors, usually papillomas and carcinomas, at the point of application to the skin are seen only with ultimate or primary carcinogens unless a chemical has such a structure as procarcinogen that it can be metabolized by the skin to an active ultimate carcinogen. For example, the polycyclic aromatic hydrocarbons fall into this class. Mouse skin is an ideal test system for such chemicals, since this tissue appears to possess activating but only limited detoxifying capacity. Cutaneous application of many products also may lead to their resorption. Thus, they can cause adverse effects and cancer in tissues remote from the point of application. It is imperative, therefore, to perform complete autopsies and examine all tissues for lesions even when the chemical is applied to the skin unless it has been determined that a remote effect does not exist.

Subcutaneous Injection. The active principles in coal tar, the polycyclic aromatic hydrocarbons, were first found to be carcinogenic by this technique. Thus, this mode has historic interest and is still practiced widely. It will detect primary and ultimate carcinogens with the proper reactivity by producing injection site sarcomas. At the same time, because many chemicals are resorbed from the injection area, information is obtained on possible effects in remote organs. However, the *in vivo* circulation after subcutaneous injection may differ substantially from that seen after other modes, such as intraperitoneal or intravenous injection, and after oral intake. This circulation can, in turn, affect the metabolic activation and detoxification sites and the relative tissue concentrations, and therefore, in many instances, it controls the effective key target organ. For example, N-dibutylnitrosamine given to rats subcutaneously yields only bladder carcinomas whereas orally it induces liver and esophageal cancer in addition (*64, 65*).

Intraperitoneal Injection. This mode is a convenient way of introducing test chemicals, even repeatedly over long periods of time, provided they are not too insoluble by themselves or their vehicle does not accumulate. Oils tend to be absorbed poorly from the peritoneal cavity. However, even fairly water-insoluble chemicals are resorbed amazingly well after intraperitoneal injection into rodents. This point needs to be ascertained in each individual case.

With direct-acting primary carcinogens local tumor production in the form of sarcomas is often seen. With agents requiring chemical or biochemical activation the tumor spectrum obtained usually is similar to that noted upon oral intake.

Intravenous Injection. This technique is somewhat more delicate to execute, especially for multiple dosing. It permits the rapid widespread distribution of a test chemical to many organs, especially if it is relatively miscible in aqueous phase. Even so, the specific organ affinity of carcinogens is maintained. Injection of suspensions, on the other hand, tend to be filtered out by the vascular system in select organs such as the lung, and cancer may develop primarily there.

Respiratory Exposure. This mode is potentially very important inasmuch as man inhales many agents such as air pollutants, volatile chemicals, pesticides, dust, tobacco smoke, and the like (*36, 66, 67, 68*). However, the anatomy and physiology of animals used in experimental toxicology, particularly rodents, need to be considered in the design and evaluation of results. Animals exhibit an involved filtering system in the nasal cavity. Also, the cavity and upper respiratory tract is further protected by layers of mucous secretions in which inhaled chemicals are retained and expelled or transferred to the digestive tract. Unless chemicals are completely gasous, they do not reach the lower parts of the respiratory tract. Colloids or dusts more often than not are filtered in the nasal cavity and may not reveal adverse effects in the lower respiratory tract and lung. This behavior is distinct from that of man, who inhales air pollutants, tobacco smoke, and the like through the mouth, bypassing the nasal filtering system which is less developed than in animals.

Preliminary Toxicology

Once the mode of administration, the species, and strain of animals have been selected, the maximum tolerated dose under the precise experimental conditions must be determined. Typically five males and five females are administered a range of dose levels by the route selected. These tests need to mimic the definitive experiment. Thus, if the protocols call for a single dose, a classical LD_{50} acute toxicity can be determined. A few chemicals can be carcinogenic after single dose if the animals are subsequently held for their lifetimes. Most chemicals are not active except upon repeated exposure. Also, more often than not, man is exposed chronically, so most studies involve determination of a maximum tolerated dose over a six- to eight-week period which gives a fair indication of dose levels tolerated for lifespan tests. The dose levels are selected on the basis of mortality and weight gain in relation to vehicle or untreated controls. The maximum tolerated dose is one which leads to low mortality in the eight week test and may depress the weight gain of animals 5–20% with an optimal depression of approximately 10%. Except for special cases where tests involve newborn animals or in more recent times with a two-generation study, it is customary to begin such tests when rodents are six weeks old.

The importance of correctly selecting the maximum tolerated dose level cannot be overemphasized. In some cases where the first set of tests has given inadequate indication, it is useful to conduct a second series using doses centered around the area which seems to be appropriate from the data obtained in the first series.

It is expensive and wasteful to conduct tests on large groups of animals only to discover at the end of two years that the dosages used were too low and produced uninterpretable results. Doses on the high side will be noted readily by inadequate weight gain or mortality. If the latter is not excessive a downward adjustment in dosage can be made promptly.

The question has sometimes been asked why carcinogen bioassays are conducted at high dose levels. First, carcinogens, like other pharmacologic agents, exhibit a dose–response curve *(33, 69, 70, 71)*. This means that the higher the dose level, the more elevated will be the response—in this instance, tumor induction. In addition, the higher the dose, the shorter the time to tumor production. Chemical carcinogens of strong or moderate potency exhibit this additional distinct parameter from the customary drug reaction. Thus, with a carcinogen, a positive result is seen in a shorter time with a high dose, with a consequent saving in cost. With two different chemicals exhibiting identical tumor yields, it can be stated that the one inducing tumors faster is the more powerful agent.

This problem of dose levels is sometimes confused. When cancer develops in man as a result of exposure to a chemical carcinogen (for example, as an occupational risk) it is difficult, if not impossible, to arrive at the dosages involved. Indeed, cancer often develops many years after a variable exposure index. However, in some cases levels have been reasonably accurately evaluated. When urinary bladder cancer has developed subsequent to known exposure to a drug like chlornaphazin, it has been possible to gather such information from hospital records. Lung cancer incidence in cigarettte smokers increases within a shorter latent period the higher the number of cigarettes smoked per day *(2)*. Recently, prepubertal girls were found to have a rare form of vaginal cancer after their mothers were treated with high, but not low, doses of a hormone, diethylstilbestrol (58). 2-Naphthylamine is a recognized human carcinogen. High dosages of this chemical were required to reproduce in an animal system the condition found in man.

On the basis of these considerations, it would seem logical to recommend the administration of as high a dosage as tolerated to enable survival of the animals for carcinogen bioassay. The question can be asked whether administration of such high dose levels might not cause cancer induction as an artifact resulting from the dose levels used. However, in most instances, there is probably little chance of this eventuality. Many noncarcinogenic chemicals have been administered at high dose levels without eliciting evidence of a neoplastic response.

Careful analysis must be given where treatment of animals with high dose levels of a chemical has yielded a carcinogenic response and, at the same time, other abnormalities which most likely were actually responsible for the neoplastic response. For example, it seems established that the presence of foreign bodies in the kidney, renal pelvis, or urinary bladder may by itself elicit a neoplastic response (24, 25, 63, 72). Thus, where administration of a chemical leads to crystalluria and the deposition of stones in the excretory organs as a primary response, the possibility must be considered that the cancer induction is secondary to this phenomenon and not necessarily indicative of a carcinogenic effect of the chemical. Man may respond identically, as suggested by the fact that cancer in gall or urinary bladder has been found associated with stones.

Another problem which requires thorough analysis is the induction of tumors in the endocrine system consequent to the application of high doses of chemicals with hormonal properties over an extended period. Chemicals or drugs of this type may very likely induce cancer in the endocrine system if their administration leads to hormonal imbalance in the animal system. Indeed, it is thought that cancer in endocrine-responsive organs in man may stem from such imbalances. Current views are that such chemicals cannot be evaluated properly for carcinogenic potential in a rodent system which does not have an estrus cycle comparable with that of the human female (35, 73). However, drugs of this type can be tested for possible carcinogenic effect in non-endocrine target organs. For example, diethylstilbestrol leads to renal carcinoma in male hamsters by some as yet unknown mechanisms (42).

Definitive Bioassays

Depending on the ultimate refinement of data evaluation which is necessary, the number of animals started for the definitive experiments range from 25 males and 25 females per dose level to as many as 100 per group. More animals are occasionally required to answer special types of questions on widely used environmental chemicals. With known carcinogens serving as positive controls under known conditions, a smaller number may suffice, although there should never be fewer than 15 females and 15 males. Where it is known that males and females will respond identically, studies involving only one sex may be permissible but with an increased number per group, for example, 25–35. This is true mainly for known agents and often cannot be predicted with new chemicals.

If despite careful preliminary toxicology the weight gain of the animals in the definitive experiment appears inappropriate, *i.e.* too high like the controls or too low reflecting severe toxicity, it is permissible to adjust the dose levels even in these tests. However, such changes should be conducted relatively early, within the first 10 weeks of the test. If by chance inadequate dose selection results in severe mortality early in the test or inappropriate dose selection is noted after the 10-week period, it is best to discontinue the entire test and begin again with properly adjusted experimental conditions. We found that belated alteration in dosages, when mortality was not a factor but when the weights reflected inadequate dosing, often failed to yield an adequate change in the weight curves.

In the definitive experiments animals are maintained on test (1) until adverse effects are noted, (2) for a 90-week period for mice to a 104-week period for hamsters and rats, or (3) for lifetime. While some investigators favor lifetime studies, we believe this is feasible only under properly controlled conditions where the aged animals are carefully watched and examined frequently. This requires above average quality and quantity of staff. In most instances, especially in large-scale test series involving thousands of animals, it seems more efficient to terminate the experiment after a predetermined time. Under these conditions comparisons between various experimental and control groups as well as the statistical evaluation is considerably facilitated. Also, the quality of the tissues collected and fixed fresh and eventually studied microscopically is bound to be much better, and thus the interpretation of the experiment more reliable. Further, it is reasonable to assume that a two-year period in rodents under adequately designed and controlled conditions would detect virtually all agents which might represent a carcinogenic risk to man.

In the course of these definitive experiments it is important to inspect the animals daily or even twice a day to isolate animals which appear to be ill and to pay particular attention to such animals. Nothing is gained by attempts to maintain animals which appear to have evidence of adverse effect for another few days or even weeks. If cancer is present it will not grow much more, or if cancer is absent it is not likely to develop in a short time. It is useful to consider autopsy when an older animal either exhibits overt cancer, shows weight loss, or poor clinical appearance indicative of diminishing health.

Evaluation of Results

Throughout the experiment, careful records must be kept of weight gain, of any grossly visible neoplastic lesions, and/or of the location and multiplicity of any lesion. Regression of benign lesions such as papillomas or adenomas is of interest. Their location, time sequence of events, and related facts must be recorded.

Dead animals need to be autopsied by competent, highly trained personnel experienced in experimental pathology or under the immediate supervision or direction of a qualified pathologist. Tissues immersed in adequate amounts of the appropriate fixative solution need to be fixed carefully, and void bodies such as the urinary bladder need to be tied off and filled with fixative to avoid artifact formation and possibly misleading interpretations. After fixation the tissues are processed by conventional histopathologic techniques, and the sections studied using accepted criteria for the diagnosis of neoplastic and nonneoplastic diseases.

The results are tabulated by listing lesions according to types for every tissue. In some organs such as the mammary gland, mouse lung, and intestinal tract, the multiplicity of the lesions is a more sensitive indicator of relative carcinogenicity than the eventual listing of percent of animals with cancer at a given site. More can be learned by examining the data for each tissue or target site than a record of the overall cancer incidence. Combining the results for all tissues and organs is not very instructive, except when there is a clear-cut increase over controls and several different tissues show cancer. In fact, cases are known where the incidence of tumors in one tissue was increased and in another tissue it was decreased, so that the overall incidence, compared with controls, was almost identical (74, 75).

In all such tests simultaneous control groups are very important, for the animal used may exhibit spontaneous and nonneoplastic lesions, especially in lifetime assays. The data obtained serve as key reference points against which any effect in the experimental groups is gaged. Where a vehicle is used, there must be vehicle controls involving the same number of animals as in an experimental group. However, where a number of unknown chemicals are studied simultaneously, one control group may serve for a number of contemporary experimental groups. As a matter of logistics it is rare, however, that more than five to ten chemicals can be studied simultaneously, as exemplified by the numbers shown in the hypothetical protocol, Table III.

The advice of statisticians is necessary in assisting with the development of the specific experimental protocols as well as in the evaluation of results (76, 77). Participation of such professionals in bioassay tests will optimize the experimental design, enable the experiment to be conducted most economically, and ensure that data are obtained which yield valid, significant, and meaningful results. It is important to realize that studies conducted in groups of 50 or 100 animals are used to define a carcinogenic risk which may be applied or extended to billions of people.

Short Term Bioassays

Over the years there have been many attempts to assess the possible carcinogenic risk of chemicals by methods avoiding the time, effort, and expense inherent in the classic carcinogen bioassay tests described above. For example, certain polycyclic aromatic hydrocarbons quickly lead to epidermal thickening and atrophy of the sebaceous glands in mouse skin or hyperplasias of mouse ear skin. Such an assay system has been proposed for it can be read in a matter of days. However, many inactive chemicals may also yield similar positive endpoints, so the system has the disadvantage of false positives.

Table III. Hypothetical Test Protocols for 15 Chemicals, Using Identical Vehicle for Formulation[a]

	Groups	Total Numbers
Series A	5 chemicals @ 200 animals each/2 dose levels	1000
	1 vehicle control	100
	1 untreated control	50
Series B	5 chemicals @ 200 animals each	1000
	1 vehicle control	100
	1 untreated control	50
	1 positive control	100
Series C	5 chemicals @ 200 animals each	1000
	1 vehicle control	100
	1 untreated control	50

[a] Series A, B, and C are started one to two months apart and phased out in the same order. With a chemical of moderate to high carcinogenicity, termination earlier than 90–104 weeks will occur depending on the species. Samples of the control population should be taken at such earlier periods. The positive control group is given a known carcinogen which is related in structure or function to the unknowns tested. This control is administered in two doses; the higher resulting in quick tumor development to 30 animals (15 males, 15 females) and the lower mimicking a weak effect to 70 animals.

In recent years, much fundamental knowledge has been accrued on the nature of the chemical structures with demonstrated carcinogenic effect, as discussed elsewhere in this article. Some chemicals with alkylating properties are direct-acting carcinogens while others require biochemical activation by the host. The interaction between such activated carcinogens and select cellular and molecular receptors is becoming clearer, although the key targets for carcinogenicity have not been resolved definitively. However there is hope that based on such fundamental knowledge, indicator systems can be designed which rationally mimic the complex *in vivo* molecular receptors. Such systems, exposed to properly activated carcinogens, may be able to translate an interaction into a signal which reliably reflects the presence or absence, or indeed, the quantity of carcinogenic potential. Currently, large scale efforts are underway in a number of laboratories in the United States and in other countries to assess the value of several distinct systems designed to serve for short-term carcinogen bioassay. We have recently reviewed this area in detail (78). Thus, only brief mention will be made here of the several approaches.

Transformation of Cell Cultures. Recent developments have provided two different rapid and economic approaches which may yield information, not definitive enough to establish direct extrapolation to a carcinogenic risk for man, but sufficiently indicative to serve as a prescreen for more definitive experiments to be performed in rodent systems.

Cell culture systems derived from tissues from a variety of rodent species have been "transformed" relatively rapidly by certain chemical carcinogens (79–84). The resulting abnormal cells have produced tumors when reinserted into a syngeneic host. Currently such cell systems are being evaluated intensively with varied classes and types of carcinogens. It is hoped that they can be developed as reasonably accurate forecasters of potential carcinogenic risk. Many of the cell systems do respond positively with the powerful carcinogenic polycyclic aromatic hydrocarbons. The question will be whether the large class of other procarcinogens would be detected equally satisfactorily, especially agents which are not as potent carcinogens active as the hydrocarbon series. In part, the susceptibility of the system will depend on the presence of the biochemical activation machinery which is necessary to transform the procarcinogens to the ultimate carcinogens. Another point to be considered in this and other *in vitro* systems is that they may have the proper activation system but be much less adequately endowed with available *in vivo* detoxification systems (17, 85, 86, 87). Thus, in some instances a positive response is obtained with a chemical which would not be carcinogenic under *in vivo* conditions.

Recently, the problem of biochemical activation by cell systems has been elegantly developed by administering a carcinogenic compound to a pregnant female animals and explanting cells from the fetuses into tissue culture. They quickly gave evidence of transformation (79, 88).

Mutagenicity Tests as Prescreens for Carcinogens. Scientific achievements of the last few years in chemical carcinogenesis and in molecular biology have underwritten the concept that chemicals suitably activated either by chemical or biochemical means were both mutagenic and carcinogenic (62, 89, 90, 91, 92). Historically, these two fields were distinct until it was realized that tests of most chemical carcinogens had not developed evidence of mutagenicity because the indicator organisms to detect mutagenicity were not capable of transforming a procarcinogen to the active, ultimate carcinogen in the form of an electrophilic or one-electron reagent. Provided such activation reactions can be achieved either under *in vitro* conditions or by the host mediated assay, it would seem that mutagenesis may be a useful indicator of possible carcinogenicity (78, 85, 86, 87, 93, 94, 95). Such tests can be conducted in a matter of weeks rather than years.

The importance of securing intimate contact between the activated carcinogen and the indicator organisms cannot be overemphasized. For example, in a host-mediated assay, the intraperitoneal injection of an indicator organism followed by oral administration of the carcinogen, dimethylnitrosamine, failed to yield detectable mutants. However, a positive response was noted when the indicator organism was injected through the portal vein into the liver. The half-life of the active intermediate from dimethylnitrosamine is apparently so short that it does not escape from the liver.

Not all mutagens are carcinogens. Thus, evidence of mutagenicity, even reliably obtained, is only a suggestive but not definitive argument for carcinogenic risk. Other collateral studies are required to delineate the carcinogenicity more fully.

Sedimentation Analysis of DNA and DNA Repair Synthesis. More direct evidence for an alteration of DNA can be secured through methodology now being developed. Two approaches seem promising. One involves sedimentation analyses of potential target tissues where damage to the DNA either as single strand or double strand breaks is detected. High speed centrifugation of DNA in an alkaline sucrose gradient may yield significant information on the type of DNA break induced by carcinogens which is different from such alterations produced by noncarcinogens (*95, 96, 97, 98, 99*).

Recent developments also involve the study of DNA repair processes in tissues in cells after the introduction of chemical carcinogens (*100, 101, 102*). Such new techniques may yield quite significant information in relation to carcinogenicity if, indeed, it can be established that such alterations in the structure, function, and rates of synthesis of DNA are specifically the result of attacks by activated carcinogens of several classes.

Fetal Proteins or Antigens as Indicators. Over the last few years, it was discovered that patients with specific cancers exhibited abnormal serum protein patterns in their blood serum. Patients with liver cancer presented a protein called α-fetoprotein, which was deemed characteristic of liver cancer and in a few instances of teratoma (*103*). Patients with cancer of the colon had a carcinoembryonic antigen (*104, 105, 106*). More recent studies suggest that that carcinoembryonic antigen was typical, not only of colon, but also of certain other types of cancer and, in fact, also of a few non-neoplastic diseases.

Administration of high levels of a number of hepatocarcinogens to rats led to the precocious appearance in the serum of α-fetoprotein long before liver cancer was apparent (*107, 108, 109*). Related noncarcinogens failed to do this. This discovery may form the basis for rapid, quite specific bioassays which can be conducted semiquantitatively by sensitive radioimmunoassays for the fetal antigens.

Comment. Systems now under intensive development may be useful and widely applicable prescreens to obtain a quick indication of possible carcinogenic risks for the great variety of environmental chemicals to which man is potentially exposed (*110, 111*). Thus, information on a possible risk for man which is available sufficiently early in the development of such chemicals for practical use may assist in minimizing unnecessary effort and expenditures. Such tests hopefully will also find broad application in detecting carcinogenic hazards among naturally occurring chemicals which may be responsible for the major forms of human cancers. They should aid in selecting interesting fractions during the separation of complex mixtures and obtain reliable information on individual carcinogenic substituents therein. Thus, mankind may be in a position to remove such chemicals and mixtures from the environment, or at least diminish their effect, so that the ultimate goal of all such experiments and tests, the reduction of cancer incidence and prevention of neoplastic disease, may be closer.

Acknowledgment

I am indebted to Frances M. Williams and Muriel Mervis for dedicated and excellent editorial assistance. Research by the author is supported in part by U.S. Public Health Service grants CA-12376, CA-14298, CA-15400, CA-17613 and contract CP-33208 from the National Cancer Institute of the National Institutes of Health.

Literature Cited

1. Higginson, J., "Environment and Cancer," R. L. Clark, Ed., p. 69, Williams and Wilkins, Baltimore, 1972.
2. Wynder, E. L., Mabuchi, K., *Prev. Med.* (1972) **1**, 300.
3. Shimkin, M. B., Triolo, V. A., *Prog. Exp. Tumor Res.* (1969) **11** (1), 1.
4. Doll, R., Morgan, L. G., Speizer, F. E., *Br. J. Cancer* (1970) **24**, 623.
5. Friedell, G. H., *J. Natl. Cancer Inst.* (1969) **43**, 215.
6. Hueper, W. C., "Occupational and Environmental Cancers of the Urinary System," Yale University, New Haven and London, 1969.
7. Lilienfeld, A. M., Levin, M. L., Kessler, I. I., "Cancer in the United States," Harvard University, Cambridge, 1972.
8. Shimkin, M. B., *Methods Cancer Res.* (1967) **1**.
9. Silverberg, E., Holleb, A. I., *Ca, A Cancer J. Clin.* (1974) **24**, 2.
10. Eckardt, R. E., "Environment and Cancer," p. 93, Williams and Wilkins, Baltimore, 1972.
11. Weisburger, E. K., Weisburger, J. H., *Adv. Cancer Res.* (1958) **5**, 333.
12. Miller, J. A., Miller, E. C., *J. Natl. Cancer Inst.* (1971) **47**, V.
13. Farber, E., *Curr. Res. Oncol. Lect.* (1973) 95.
14. Weisburger, J. H., "Cancer Medicine," J. F. Holland and E. Frei, Eds., p. 45, Lea and Febiger, Philadelphia, 1973.
15. Weisburger, J. H., Weisburger, E. K., *Pharm. Rev.* (1973) **25**, 1.
16. Grover, P. L., Hewer, A., Sims, P., *Biochem. Pharmacol.* (1974) **23**, 323.
17. Oesch, F., *Xenobiotica* (1972) **3**, 305.
18. Sugimura, T., Kawachi, T., *Methods Cancer Res.* (1973) **7**, 245.
19. Wattenberg, L. W., *Toxicol. Appl. Pharmacol.* (1972) **23**, 741.
20. Conney, A. H., Burns, J. J., *Science* (1972) **178**, 576.
21. Hill, M. J., *Cancer* (1974) **33**.
22. Laqueur, G. L., "Carcinoma of the Colon and Antecedent Epithelium," W. J. Burdette, Ed., p. 305, Charles C. Thomas, Springfield, 1970.
23. Weisburger, J. H., *Proc. Natl. Cancer Conf., 7th* (1973) 465.
24. Chapman, W., *Cancer Res.* (1973) **33**, 1225.
25. Kuntz, R. E., Cheever, A. W., Myers, B. J., *J. Natl. Cancer Inst.* (1972) **48**, 223.
26. Wynder, E. L., Hoffmann, D., "Tobacco and Tobacco Smoke," Academic, New York, 1967.
27. Van Duuren, B. L., Katz, C., Goldschmidt, B. M., *J. Natl. Cancer Inst.* (1973) **51-2**, 703.
28. Saffiotti, U., *Prog. Exp. Tumor Res.* (1969) **11**, 302.

29. "Survey of Compounds Which Have Been Tested for Carcinogenic Activity," National Institutes of Health, Public Health Service Publication No. 149, Government Printing Office, Washington, D.C., 1971–72.
30. Hecker, E., *Methods Cancer Res.* (1971) **6,** 439.
31. Boutwell, R. K., *Crit. Rev. Toxicol.* (1974) 419–443.
32. Sivak, A., Van Duuren, B. L., *Chem. Biol. Interact.* (1971) **3,** 401.
33. Arcos, J. C., Argus, M. F., "Chemical Induction of Cancer, Structural Bases and Biological Mechanisms," Academic, New York, 1968.
34. Magee, P. N., *Methods Toxicol.* (1970), 158.
35. Weisburger, J. H., Weisburger, E. K., *Methods Cancer Res.* (1967) **1,** 307.
36. Miller, E. C., Miller, J. A., "Environment and Cancer," R. L. Clark, Ed., pp. 5–39, Williams and Wilkins, Baltimore, 1972.
37. Weisburger, J. H., Rall, D. P., "Environment and Cancer," R. L. Clark, Ed., p. 437, Williams and Wilkins, Baltimore, 1972.
38. Truhaut, R., "Potential Carcinogenic Hazards from Drugs," *UICC Monograph Ser.* **7.**
39. Clayson, D. B., *Drug-induced Dis.* (1972) **4.**
40. Vessilinovitch, S. D., Mihailovich, N., Wogan, G. N., Lombard, L. S., Rao, K. V. N., *Cancer Res.* (1972) **32,** 2289.
41. Staats, J., *Cancer Res.* (1968) **28,** 391.
42. Homburger, F., *Prog. Exp. Tumor Res.* (1972) **16.**
43. "Guide for the Care and Use of Laboratory Animals," Institute of Laboratory Animal Resources, National Research Council, U.S. Department of Health, Education and Welfare, Washington, D.C., 1972.
44. Huggins, C., Grand, L., Fukunishi, R., *Proc. Natl. Acad. Sci. U.S.* (1964) **51,** 737.
45. Griswold, D. P., Casey, A. E., Weisburger, E. K., Weisburger, J. H., *Cancer Res.* (1968) **28,** 924.
46. Hadidian, Z., Fredrickson, T. N., Weisburger, E. K., Weisburger, J. H., Glass, R. M. Mantel, N., *J. Natl. Cancer Inst.* (1968) **41,** 985.
47. Reuber, M. D., Glover, E. C., *J. Natl. Cancer Inst.* (1970) **44,** 419.
48. Shimkin, M. B., Weisburger, J. H., Weisburger, E. K., Gubareff, N., Suntzeff, V., *J. Natl. Cancer Inst.* (1966) **36,** 915.
49. Innes, J. R. M., Ulland, B. M., Valerio, M. G., Petrucelli, L., Fishbein, L., Hart, E. R., Pallotta, A. J., Bates, R. R., Falk, H. L., Gart, J. J., Klein, M., Mitchell, I., Peters, J., *J. Natl. Cancer Inst.* (1969) **42,** 1101.
50. Tomatis, L., Partensky, C., Montesano, R., *Int. J. Cancer* (1973) **12,** 1.
51. Shubik, P., *Prog. Exp. Tumor Res.* (1972) **16,** 176.
52. Homburger, F., Hsueh, S. S., Kerr, C. S., Russfield, A. B., *Cancer Res.* (1972) **32,** 360.
53. Hanna, M. G., Nettesheim, P., Richter, C. B., Tennant, R. W., *Israel J. Med. Sci.* (1973) **9,** 229.
54. Ross, M. H., Bras, G., *J. Nutr.* (1973) **103,** 944.
55. Toth, B., *Cancer Res.* (1968) **28,** 727.
56. Della Porta, G., Terracini, B., *Prog. Exp. Tumor Res.* (1969) **11,** 334.
57. Tomatis, L., Mohr, V., Davis, W., Eds., "Transplacental Carcinogenesis," Scientific Publication No. 4, International Agency for Research on Cancer, Lyon, 1973.
58. Herbst, A. L., *Cancer* (1972) **22,** 292.
59. Bryson, G., Bishoff, F., *Progr. Exp. Tumor Res.* (1969) **11,** 100.
60. Grasso, P., *Food Cosmet. Toxicol.* (1971) **9,** 463.
61. Hooson, J., Grasso, P., Gangolli, S. D., *Br. J. Cancer* (1973) **27,** 230.
62. Weisburger, J. H., "Toxicology," L. Casarett, J. Doull, Eds., McMillan, New York, 1975.
63. Clayson, D. B., *J. Natl. Cancer Inst.* (1974) **52,** 1685.
64. Druckrey, H., Preussmann, R., Ivankovic, S., Schmähl, D., *Z. Krebsforsch.* (1967) **69,** 103.

65. Druckrey, H., *Xenobiotica* (1973) **3**, 271.
66. Hanna, M. G., Nettesheim, P., Gilbert, J. R., "Inhalation Carcinogenesis," *AEC Symp. Ser.* (1970) **18**.
67. Nettesheim, P., Hanna, M. G., Deatherage, J. W., Jr., "Morphology Of Experimental Respiratory Carcinogenesis," *AEC Symp. Ser.* (1970) **21**.
68. Hoffmann, D., Wynder, E. L., this volume, chapter 7.
69. Bingham, E., *Arch. Environ. Health* (1971) **22**, 692.
70. Weisburger, J. H., Weisburger, E. K., *Food Cosmet. Toxicol.* (1968) **6**, 235.
71. Druckrey, H., "Potential Carcinogenic Hazards From Drugs," *UICC Monograph Ser.* (1967) **7**, 60.
72. Saffiotti, U., Cefis, F., Montesano, R., Sellakumar, A. R., "Bladder Cancer, A Symposium," W. B. Deichman and K. F. Lampe, Eds., p. 129, Aesculapius, Birmingham, 1967.
73. Leonard, B. J., "Pharmacological Models to Assess Toxicity and Side Effects of Fertility Regulating Agents," *Excerpta Med. Found.* (1973), 1.
74. Toth, B., *J. Natl. Cancer Inst.* (1969) **42**, 469.
75. Yamamoto, R. S., Weisburger, E. K., Korzis, J., *Proc. Soc. Exp. Biol. Med.* (1969) **124**, 1217.
76. Mantel, N., *Prog. Exp. Tumor Res.* (1969) **11**, 431.
77. Schneiderman, M. A., Mantel, N., *Prev. Med.* (1973) **2**, 165.
78. Stoltz, D. R., Poirier, L. A., Irving, C. C., Stich, H. F., Weisburger, J. H., Grice, H. C., *Toxicol. Appl. Pharmacol.* (1975) **29**, 157.
79. DiPaolo, J. A., Nelson, R. L., *Arch. Pathol.* (1973) **95**, 380.
80. Heidelberger, C., "Proceedings of the World Symposium on Model Studies in Chemical Carcinogenesis," P. O. P. Ts'o, and J. A. DiPaolo, Eds., Marcel Dekker, New York, 1974.
81. Schindler, R., *Food Cosmet. Toxicol.* (1969) **7**, 233.
82. Gelboin, H. V., Kinoshita, N., Wiebel, F. J., *Fed. Proc. Fed. Amer. Soc. Exp. Biol.* (1972) **31**, (4) 1298.
83. Williams, G. M., Elliot, J. M., Weisburger, J. H., *Cancer Res.* (1973) **33**, 606.
84. Katsuta, H., Takoka, T., "Topics in Chemical Carcinogenesis," *Proc. Int. Symp. Princess Takamatsu Cancer Res. Fund, 2nd* (1972), 389.
85. Hathway, P. E., "Foreign Compound Metabolism in Animals," The Chemical Society, London, 1970, 1972.
86. Fishman, W. H., "Metabolic Conjugation and Metabolic Hydrolysis," Academic, New York, 1970.
87. Grover, P. L., Sims, P., Hubermann, E., Marquart, H., Kuroki, T., Heidelberger, C., *Proc. Natl. Acad. Sci. USA* (1971) **68**, 1098.
88. Shabad, L. M., Kolesnichenko, T. S., Ye, E., *J. Natl. Cancer Inst.* (1971) **47**, 987.
89. Hollander, A., "Chemical Mutagens," 2 volumes, Plenum, New York, 1971.
90. Miller, E. C., Miller, J. A., "Chemical Mutagens," A. Hollander, Ed., p. 83, Plenum, New York, 1971.
91. Vogel, F., Röhrborn, G., "Chemical Mutagenesis In Mammals and Man," Springer, Berlin-Heidelberg-New York, 1970.
92. De Serres, F. J., *Proc. Int. Congr. Pharmacol. 5th* (1972) **2**, 150.
93. Garner, R. C., Miller, E. C., Miller, J. A., *Cancer Res.* (1972) **32**, 2058.
94. Nichols, W. W., *Ag. Actions* (1973) **3**, 86.
95. Legator, M. S., Flamm, W. G., *Ann. Rev. Biochem.* (1973) 683.
96. Stich, H. F., Laishes, B. A., *Pathobiology Ann.* (1973).
97. Cox, R., Damjanov, I., Abanobi, S. E., Sarma, D. S. R., *Cancer Res.* (1973) **33**, 2114.
98. Hennings, H., Michael, D. M., Eaton, S. D. A., Morgan, D. L., *J. Invest. Dermatol.* (1974) **62**, 480–484.
99. Goodman, J. I., Potter, V. R., *Cancer Res.* (1972) **32**, 766.
100. Stich, H. F., San, R. H. C., *Proc. Soc. Exp. Biol.* (1973) **142**, 155.
101. Irving, C. C., *Methods Cancer Res.* (1973) **7**, 189.

102. Cleaver, J. E., *J. Invest. Dermatol.* (1973) **60,** 374.
103. Abelev, G. I., *Adv. Cancer Res.* (1971) **14,** 295.
104. Gold, P., *Prog. Exp. Tumor Res.* (1971) **14,** 43.
105. Moore, T. L., Kupchik, H. Z., Marcon, N., Zamcheck, N., *Am. J. Dig. Dis.* (1972) **16,** 1.
106. Anderson, N., *Cancer Res.* (1974) **34,** 2021.
107. Kroes, R., Williams, G. M., Weisburger, J. H., *Cancer Res.* (1973) **33,** 613.
108. Watabe, H., *Cancer Res.* (1971) **31,** 1192.
109. Nechaud, B. de, Uriel, J., *Int. J. Cancer* (1973) **11,** 104.
110. Grice, H. C., Ed., "The Testing of Chemicals for Carcinogenicity, Mutagenicity, Teratogenicity," Canadian Ministry of Health and Welfare, Ottawa, 1973.
111. Lee, D. H. K., Kotin, P., Eds., "Multiple Factors in the Causation of Environmentally Induced Disease," Academic, New York, 1972.

Chapter

2

Tumor-Promoting and Co-carcinogenic Agents in Chemical Carcinogenesis

Benjamin L. Van Duuren, Laboratory of Organic Chemistry and Carcinogenesis, Institute of Environmental Medicine, New York University Medical Center, New York, N. Y. 10016

ALTHOUGH FIRST DISCOVERED in 1941, the exact chemical nature of tumor promoters and their biological mode of action only recently have become the subject of intensive study in many laboratories. The first major advance in this area was the isolation and identification of the phorbol esters which are active principles of croton oil, the classical tumor promoter. Since then the biochemical and biological effects of these and related materials have been studied in a variety of test systems. Not all of these biological effects are necessarily related to the process of tumor promotion, but they may help to elucidate the mode of action of tumor promoters; hence, they are also discussed in this report. The word "tumor promoter" is used at times interchangeably with co-carcinogen, accelerating agent, and so forth. However, there is a clearcut distinction in the method of biological testing for tumor promoters and for co-carcinogens. This may apply to their mode of action. The title for this article is based on this observation.

There have been a number of recent reviews on tumor promoters (*1*, *2*, *3*, *4*). This article gives a brief historical review of the unfolding of this fascinating area of cancer research. Emphasis is on a critical discussion of recent biochemical and biological studies on tumor promoters and co-carcinogens and their possible mode of action.

Historical

Croton oil is obtained from the seeds of the plant *Croton tiglium L.* (*Euphorbiaceae*), which is indigenous to India and Ceylon. Since 1930 Flaschenträger and co-workers (*5*, *6*, *7*), Kauffmann and co-workers (*8*, *9*), Cherbuliez and co-workers (*10*, *11*), and Bernhard (*12*) have studied the toxic, vesicant, irritant properties, and chemistry of croton oil. At that time, croton oil was used as a cathartic in veterinary medicine, and nothing was known about its role in chemical carcinogenesis.

Rous and co-workers (13, 14) examined the role of irritation, wounding, and the stimulation of cell division in tumor induction. Rous suggested the term initiation to describe the first event which led to cancer in rabbit ears when the initial treatment was followed by treatment with a secondary agent which he called a tumor promoter.

Berenblum studied the effects of irritation in chemical carcinogenesis. He discovered that croton resin, a concentrate of the active fractions of croton oil obtained by solvent fractionation, together with low doses of benzo(a)-pyrene enhanced tumor induction much more than benzo(a)pyrene alone (15). Subsequently, Mottram (16) found that a single application of benzo-(a)pyrene followed by repeated applications of croton oil elicited many skin tumors in mice. These early experiments are summarized in Table I. These historic findings stimulated many years of research on what became known as initiation–promotion experiments or two-stage carcinogenesis (1, 2, 3, 4). As initiating agents, low doses of skin carcinogens (e.g., benzo(a)pyrene or 7,12-dimethylbenz(a)anthracene) were used, and croton oil or croton resin was the universal tumor promoter.

There were many studies concerning dose response of initiator with constant dose of croton oil and vice-versa, the high frequency of tumor regression with croton oil as promoter, the role of mouse skin inflammatory responses in tumor promotion, and the induction of tumors by croton oil alone. All these experiments were done on mouse skin. These early studies with croton oil generated controversy among workers concerning the role of croton oil in mouse skin carcinogenesis, and much of this controversy and experimentation

Table I. Tumor Promotion and Co-carcinogenesis with Croton Oil and Croton Resin (15, 16)

Treatment[a]	Duration (weeks)	Mice with Tumors / Total Mice	Weeks to First Tumor
BP, 0.05%[b]	28	5/112	17
BP, 0.05% + CO, 0.5%[b]	29	15/31	10
CO, 0.5%[b]	24	0/36	—
CR, 1%[b]	22	0/20	—
BP, 0.3%, three applications[c]	20	0/6	—
BP, 0.3%, three applications followed by CO (three times weekly)[c]	20	5/6	8
BP, 0.3%, one application followed by CO (three times weekly)[c]	20	11/12	8

[a] Abbreviations: BP, benzo(a)pyrene; CO, croton oil; CR, croton resin.
[b] Ref. 15, treatment once weekly.
[c] Ref. 16.

Table II.   Structural Features of Phorbol ($C_{20}H_{28}O_6$)
According to Flaschenträger (*5, 6, 7*)

Five hydroxyl groups
One isolated double bond
One: C=C—C=O

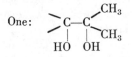

One:

could have been avoided if the active tumor-promoting agents had been available earlier. These earlier controversial aspects have been reviewed (*1*).

Flascheträger and co-workers (*5, 6, 7*) isolated a compound which he named phorbol; molecular formula: $C_{20}H_{28}O_6$. They suggested that this compound contains a cyclic terpene nucleus. With no instrumental methods, so commonly assumed to be essential in a modern chemical laboratory, Flaschenträger deduced several essential structural features of the phorbol molecule as shown in Table II. All of these were subsequently proved to be correct.

In the early 1960's Van Duuren and co-workers (*17, 18*) and Hecker and co-workers (*19, 20*) independently reported the isolation and partial characterization of various active compounds from croton oil. All of these materials were potent tumor-promoting agents and were diesters of phorbol which was isolated and partially characterized many years earlier by Flaschenträger and co-workers (*5, 6, 7*). The detailed chemical structures of the active agents were determined by x-ray analysis of suitable bromo derivatives and were published independently and simultaneously by Pettersen and co-workers (*21*) in England and by Hoppe and co-workers (*22*) in Germany. Based on these x-ray analyses, the detailed structure and stereochemistry of the most widely used diester of phorbol—phorbol myristate acetate (PMA)— is that shown in Structure 1. As far as the known diesters of phorbol that have been tested, PMA is the most active agent known in two-stage carcino-

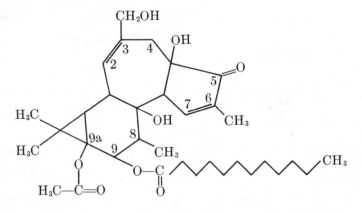

1

genesis experiments on mouse skin (*1, 2*). In subsequent studies Hecker (*3*) reported the isolation of additional diesters of phorbol from croton oil. Crombie and co-workers (*23*) detailed their studies on the structure and stereochemistry of phorbol and derivatives. Recently, we described a rapid method for preparing highly purified PMA from croton oil (*24*). Starting with phorbol, Bresch *et al.* (*25*) prepared a semisynthetic PMA. They also described the preparation of an extensive series of other di- and triesters of phorbol (*25*). Some of these esters are described in the section on structure–activity relationships below.

There has been some disparity in the nomenclature used for phorbol, its diesters, and other derivatives. This author has used the trivial name phorbol myristate acetate (PMA) since 1965 (*18*). Hoppe *et al.* (*22*) used an arbitrary numbering system for the phorbol ring system. Another nomenclature was used by Crombie *et al.* (*23*). This author urges that *Chemical Abstracts (CA)* nomenclature be used by all authors and that the trivial name phorbol myristate acetate be used in titles and texts of papers dealing with this compound because of the unwieldy length of the correct *Chemical Abstracts* nomenclature (*25a*). This numbering system is shown in Structure **1.** The correct *CA* name for PMA is: myristic acid, 9-ester with 1,1aα,1bβ,-4,4a,7aα,7b,8,9,9a-decahydro-4aβ,7bα,9β,9aα-tetrahydroxy-3-(hydroxymethyl)-1,1,6,8α-tetramethyl-5*H*-cyclopropa[3,4]benz[1,2-*e*]azulen-5-one 9a-acetate. (*CA* Registry Number 20839-11-6). *CA* nomenclature is the most widely used throughout the world. In addition, each chemical it lists carries a *CA* registry number. This name is also the preferred IUPAC nomenclature for organic compounds.

Other tumor-promoting agents of historical interest are: phenol (*26*), Tween and Span compounds (*27, 28*), anthralin (*29, 30*), and dodecane (*27*). They are discussed under structure–activity relationships.

Definitions

To date all experiments involving initiating and promoting agents—*i.e.*, two-stage carcinogenesis—have been done on mouse skin. Most co-carcinogenesis experiments have also been carried out on mouse skin.

At present it is not possible to define initiating and promoting agents which are involved in two-stage carcinogenesis in terms of their mechanism of action since little is known about this aspect. For the present purposes, they are described in operational terms.

Two-stage carcinogenesis on mouse skin involves an initiating agent and promoting agent. An initiator or initiating agent is one which results in induction of benign and malignant tumors when applied on mouse skin in a single dose followed by repeated applications of a promoting agent. The initiating agent alone is given in such a dose that it does not result in skin tumors at the site of application during the lifespan of the animal. Many initiating agents used in two-stage carcinogenesis are carcinogenic, *e.g.*, the aromatic hydrocarbons, benzo(*a*)pyrene, and 7-12-dimethylbenz(*a*)anthracene. Some noncarcinogenic mouse skin initiating agents are known (Table

Table III.   Initiating Agents Which Are Not Carcinogenic on Mouse Skin

Compound	Reference for Carcinogenicity Assay on Mouse Skin	Reference for Initiating Activity
Dibenz (a,c) anthracene	38	31
Chrysene [a]	38	34
Benz (a) anthracene [a]	38	31, 35
Urethane [b]	33	32, 33, 35
Triethylenemelamine	35	35
1,4-Dimethanesulfonoxy-2-butyne	37	37
Epichlorohydrin [c]	39	39
Chloromethyl methyl ether [c]	36	36

[a] These are considered borderline carcinogens by some.
[b] Causes lung tumors in mice.
[c] Induces sarcomas in mice by subcutaneous injection (39).

III). Urethane is not carcinogenic for mouse skin but has been used widely in two-stage carcinogenesis as an initiator either when applied topically or when given by subcutaneous or intraperitoneal injection in high doses (32, 33). Urethane, however, does induce lung tumors in mice (33). However, not all chemical carcinogens are initiating agents. These are usually carcinogens which have to be metabolized *in vivo* to activated carcinogenic intermediates.

A promoting agent is one which is applied repeatedly after a single dose of an initiating agent and results in benign and malignant tumors. All known

Table IV.   Dose–Response Studies with Phorbol Myristate Acetate (24) [a]

Dose PMA, μg in 0.1 ml Acetone [b]	Number of Mice with Papillomas	Total Number of Papillomas	Number of Mice with Squamous Carcinoma	Days to First Tumor
25.0 [c]	20	245	11	27
5.0	20	155	9	35
2.5	19	127	4	41
0.5	13	54	3	36
0.1	0	0	0	—

[a] Twenty female ICR/Ha Swiss mice were in each group; results at 365 days; median survival time was greater than 365 days except where noted. Control groups not shown were: (a) DMBA once, followed by acetone three times weekly; (b) acetone only three times weekly; (c) a no-treatment group. No skin tumors were observed in any of these groups. For the test groups, there were 17 to 20 survivors at the times of first appearance of tumors.
[b] Single treatment of 5 μg 7,12-dimethylbenz(a)anthracene was given 14 days prior to the beginning of treatment with PMA. PMA was applied at the dosages indicated three times weekly.
[c] Median survival time was 246 days.

promoting agents also have weak tumorigenic activity (1). The two terms, initiator and tumor promoter, are mechanistically and temporally interrelated and cannot be separated. When the sequence of applications is reversed, few if any tumors appear.

In co-carcinogenesis experiments two agents are administered simultaneously and usually repeatedly and result in significantly higher tumor incidences than either agent alone. Thus, there is an operational difference and probably a real difference in mode of action since not all co-carcinogens are tumor promoters and vice-versa (40, 41, 42, 43). This aspect is described below.

Several features are unique to two-stage carcinogenesis. These are depicted in Table IV and Figure 1 (24) for PMA. Tumors appear very rapidly after promoting treatment begins, ~ 35 days. In the dosage range 2.5–25 µg, PMA applied three times weekly results in papillomas on most or all of the

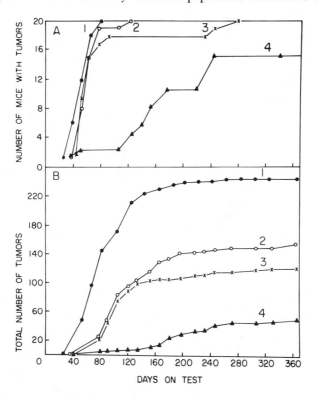

Figure 1. Rate of tumor appearance in two-stage carcinogenesis.

A single dose of 5 µg 7,12-dimethylbenz(a)anthracene applied to the dorsal skins of mice was followed 14 days later by three-times weekly applications of PMA at various doses in 0.1 ml acetone per application. Curve 1, 25 µg; curve 2, 5.0 µg; curve 3, 2.5 µg; curve 4, 0.5 µg. There were 20 female ICR/Ha mice per group.

animals, and 20–55% of these animals also bear squamous carcinomas of the skin after one year on test. Each animal shows multiple tumors as noted in Table IV. These papillomas are so numerous that they coalesce, and some of these coalesced tumors proceed to squamous carcinomas of the skin. Based on these data and those in which PMA was applied once weekly (24), a dose–response curve was plotted. At weekly doses above 7.5 μg, there is no decrease in t_{50}, *i.e.*, the time required for 50% of the animals to develop papillomas, with increasing dose levels. Below this value, the t_{50} increases directly as a function of the weekly dose, regardless of application frequency, reaching an apparent threshold at $\sim$ 0.3–0.5 μg PMA per week (24).

Because tumors can be rapidly induced in mouse skin by the two-stage carcinogenesis method with PMA as promoter, this procedure is being used in our laboratory to screen for potential carcinogens (39) since some carcinogens are initiating agents.

[↓, Initiation, 20µg DMBA, once only; ↳ Promotion, 2.5µg PMA, three times weekly]

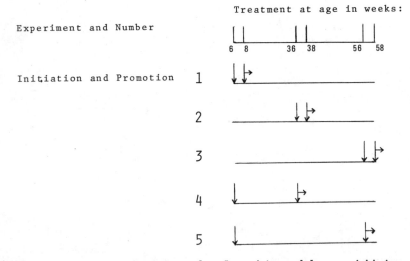

Figure 2. Protocol for determining the effect of interval between initiation and promotion and the effect of aging of mice in two-stage carcinogenesis

The early tumor appearance with PMA or other phorbol esters as promoting agents was mentioned above. Our studies found that this rapid appearance of tumors is independent of the dose of 7,12-dimethylbenz(a)anthracene whether it is 300 or 150 (1) or as low as 5 μg as in the dose–response studies described above (24). This time to first tumor, $\sim$ 35 days, and its independence from dose of initiator (5–300 μg) or promoter (PMA, 0.5–25 μg), raise interesting questions concerning the biological events during the promoting treatment. For example, this time might be required for a certain

Table V.   Permanence of Initiating Treatment (44)

Group Number	Age at Primary Treatment (weeks)	Interval to Secondary Treatment (weeks)	Number of Mice[a]	% Mice with Papillomas	% Mice with Squamous Carcinoma
1	6	2	120	100	50
2	44	2	20	100	30
3	56	2	50	56	6
4	6	36	35	90	25
5	6	56	35	57	11

[a] Female ICR/Ha Swiss mice.

Cancer Research

critical number of tumor cells to be formed before papillomas become visible to the naked eye. This regimen, *i.e.*, 7,12-dimethylbenz(*a*)anthracene followed by PMA, results in the appearance of papillomas much earlier and in larger numbers than any known mouse skin carcinogen if the latter is applied repeatedly without a promoter. In addition, in two-stage carcinogenesis experiments squamous skin carcinomas appear very early, in 15–20 weeks.

Another interesting feature in two-stage carcinogenesis is the permanence or persistence of the initiating effect—*i.e.*, a single treatment with the initiator followed much later, up to 58 weeks, by the promoting treatment. The earlier data have been reviewed before (*1*). Since then a definitive study was done in our laboratory (*44*) using the procedure shown in Figure 2. Not shown are the appropriate control groups—*i.e.*, one agent only given at the various time intervals. Such control groups were included in the experiments described (*44*). The results are summarized in Table V. The carcinoma incidences observed are illustrated in Figure 3. These results show that skin carcinomas are induced whether the interval between initiation and promotion

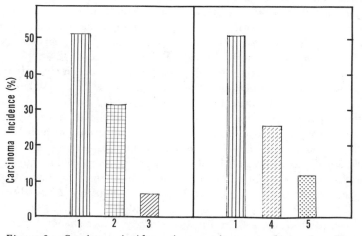

Figure 3.   Carcinoma incidence for experiment numbers referred to in Figure 2. The group sizes are given in Table V.

is 2, 36, or 56 weeks. The carcinoma incidences are significantly lower in groups 3 and 5 where the secondary treatment was started when the animals were 58 and 62 weeks old, respectively.

The weak tumorigenic activity of phorbol esters and other tumor promoters on mouse skin has been referred to above and was reviewed earlier (1). This property does not detract from their remarkable promoting activity. The tumorigenicity of phorbol esters can be reasonably interpreted if one assumes that in any group of animals there will be some which have latent tumor cells, either by earlier exposure to an external initiating agent or by spontaneous conversion of normal cells into latent tumor cells. If this explanation is accepted, the question about "pure" promoting agents should become obsolete. Latent tumor cells should precede the occurrence of clusters of tumor cells in the development of spontaneous cancer. This factor is of central importance concerning the role of exogenous and endogenous tumor-promoting agents.

Prehn (45) in his description of the clonal selection theory of carcinogenesis pointed out that pure promoting agents will never be found because of the spontaneous occurrence of clones of variants.

Structure–Activity Relationships of Tumor-Promoting Agents

Phorbol myristate acetate is by far the most active of the many phorbol diesters prepared to date (1, 3, 46). Several workers (3, 46) examined the effect of ester chain length at positions 9 and 9a of the phorbol moiety. Phorbol diacetate, phorbol dibenzoate, and phorbol are inactive or very weakly active as promoters in Charles River mice; phorbol didecanoate is an active but not very potent promoter (46). The earlier work (1, 3, 46) shows that one short-chain ester function and one long-chain ester function at the C-9a and C-9 positions of phorbol and a free hydroxymethyl group at the C-3 position are important for biological activity. In the 11 natural phorbol diesters from croton oil the short-chain acid is either acetate or isobutyrate, and the long-chain acids are straight-chain saturated acids from C_8 to C_{14}. We considered the lipophilic–hydrophilic (amphiphatic) nature a significant aspect of these phorbol esters (1) in relation to their biological activity. This is discussed in greater detail below. However, lipophilic–hydrophilic molecules, such as the monolaurates of catechol, resorcinol, hydroquinone, and pyrogallol, are inactive as tumor promoters (47). Hecker has isolated a number of compounds containing the phorbol or a related moiety from *Euphorbia* and other plant species (3). Some of these compounds have weak tumor-promoting activity, but none showed activity comparable with that of PMA.

Many compounds have been tested as tumor-promoting agents (26, 27, 28, 29, 30, 47) using either 7,12-dimethylbenz(a)anthracene, benzo(a)pyrene, or urethane as the initiator. Of these only a few showed noteworthy activity. They are: anthralin (1,8-dihydroxy-9-anthrone), Structure 2 (29, 30), phenol (26, 47), n-dodecane (27, 42, 48), lauric acid (49), methyl-12-oxo-*trans*-10-octadecenoate, Structure 4, and methylhydroxyoctadecadienoate, Structure 5 (50). Tween and Span compounds were tested by Setälä for tumor-promoting activity (28). The latter compounds as tested were not pure and were active only in massive doses. Thus, Setälä's findings are probably not relevant to tumor promotion.

Of the compounds listed above, anthralin is the most active tumor promoter after the phorbol esters. Anthralin was formerly assigned the tautomeric structure 1,8,9-trihydroxyanthracene (Structure **3**) in chemistry texts. Studies in our laboratory *(30)* showed that it is in the anthrone form.

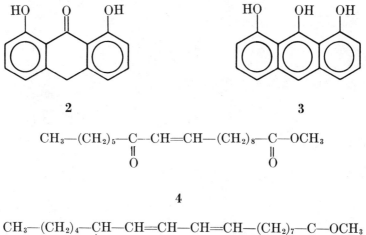

$$CH_3—(CH_2)_5—\underset{\underset{O}{\|}}{C}—CH=CH—(CH_2)_8—\underset{\underset{O}{\|}}{C}—OCH_3$$

4

$$CH_3—(CH_2)_4—\underset{\underset{OH}{|}}{CH}—CH=CH—CH=CH—(CH_2)_7—\underset{\underset{O}{\|}}{C}—OCH_3$$

5

Our studies on the tumor-promoting activity of anthralin showed that close analogs of anthralin were inactive tumor promoters. These included 1,8-dihydroxyanthraquinone, 1,8-dihydroxyanthracene, anthrone, and a dimer of anthralin (Structure **6**) which is formed spontaneously from anthralin in

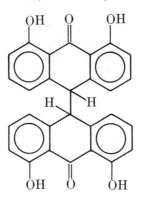

a

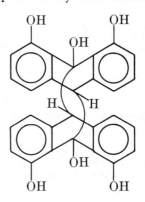

b

6

Table VI.   Tumor-Promoting Activity of Anthralin and Related Compounds (30)[a]

Primary Treatment[b]	Secondary Treatment and Dose in μg/0.1 ml of Acetone[c]		Days to First Papilloma	Number of Mice with Tumors[d] Total Number of Tumors
DMBA	1,8-dihydroxy-9-anthrone	80.0	59	18/94[e] (9)
None	1,8-dihydroxy-9-anthrone	80.0	287	1/1
DMBA	1,8-dihydroxyanthraquinone	170.0	—	0
None	1,8-dihydroxyanthraquinone	170.0	—	0
DMBA	anthralin dimer	80.0	—	0
None	anthralin dimer	80.0	—	0
DMBA	1,8-dihydroxynaphthalene	60.0	—	0
None	1,8-dihydroxynaphthalene	60.0	—	0
DMBA	anthrone	70.0	—	0
None	anthrone	70.0	—	0
DMBA	phorbol myristate acetate	2.5	54	20/278[f] (13)
None	phorbol myristate acetate	2.5	361	2/2
DMBA	acetone		—	0
None	acetone		—	0
No treatment[g]			—	0

[a] 20 ICR/Ha female Swiss mice per group. Results are at 490 days when the experiment was terminated. Median survival time was >490 days, except where noted.
[b] DMBA: 7,12-dimethylbenz(a)anthracene, 20 μg in 0.1 ml of acetone once only by micropipet.
[c] Promoters applied three times a week at doses indicated beginning 14 days after primary treatment.
[d] Squamous papilloma; number of mice with squamous carcinoma in parenthesis.
[e] The median survival time was 348 days.
[f] The median survival time in this group was 305 days.
[g] 100 mice.

Journal of Medicinal Chemistry

acetone solution (30). The exact structure of this compound—i.e., **6a** or **6b** remains to be determined. In these experiments PMA was used as a positive control which allows a direct comparison of the tumor-promoting activity of PMA and anthralin. These findings are summarized in Table VI.

Comparison of Tumor-Promoting and Co-carcinogenic Agents

Several reports have indicated that n-dodecane and mineral oil (48, 51) are co-carcinogens when applied repeatedly on mouse skin together with varying doses of benzo(a)pyrene. Similar experimental findings were obtained when mineral oil was applied simultaneously with varying doses of 7,12-dimethylbenz(a)anthracene (52). Hoffmann and Wynder (43) found that the noncarcinogenic aromatic hydrocarbons, pyrene and fluoranthene, resulted in co-carcinogenic activity when applied on mouse skin together and repeatedly with a low dose of benzo(a)pyrene. In a recent study we found that linalyl oleate and linalyl acetate are weak co-carcinogens (40). In the same series of tests (40) phenol, earlier shown to be a weak tumor-promoting agent (26, 47), was an inhibitor when tested as a co-carcinogen together with repeated applications of 5 µg of benzo(a)pyrene at the same dosage used in the earlier two-stage carcinogenesis experiments, *i.e.*, 3 mg per application, three times weekly (47). Because of these findings we tested an extensive series of compounds for co-carcinogenic activity. The results of some of these experiments are given in Table VII (42). The rates of tumor appearance for a few of these tests are shown in Figure 4, and some of the findings of these experiments are illustrated in Figure 5.

Table VIII compares some of the known tumor-promoting agents and co-carcinogens; clearly, not all tumor promoters are co-carcinogens and vice-versa. The two most potent tumor promoters, PMA and anthralin, have both properties and so does *n*-dodecane.

Of great interest in this work (42) is that catechol has remarkable co-carcinogenic activity but is inactive when tested as a tumor promoter. This is important in tobacco carcinogenesis which is discussed in another part of this article. Also, the isomer of catechol (*i.e.*, resorcinol) and the related

Table VII. Co-carcinogenesis on Mouse Skin (42) [a]

Carcinogen[b]	Co-carcinogen and Dose (mg)	Days to First Papilloma	Mice with Papillomas — Total Number of Papillomas	Mice with Squamous Carcinomas
B(a)P	phenol, 3	267	7/9	3
None	phenol, 3	355	1/1	0
B(a)P	eugenol, 10	299	4/4	2
None	eugenol, 10	—	0	0
B(a)P	pyrene, 0.004	250	12/14	6
B(a)P	pyrene, 0.012	186	26/42	20
None	pyrene 0.012	—	0	0
B(a)P	benzo(g,h,i)perylene, 0.007	238	19/31	10
B(a)P	benzo(g,h,i)perylene, 0.021	222	20/39	18
None	benzo(g,h,i)perylene, 0.021	—	0/0	0
B(a)P	benzo(e)pyrene, 0.005	249	24/33	9
B(a)P	benzo(e)pyrene, 0.015	246	33/79	27
None	benzo(e)pyrene, 0.015	—	0	0
B(a)P	catechol, 2	229	36/90	31
None	catechol, 2	292	1/1	1
B(a)P	resorcinol, 10	249	5/6	2
None	resorcinol, 10	—	0	0
B(a)P	anthralin, 0.080	159	25/58	15
None	anthralin, 0.080	307	2/2	0
B(a)P	P.M.A., 0.0025	60	45/260	37
None	P.M.A., 0.0025	174	5/5	0
B(a)P	acetone, 0.1 ml	251	14/16	10
No treatment (100 mice)		—	0	0

[a] 50 female ICR/Ha mice per group; results at 368 days.
[b] B(a)P: 5 µg benzo(a)pyrene, applied simultaneously in the same solution with cocarcinogen three times weekly in 0.1 ml acetone per application.

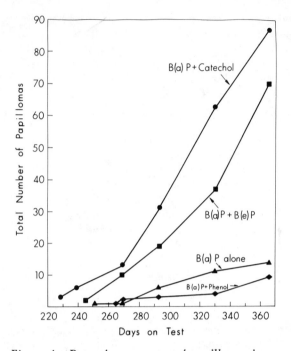

Figure 4. Rate of appearance of papillomas in co-carcinogenesis experiments. Dose of benzo(a)pyrene (B(a)P) was 5 μg per application in all cases. Doses of cocarcinogens applied simultaneously three times per week were: Benzo(e)pyrene (B(e)P): 15 μg; phenol: 3 mg; catechol: 2 mg. All solutions were applied in 0.1 ml acetone. Fifty female ICR/Ha mice per group.

phenol (eugenol) are inactive as co-carcinogens. The finding that noncarcino-genic aromatic hydrocarbons such as pyrene and benzo(e)pyrene have potent co-carcinogenic activities at low doses is important in relation to tobacco carcinogenesis discussed below.

Biochemical Studies on The Mode of Action of Tumor-Promoting Agents: in Vitro and in Vivo

Numerous studies have been carried out within the past few years con-cerning the mode of action of tumor promoters. Most of these studies have focused on the use of PMA and a few related compounds. As a result, a variety of divergent concepts have been proposed concerning the mode of action of PMA. Some of these findings are described below. Since it is too early to pinpoint mode of action of tumor promoters, no attempt is made to present a unifying concept; instead we point out which features researchers in this field consider important.

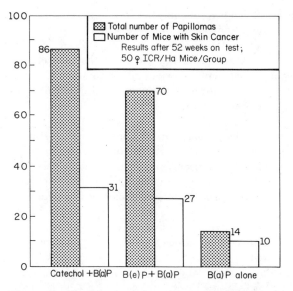

Figure 5. Papilloma and carcinoma incidences for same experiments shown in Figure 4

These studies are complicated by the fact that in two-stage carcinogenesis an initiating event whose exact nature is unclear is also involved. Some workers believe that initiation involves covalent interaction with DNA, *i.e.*, a

Table VIII.   Comparison of Tumor-Promoting and Co-carcinogenic Activities[a]

Compound	Tumor-Promoting Activity	Cocarcinogenic Activity
Phorbol myristate acetate	+	+
Anthralin	+	+
n-Dodecane	+[b]	+[c]
Linalyl oleate	−[d]	+[d]
Phenol	+	−
Catechol	−	+
Resorcinol	−	−
Hydroquinone	−	−
Eugenol	−[e]	−[e]
Pyrogallol	−	+
Pyrene	−[f]	+[f]
Fluoranthene	−[f]	+[f]
Benzo (e) pyrene	?	+

[a] From Ref. *42,* except where noted.
[b] Ref. *27.*
[c] Ref. *48* and *51.*
[d] Ref. *40.*
[e] Ref. *34.*
[f] Ref. *42.*

permanent heritable change in the genome of the cell. The promoting agent then allows this initial change to be expressed.

When PMA was isolated in this laboratory (*17, 18*), its lipophilic–hydrophilic nature suggested that an interaction at the plasma membrane of the cell might be important, and we began *in vivo* mouse skin experiments using tritiated phorbol ester. However, because of the difficulties associated with biochemical studies in mouse skin, *in vitro* experiments in cell culture were also done.

In the mouse skin localization experiments we determined (*1*) that at 3–6 hr after skin application the keratin layer just above the basal cells was highly labeled, and the sebaceous glands and hair follicles were moderately labeled. After 48 hr there was still some labeling in the sebaceous glands and hair follicles. The half-life of the labeled promoter was close to 24 hr.

Following these observations Weissmann *et al.* (*53*) observed that PMA releases several rabbit liver lysosomal enzymes *in vitro*. However, this occurred only at high concentrations ($\sim 50\ \mu g/ml$) compared with the very low doses required for effective tumor-promoting activity on mouse skin. Subsequent studies in this laboratory (*54*) showed that the lysosomes of mouse epidermal cells as well as of normal and SV 40-transformed 3T3 cells were resistant to labilization of lysosomal enzymes. The enzymes assayed were acid phosphatase and β-glucuronidase. These and related findings (*54*) suggested that while the release of lysosomal enzymes *in vitro* in rabbit (*53*), mouse, and rat liver (*54*) is of interest, it is probably not a critical event in tumor promotion (*1*).

An earlier *in vitro* study in 3T3 mouse embryo fibroblasts from this laboratory (*1, 55*) had also yielded interesting new findings which showed that cells in culture can be released from contact inhibition by PMA. Mixed populations of 10,000 3T3 cells and 100 virus-transformed 3T3 cells were exposed to the phorbol ester at 1.0 $\mu g/ml$ of medium (*55*). In contrast to control groups not exposed to the phorbol ester, there was a marked increase in the number of transformed clones that grew out in the mixed culture exposed to phorbol ester. In a subsequent study this mixed culture system was evaluated further for use in assessing tumor-promoting activity rapidly (*56*).

In another study we examined the binding pattern of [³H]-PMA to a stationary monolayer of 3T3 cells at various time intervals (*57*). In the continued presence of PMA a binding plateau is reached in about 18 hr and remains constant for an additional day. From the autoradiographs of formalin-fixed cells it was clear that the binding was primarily nonnuclear and that most of the binding probably was in membrane-rich areas of the cell. By contrast, when the cells were methanol fixed, no binding could be observed using the same autoradiographic techniques. Thus, organic solvent effects should be considered carefully in studies dealing with the effect of PMA on cell membranes or membrane-associated phenomena. In these studies on binding of tritium-labeled PMA to mouse skin and to 3T3 cells in culture (*57*), one could not be sure that binding of intact PMA was involved. We expected that PMA metabolism would be occurring and that this metabolism might be rapid. To date few studies on the metabolism of the phorbol esters have been described, and these are detailed below.

Other findings from this laboratory that relate to interaction of PMA at the plasma membrane were that PMA decreases the ability of both normal and virus-transformed 3T3 cells to exclude the dye, trypan blue, without causing lysis or cell disruption (*54*). In another experiment (*54*), contact-inhibited monolayer cultures of normal 3T3 cells were exposed to PMA for 18–72 hr. The control culture—*i.e.*, untreated cells that had been at mono-layer for one week—were granular and vacuolated, and their external membranes were diffuse and unrefractile. Treatment with PMA resulted in a rapid and dramatic change in the configuration of the cells in the culture. The cells resumed their characteristic fibroblast morphology, and the cell membranes were refractile and discrete as in a growing culture not at mono-layer. PMA also increased the specific activities of the cell membrane enzymes Na^+–K^+ATPase and $5'$-nucleotidase in microsomal preparations from sta-tionary cultures of Balb/c-3T3 mouse embryo fibroblasts (*58*).

Although these studies were incomplete and indirect, we proposed (*1*, *54*) that PMA and possibly other tumor promoters interact with the external cell membrane in such a way that unusual exchanges of various macromole-cules and/or metal ions occur. Alterations in intracellular constituents in-duced this way can in turn change control mechanisms inside the cell in undefined ways.

The possible role of interaction of phorbol esters with cell membranes has received recent attention from other laboratories (*59, 60*). The latter studies showed that in cesium chloride equilibrium density gradients, tritium-labeled phorbol didecanoate co-sediments with rat liver microsomal and nuclear membranes. Furthermore, there are changes in the membranes thus treated, including changes in density and in the ability of the membrane to bind DNA. By comparison the parent compound phorbol, which is inactive as a tumor promoter, does not affect any of these properties of rat liver microsomal membranes *in vitro*. From their work the authors tentatively concluded that PMA binds to membrane sites that control DNA synthesis and cell division (*60*).

In 1970 a report from this laboratory (*61*) described the enhancement of RNA synthesis by PMA in stationary cultures of 3T3 mouse embryo fibroblasts. Cultures that had grown to saturation density were allowed to remain there for at least three days before PMA was added. The cultures were therefore stationary in the G_0 phase of the cell cycle where DNA synthesis and cell division had essentially stopped and RNA synthesis was considerably reduced. It was found also (*61*) that in virally or chemically transformed cell lines, RNA synthesis was not affected. Actinomycin D did not completely inhibit the synthesis of RNA in the presence of PMA in these experiments (*61*).

Several recent reports concerning the effects of PMA on the synthesis of DNA, RNA, and proteins *in vivo* or *in vitro* have appeared (*62, 63, 64, 65*).

There was some indication that the stimulation of macromolecular synthesis in mouse skin correlated with tumor-promoting activity (64). The same workers (66) showed that a single topical application of PMA resulted in a stimulation of the phosphorylation of mouse epidermal histones. When phorbol dibenzoate, a weak promoter, or phorbol was used instead of PMA, stimulation of histone phosphorylation was slight or nonexistent. However, the role of increased macromolecular synthesis or stimulation of mouse epidermal histone phosphorylation induced by PMA in the mechanism of tumor promotion has yet to be explained.

PMA was shown to stimulate DNA synthesis *in vitro* in rat thymic lymphoblasts (63) at a very low concentration (0.05 μg/ml). Furthermore, this stimulatory effect of PMA was calcium dependent since it did not stimulate the initiation of DNA synthesis or proliferation when calcium was omitted from the medium. This calcium dependency was not the result of a general cellular deficiency since other stimulants of DNA synthesis in thymic lymphoblasts such as prostaglandin E_1 and cyclic AMP enhanced DNA synthesis in the same calcium-deficient medium (63).

Recent studies (67) have shown that phytohemagglutinin (PHA), a mitogenic agent, does not have to enter lymphocytes to enhance cell proliferation. By using PHA covalently bound to Sepharose beads, other workers (68) suggested that a mitogenic signal is produced at the cell membrane when certain plant lectins are allowed to interact with lymphocytes. This mitosis induction is accompanied by a marked increase in intracellular cyclic-3',5'-guanosine monophosphate (cGMP). Based on these observations, Estensen and associates (69) examined the effects of PMA on cGMP synthesis *in vitro* in Balb/c-3T3 cells and in human lymphocytes. Confluent monolayers of 3T3 cells were exposed to 0.1 μg/ml of PMA, and intracellular cGMP was measured at various time intervals between 15 and 60 sec after exposure to PMA. There was a rapid increase in cGMP within seconds, amounting to a 20-fold increase 45 sec after exposure began. The cGMP levels returned to control levels by 3 min. Cyclic adenosine monophosphate (cAMP) levels did not show any effect in this time interval. Other mitogenic agents which cause increases in intracellular cGMP do so only after longer time intervals (70).

Other workers (71) have examined the effect of PMA on cAMP in mouse skin. A single dose of PMA, 15 μg, was applied to mouse skin, the skins were removed after several time intervals, and cAMP measured. There was a rapid decrease in whole mouse skin cAMP within 1–2 hr. That level was maintained for ~ 24 hr, and by 48 hr the cAMP levels had returned to normal.

These effects of PMA on intracellular cGMP and cAMP are by no means unique since other agents are known to cause similar effects. The role of these effects in tumor promotion thus remains to be clarified, but they add to the body of evidence which will eventually lead to an understanding of the mode of action of tumor promoters.

Several reports have suggested that tumor promoters function by inhibiting DNA-repair mechanisms (*72, 73, 74*). These studies were carried out in human lymphocytes (*72, 73*) and in Hela cells (*74*). Inhibition of DNA repair mechanisms as the mode of action of tumor promoters, as suggested (*72, 73*), is most unlikely in view of the persistence of the initiating effect described earlier. Furthermore, there appears to be no correlation between tumor-promoting activity and concentrations required to produce 50% inhibition of repair. The Tween and Span compounds have borderline, if any, tumor-promoting activity *in vivo*, but they produce 50% inhibition of repair at very low concentrations (*72*).

Because of its structural complexity phorbol has not yet been synthesized. Therefore ^{14}C-labeled phorbol is not available for studies on its metabolism or active tumor-promoting diesters. However, tritiated PMA has been prepared from PMA (*57, 75, 76*) and used for mouse skin and cell culture localization studies (*57*).

We synthesized phorbolol myristate acetate (Structure **7**) from PMA by reducing its C-5 carbonyl group (*76*). This compound is a metabolite of PMA in mouse skin (*76*). PMA exerts tumor-promoting activity without prior conversion to an activated metabolic intermediate. This supposition is based solely on the high structural specificity that is so important for the tumor-promoting activity of PMA.

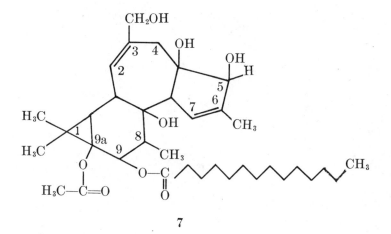

7

We found that PMA bound to rat liver plasma cell membranes suspended in phosphate-buffered saline changed both the intrinsic membrane fluorescence and that of 1-anilinonaphthalene-8-sulfonate, a hydrophobic fluorescent probe (*82*). The fluorescence probe technique is a useful way of studying conformational changes in membranes induced by PMA and other tumor promoters.

In early experiments carried out with PMA dissolved in organic solvents such as ethanol or dimethyl sulfoxide, it was observed that the solvent also affected membrane fluorescence. Concentrations of 0.05% ethanol or dimethyl sulfoxide in the membrane suspension had specific effects on membrane fluorescence which were distinct from those of PMA. These solvent effects on membranes should be kept in mind in studies on the mode of action of PMA, because they may result in effects that are unrelated to the mode of action of PMA or other tumor promoters.

Other Biological Effects of Tumor-Promoting Agents

The irritant effects of croton oil and of PMA have been discussed by many workers and reviewed (1). Using pure PMA, it was shown that the degree of inflammation is dose related and that maximal inflammation occurs within 24 hr after a single application of 2.5 μg PMA (24). At that stage there are many neutrophils and focal sloughing of epidermis. Single doses of 0.5, 0.1, or 0.02 μg cause mild inflammation in which most of the inflammatory cells are lymphocytes. The continued use of 2.5-μg applications of PMA three times weekly maintained a diffuse low-level epidermal hyperplasia persisting until the first papilloma appears. One year after the promoting treatment began, tissue sections revealed that papillomas can occur in essentially normal skin where neither a general inflammatory response nor epidermal hyperplasia was evident (Figure 6). This suggested that the induction of

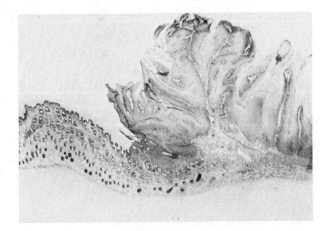

Figure 6. Squamous papilloma of mouse skin with adjacent normal skin, X 40. Induced by 7,12-dimethylbenz(a)anthracene followed by PMA.

papillomas by PMA does not require the concomitant occurrence of tissue damage (24). Other workers suggest that the inflammatory effects of PMA may be related to the mechanism of tumor promotion (77).

PMA is a human blood platelet aggregating agent (78). Low concentrations of PMA aggregated human platelets slowly at first, but then more rapidly as adenosine diphosphate (ADP) was released. ADP alone also induced platelet aggregation, but unlike ADP-induced aggregation the PMA-induced effect could be readily inhibited by chelation of calcium ions. Phorbol, the parent alcohol, which is not a tumor promoter did not aggregate platelets even at much higher concentrations than PMA (*79*). Furthermore, when ethylenediaminetetraacetic acid chelated the divalent cations (*e.g.*, Ca^{2+}), the PMA platelet-aggregating effect was inhibited. Platelets contain a high concentration of a contractile protein, actomyosin, and it was suggested (*79*) that the PMA-aggregating effect was mediated by platelet actomyosin. The ultrastructural features of PMA-induced platelet aggregation were also studied (*80, 81*). The blood platelet-aggregating effect is probably not related to the tumor-promoting activity of PMA; however, it is of interest in the general phenomenon of cell aggregation.

Environmental Factors

Although it is impossible to extrapolate from two-stage carcinogenesis and co-carcinogenesis experiments on mouse skin to human health hazards, it is worthwhile to consider some of the possible implications of laboratory experiments to the human environment.

One area that has received attention is air pollution. Carcinogenic aromatic hydrocarbons occur in urban polluted air (*83*), but little is known about the nature of tumor-promoting or co-carcinogenic agents in polluted air. However, it is expected that phenols and long-chain aliphatic hydrocarbons occur. These are known co-carcinogenic and/or tumor-promoting agents. For example, catechol is a potent co-carcinogen formed in the incomplete combustion of plant products (*84*). The role of irritants (*e.g.*, oxides of nitrogen and sulfur in polluted air) as contributing factors in human lung cancer is unknown. However, rats exposed to benzo(*a*)pyrene and sulfur dioxide by inhalation develop squamous carcinoma of the lung (*85*). Noncarcinogenic aromatic hydrocarbons, such as pyrene and fluoranthene, are potent co-carcinogens and contribute to the overall carcinogenicity of polluted air, as described earlier.

Much work remains to be done on the volatile organic components of polluted air which are expected to contain co-carcinogenic agents. To date most of the research and measurement of air pollutants have dealt with sulfur and nitrogen oxides and the particulate phase of polluted air. However, some of the volatile agents (*e.g.*, phenols and aliphatic or olefinic hydrocarbons) may be co-carcinogenic agents with carcinogenic aromatic hydrocarbons in human lung cancer caused by polluted air.

Cigarette smoke is a complex mixture of organic compounds. Approximately 1200 compounds in its condensate have been identified (*86*), and many more remain to be characterized. A number of carcinogenic aromatic hydrocarbons have been characterized in cigarette smoke (*87*), but these compounds do not account for the carcinogenicity of tobacco tars in mouse skin (*88*). For many years researchers examined the tumor-promoting activity of tobacco tars (*87, 89*) and various known tobacco tar components (*47*). The tumor-promoting activity observed with cigarette smoke con-

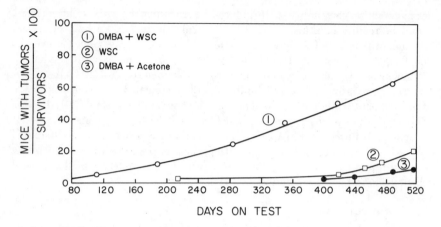

Figure 7. Tumor-promoting activity of cigarette smoke condensate (WSC) after single application of 7,12-dimethylbenz(a)anthracene (50 μg). WSC applied five times weekly, 40 mg in 0.1 ml acetone per application. Sixty female ICR/Ha mice per group.

densate in the classical two-stage mouse skin experiment is illustrated in Figure 7 (*89*). Since cigarette smoking constitutes simultaneous exposure to carcinogenic aromatic hydrocarbons and a variety of agents, some of which may be co-carcinogens, it was important to test known tobacco tar components such as phenols (catechol, resorcinol, and so forth) and noncarcinogenic aromatic hydrocarbons by simultaneous application of low doses of a carcinogenic hydrocarbon with the suspected co-carcinogenic agents. These findings (*41, 42*) are presented in an earlier part of this review. Catechol is the most abundant phenol in cigarette smoke, amounting to ~ 0.5 mg from one nonfilter cigarette (*90*). It is not present in tobacco but is formed in the pyrolytic process (*84*). These findings may help workers to develop a less hazardous cigarette if the known or suspected precursors of compounds (*e.g.*, catechol) (*84*) are removed from the plant or more effective cigarette filters devised.

Some potent plant or other natural product carcinogens have been uncovered and are described in other chapters of this book. However, little is known about natural product co-carcinogens and tumor promoters other than PMA and its analogs. Essential oils and other plant products are regularly used as part of the human diet. However, little is known about their chronic toxic effects. Some evidence indicated that lime oil is a tumor-promoting agent in the forestomach of the mouse (*91*).

Tumorigenesis Inhibition

The inhibition of tumor induction was reviewed recently (*92, 93*). The inhibition of two-stage carcinogenesis is of particular interest since some of the experiments may pertain to modes of action of initiators and promoters in two-stage carcinogenesis.

Because endogenous proteases may play a role in the mechanism of action of tumor promoters, three known protease inhibitors were tested for their inhibitory effects in two-stage carcinogenesis (*94*). The protease inhibitors used were tosyl lysine chloromethyl ketone, tosyl phenylalanine chloromethyl ketone, and tosyl arginine methyl ester. These agents were applied to mouse ears after initiation with a single dose of 7,12-dimethylbenz(*a*)anthracene followed by promotion with croton oil or PMA. The inhibitors were applied three times weekly immediately after application of the promoting agent. The protease inhibitors delayed the appearance of first tumors, changed the general pattern of rate of tumor appearance, and caused some decrease in tumor incidences.

Several anti-inflammatory steroid hormones—dexamethasone (*95, 96*), prednisolone, hydrocortisone, and cortisone (*95*)—were recently tested for tumor-inhibitory action. Dexamethasone appears to be the most active inhibitory agent (*95*). Theophylline also inhibited two-stage carcinogenesis on mouse skin (*71*).

Berenblum (*97, 98, 99*) showed earlier that sulfur mustard, bis(*β*-chloroethyl)sulfide, inhibited coal-tar carcinogenesis. We showed that low dosages of sulfur mustard completely inhibited two-stage carcinogenesis in mouse skin (*100*). These findings are summarized in Table IX.

Many attempts have been made to study the processes of two-stage carcinogenesis and co-carcinogenesis by the intervention of a third or fourth chemical. However, such studies are complicated by the variety of effects that such additional agents may have, as discussed in earlier reviews (*92, 93*). Such studies must be continued because of the importance of tumorigenesis inhibition to cancer prevention.

Table IX.   Inhibition of Two-stage Carcinogenesis by Bis(*β*-chloroethyl)sulfide (*100*) [a]

Initiator [b]	Promoter [c]	Inhibitor [c]	Mice with Papillomas	Days to First Tumor
DMBA	PMA	BCS (twice weekly)	1	90
DMBA	PMA	BCS (thrice weekly)	2	209
DMBA	PMA	none	27[d]	40
None	PMA	none	4	218
DMBA	none	BCS (twice weekly)	1	385
DMBA	none	BCS (thrice weekly)	0	—
None	none	BCS (thrice weekly)	1	323
DMBA	acetone	none	1	219
None	acetone	none	0	—
None	none	none	0	—

[a] 30 female ICR/Ha mice per group, results at 400 days.
[b] DMBA, 7,12-dimethylbenz(*a*)anthracene, 20 µg/0.1 ml acetone, once only.
[c] PMA, phorbol myristate acetate, 2.5 µg/0.1 ml acetone, thrice weekly; BCS, bis(*β*-chloroethyl)sulfide, 20 µg/0.1 ml acetone, beginning 14 days after initiator.
[d] Sixteen animals with squamous cell carcinomas.

Conclusions

Notable progress has been made in recent years in studies of two-stage carcinogenesis and co-carcinogenesis. They are:

1. The elucidation of the structures of the most potent tumor-promoters, the phorbol esters, from croton oil and the establishment of structure–activity relationships in this series of compounds. PMA is the most potent tumor promoter of the known natural product and semisynthetic diesters of phorbol. After the phorbol esters, anthralin is the most potent tumor promoter.

2. Biochemical studies have revealed that binding at the plasma membrane is a primary interaction of importance in tumor promotion.

3. PMA stimulates mitosis accompanied by increased intracellular synthesis of DNA, RNA, and proteins and stimulates *in vivo* phosphorylation of mouse skin epidermal histones. The relevance of the stimulation by PMA of macromolecular synthesis to the mechanism of tumor promotion remains to be established.

4. PMA stimulates a rapid, but short-lived, increase in cyclic GMP in cells in culture.

5. In operational terms a clearcut distinction can be made between two-stage carcinogenesis and co-carcinogenesis. Enough compounds were tested by both methods to suggest that not all promoters are co-carcinogens and vice-versa. The two most potent types of tumor promoters, *i.e.*, the phorbol esters and anthralin, have both types of activity.

6. Several new co-carcinogenic agents have been uncovered. These include phenols such as catechol and polycyclic aromatic hydrocarbons such as pyrene and fluoranthene. These agents are not carcinogenic by themselves. These new findings may have important implications in air pollution and tobacco carcinogenesis.

7. Several agents, notably sulfur mustard and dexamethasone, inhibit two-stage carcinogenesis. The mechanism of action of these agents remains largely unknown.

Acknowledgments

The work of this author and his associates on tumor promotion and co-carcinogenesis, some of which was referred to in this article, was supported by USPHS grants CA-14211, CA-15095, USPHS contract NO1 CP 3-3241, and USPHS Center grant ES-00260. The author is indebted to the following people who collaborated with him in studies related to tumor promotion and co-carcinogenesis in the Laboratory of Organic Chemistry and Carcinogenesis: B. M. Goldschmidt, C. Katz, S. Melchionne, A. Segal, A. Sivak, and G. Witz.

Literature Cited

1. Van Duuren, B. L., "Tumor-Promoting Agents in Two-Stage Carcinogenesis," *Prog. Exp. Tumor Res.* (1969) **11**, 31–68.
2. Van Duuren, B. L., Sivak, A., "Tumor-Promoting Agents from *Croton tiglium L.* and Their Mode of Action," *Cancer Res.* (1968) **28**, 2349–2356.

3. Hecker, E., "Cocarcinogens From *Euphorbiaceae* and *Thymeleaceae*," in Symposium on Pharmacognosy and Phytochemistry," pp. 147–165, Springer Verlag, Berlin/New York, 1971.
4. Berenblum, I., "A Re-evaluation of the Concept of Cocarcinogenesis," *Prog. Exp. Tumor Res.* (1969) **11**, 21–30.
5. Flaschenträger, B., "Über den Giftstoff im Crotonöl, Versammlungsberichte," *Z. Angew. Chem.* (1930) **43**, 1011–1012.
6. Flaschenträger, B., Falkenhausen, F. V., "The Poisons in Croton Oil. II. The Constitution of Krotophorbolone," *Justus Liebigs Ann. Chem.* (1934) **514**, 252–260.
7. Flaschenträger, B., Wigner, G., "The Poisons in Croton Oil. V. The Isolation of Croton Resin, Thin Oil and Phorbol from Croton Oil by Alcoholysis," *Helv. Chim. Acta* (1942) **25**, 569–581.
8. Kauffmann, T., Neumann, H., "Zur Konstitution des Phorbols. I. Über die reduzierende Gruppe des Phorbols," *Chem. Ber.* (1959) **92**, 1715–1726.
9. Kauffmann, T., Eisinger, A., Jasching, W., Lenhardt, K., "Zur Konstruktion des Phorbols. II. Über die α-Glykolgruppe des Phorbols," *Chem. Ber.* (1959) **92**, 1727–1738.
10. Cherbuliez, E., Ehninger, E., Bernhard, K., "Recherches sur la Graine de Croton. II. Le Principe Vesicant," *Helv. Chim. Acta* (1932) **15**, 658–670.
11. Cherbuliez, E., Bernhard, K., "Recherches sur la Graine de Croton. I. Sur le Crotonoside (2-Oxy-6-amino-purine-*d*-ribose)," *Helv. Chim. Acta* (1932) **15**, 464–471.
12. Bernhard, K., "Recherches sur la Graine de Croton (*Croton Tiglium L.*)," *J. Guerny*, Geneva, 1932.
13. Rous, P. Kidd, J. G., "Conditional Neoplasms and Sub-threshold Neoplastic States: A Study of the Tar Tumors of Rabbits," *J. Exp. Med.* (1941) **73**, 365–390.
14. Friedewald, W. F., Rous, P., "The Initiating and Promoting Elements in Tumor Production. An Analysis of the Effects of Tar, Benzpyrene, and Methylcholanthrene on Rabbit Skin," *J. Exp. Med.* (1944) **80**, 101–126.
15. Berenblum, I., "The Cocarcinogenic Action of Croton Resin," *Cancer Res.* (1941) **1**, 44–47.
16. Mottram, J. C., "A Developing Factor in Experimental Blastogenesis," *J. Pathol. Bacteriol.* (1944) **56**, 181–187.
17. Van Duuren, B. L., Orris, L., Arroyo, E., "Tumor-Enhancing Activity of the Active Principles of *Croton tiglium L*," *Nature* (1963) **200**, 1115–1116.
18. Van Duuren, B. L., Orris, L., "The Tumor-Enhancing Principles of *Croton Tiglium L.*," *Cancer Res.* (1965) **25**, 1871–1875.
19. Hecker, E., "Über das toxische, entzündliche und cocarcinogene Prinzip des Crotonöls," *Angew. Chem.* (1962) **74**, 722.
20. Hecker, E., Kubinyi, H., Bresch, H., "A New Group of Cocarcinogens from Croton Oil," *Angew. Chem. Int. Ed.* (1964) **3**, 747–748.
21. Pettersen, R. C., Ferguson, G., "The Structure and Stereochemistry of Phorbol, Diterpene Parent of Co-carcinogens of Croton Oil," *Chem. Commun.* (1967), 716–717.
22. Hoppe, W., Brandl, F., Strell, I., Röhrl, M., Gassmann, J., Hecker, E., Bartsch, H., Kreibich, G., Szczepanski, Ch. v., "Röntgenstrukturanalyse des Neophorbols," *Angew. Chem.* (1967) **79**, 824.
23. Crombie, L., Games, M. L., Pointer, D. J., "Chemistry and Structure of Phorbol, the Diterpene Parent of the Co-carcinogens of Croton Oil," *J. Chem. Soc., C* (1968), 1347–1362.
24. Van Duuren, B. L., Sivak, A., Segal, A., Seidman, I., Katz, C., "Dose-Response Studies with a Pure Tumor-Promoting Agent, Phorbol Myristate Acetate," *Cancer Res.* (1973) **33**, 2166–2172.

25. Bresch, H., Kreibich, G., Kubinyi, T., Schairer, H.-U., Thielmann, H. W., Hecker, E., "Über die Wirkstoffe des Crotonöls, IX. Partialsynthese von Wirkstoffen des Crotonöls," *Z. Naturforsch., B* (1968) **23**, 538–546.

25a. *Chemical Abstracts Registry Number Index,* "C.A. Reg. No. 20839-11-6, Molecular Formula $C_{36}H_{56}O_8$," (1970) **72–73**, 536 N.

26. Boutwell, R. K., Bosch, D. K., "The Tumor-Promoting Action of Phenol and Related Compounds for Mouse Skin," *Cancer Res.* (1959) **19**, 413–424.

27. Saffiotti, U., Shubik, P., "Studies on Promoting Action in Skin Carcinogenesis," *Natl. Cancer Inst., Monogr.* (1963) **10**, 489–507.

28. Setälä, H., "Tumor-Promoting and Co-carcinogenic Effects of Some Nonionic Lipophilic-Hydrophilic (Surface Active) Agents. An Experimental Study on Skin Tumors in Mice," *Acta Pathol. Microbiol. Scand., Suppl.* (1956) **115**, 7–91.

29. Bock, F. G., Burns, K., "Tumor-Promoting Properties of Anthralin (1,8,9-Anthratriol)," *J. Natl. Cancer Inst.* (1963) **30**, 393–398.

30. Segal, A., Katz, C., Van Duuren, B. L., "Structure and Tumor-Promoting Activity of Anthralin (1,8-Dihydroxy-9-anthrone) and Related Compounds," *J. Med. Chem.* (1971) **14**, 1152–1154.

31. Van Duuren, B. L., Sivak, A., Goldschmidt, B. M., Katz, C., Melchionne, S., "Initiating Activity of Aromatic Hydrocarbons in Two-Stage Carcinogenesis," *J. Natl. Cancer Inst.* (1970) **44**, 1167–1173.

32. Van Duuren, B. L., Sivak, A., Langseth, L., "The Tumor-Promoting Activity of Tobacco Leaf Extract and Whole Cigarette Tar," *Br. J. Cancer* (1967) **21**, 460–463.

33. Salaman, M. H., Roe, F. J. C., "Incomplete Carcinogens: Ethyl Carbamate (Urethane) as an Initiator of Skin Tumor Formation in the Mouse," *Br. J. Cancer* (1953) **7**, 472–481.

34. Van Duuren, B. L., Sivak, A., Segal, A., Orris, L., Langseth, L., "The Tumor-Promoting Agents of Tobacco Leaf and Tobacco Smoke Condensate," *J. Natl. Cancer Inst.* .(1966) **37**, 519–526.

35. Roe, F. J. C., Salaman, M. H., "Further Studies on Incomplete Carcinogenesis. Triethylene Melamine (TEM), 1,2-Benzanthracene and β-Propiolactone as Initiators of Skin Tumor Formation in the Mouse," *Br. J. Cancer* (1955) **9**, 177–203.

36. Van Duuren, B. L., Sivak, A., Goldschmidt, B. M., Katz, C., Melchionne, S., "Carcinogenicity of Halo-Ethers," *J. Natl. Cancer Inst.* (1969) **43**, 481–486.

37. Roe, F. J. C., "Tumor Initiation in Mouse Skin by Certain Esters of Methanesulfonic Acid," *Cancer Res.* (1957) **17**, 64–69.

38. Hartwell, J. N., "Survey of Compounds Which Have Been Tested for Carcinogenic Activity," 2nd ed., Public Health Publication No. 149, U.S. Govt. Printing Office, Washington, D.C., 1951.

39. Van Duuren, B. L., Goldschmidt, B. M., Katz, C., Seidman, I., Paul, J., "The Carcinogenic Activity of Alkylating Agents," *J. Natl. Cancer Inst.* (1974) **53**, 695–700.

40. Van Duuren, B. L., Blazej, T., Goldschmidt, B. M., Katz, C., Melchionne, S., Sivak, A., "Cocarcinogenesis Studies on Mouse Skin and Inhibition of Tumor Induction," *J. Natl. Cancer Inst.* (1971) **46**, 1039–1044.

41. Van Duuren, B. L., Katz, C., Goldschmidt, B. M., "Brief Communication: Cocarcinogenic Agents in Tobacco Carcinogenesis," *J. Natl. Cancer Inst.* (1973) **51**, 703–705.

42. Van Duuren, B. L., Goldschmidt, B. M., "Cocarcinogenic and Tumor-Promoting Agents in Tobacco Carcinogenesis," *J. Natl. Cancer Inst.* (1976) **56**, 1237–1242.

43. Hoffmann, D., Wynder, E. L., "Studies on Gasoline Engine Exhaust," *J. Air Pollut. Contr. Ass.* (1963) **13**, 322–327.

44. Van Duuren, B. L., Sivak, A., Katz, C., Seidman, I., Melchionne, S., "The Effect of Aging and Interval Between Primary and Secondary Treatment

46. Baird, W. M., Boutwell, R. K., "Tumor Promoting Activity of Phorbol and Four Diesters of Phorbol in Mouse Skin," *Cancer Res.* (1971) **31**, 1074–1079.

47. Van Duuren, B. L., Sivak, A., Langseth, L., Goldschmidt, B. M., Segal, A., "Initiators and Promoters in Tobacco Carcinogenesis," *Natl. Cancer Inst., Monogr.* (1968) **28**, 173–180.

48. Horton, A. W., Denman, D. T., Trosset, R. P., "Carcinogenesis of the Skin. II. The Accelerating Properties of Aliphatic and Related Hydrocarbons," *Cancer Res.* (1957) **17**, 758–766.

49. Holsti, P., "Tumor Promoting Effects of Some Long Chain Fatty Acids in Experimental Skin Carcinogenesis in the Mouse," *Acta Pathol. Microbiol. Scand.* (1959) **46**, 51–58.

50. Arffmann, E., Glavind, J., "Carcinogenicity in Mice of Some Fatty Acid Methyl Esters," *Acta Pathol. Microbiol. Scand., A* (1974) **82**, 127–136.

51. Bingham, E., Falk, H. L., "Environmental Carcinogens. The Modifying Effect of Cocarcinogens on the Threshold Response," *Arch. Environ. Health* (1969) **19**, 779–783.

52. Frei, J. V., Kingsley, W. F., "Observations on Chemically Induced Regressing Tumors of Mouse Epidermis," *J. Natl. Cancer Inst.* (1968) **41**, 1307–1313.

53. Weissmann, G., Troll, W., Van Duuren, B. L., Sessa, G., "A New Action of Tumor-Promoting Agents: Lysis of Cell and Intracellular Membranes," *J. Cin. Invest.* (1967) **46**, 1131.

54. Sivak, A., Ray, F., Van Duuren, B. L., "Phorbol Ester Tumor-Promoting Agents and Membrane Stability," *Cancer Res.* (1969) **29**, 624–630.

55. Sivak, A., Van Duuren, B. L., "Phenotypic Expression of Transformation: Induction in Cell Culture by a Phorbol Ester," *Science* (1967) **157**, 1443–1444.

56. Sivak, A., Van Duuren, B. L., "A Cell Culture System for the Assessment of Tumor-Promoting Activity," *J. Natl. Cancer Inst.* (1970) **44**, 1091–1097.

57. Sivak, A., Van Duuren, B. L., "Cellular Interactions of Phorbol Myristate Acetate in Tumor Promotion," *Chem. Biol. Interact.* (1971) **3**, 401–411.

58. Sivak, A., Mossman, B. T., Van Duuren, B. L., "Activation of Cell Membrane Enzymes in the Stimulation of Cell Division," *Biochem. Biophys. Res. Commun.* (1972) **46**, 605–609.

59. Rohrschneider, L., Boutwell, R. K., "The Early Stimulation of Phospholipid Metabolism by 12-O-Tetradecanoyl-phorbol-13-acetate and its Specificity for Tumor Promotion," *Cancer Res.* (1973) **33**, 1945–1952.

60. Kubinski, H., Strangstalien, M. A., Baird, W. M., Boutwell, R. K., "Interactions of Phorbol Esters with Cellular Membranes *in Vitro*," *Cancer Res.* (1973) **33**, 3103–3107.

61. Sivak, A., Van Duuren, B. L., "RNA Synthesis Induction in Cell Culture by a Tumor Promoter," *Cancer Res.* (1970) **30**, 1203–1205.

62. Baird, W. M., Melera, P. W., Boutwell, R. K., "Acrylamide Gel Electrophoresis Studies of the Incorporation of Cytidine-³H into Mouse Skin RNA at Early Times After Treatment with Phorbol Esters," *Cancer Res.* (1972) **32**, 781–788.

63. Whitfield, J. F., MacManus, J. P., Gillan, D. J., "Calcium-Dependent Stimulation by a Phorbol Ester (PMA) of Thymic Lymphoblast DNA Synthesis and Proliferation," *J. Cell. Physiol.* (1973) **82**, 151–156.

64. Baird, W. M., Sedgwick, J. A., Boutwell, R. K., "Effects of Phorbol and Four Diesters of Phorbol on the Incorporation of Tritiated Precursors into DNA, RNA and Protein in Mouse Epidermis," *Cancer Res.* (1971) **31**, 1434–1439.

65. Frankfurt, O. S., Raitcheva, E., "Fast Onset of DNA Synthesis Stimulated by Tumor Promoter in Mouse Epidermis at the Initiation Stage of Carcinogenesis," *J. Natl. Cancer Inst.* (1973) **51**, 1861–1864.

65. Frankfurt, O. S., Raitcheva, E., "Fast Onset of DNA Synthesis Stimulated by Tumor Promoter in Mouse Epidermis at the Initiation Stage of Carcinogenesis," *J. Natl. Cancer Inst.* (1973) **51**, 1861–1864.

66. Raineri, R., Simsiman, R. C., Boutwell, R. K., "Stimulation of the Phosphorylation of Mouse Epidermal Histones by Tumor-Promoting Agents," *Cancer Res.* (1973) **33**, 134–139.

67. Greaves, M. F., Bauminger, S., "Activation of T and B Lymphocytes by Insoluble Phytomitogens," *Nature, New Biol.* (1972) **235**, 67–70.

68. Hadden, J. W., Hadden, E. M., Haddox, M. K., Goldberg, N. D., "Guanosine 3′:5′-Cyclic Monophosphate: A Possible Intracellular Mediator of Mitogenic Influences in Lymphocytes," *Proc. Natl. Acad. Sci. U.S.* (1972) **69**, 3024–3027.

69. Estensen, R. D., Hadden, J. W., Hadden, E. M., Touraine, F., Touraine, J. L., Haddox, M. K., Goldberg, N. D., "Phorbol Myristate Acetate. Effects of a Tumor Promoter on Intracellular Cyclic GMP in Mouse Fibroblasts and as a Mitogen on Human Lymphocytes," *Control of Proliferation in Animal Cells, Cold Spring Harbor Conferences on Cell Proliferation*, Eds. B. Clarkson, R. Baserga, Cold Spring Harbor, New York, 1974, **Vol. 1**, pp. 627–634.

70. Goldberg, N. D., Haddox, M. K., Dunham, E., Lopez, C., Hadden, J. W., "The Yin Yang Hypothesis of Biological Control: Opposing Influences of Cyclic GMP and Cyclic AMP in the Regulation of Cell Proliferation and Other Biological Processes," *Control of Proliferation in Animal Cells, Cold Spring Harbor Conferences on Cell Proliferation*, Eds. B. Clarkson, R. Baserga, Cold Spring Harbor, New York, 1794, **Vol. 1**, pp. 609–625.

71. Belman, S., Troll, W., "Phorbol-12-Myristate-13-Acetate Effect on Cyclic AMP Levels in Mouse Skin: Inhibition of Phorbol-Myristate-Acetate Promoted Tumorigenesis by Theophylline," *Cancer Res.* (1974) **34**, 3446–3455.

72. Gaudin, D., Gregg, R. S., Yielding, K. L., "DNA Repair Inhibition: A Possible Mechanism of Action of Cocarcinogens," *Biochem. Biophys. Res. Commun.* (1971) **45**, 630–636.

73. Gaudin, D., Gregg, R. S., Yielding, K. L., "Inhibition of DNA Repair by Cocarcinogens," *Biochem. Biophys. Res. Commun.* (1972) **48**, 945–949.

74. Teebor, G. W., Duker, N. J., Ruacan, S. A., Zachary, K. J., "Inhibition of Thymine Dimer Excision by the Phorbol Ester, Phorbol Myristate Acetate," *Biochem. Biophys. Res. Commun.* (1973) **50**, 66–70.

75. Kreibich, G., Hecker, E., "On the Active Principles of Croton Oil. X. Preparation of Tritium Labelled Croton Oil Factor A_1 and Other Tritium Labelled Phorbol Derivatives," *Z. Krebsforsch.* (1970) **74**, 448–456.

76. Segal, A., Van Duuren, B. L., Maté, U., "The Identification of Phorbolol Myristate Acetate as a New Metabolite of Phorbol Hyristate Acetate in Mouse Skin," *Cancer Res.* (1975) **35**, 2154–2159.

77. Janoff, A., Klassen, A., Troll, W., "Local Vascular Changes Induced by the Cocarcinogen, Phorbol Myristate Acetate," *Cancer Res.* (1970) **30**, 2568–2571.

78. Puszkin, E. G., Zucker, M. B., "Enhancement of Platelet and Muscle Actomyosin ATPase Activity and Superprecipitation by the Tumor-promoter 12-O-Tetradecanoyl-phorbol-13-acetate (PMA)," *Nature, New Biol.* (1973) **245**, 277–280.

79. Zucker, M. B., Troll, W., Belman, S., "The Tumor-Promoter Phorbol Ester (12-O-Tetradecanoyl-phorbol-13-acetate), A Potent Aggregating Agent for Blood Platelets," *J. Cell Biol.* (1974) **60**, 325–336.

80. Estensen, R. D., White, J. G., "Ultrastructural Features of the Platelet Response to Phorbol Myristate Acetate," *Amer. J. Pathol.* (1974) **74**, 441–452.

81. White, J. G., Rao, G. H. R., Estensen, R. D., "Investigation of the Release Reaction in Platelets Exposed to Phorbol Myristate Acetate," *Amer. J. Pathol.* (1974) **75**, 301–314.
82. Witz, G., Van Duuren, B. L., Banerjee, S., "The Interaction of Phorbol Myristate Acetate, A Tumor Promoter, with Rat Liver Plasma Membranes: A Fluorescence Study," *Proc. Amer. Assoc. Cancer Res.* (1975) **16**, 30.
83. Committee on Biologic Effects of Atmospheric Pollutants, "Particulate Polycyclic Organic Matter," National Academy of Sciences, Washington, D.C., 1972.
84. Chortyk, O. T., Schlotzhauer, W. S., "Studies on the Pyrogenesis of Tobacco Smoke Constituents (A Review)," *Beitr. Tabakforsch.* (1973) **7**, 165–178.
85. Kuschner, M., "The J. Burns Amberson Lecture. The Causes of Lung Cancer," *Amer. Rev. Resp. Dis.* (1968) **98**, 573–590.
86. Stedman, R. L., "The Chemical Composition of Tobacco and Tobacco Smoke," *Chem. Rev.* (1968) **68**, 153–207.
87. U.S. Dept. Health, Education, and Welfare, "Smoking and Health. Report of the Advisory Committee to the Surgeon General of the Public Health Service," PHS Publ. No. 1103, U.S. Govt. Printing Off., Washington, D.C., 1964.
88. Orris, L., Van Duuren, B. L., Kosak, A. I., Nelson, N., Schmitt, F. L., "The Carcinogenicity for Mouse Skin and the Aromatic Hydrocarbon Content of Cigarette-Smoke Condensates," *J. Natl. Cancer Inst.* (1958) **21**, 557–561.
89. Van Duuren, B. L., Sivak, A., Katz, C., Melchionne, S., "Cigarette Smoke Carcinogenesis: Importance of Tumor Promoters," *J. Natl. Cancer Inst.* (1971) **47**, 235–240.
90. Waltz, P., Häusermann, M., Krull, A., "Methoden der quantitativen Bestimmung des Brenzcatechins im Cigarettenrauch," *Beitr. Tabakforsch.* (1965) **3**, 263–277.
91. Roe, F. J. C., Field, W. E. H., "Chronic Toxicity of Essential Oils and Certain Other Products of Natural Origin," *Food Cosmet. Toxicol.* (1965) **3**, 311–324.
92. Falk, H. L., "Anticarcinogenesis—an Alternative," *Prog. Exp. Tumor Res.* (1971) **14**, 105–137.
93. Van Duuren, B. L., Melchionne, S., "Inhibition of Tumorigenesis," *Prog. Exp. Tumor Res.* (1969) **12**, 55–101.
94. Troll, W., Klassen, A., Janoff, A., "Tumorigenesis in Mouse Skin: Inhibition by Synthetic Inhibitors of Proteases," *Science* (1970) **169**, 1211–1213.
95. Belman, S., Troll, W., "The Inhibition of Croton Oil–Promoted Mouse Skin Tumorigenesis by Steroid Hormones," *Cancer Res.* (1972) **32**, 450–454.
96. Scribner, J., Slaga, T. J., "Multiple Effects of Dexamethasone on Protein Synthesis and Hyperplasia Caused by a Tumor Promoter," *Cancer Res.* (1973) **33**, 542–546.
97. Berenblum, I., "The Modifying Influence of Dichloroethyl Sulphide on the Induction of Tumors in Mice by Tar," *J. Pathol. Bacteriol.* (1929) **32**, 425–434.
98. Berenblum, I., "The Anti-carcinogenic Action of Dichlorodiethylsulphide (Mustard Gas)," *J. Pathol. Bacteriol.* (1931) **34**, 731–746.
99. Berenblum, I., "Experimental Inhibition of Tumour Induction by Mustard Gas and Other Compounds," *J. Pathol. Bacteriol.* (1935) **40**, 549-558.
100. Van Duuren, B. L., Segal, A., "Inhibition of Two-Stage Carcinogenesis in Mouse Skin with Bis(2-chloroethyl)sulfide," *Cancer Res.* (1976) **36**, 1023–1025.

3

Endocrine Aspects of Carcinogenesis

J. W. Jull,[1] Cancer Research Centre, University of British Columbia, Vancouver 8, Canada

HORMONES ARE SUBSTANCES secreted directly into the bloodstream by specific tissues. They are then carried to distant sites where they exert their effects. Many compounds may be defined as hormones, and their interrelationships in modulating differentiation, metabolism, and function in various tissues of the body are so complex that it is impossible to summarize them. For a comprehensive account of most aspects of endocrinology, the reader is referred to the excellent presentation of Turner and Bagnara (1).

The relation of hormones to cancer was critically reviewed by Clayson (2). Noble presented a comprehensive index of work in this field up to 1964 (3). The account of tumorigenesis in endocrine glands (4) and the recent discussion by Bischoff (5) of the carcinogenic effects of steroids are authoritative works in this area.

This exposition concentrates on the protein hormones of the anterior pituitary and the steroid hormones of the ovary, testis, and adrenal. The normal situation is first summarized, followed by an outline of the neoplastic lesions induced by endogenous hormones in certain experimental conditions, the effects of exogenous hormones on cancer induction, and an indication of the effects of hormonal factors on other carcinogenic agents. The treatment is very selective, but it introduces a major parameter whose expansion must constitute a fundamental plank in understanding the mechanisms concerned in carcinogenesis.

Normal Endocrine Function

The Pituitary. This gland is situated in the sella turcica at the base of the brain. Anatomically, in the majority of mammals, it is divided into the posterior lobe, the intermediate lobe, and the anterior lobe. The origin

[1] Deceased

of the blood supply to these lobes is functionally significant. The major vascular route to the anterior lobe is through the hypophyseal portal system, which comes from the median eminence, and is largely independent of the blood supply to other parts of the pituitary.

In contrast to the posterior lobe, the anterior lobe of the pituitary is virtually devoid of any nervous connection. Its function is controlled entirely by hormonal factors. Those delivered from the median eminence *via* the portal system are of the greatest importance.

Anterior pituitary hormones are protein or glycoprotein in nature, and their amino acid sequences are elucidated for some species. Somatotrophin (STH, growth hormone, GH) was initially identified as an anterior pituitary secretion because of its marked stimulation of skeletal and body growth. STH has profound influences on metabolic activity, promoting the incorporation of amino acids into protein; the mobilization of fat, causing an increase in circulating fatty acids; and opposing the action of insulin, resulting in an increase in blood glucose concentration.

STH has growth stimulating and lactogenic activities in mammary tissues, although these functions may be only synergistic with prolactin and require other hormones for completion. In general the action of other pituitary trophic hormones and the normal function of most organs require the presence of somatotrophin. It seems likely that most if not all the actions of STH are mediated through the induction of somatomedin synthesis (6) by the liver. Prolactin (luteotrophin, LTH) was first recognized by its activity in the secretion of crop milk in pigeons. Subsequently, its fundamental activity was shown in breast growth and lactation in mammals (7, 8). It has an extensive range of functions (9) in many species and overlaps with STH in its actions on the breast. Recently the identification of prolactin in man (10) has opened up a new area of research into its physiological and possibly pathological functions. Prolactin stimulates secretion by the corpus luteum in the rat and has various effects on the metabolism of steroids in the testis and the adrenal.

Thyrotrophic hormone (TSH) stimulates thyroid growth and the secretion of the thyroid hormones, of which thyroxine is the most important. Adrenocorticotrophic hormone (ACTH) mainly stimulates growth and steroid secretion by the fasciculate zone of the adrenal cortex. It probably has a synergistic effect on steroid synthesis by the glomerulosa. Follicle-stimulating hormone (FSH) and luteinizing hormone (LH) are responsible for the development of the ovarian follicle and its conversion to a corpus luteum in the female. In the male they stimulate the germinal epithelium and the development and steroid secretion of the interstitial cells of the testis.

Steroid hormones are synthesized from cholesterol in the ovary, the testis, and the adrenals *via* the pathways illustrated in Figure 1. The major steroids produced by these tissues are summarized in Table I.

Control of Pituitary Secretion. Those pituitary hormones which have specific target tissues (TSH, ACTH, FSH, and LH) in which they stimulate growth and secretion are normally released in amounts reciprocally related

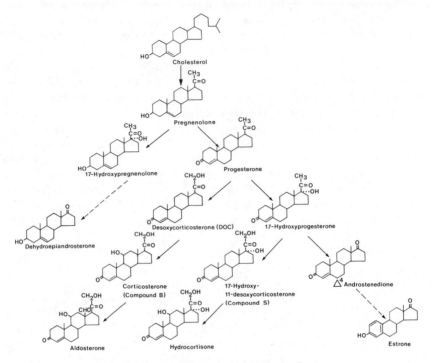

Figure 1.   Pathways of steroid biosynthesis

Table I.   Steroid Hormones Secreted by Various Organs

	Secretion	
Organ	*Nature*	*Example*
Testis	androgens	testosterone
	estrogens	estradiol
Ovary	estrogens	estradiol
	progestins	progesterone
	androgens	androstenedione
Adrenal cortex		
glomerulosa	mineralocorticoids	aldosterone
fasciculata	glucocorticoids	corticosterone
		cortisol
	androgens[a]	androstenedione
		dehydroepiandrosterone
	estrogens[a]	estrone
		estradiol

[a] Small amounts only from normal tissue.

to hormone production of the organ they stimulate. Thus release of TSH from the anterior pituitary into the blood increases the secretion of thyroxine by the thyroid gland. The increase in blood concentrations of the thyroid hormone depresses the factors responsible for TSH synthesis and release so that the blood level of the trophic hormone falls. With less circulating TSH, thyroid stimulation is reduced, thyroid hormones are diminished, and thus the inhibition to TSH production is removed. Thyroid hormones therefore exert a feedback inhibition of the thyrotrophic hormone TSH.

A similar relationship exists between ACTH and adrenal function. Elevated ACTH levels increase steroid secretion by the fasciculate zone of the adrenal cortex, and increased levels of the 11-oxygenated steroids produced there inhibit ACTH synthesis and release.

The relationship between the gonadotrophic follicle-stimulating hormone (FSH) and luteinizing hormone (LH) and the ovary is more complex. In this case FSH with low levels of LH is necessary for follicle development and the induction of estrogen secretion. When the follicle matures, however, and the ovum is ready to be shed, a sharp increase in LH occurs with rupture of the follicle, escape of the ovum, and multiplication and differentiation of the follicular thecal and granulosa cells to form the corpus luteum. Formation of the corpus luteum involves changes, qualitatively and quantitatively, in steroid hormone production. Progesterone is now a major product as well as estrogen. Both progesterone and estrogen can inhibit LH and FSH release by the anterior pituitary. In the absence of pregnancy this interaction between the hormones produced by the ovary and their inhibition of LH and FSH release constitutes the basic rhythm which outlines the cyclic function of the ovary. In the case of some pituitary hormones, such as prolactin or STH, there is no evidence of systemic feedback inhibition.

The reciprocal relationship between the anterior pituitary secretion of trophic hormones and the hormones of their target organs is, however, simply one facet of a complex control system which is responsive to many neural, hormonal, metabolic, and environmental stimuli which affect the function of the endocrine glands.

In specific cases hormones released by the target tissue can also exert a positive feedback in stimulating trophic hormone release by the anterior pituitary. Psychic and sensory stimuli mediated through higher neural centers may override the direct hormonal interactions. The stimulation of prolactin release by a direct action of estrogen on the anterior pituitary is a major factor in the physiological action of this steroid. This effect must be borne in mind when considering the carcinogenic action of estrogens which is detailed later.

Neural Control of Anterior Pituitary Function. Hormone secretion can be induced by direct nervous stimulation in the case of the adrenal medulla. In this tissue adrenalin and noradrenalin are secreted directly into the systemic circulation and carried to the many distant sites where they exert their effects. The complex area of neural–hormonal relationships in general has been admirably detailed by Donovan (*11*). The neural–endocrine control of anterior pituitary secretion is, however, a specialized aspect of this subject which is fundamental to the understanding of hormone control with regard to growth and function.

The hypothalamic area of the brain assimilates and transforms the many stimulatory and inhibitory factors in an animal's environment. At the level of the median eminence these various interacting moderators control anterior pituitary function by varying the secretion of "releasing factors" which are passed directly into the hypophyseal portal system of blood vessels (Figure 2) and then to the anterior pituitary.

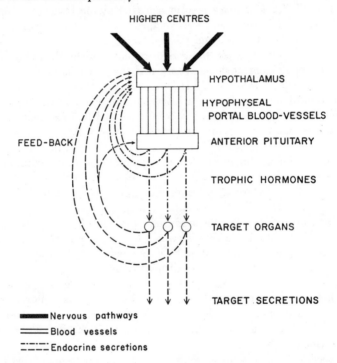

Figure 2.   Pathways controlling anterior pituitary secretion

Specific releasing factors have been demonstrated for each of the anterior pituitary trophic hormones, *i.e.*, growth hormone or somatotrophin releasing factor, corticotrophin releasing factor, thyrotrophin releasing factor, luteinizing hormone releasing factor, and follicle stimulating hormone releasing factor.

Tumor Induction by Hormones

Hormonal factors, especially those of the anterior pituitary and the steroids, are intimately concerned with the stimulation of growth and differentiation in many tissues. Pituitary secretion and steroids act synergistically in the development of the secondary sex organs in the male and female. In the absence of complete growth carcinogens may not be able to act. Therefore, in experimental tumor induction, it is difficult to dissociate the effects of the hormones themselves and the effects of other physical, chemical, or viral agents which might be present in the environment.

Not only can hormones provide synergistic activity necessary for the carcinogenic activity of other compounds, but cancer-inducing agents may disturb the hormonal balance, so that hormonal factors are the effective inducers of neoplasia. Hormones may therefore precipitate neoplasia by:

1. direct carcinogenic action,

2. stimulating the production of other hormonal factors which, in excess, cause cancer,

3. acting synergistically to promote growth in tissues affected by a physical, chemical, or viral carcinogen,

4. modifying the metabolism of chemical agents so that they become active carcinogens.

Tumors Induced by Hormonal Imbalance. The close relationship between the amounts of pituitary trophic hormones produced and secretion by their target organs was outlined above. Positive and negative feedback modification of trophic hormone secretion is a dominant characteristic of this interaction. If there is interference in the balance between pituitary stimulation and organ response, tumorigenesis may result. In these circumstances exogeneous agents are not necessarily involved.

OVARIAN TUMORS. Early observations suggested that the liver is able rapidly to inactivate steroid hormones (*12, 13, 14*), and this was confirmed by Biskind (*15*). He showed that pellets of estradiol implanted subcutaneously in rats induced constant estrus. If they were implanted into the spleen, from which the blood flows directly to the liver, no biological activity was seen. Extirpation of the estrogen-containing spleen and its systemic implantation, however, caused estrus-inducing activity to resume.

Biskind and Biskind (*16*) then found that tumors developed if ovaries were transplanted to the spleens of ovariectomized rats. These observations in rats were confirmed (*17, 18, 19*), and ovarian tumors were also found after similar operations in mice (*20–26*). Significantly, where adhesions had occurred between the splenic implant and the systemic circulation, estrus was observed and no ovarian tumors developed. Thus, the estrogens produced by the intrasplenic ovary must have been rapidly inactivated by the liver (Figure 3), causing a hormonal imbalance (*16, 27*). As a result of the absence of inhibition by ovarian hormones the pituitary secretion of gonadotrophins remained high. The chronic excess of these gonadotrophins was presumed to be responsible for ovarian tumor development. If exogenous estrogens or androgens were injected systemically, no tumors arose in the intrasplenic grafts even though hormone administration was delayed for up to 136 days after the initial implantation of the ovary into the spleen (*28*). The course of events culminating in tumorigenesis is, therefore, not complete at an early stage.

The follicles and the ova they contained were rapidly eliminated from the intrasplenic ovaries (*22*). Histological evidence of neoplasia only became

a.

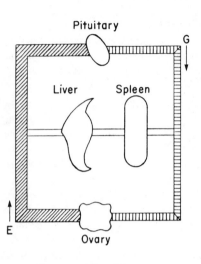

b.

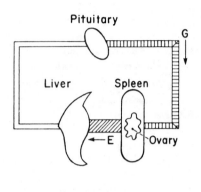

G – gonadotrophins
E – estrogens

*Figure 3.   Mechanisms involved in tumorigenesis in intrasplenically implanted
ovary*

*(a) Normal situation—gonadotrophin (G) stimulates estrogen secretion (E) by ovary
which feeds back to inhibit pituitary secretion of G. (b) Intrasplenic ovary is stimulated by gonadotrophin (G) to secrete estrogen (E) which is directly transported to
the liver where it is metabolized to products which cannot inactivate secretion of G.*

marked after their complete disappearance. A similar rapid depletion of
viable oocytes and follicles can also be achieved experimentally by other
means. Thus irradiation by various sources eliminates oocytes and their
containing follicles (*29*). The emergence of ovarian tumors after exposure
of mouse ovaries to a sufficient radiation dose has been documented extensively
(*30–36*).

The chemical carcinogen 7,12-dimethylbenz(*a*)anthracene (DMBA) has
a marked ability to induce granulosa-cell tumors of the mouse ovary (*37*)
when administered by various routes, *e.g.*, intragastric (*38, 39*), intraperitoneal (*40, 41*), intravenous (*41, 42*), subcutaneous (*43*), or direct application to the ovary (*41*). Oocyte and follicular disruption are also caused by
exposure to DMBA *in vitro*, and ovaries treated in this way develop granulosa-
cell tumors after reimplantation into an ovariectomized mouse. Ovaries
exposed to culture medium alone *in vitro*, however, develop normally when
reimplanted into ovariectomized mice (*44, 45*).

In ovarian tumors after DMBA administration, Marchant showed that
pituitary secretions are necessary for tumors to arise (*46*). Conversely (*47,
48*), normal ovarian tissue is completely inhibitory to ovarian tumor devel-

opment after exposure to DMBA, and a similar inhibition is exerted by normal ovarian tissue on tumorigenesis in irradiated ovaries (*34, 36*). Inhibition of tumor formation occurs in intrasplenic grafts if a normal ovary is present *in situ* (*17, 18*).

Tumor development in intrasplenic grafts requires no external agent. The major disturbance is in the levels of gonadotrophic hormones. The only possible agent, other than hormones, which could be involved is a virus which so far has not been detected. When ovarian tumors follow irradiation or exposure to a chemical carcinogen, however, it is possible that some direct initiating action occurs which converts some ovarian cells to latent tumor cells. Pederson and Krarup (*49*) showed the basic necessity for oocyte elimination in tumor induction by x-rays and DMBA, so that hormonal imbalance induced by follicular damage appears to be the overriding factor in all cases.

There are other experimental situations where hormonal imbalance leads to ovarian tumorigenesis without the intervention of external agents. Mühlbock (*50*) showed that parabiosis of intact mice to castrated partners induced high levels of gonadotrophins in the intact animal and a tendency to ovarian tumor development. Unique observations on a strain of mice with a congenital lack of oocytes (*51, 52*) demonstrated that ovarian tumors occur spontaneously after a long period. In these mice no external factor or manipulation is used, so that the course of events in the ovary is uncomplicated by side reactions to chemical or physical agents. Since ovaries containing a full complement of ova develop normally in ovariectomized deficient mice (*53*), it is the abnormality in the target organ which is responsible for the hormonal imbalance resulting in tumors.

ADRENAL CORTEX TUMORS. There is a close relationship between the ovary, the testis, and the adrenal cortex, not only in their embryological origin but also in the nature of the steroids they secrete. The principal adrenal steroids differ fundamentally from those of the ovary and the testis in their structure and function. There is, however, overlap in the capacity of these tissues to produce certain steroids. Thus the ovary and the testis in some species can secrete the 21-hydroxysteroid, 11-deoxycorticosterone. In contrast, estrogens and testosterone can be secreted by the normal adrenal and are often produced in large amounts by adrenal tumors.

A stimulating effect of LH to cause hypertrophy of the X-zone of the mouse adrenal (a juxtamedullary zone) has been known for many years (*54*), and there may be an analogy between this and the relationship of human fetal adrenal hypertrophy to placental gonadotrophin. It is possible that gonadotrophic hormones can act physiologically on the normal adrenal. A pathological action of elevated levels of gonadotrophins on the adrenal cortex might, therefore, be expected.

Spontaneous tumors of the adrenal cortex are uncommon in most strains of mice except for the NH strain (*55, 56, 57*). They are also extremely rare in rats, except for the Osborne–Mendel line (*58*). In Syrian hamsters, however, adrenocortical tumors are not uncommon (*59, 60*).

Woolley *et al.* *(61)* found a high incidence of adrenal tumors in dba mice which had been ovariectomized just after birth. The tumorous adrenals secreted sufficient sex hormones to replace ovarian function in the genesis of mammary tumors. Similar adrenal lesions were studied in other mouse strains *(62)*. In the Ce strain the incidence may be 100% *(63)*. Males are also susceptible to adrenal tumor induction after castration, but the neoplastic development is slower than in ovariectomized females *(64)*.

The development of breast hypertrophy and the stimulation of other estrogen-dependent tissues were observed in association with these adrenal tumors *(61, 65, 66)*, and evidence for androgen secretion was reported *(56, 67, 68, 69, 70)*. Much of the evidence for the type of hormone production was based on morphological changes in tissues, *e.g.*, the salivary glands and kidney. There is little evidence of the chemical nature of the steroids produced.

Post-castration adrenal tumors in mice were shown to arise as downgrowths from the capsule which surrounds the adrenal. This capsule is the source of regenerating tissue when the adrenal is damaged, but it is not implicated as a source of steroid hormone synthesis. The morphology and histogenesis of these adrenal tumors are distinct from those of adrenal tumors induced in rats by estrogen administration (p. 64), but histological studies of the latter are not well documented.

The marked differences in susceptibility of different mouse strains to adrenal tumor formation following gonadectomy *(62)* might depend considerably on genetic variations in anterior pituitary function. However, there is a definite genetic component in the adrenal itself. Hybrid mice were produced by mating an insusceptible strain to a susceptible one *(71)*. Adrenals from each parent strain were grafted subcutaneously into adrenalectomized, gonadectomized recipient hybrids. Adrenal tumor induction in the hybrids was similar to that in gonadectomized mice of the strain from which the adrenal grafts were obtained.

Dependence of adrenal tumor induction on pituitary secretion is demonstrated by their failure to occur in hypophysectomized, gonadectomized mice *(72, 73)*. The appearance of post-castration adrenal tumors can also be prevented by grafting ovaries *(74)* or administering estrogens and androgens *(63)* but not by 11-deoxycorticosterone or progesterone. Monsen *(75)* found complete inhibition of adrenal tumors in castrates by the injection of testosterone. However, cortisone administration, which induced adrenal atrophy, did not inhibit tumorigenesis, suggesting that ACTH is not involved. Houssay *et al.* *(76)* found that estrogen secretion in gonadectomized, hypophysectomized rats was stimulated by gonadotrophin but not by ACTH. A high incidence of pituitary basophil adenomas occurred in rats after gonadectomy *(77)*. Cytologically the tumor cells were similar to the gonadotrophin secreting cells of the normal pituitary.

LH appears to be the effective agent in this form of tumorigenesis which depends on hormonal imbalance. This possibility should be borne in mind in contrast to the adrenal tumorigenesis in rats following estrogen administration (p. 64), a situation in which LH must be depressed.

TUMORS OF THE TESTIS. The interstitial cells of the testis depend on the LH component (ICSH) of the anterior pituitary secretion, and androgens produced with this stimulation inhibit gonadotrophin secretion. It might be expected by analogy with the ovary that disturbance of this reciprocal control mechanism in the male would result in tumors of the interstitial cells. Tumors of the testis have in fact been reported after transplanting testicular tissue into the spleens of gonadectomized adult male or female rats (*78, 79*). Tumors did not occur if transplants were made into the spleens of intact rats. No tumors occurred, however, in similar experiments with A strain mice (*80*).

Hepatic inactivation of the testicular secretion is presumably involved in maintaining high levels of systemic LH in the experimental situation. This should be contrasted with the induction of interstitial cell tumors in mice (p. 65) by the exogenous administration of estrogen. High levels of LH (or ICSH) cannot be invoked as a causative factor in that case.

THYROID TUMORS. Tumors of the thyroid gland arise in experimental or environmental situations in which there is an imbalance between thyroxine secretion and pituitary TSH release. Bielschowsky (*81*) reviewed the literature up to 1955, and his conclusions regarding the mechanisms of the genesis of these lesions are still valid.

Thyroid tumorigenesis is difficult to interpret because the malignancy of tumor nodules cannot be diagnosed with certainty unless they have metastasized or invaded locally. These tumors often depend on continued hormonal stimulation for a long time. The splenic implantation technique, used successfully to produce ovarian and testicular tumors, is ineffective when applied to thyroid tissue. This is not surprising since thyroid extracts are very active when given by mouth; hence, inactivation of the thyroid hormone cannot be very great.

Procedures which markedly reduce functional thyroid tissue have been used successfully to induce thyroid tumors. Simple surgical ablation of most of the thyroid gland caused both adenomas and carcinomas in rats (*82*), although similar experiments in mice did not induce neoplasia.

Goitrogenic drugs inhibit the synthesis of thyroxine by the thyroid, thus increasing secretion of TSH by the pituitary. As for gonadectomized mice, sustained increases in pituitary activity frequently lead to pituitary adenomas which are potentially neoplastic.

In mice hyperplasia of the thyroid was the initial reaction to goitrogens, but after a year or more small islands of thyroid tissue appeared in the lungs (*83, 84, 85, 86, 87*). These distant foci of thyroid tissue were neoplastic, because they grew ectopically. They were not autonomous, however, because they disappeared when treatment was stopped. Subsequently thyroid nodules produced by goitrogen treatment were serially transplanted into mice treated with thiouracil (*88, 89*). Independent tumor growth was achieved after the third transplant generation in one line and after the ninth generation in another. Simultaneous exposure to a transplanted TSH-producing pituitary tumor caused the hyperplasia induced in the mouse thyroid by thiouracil treatment to become malignant (*90*).

A goitrogen combined with the potent carcinogen 2-fluorenylacetamide (FAA) induced multiple adenomas, two of which were malignant, in rat thyroids (91). Administration of thyroxine equivalent to the daily requirement of the hormone suppressed formation of thyroid tumors in rats fed thiouracil (81).

Iodine deficiency causes thyroid hyperplasia (goiter) in man where iodine is deficient in the local environment. Rats raised in iodine-deficient areas develop adenomas of the thyroid which may become malignant (92). Initial nodular hyperplasia can be inhibited, however, by administering iodide in the water (93).

Axelrad and Leblond (94) found thyroid tumors, some of which were malignant, in rats after a year on a low iodine diet. Thyroid tumors are not produced in mice by a low iodine diet.

The radiation from an atomic bomb (95) and from neutrons (96) caused thyroid tumors in mice. In rats local irradiation induces a greater incidence of malignant thyroid tumors than occur spontaneously (97).

Radioactive iodine, which is selectively concentrated in the thyroid, effectively destroys that tissue. In mice this ablation may be complete with high doses. After the tissue is destroyed, the pituitary is hyperstimulated and pituitary tumors develop. Lower doses which leave some thyroid tissue intact do not result in thyroid tumors, possibly because of associated stromal damage (98). In rats on the other hand, ^{131}I may induce metastatic carcinoma of the thyroid (99), but pituitary tumors do not develop.

[131]I combined with methylthiouracil in rats increases the incidence of thyroid adenomas over that produced by the goitrogen alone. The dose of ^{131}I is critical. Doses exceeding 30 μ Ci may actually reduce the hyperplasia caused by the drug (100, 101). Therefore, a delicate balance exists between thyroid destruction sufficient to trigger increased TSH secretion and avoidance of extreme thyroid damage which will destroy the ability of this tissue to respond to stimulation by the trophic hormone.

The common factor in tumor induction is deficiency of the thyroid secretion, despite the experimental necessity for the intervention of external agents in some cases for neoplasia to become evident. The fundamental mechanism is reaction by the pituitary to liberate excessive quantities of TSH. The sequence of thyroid lesions induced by increased stimulation is initially hyperplasia, then adenoma, and finally neoplasia. In some situations where exogenous agents are used, possibly these external factors cause local changes in the target tissue which then progress to malignancy. The fact that a similar sequence of change is induced by thyroid ablation or iodine deficiency in some cases argues strongly that hormonal imbalance is the effective mechanism and that external agents only exacerbate this.

PITUITARY TUMORS. Secretion of trophic hormones by the pituitary is necessary for tumors to develop in the gonads, adrenals, and thyroid. The work outlined above suggested that the essential step in the genesis of these tumors in the target glands is an imbalance between their secretions and that of the pituitary. If there is an imbalance at the level of the target organ, this must involve a complementary imbalance at the level of the pituitary.

Gonadectomy may be followed in some strains of mice by adrenocortical tumors, and these are usually associated with basophilic pituitary adenomas (*64, 102*). Similar pituitary lesions occurred in castrated rats (*76*).

Thyroid function deficiencies responsible for thyroid neoplasia and complete thyroid ablation, possibly leading to thyroid hyperplasia, may result in pituitary tumors. Thus in mice surgical thyroidectomy (*103, 104*), goitrogens (*105, 106*), or radioactive iodine (*105, 107, 108*) result in pituitary tumors. In rats iodine deficiency (*94*) and partial thyroidectomy (*82*) are followed by pituitary tumor growth. Although goitrogens or ^{131}I are not clearly tumor-inducing alone, they are synergistic with other treatments.

Estrogens have been extensively investigated in relation to pituitary tumor induction. Mice are extremely susceptible to this form of tumorigenesis but there are marked strain differences (*105, 109–113*). Both natural and synthetic estrogens are effective. Estrogens readily induce pituitary tumors in rats but there are also marked strain differences in susceptibility, as in mice (*114, 115, 116*). The tumors in mice and rats are often functional and may produce effects similar to STH, prolactin, TSH, or ACTH. Pituitary tumors which secrete FSH or LH have not been reported. The tumors are chromophobe adenomas and usually depend on estrogenic stimulation initially for growth. On serial transplantation they often become autonomous.

Pituitary tumors may develop after long latent periods when the gland is transplanted to a remote site in rats or mice (*117, 118, 119*). It is probably significant that such tumors show ample evidence of prolactin secretion. Severance of the anterior pituitary removes the stimuli caused by the releasing factors of the hypothalamus, but concurrently the gland is removed from the prolactin inhibiting factor. The release of this inhibition is probably fundamental to the development of secretion and tumor formation in the isolated gland.

The target organs secrete hormones which control the activity of releasing factors which in turn stimulate secretion by the pituitary gland. Thus the anterior pituitary can be hyperstimulated by hypothalamic factors which may result in tumor formation in a way similar to that in which its own secretions may cause hyperstimulation of distant tissues. The difference here is that the hypothalamic hormones are carried directly to their target tissue by the hypophyseal portal system.

Tumors Induced by Estrogens. Endogenous estrogens play a fundamental role in the development of the female, in which they are produced cyclically by the ovary. They may also be secreted by the adrenal cortex and the testis, and certainly there is a low level of production in males. Exogenous estrogen administration to either sex has marked effects. In the male it raises the circulating level beyond that encountered physiologically. In the female increased estrogens cause hyperstimulation of the tissues which normally depend on them, such as the uterus and the breast. A constant supply of the hormone eliminates the normal cyclic variations of estrogen levels.

The initial result of hyperestrogenization in both sexes is the complete depression of anterior pituitary secretion of FSH and LH, resulting in gonadal atrophy. The effects of estrogen on anterior pituitary function are also direct, however, with stimulation of prolactin synthesis and release by a local action on the gland (120, 121), in addition to other effects mediated via the hypothalamus. Species and strain susceptibilities vary, but in general the degree of response of the anterior pituitary to chronic estrogen stimulation is proportional to time.

Pituitary tumors which may be the end result of chronic estrogen treatment have been referred to above. The predominant secretion of these tumors is prolactin, but growth-promoting properties are also common, and ACTH-like effects have been reported (122, 123, 124).

In view of the marked effects of pituitary secretions on growth generally and the common sequel of pituitary hyperfunction with estrogen treatment, the tumorigenic activity of estrogen in other tissues cannot be ascribed to the actions of that hormone alone. The relative importance of direct actions of estrogens and the accompanying disturbances of pituitary function involving nonphysiological levels of anterior pituitary hormones is a facet of cancer research which is unexplored.

ADRENAL TUMORS. These tumors are readily induced by estrogens in rats although some strains are more susceptible than others (125, 126). Sensitivity to estrogen seems to be a dominant factor in hybridization experiments.

The adrenal tumors reported by Noble (126) occur in about 20% of rats of a hooded strain which are implanted with a pellet of estrone/cholesterol (9:1). They are unusual because they are readily transplantable into estrogen-treated rats but not into unestrogenized animals. This hormone dependence was maintained through many transplant generations.

Recent experiments have thrown considerable light on the hormones responsible for the growth of these estrogen-dependent, transplanted rat adrenal tumors. In adrenal tumor grafts in estrogen-pelleted rats, specific enzymes associated with DNA synthesis decreased sharply when the estrogen pellet was removed (127). The levels of these enzymes were maintained, however, if prolactin was injected daily after estrogen removal (128). In rats receiving ACTH only replacement with ACTH after estrogen removal maintained the enzymes for a period of two days, but the enzyme levels fell after seven days to the levels found in regressing tumors. In parallel experiments with a dependent mammary tumor with faster rate of regression without estrogen, administration of prolactin increased tumor size. The growth of adrenal tumor transplants was not fast enough for this to be significant.

These observations demonstrate that prolactin is effective in maintaining DNA synthesis and, by inference, cellular multiplication in these adrenal tumors. It cannot be concluded yet that prolactin is the causative agent in the original genesis of the adrenal neoplasia; however, the association of tumorigenesis with pituitary hyperplasia and abundant biological evidence of prolactin secretion is highly suggestive. The alternative possibility—that estrogen acts directly on the adrenal or its neoplasms—has no direct evidence to support it, but its possible role could be resolved with present techniques.

Adrenal hyperplasia is induced by estrogens in mice, but adrenal tumors have not been reported with this agent. The species differences in susceptibility of rats and the insensitivity of mice to this form of tumor induction suggest that there is a genetic component at the level of the adrenal tissue which is a dominant factor in its responsiveness to estrogen.

TUMORS OF THE TESTIS. Spontaneous interstitial cell tumors of the testis occur infrequently in mice of most strains; however, in the Balb/c strain the incidence is about 1% in old mice *(109)*, and in the H strain *(129)* the males have a high incidence of impaired fertility associated with interstitial cell hyperplasia.

Chronic estrogen treatment of male mice of the Balb/c, A, and C strains induces interstitial cell hyperplasia and eventual tumor formation *(130, 131, 132, 133)*. Both natural and synthetic estrogens are effective in tumor induction. As with the adrenal there is a genetic factor in the testicular tissue which determines response by tumor formation.

The induced interstitial cell tumors usually depend on estrogen stimulation for successful transplantation *(134, 135, 136)*. Most transplanted tumors show some androgen production, but there is no clear correlation between the type of secretion and the hormonal requirements for growth *(137)*. Estrogens may be produced by some tumors *(138)*—an interesting correlation with the rare feminizing interstitial cell tumors of man. The production of 11-deoxycorticosterone and 11-oxygenated pregnane and androstane derivatives by interstitial cell tumors of Balb/c mice has been extensively investigated *(139)*. This capacity for steroid 11- and 21-hydroxylation may have some significance because these functions are normally confined to the adrenal cortex. The susceptibility of testicular tissue and adrenal tissue to tumor induction by estrogens and the capacity of tumors from both tissues to produce specific steroid metabolites are presumably related to their similar embryological origin. Genetic susceptibility to estrogen-induced adrenal tumorigenesis and testicular tumorigenesis appears to be inversely related. Thus the rat adrenal is susceptible, but the testis is relatively insensitive; conversely, the mouse adrenal does not become tumorous with estrogen treatment, but the testis does so readily.

Although interstitial cell tumors of the rat testis may occur spontaneously *(140)*, it is only recently that such tumors have been reported in rats after long exposure to implanted estrogen pellets. One tumor was transplantable into males and females treated with estrogen but not into nonestrogenized rats. Other morphologically similar tumors have been observed with estrogen in the same strain. This transplanted estrogen-induced rat tumor produced large amounts of 3α- and 3β-androstanediols but not testosterone, the normal hormone of the testis. The secretion of these compounds accounts for the extremely marked androgenic stimulation found in rats bearing grafts, in which the biological effects of the continued estrogen treatment are completely reversed as tumor growth commences. Despite this neutralization of estrogenic activity by the tumor secretion, both growth and secretion of the neoplasm cease if the estrogen is withdrawn.

RENAL TUMORS. These tumors have unusual morphology and are induced in the hamster kidney after long-term estrogen treatment (*141–150*). The tumors appear to arise from kidney tubules (*143*), but their exact origin is not clear.

The tumors can be induced in male hamsters or castrated males or females, but they regress if estrogen treatment is stopped. Tumor induction is opposed by simultaneous treatment with testosterone, deoxycorticosterone, or progesterone. The secretion of the last hormone appears to be related to the conditions responsible for the inhibition of tumor development in intact females. Estrogen induced tumors in intact females if treatment was started at an early age or if progesterone secretion was low (*146*), as for example after neonatal testosterone injection.

The lesions must be regarded as completely hormone-dependent neoplasms. The fact that they have been induced only in the hamster suggests specific endocrine factors peculiar to that species whose nature is unknown. Alternatively there could be a specific genetic factor in the kidney which leads to these lesions.

TUMORS IN THE FEMALE GENITAL TRACT. Fibromyomas, which are essentially nonmalignant lesions, were induced in guinea pigs by estrogen administration (*151, 152*). Carcinomas of the endometrium were reported in mice but only rarely (*153, 154*). It was suggested in a review (*155*) that estrogens have only a developmental role in this tissue and that some other agent is necessary to initiate tumor growth. Tumors of the cervix were reported in a number of mouse strains after prolonged estrogen treatment (*62, 156, 157, 158*).

Vaginal tumors were induced in one strain of mice (*159*) by the local implantation of diethylstilbestrol (DES), but other strains of mice were not susceptible. This experimental model should be investigated further because of the suspected association between clear-cell carcinomas of the vagina, which have been reported in women aged 15–22 years, and exposure to DES *in utero*. Their mothers were given this drug during pregnancy (*160, 161*) to inhibit spontaneous abortion. As a result of these findings, it is possible that the commercial use of DES in cattle production for human consumption might constitute a hazard. Substances with estrogenic activity occur in a number of plants, and possible carcinogenic hazards of these are discussed in Chapter 12.

Tumors Induced by Testosterone. Uterine tumors following the subcutaneous implantation of testosterone pellets were described in mice (*162, 163, 164*). These tumors were locally infiltrating and in some cases metastasized to the lungs. Anatomically they were restricted to the cervix and the unpaired portion of the uterus. They were considered similar to the proliferation observed in the uterus in early pregnancy. Initial transplants of the tumor into other mice depended on androgen stimulation for growth.

Tumors Induced by Progestational Compounds. Elevated levels of progesterone or synthetic progestational agents inhibit follicular development, ovulation, and the development of the corpus luteum. The inhibitory effect is probably mediated by suppression of pituitary FSH and LH secretion, but direct action on the ovary cannot be ruled out.

In a study of fertility suppression in mice (*165*), ovarian tumors ranging from 4 mg to 1.24 g were found among Balb/c mice subjected to implantation with subcutaneous pellets of 19-norprogesterone for 395 days or more. Subsequently (*166*), ovarian tumors were found in 13 of 45 mice of the same strain implanted with norethindrone (17α-ethinyl-19-nortestosterone) and in 2 of 24 mice which had norethynodrel (17α-ethinyl-$\Delta^{5\text{-}10}$-19-nortestosterone). A much smaller incidence of tumors was obtained with progesterone (*167*).

Although they were classified as granulosa-cell tumors, the lesions appeared to be derived from downgrowths of the germinal epithelium. There seemed to be a significant genetic factor associated with the Balb/c strain in this type of tumorigenesis (*168*). The phenomenon is of considerable interest in view of the use of steroids of this type as contraceptive agents.

Breast Cancer

Cancer of the breast is the most common form of cancer in women and for this reason has been the subject of intense study. It also occurs spontaneously in many other animals especially the dog, the rat, and the mouse. Because of their convenience the last two species have been the most commonly used for laboratory investigations. There is such a vast literature describing the effects of hormones on mammary tumorigenesis that a comprehensive survey is not possible. Many aspects of the earlier experimental work have been succinctly summarized (*3, 4, 169*), however, and the pathological aspects of the disease in man have been described (*170*). An attempt is made here to summarize some aspects of hormonal interactions in mammary carcinogenesis, but for clarity the work referred to is limited. In all cases the advances in knowledge which are outlined were based on much meticulous work by many people not mentioned specifically. Consultation of the reports quoted provides a wider access to the literature.

Normal Breast Development. The breast originates embryologically as an ectodermal outgrowth and can be regarded as a modified sweat gland. In its rudimentary state, in most males and immature females, it consists of a simple duct opening to the surface of the skin at the nipple (Figure 4A). With appropriate hormonal stimulation the primary duct becomes extended and ramifies to form a complex branching system (Figure 4B). Qualitative changes in the hormonal environment cause outgrowth of clusters of acini from the ducts (Figure 4C). This basic structure of the ducts and acini varies in extent according to the degree of hormonal stimulation, but it can function as a metabolic unit with milk production at any stage of proliferation. Individual breast lobules may be situated separately as distinct units, as in the mouse and rat, or they may be associated in clumps of about 20, with ducts opening to the surface as a group, as in the human.

   A detailed analysis of mammary growth and function in the Long–Evans
rat (7) incorporated much new information which, together with the efforts
of many preceding workers, established the basic hormonal requirements for
the development of mammary ducts and acini and the induction of lactation.
The experimental model used so successfully in these studies was to replace
combinations of pituitary and steroid hormones exogenously in rats from
which the pituitary, adrenals, and ovaries had been removed. It was found
that duct growth required somatotrophin (STH), estrogen, and corticoid.
For full acinar growth STH, prolactin, estrogen, corticoid, and progesterone
were required. Lactation was induced and maintained when estrogen and
progesterone were reduced and prolactin and a corticoid were given alone.
STH and thyroxine were not essential for lactation in the experiments.

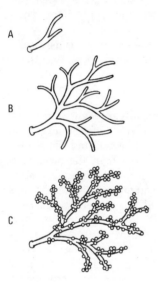

A

B

C

*Figure 4. Diagram of breast development. (A)
Rudimentary duct. (B) Duct outgrowth. (C)
Duct and acinar development.*

   In an extended series of similar experiments in hypophysectomized,
adrenalectomized, ovariectomized mice of the C3H/HeCrgl strain, Nandi
(8) found similar requirements of hormones for different stages of breast
growth and function. There were, however, some differences. Thus, duct
growth required a combination of somatotrophin, estrogen, 11-deoxycorti-
costerone (DOC), and cortisol. The proliferation of acini comparable to
that in the adult virgin mouse required estrogen, progesterone, and prolactin
or STH. For acinar proliferation comparable with early pregnancy, estrogen,
progesterone, DOC, and prolactin or STH were required. The fuller acinar
growth of late pregnancy could be induced either by estrogen, progesterone,
DOC, cortisol, and STH or by estrogen, progesterone, DOC, STH, and prolactin (*i.e.*, without cortisol). Lactogenesis could be induced in the developed
gland with either prolactin or STH in combination with cortisol but was
more complete with both prolactin and STH combined with cortisol. DOC
was not an effective substitute for cortisol in lactogenesis.

Normal growth of breast epithelial tissue occurs only in a stroma of white fat. Thus proliferation of the *in situ* breast is confined to the local fat pad. Mammary cancer differs fundamentally from the normal tissue in its ability to grow without a local environment of stromal fat cells and can be transplanted subcutaneously or into many other tissues.

Normal mammary epithelium is a target organ for many hormonal stimuli; although it produces secretions, there is no evidence that the quantity of breast tissue exerts any feedback inhibition of its own growth. Whole breast lobules are readily removed and transplanted, but in experimental situations there is no evidence that diminution or increase of the total amount of mammary tissue influences the degree of proliferation (*171*).

Breast Tumor Induction. Mammary cancer can be induced in mice by a variety of agents which fit generally into four groups—viral, chemical, radiation, and hormonal. In all cases a prerequisite for the initiating action of any agent is the presence of a developed mammary epithelial system. The interaction of hormonal factors in tumor induction has been reviewed frequently (*4, 169, 172, 173*). The actions of viruses, chemicals, and radiation as agents which cause cancers with adequate hormonal stimulation is well established, but the possibility that hormonal stimulation alone can induce neoplasia is less certain.

VIRUSES. The role of viral agents in mammary cancer induction in mice could not have been established without the prior development of highly inbred strains with reproducible genetic characters and tumor incidences. Certain strains have a high incidence of "spontaneous" breast cancer, but it is very low in others. Crossbreeding experiments showed that the tendency for breast tumors to occur was not inherited in the manner expected of a genetically controlled character. In reciprocal crosses between a high and a low breast cancer strain, the tumor incidence was only high if the mother was a high cancer strain. When a male from the high cancer strain was the parent, the incidence was much lower. As the genetic makeup of the first generation females was the same, irrespective of the mother's strain, it was concluded that an extra-chromosomal factor was involved. Bittner (*174, 175*) showed that a tumor-inducing agent was transferred in the milk by a female to her young. The milk agent is now accepted as a mammary tumor virus (MTV), and it is present in many tissues (*176*).

Even when the MTV is present there may be marked differences in the virgin incidence of breast tumors as opposed to that in breeding mice. Thus in female A strain mice the virgin breast tumor incidence is low, but virgin female C3H mice have a high incidence (Table II). Breeders of both A and C3H strains have a high incidence. Hybrid A × C3H females develop high incidences of breast cancer in both virgins and breeding females. The dominant hormonal pattern involved in this susceptibility was termed the "inherited hormonal influence" (*177*). It was suggested (*178*) that there might be a correlation between the inherited hormonal influence and the susceptibility of mice to develop adrenal cortical hyperplasia after castration (*cf.* p. 60). Although this correlation held in some instances, it was not absolute. In other transplantation experiments, in which ovaries from strains

Table II. Mammary Cancer Incidence (%) in Female Mice of A and C3H Strains Possessing Milk Agent and Their Hybrids (177)

Strain	Virgins	Breeders
A	4	84
C3H	66	95
A X C3H	89	94

Annals of the New York Academy of Science

with or without the hormonal influence were transplanted into ovariectomized hybrid recipients, there was little difference in tumor incidence in the hybrids irrespective of the parent strain from which the transplanted ovaries were obtained.

The mammary glands of virgin mice possessing the inherited hormonal influence have a copious development of acini as compared with the breasts of mice without the influence. In addition the ovaries of susceptible mice have many more corpora lutea (179). The presence of breast acini suggests that progesterone is available in the virgin mice which possess them, despite the fact that the estrus cycle of the mouse has no active luteal phase (173). It is known that pseudopregnancy occurs frequently in mice of some strains under the influence of various stimuli such as smell or association with other mice of either sex (180). Pseudopregnancy results in the active luteal secretion of progesterone. It can be prevented by isolation or removal of the olfactory lobes. Tendency to become pseudopregnant varies greatly from strain to strain and could account for the variations in the virgin structure of the breast and the associated mammary tumor incidence (181).

Genetic Factors in Hormone Requirements. A major contribution to the understanding of breast cancer susceptibility of virgin mice of different strains was made by Nandi and Bern (182). They found that after hypophysectomy and ovariectomy all strains of mice responded (by mammary duct and acinar growth) to hormonal treatment with estrogen, progesterone, and prolactin. Subsequent treatment with cortisol and prolactin induced lactation. Strains of mice, such as the C3H, which have a high virgin incidence of breast cancer also had full breast development when prolactin was replaced by somatotrophin (STH) (i.e., estrogen, progesterone, and STH) and then lactated when just cortisol and STH were given. Hypophysectomized mice with a low virgin incidence of mammary cancer (e.g., A strain), reacted to the latter combination with duct growth only, and lactation was not induced by subsequent treatment with cortisol and STH. The responses of a number of strains of mice to prolactin (mammotrophin) or STH (somatotrophin) are shown in Table III.

Convincing additional evidence for a genetic difference in the breast tissue between A and C3H strain mice was forthcoming (183). Breasts from A and C3H mice were transplanted into the fat pads of hybrid C3H X A mice. The hosts were hypophysectomized, ovariectomized, and treated with estradiol, progesterone, and STH. Some were given additional treatment with cortisol and STH alone. There was little acinar development and no lactation in breasts transplanted from A strain mice. The breasts of mice from the C3H strain had copious acinar development and full milk secretion with the addition of cortisol and STH. A similar difference in the susceptibility of mammary tissue was demonstrated in organ culture *in vitro* (*184*). Therefore, (*185*) one major component of differences in susceptibility of various strains to breast cancer is a genetic factor in the mammary tissue itself which determines the proliferative and secretory response to STH.

Stages of Tumor Development. By the introduction and perfection of many elegant new techniques, the process of tumor induction by viruses in mice has been developed into a model system which has been exploited to answer specific questions regarding the mechanisms involved (*158, 186, 187*). The fact that the origin of mammary tumors in mice is associated with the previous development of hyperplastic alveolar nodules (*188*) is well established (*173, 189*). Their occurrence in mice lacking the MTV offered difficulties in determining their association with viral infection until a separate nodule-inducing virus (NIV) was discovered in some strains of mice (*187, 190*). The NIV, unlike the MTV, is not transmitted in the milk but through the germ cells. Both MTV and NIV can induce hyperplastic nodules, but the tumorigenic potential of NIV-induced lesions is much lower.

Hormonal factors which will cause the transformation of normal mammary glands through an intermediate stage of nodule formation to a fully autonomous carcinoma were identified in the C3H mouse (Table IV) (*169, 182*). Essentially the hormone requirements for preneoplastic nodule induc-

Table III.   Relation of Bittner's Inherited Hormonal Influence to Mammary Gland Responses of Female Mice, Hypophysectomized–Ovariectomized at 12 Weeks of Age (*169*)

Strain (Crgl)	Mammary Tumor Incidence		Lobulo-Alveolar and Lactogenic Response[a]		Inherited Hormonal Influence (*177*)
	Virgins	Breeders	Mammo-trophin	Somato-trophin	
C3H	high	high	+	+	+
R111	high	high	+	+	+
DBA	high	high	+	+	+
BALB/c	low	low	+	+	+
	(high if MTA +)				
A	low	high	+	−	−
A/3	low	high	+	−	−
F₁ (A x C3H)[b]	high	high		+	+
C57BL	low	low	+	±	−
	(low if MTA +)				

[a] Injected daily for 21 days with 1μg estradiol–17β, 1000 μg progesterone, and somatotrophin or mammotrophin for 21 days followed by 5 days of treatment with somatotrophin or mammotrophin and 125 μg cortisol acetate. Daily dose of somatotrophin or mammotrophin: 100 μg, one to seven days; 500 μg, 15–26 days.
[b] Hypophysectomized–ovariectomized at seven weeks of age.

Table IV. Summary of Minimum Experimental Hormonal Combinations for Mammary Development in the C3H/Crgl Mouse (169)

	Estra-diol	Pro-gest-erone	Deoxy-corti-cost-erone	Cortisol	Mam-mo-tropin	Somato-tropin
Normal mammary gland:						
ductal development	+	+ or +				+ or +
lobulo–alveolar development	+	+ or +				+ or +
lactation				+		+ or +
Hyperplastic alveolar nodules:						
induction	+	+ or +				+ or +
maintenance		+ or		+		+ or +
adenocar-cinomatous change			+			+ or +

tion are the same as for normal mammary growth. Their maintenance and transformation to carcinoma, however, require only a corticoid (11-deoxy-corticosterone or cortisol) and prolactin or STH. Fully developed carcinomas are independent of both ovarian and pituitary secretion.

A nodule outgrowth which contained neither MTV nor NIV was investigated in transplants in Balb/cCrgl mice. Addition of MTV or NIV considerably increased the origin of tumors from the nodules. Prolonged stimulation of the nodules by pituitary isografts significantly potentiated the effects of both viruses, but the hormonal stimulation alone had no effect on nodule transformation to cancer (191, 192).

CHEMICALS. Many chemical compounds will induce cancer of the breast in mice or rats. Certain aromatic amines are potent carcinogenic agents in many tissues, e.g., 2-fluorenylactamide induces breast cancer in mice (193) and rats (194). The polycyclic hydrocarbons were more widely used to study the relationship of hormones to cancer induction by chemicals. The earlier literature has been reviewed for mice (170) and rats (172).

Observations of mammary cancer induction by chemicals in mice must be evaluated carefully to determine whether the compound is acting directly on the breast or whether it is modifying the action of endogenous viral agents. There are nevertheless mouse strains which are not known to carry a viral mammary tumor agent, and no viral agent has been implicated in the genesis of breast tumors in rats.

Dosage. The route of administration of polycyclic hydrocarbons appears to be immaterial in tumor induction provided a sufficient concentration reaches the breast tissue. Thus in mice 3-methylcholanthrene is effective when painted on the skin (*195*), injected subcutaneously (*196*), implanted locally (*197*), or given by gavage (*38*). In rats polycyclic hydrocarbons applied to the skin (*198*), given by gavage (*199*), or injected intravenously (*200*) are equally effective. Induction of breast cancer by a single administration of a chemical carcinogen (*172, 200*) is an invaluable technique for investigating the role of hormonal factors in this form of tumorigenesis.

Dao *et al.* (*201*) gave a single dose of 7,12-dimethylbenz(*a*)anthracene (DMBA) to a donor rat, and the breast tissue was subsequently transplanted to an untreated female of the same strain. Carcinomas arose only in the transplanted breast, and their incidence was high even when the interval between treatment of the donor and transplantation was as little as 4 hrs. This clearly demonstrates the early effect of the chemical on the mammary tissue, and that only a limited exposure is necessary to induce the changes leading to cancer upon subsequent hormonal stimulation.

Effect of the Ovary. Mammary cancer cannot be induced in male mice by chemicals alone, but breast tumors do appear if the males also bear a transplanted ovary (*202*). If female mice are ovariectomized after exposure to a carcinogen, the incidence of breast cancer is reduced and is proportional to the time the ovaries remain *in situ* (*170*) (Table V). Castrated male rats which were given a carcinogen and grafted with an ovary at the same time (*203*) developed a high incidence of breast cancer, but the incidence of tumors was not elevated above control levels if ovarian implantation was delayed for 25 days. Similar results were obtained after the exposure of ovariectomized female rats to a carcinogen coupled with grafting of an ovary (Table VI). Breast tumors were induced if the chemical was given 7 or 15 days after castration but not if it was delayed for 30 days. Delaying ovarian transplantation for periods up to 30 days after the carcinogen did not diminish the number of breast tumors induced.

Pregnancy and Lactation. Pregnancy without lactation or pseudopregnancy induced by mating with vasectomized males increases the incidence of breast tumors induced by chemical carcinogens in mice which have only a low incidence of tumors in virgins treated with the chemical (*204*).

Mice which are susceptible to chemical induction of mammary cancer do not develop breast tumors if they are exposed to the carcinogen and

Table V. Incidence of Breast Cancer in Female IF Mice Treated with 3-Methylcholanthrene and Then Ovariectomized at Different Times after Application (*170*)

Interval before Ovariectomy (weeks)	No. of Mice	No. with Breast	Cancer (%)
8	30	1	3
12	10	1	10
15	11	2	18
18	12	4	33
Not done	39	17	39

Human and Experimental Breast Cancer

**Table VI.   Effects of Ovarian Grafts on Incidence of Breast Cancer
in Castrated Female Rats Receiving a Single Dose of 20 mg
7,12-Dimethylbenz[a]anthracene (DMBA) (201)**

Groups	Rats Fed DMBA 7 Days after Castration		Rats Fed DMBA 15 Days after Castration		Rats Fed DMBA 30 Days after Castration
	No. Rats with Tumors[a]	Total No. Tumors	No. Rats with Tumors[a]	Total No. Tumors	No. Rats with Tumors[a]
Control (castrated)	1/20 (5%)	1	0/20		0/20
Ov. graft 0 days after DMBA	3/7 (43%)	9	3/7 (43%)	4	0/7
Ov. graft 7 days after DMBA	2/6 (33%)[b]	4	3/7 (43%)	3	0/7
Ov. graft 15 days after DMBA	3/7 (43%)	7	2/7 (29%)	2	0/7
Ov. graft 30 days after DMBA	2/7 (29%)	2	2/7 (29%)	2	0/7

[a] No. rats with tumors/No. of rats.
[b] One rat died one week after feeding of DMBA.

National Cancer Institute Journal

allowed to lactate normally (205). That the effect of lactation is local on the individual breast was shown conclusively (204, 206, 207) by inhibition of lactation by excision of the nipples on one side of carcinogen-treated breeding mice. Breasts on the other side were allowed to lactate normally. In all experiments there was a much greater incidence of tumors in the non-lactating breasts. It is possible that inhibition of tumor induction by lactation is caused by excretion of the carcinogen in the milk. Alternatively, suppression of lactation, by cutting the nipples or removing the litters, has a local suppressive effect on the breast's metabolic activity which might make it susceptible to the stimulating action of endogenous hormones.

Ovarian Hormones. Both estrogen and progesterone are produced by the ovaries of mice and rats in pregnancy although in normal estrus cycles only estrogens are secreted. Cantarow et al. (194) showed that the injection of progesterone into rats fed 2-fluorenylacetamide greatly increased breast tumor formation. Recently Sydnor et al. (208) showed that estrogen injection alone did not restore susceptibility of the rat mammary gland to polycyclic hydrocarbon tumorigenesis after ovariectomy and adrenalectomy. Progesterone injected with estrogen restored the incidence of breast tumors to that found in intact females.

Mice are similar to rats in that estrogen alone is not a sufficient hormonal stimulus for chemical breast tumor induction (*197*). Progesterone and estrogen together resulted in a marked stimulation of mammary cancer induction by a chemical carcinogen in ovariectomized female or castrated male mice lacking both MTV and NIV (*181*). Similar results were subsequently obtained in another strain of mice lacking the MTV but presumably carrying NIV (*181*).

Thyroidectomy. This inhibits body growth generally in rats, but does not inhibit ovarian function. The incidence of breast tumors induced by DMBA was significantly reduced by surgical removal of the thyroid (*209*). Administration of thiouracil had a comparable effect (*210*). This could be caused by restriction of food intake or by decreased STH secretion in thyroid-deficient rats.

Pituitary Hormones. These are essential for cancer induction in rats and mice (*172*) but the role of the individual hormones has not been determined in detail for cancers induced by chemical agents. A pituitary tumor which secretes prolactin can increase susceptibility in mice which are refractory to the chemical induction of breast cancer (*211*). Prolactin, however, can have a direct effect on breast tissue and an indirect effect by stimulation of ovarian secretion of progesterone. Whether the major effect of prolactin is direct or indirect is not known.

IRRADIATION. This is an effective agent for inducing breast tumors in rats (*212, 213*). The tumors tend to be restricted to the mammary tissue exposed to direct radiation (*214*), and the incidence is proportional to the dose (*215*). Irradiation seems to act as a direct carcinogen and does not produce its effects by an indirect action on the ovaries or the pituitary. Hyperplastic alveolar nodules similar to those induced by viruses or chemical carcinogens in mice were produced by radiation, and are probably preneoplastic lesions. Local breast irradiation also produces mammary cancer in mice (*216*). There is no reason to suppose that the hormonal requirements for radiation-induced breast cancer differ from those necessary with other types of carcinogens.

HORMONES. Lacassagne demonstrated that prolonged injection of an estrogenic agent caused mammary cancer in male mice (*217*). It was assumed then that ovarian hormones were directly carcinogenic to the breast. The later discovery of the mammary tumor viruses completely undermined the early evidence suggesting a direct mammary cancer-inducing property of the estrogens. Male mice from strains with a low spontaneous incidence of breast cancer do not develop tumors with estrogen administration (*218, 219*).

Mammary tumors can be induced in male mice of the C3Hb strain, which lack the MTV, by chronic exposure to estrogens (*220, 221*). With the demonstration of a nodule-inducing virus (NIV) in this strain, it is no longer believed that the tumors were caused by a direct action of the estrogen or by hormonal imbalance.

Rats have never been shown to carry any viral agent associated with mammary cancer induction. That chronic treatment with estrogens induces a high incidence of breast tumors in some strains of rats is most important

(*222–228*). These tumors depend on the continued presence of estrogen for their growth (*222, 229, 230*). Complete tumor regression follows removal of the estrogen-containing pellet, and renewed growth follows its reimplantation. The tumors in the estrogen-dependent form can metastasize and kill their hosts. Complete tumor regression follows hypophysectomy. Breast tumor induction by estrogens in rats is always associated with pituitary hypertrophy and often the development of mammotrophic pituitary tumors. Biological evidence of prolactin secretion under these conditions is abundant.

The hormonal environment which exists in hyperestrogenized rats is complex. The stimulation of pituitary secretion of prolactin is of fundamental importance in the genesis of these neoplasms, not only of the breast but also of the adrenal (p. 64). Richards *et al.* (*128*) showed that the mammary tumors induced by estrogen may be maintained by prolactin injection after estrogen removal. Prolactin stimulation might not play an inciting role by itself, but it might do so in conjunction with other hormones. Unknown viral or other environmental factors could have a significant effect.

Breast tumor induction in mice was studied by the repeated subcutaneous implantation of whole pituitary glands over an extended period. Subcutaneous insertion of 20–200 pituitaries induced mammary tumors in MTV-free mice of six strains and in two hybrid strains (Table VII) (*119*). Pituitary grafts into the renal capsule were more effective (*231*).

Table VII.   Mammary Cancer Induced in Female Mice of Various Strains by the Repeated Subcutaneous Implantation of Pituitaries (*119*)

Strain	No. of Mice	No. with Mammary Tumors
C3Hf	23	22
DBAf	5	5
WLL	9	4
CBA	9	5
O20	14	11
C57BL	18	2
O20 X DBAf	20	16
C57 X DBAf	15	10

Cancer Research

Single grafts of pituitaries were effective (*232*), but hypophysectomy or ovariectomy inhibited tumor induction. Male mice grafted with pituitaries alone did not develop mammary tumors but did so if an ovary was also implanted (*214, 233*).

Leukemia

Some steroid hormones and various other humoral factors, which are concerned in the regulation of hematopoiesis, affect the development of a number of lymphoid tumors. There are also sex differences in the incidences of many of these neoplasms.

Metcalf reviewed the subject comprehensively (*234*). The more specialized topic of plasma-cell tumor induction is discussed by Hollander *et al.* (*235*).

Conclusions

Four possible mechanisms through which hormones might be involved in the process of carcinogenesis were noted. The work reviewed makes it possible to assess their relative importance.

1. A direct carcinogenic action of a hormone of any kind in the genesis of tumors has not been demonstrated although in many instances hormones are responsible for maintaining tumor growth.

2. In many experimental situations, a hormone can stimulate the secretion of a second endocrine factor which is directly or indirectly involved in carcinogenesis.

3. Hormones are essential to tumor induction in many tissues by stimulating growth and thus the presence of the cells on which other carcinogens may act (*e.g.*, mammary tissue).

4. Hormonal factors can modify the metabolism of chemical carcinogens so that active proximate agents are formed in a sufficient concentration (*236, 237*).

In considering the potential carcinogenic action of any agent, therefore, the hormonal environment may constitute a major modifying parameter which must be taken into account.

Literature Cited

1. Turner, C. D., Bagnara, J. T., "General Endocrinology," W. B. Saunders, Philadelphia, 1971.
2. Clayson, D. B., "Chemical Carcinogenesis," J. & A. Churchill, London, 1962.
3. Noble, R. L., "The Hormones," G. Pincus and K. V. Thimann, Eds., Vol. 5, pp. 559–695, Academic, New York, 1964.
4. Russfield, A. B., "Tumors of the Endocrine Glands and Secondary Sex Organs," U.S. Dept. of Health, Education, and Welfare, Washington, D.C., 1966.
5. Bischoff, F., *Adv. Lipid Res.* (1969) **7**, 165.
6. Tanner, J. M., *Nature* (1972) **237**, 433.
7. Lyons, W. R., Li, C. H., Johnson, R. E., *Recent Progr. in Horm. Res.* (1958) **14**, 219.
8. Nandi, S., *Natl. Cancer Inst. J.* (1958) **21**, 1039.
9. Bern, H. A., *Recent Progr. in Horm. Res.* (1968) **24**, 681.
10. Friesen, H., Kleinberg, D. L., Noel, G. L., "Lactogenic Hormones," G. E. W. Wolstenholme and J. Knight, Eds., pp. 83–103, Churchill, Livingstone, Edinburgh, 1972.
11. Donovan, B. T., "Mammalian Neuroendocrinology," McGraw-Hill, London, 1970.
12. Golden, J. B., Sveringhaus, E. L., *Proc. Soc. Exp. Biol. Med.* (1938) **39**, 361.
13. Long, J. A., Evans, H. M., *Mem. Univ. Calif.* (1922) **6**, 1.
14. Pfeiffer, C. A., *Amer. J. Anat.* (1936) **58**, 195.
15. Biskind, G. R., *Endocrinology* (1941) **28**, 894.
16. Biskind, M. S., Biskind, G. R., *Proc. Soc. Exp. Biol. Med.* (1944) **55**, 176.
17. Biskind, G. R., Biskind, M. S., *Science* (1948) **108**, 137.

18. Biskind, G. R., Kordan, B., Biskind, M. S., *Cancer Res.* (1950) **10,** 309.
19. Peckham, B. M., Greene, R. R., *Cancer Res.* (1952) **12,** 25.
20. Furth, J., Sobel, H., *Natl. Cancer Inst. J.* (1946) **8,** 7.
21. Gardner, W. U., *Natl. Cancer Inst. J.* (1961) **26,** 829.
22. Guthrie, M. J., *Cancer* (1957) **10,** 190.
23. Klein, M., *Natl. Cancer Inst. J.* (1952) **12,** 877.
24. *Ibid.* (1953) **14,** 77.
25. Li, M. H., Gardner, W. U., *Cancer Res.* (1947) **7,** 549.
26. *Ibid.* (1949) **9,** 35.
27. Furth, J., "Thule International Symposia: Cancer and Ageing," A. Engel and D. Larsson, Eds., Nordiska Bokhandelns, Sweden, 1967.
28. Li, M. H., Gardner, W. U., *Cancer Res.* (1952) **10,** 162.
29. Peters, H., *Adv. Reprod. Physiol.* (1969) **4,** 149.
30. Furth, J., *Proc. Soc. Exp. Biol. Med.* (1949) **71,** 274.
31. Furth, J., Furth, O. B., *Am. J. Cancer* (1936) **28,** 66.
32. Geist, S. H., Gaines, J. A., Pollack, A. D., *Am. J. Obstet. Gynecol.* (1939) **38,** 786.
33. Guthrie, M., *Cancer* (1958) **11,** 1226.
34. Kaplan, H. S., *Natl. Cancer Inst. J.* (1950) **11,** 125.
35. Lacassagne, A., Duplan, J. F., Marcovich, H., Raynaud, A., "The Ovary," S. Zuckerman, Ed., Vol. II, p. 463, Academic, London, 1962.
36. Lick, L., Kirschbaum, A., Mixer, H., *Cancer Res.* (1949) **9,** 532.
37. Marchant, J., Orr, J. W., Woodhouse, D. L., *Nature* (1954) **173,** 307.
38. Bianciflori, C., Bonser, G. M., Caschera, F., *Br. J. Cancer* (1961) **15,** 270.
39. Jull, J. W., *Can. Cancer Conf.* (1966) **6,** 109.
40. Krarup, T., *Acta Pathol. Microbiol. Scand.* (1967) **70,** 241.
41. Kuwahara, I., *Gann.* (1967) **58,** 253.
42. Jull, J. W., *Natl. Cancer Inst. J.* (1969) **42,** 961.
43. Shisa, H., Nishizuka, Y., *Br. J. Cancer* (1968) **23,** 70.
44. Jull, J. W., Hawryluk, A., Russell, A., *Natl. Cancer Inst. J.* (1968) **40,** 687.
45. Jull, J. W., Russell A., *Natl. Cancer Inst. J.* (1970) **44,** 841.
46. Marchant, J., *Br. J. Cancer* (1961) **15,** 821.
47. Jull, J. W., *Natl. Cancer Inst. J.* (1969) **42,** 697.
48. Marchant, J., *Br. J. Cancer* (1960) **14,** 514.
49. Pedersen, T., Krarup, T., *Int. J. Cancer* (1969) **4,** 495.
50. Mühlbock, O., *Acta Endocrinol.* (1953) **12,** 105.
51. Murphy, E., *Natl. Cancer Inst. J.* (1972) **48,** 1283.
52. Russell, E. S., Fekete, E., *Natl. Cancer Inst. J.* (1958) **21,** 365.
53. Russell, W. L., Russell, E. S., *Genetics* (1948) **33,** 122.
54. Chester-Jones, I., *Br. Med. Bull.* (1955) **11,** 156.
55. Frantz, M. J., Kirschbaum, A., *Proc. Soc. Exp. Biol. Med.* (1948) **69,** 357.
56. Frantz, M. J., Kirschbaum, A., *Cancer Res.* (1949) **9,** 257.
57. Kirschbaum, A., Frantz, M., Williams, W. L., *Cancer Res.* (1946) **6,** 707.
58. Snell, K. C., Stewart, H. L., *Natl. Cancer Inst. J.* (1959) **22,** 1119.
59. Dunham, L. J., Herrold, K. M., *Natl. Cancer Inst. J.* (1962) **29,** 1047.
60. Fortner, J. G., *Cancer Res.* (1961) **21,** 1491.
61. Woolley, G. W., Fekete, E., Little, C. C., *Proc. Natl. Acad. Sci.* (1939) **25,** 277.
62. Gardner, W. U., *Adv. Cancer Res.* (1953) **1,** 173.
63. Woolley, G. W., *Cancer Res.* (1950) **10,** 250.
64. Dickie, M. M., Lane, P. W., *Cancer Res.* (1956) **16,** 48.
65. Fekete, E., Woolley, G. W., Little, C. C., *J. Exp. Med.* (1941) **74,** 1.
66. Woolley, G. W., Fekete, E., Little, C. C., *Endocrinology* (1941) **28,** 34.
67. Gardner, W. U., *Cancer Res.* (1941) **1,** 632.
68. Hoffman, F. G., Dickie, M. M., Christy, N. P., *Acta Endocrinol.* (1960) **34,** 84.
69. Paschkis, K. E., Cantarow, A., Huseby, R. A., *Proc. Soc. Exp. Biol. Med.* (1954) **85,** 422.

70. Woolley, G. W., Little, C. C., *Cancer Res.* (1945) **5**, 193.
71. Huseby, R. A., Bittner, J. J., *Cancer Res.* (1951) **11**, 644.
72. Ferguson, D. J., Visscher, M. B., *Cancer Res.* (1953) **13**, 405.
73. Atkinson, W. B., Dickie, M. M., *Proc. Soc. Exp. Biol. Med.* (1958) **99**, 267.
74. Tullos, H. S., Kirschbaum, A., Trentin, J. J., *Cancer Res.* (1961) **21**, 730.
75. Monsen, H., *Cancer Res.* (1952) **12**, 284.
76. Houssay, B. A., Houssay, A. B., Cardeza, A. F., Pinto, R. M., *Schweiz. Med. Wochenschr.* (1955) **85**, 291.
77. Griesbach, W. E., Purves, H. D., *Br. J. Cancer* (1960) **14**, 49.
78. Biskind, M. S., Biskind, G. R., *Proc. Soc. Exp. Biol. Med.* (1945) **59**, 4.
79. Twombly, G. H., Meisel, D., Stout, A. P., *Cancer* (1949) **2**, 884.
80. Li, M. H., Pfeiffer, C. A., Gardner, W. U., *Proc. Soc. Exp. Biol. Med.* (1947) **64**, 319.
81. Bielschowsky, F., *Br. J. Cancer* (1955) **9**, 80.
82. Doniach, I., Williams, E. D., *Br. J. Cancer* (1962) **16**, 222.
83. Dalton, A. J., Morris, H. P., Dubnik, S. S., *Natl. Cancer Inst. J.* (1948) **9**, 201.
84. Gorbman, A., *Cancer Res.* (1946) **6**, 492.
85. *Ibid.* (1947) **7**, 746.
86. Morris, H. P., Dubnik, C. S., Dalton, A. J., *Natl. Cancer Inst. J.* (1946-47) **7**, 159.
87. Morris, H. P., Dubnik, C. S., Dalton, A. J., *Cancer Res.* (1946) **6**, 492.
88. Morris, H. P., Dalton, A. J., Green, C. D., *J. Clin. Endocrinol.* (1951) **11**, 1281.
89. Morris, H. P., Green, C. D., *Science* (1951) **114**, 44.
90. Haran-Ghera, N., Pullar, P., Furth, J., *Endocrinology* (1960) **66**, 694.
91. Bielschowsky, F., *Br. J. Exp. Path.* (1944) **25**, 90.
92. Wegelin, C., *Schweiz. Med. Wochenschr.* (1927) **57**, 848.
93. Bielschowsky, F., *Br. J. Cancer* (1953) **7**, 203.
94. Axelrad, A., Leblond, C. P., *Cancer* (1955) **8**, 339.
95. Upton, A. C., Kimball, A. W., Furth, J., Christenberry, K. W., Benedict, W. H., *Cancer Res.* (1960) **20**, 1.
96. Haran-Ghera, N., Furth, J., Buffet, R. E., Yokoro, K., *Cancer Res.* (1959) **19**, 1181.
97. Lindsay, S., Sheline, G. E., Potter, G. D., Chaikoff, I. L., *Cancer Res.* (1961) **21**, 9.
98. Furth, J., Burnett, W. T., Gadsden, E. L., *Cancer Res.* (1953) **13**, 298.
99. Goldberg, R. C., Chaikoff, I. L., *Arch. Pathol.* (1952) **53**, 22.
100. Doniach, I., *Br. J. Cancer* (1953) **7**, 181.
101. Doniach, I., Logothetopoulos, J. H., *Br. J. Cancer* (1955) **9**, 117.
102. Dickie, M. M., Woolley, G. W., *Cancer Res.* (1949) **9**, 372.
103. Dent, J. N., Gadsden, E. L., Furth, J., *Cancer Res.* (1955) **15**, 70.
104. *Ibid.* (1956) **16**, 171.
105. Kwa, H. G., "An Experimental Study of Pituitary Tumors," *in* "Genesis, Cytology, and Hormone Content," Springer-Verlag, Berlin, 1961.
106. Moore, G. E., Brackney, E. L., Bock, F. G., *Proc. Soc. Exp. Biol. Med.* (1953) **82**, 643.
107. Furth, J., Dent, J. N., Burnett, W. T., Gadsden, E. L., *J. Clin. Endocrinol.* (1955) **15**, 81.
108. Goldberg, R. C., Chaikoff, I. L., *Endocrinology* (1951) **48**, 1.
109. Andervont, H. B., Shimkin, M. B., Canter, H. Y., *Natl. Cancer Inst. J.* (1960) **25**, 1069.
110. Gardner, W. U., *Cancer Res.* (1941) **1**, 345.
111. Gardner, W. U., *Ciba Found. Colloq. in Endocrinol. (Proc.)* (1958) **12**, 239.
112. Gardner, W. U., Strong, L. C., *Yale J. Biol. Med.* (1940) **12**, 543.
113. Richardson, F. L., *Natl. Cancer Inst. J.* (1957) **18**, 813.
114. McEuen, C. S., Selye, H., Collip., J. B., *Lancet* (1936) **1**, 775.
115. Nelson, W. O., *Am. J. Physiol.* (1941) **133**, 398.

116. Segaloff, A., Dunning, W., *Endocrinology* (1945) **36,** 238.
117. Bardin, C. W., Liebelt, A. G., Lipscomb, H. S., Mountcastle, W., Liebelt, R. A., *Proc. Am. Ass. Cancer Res.* (1962) **3,** 302.
118. Gardner, W. U., "On Cancer and Hormones," p. 89, University of Chicago, Chicago, 1962.
119. Mühlbock, O., Boot, L. M., *Cancer Res.* (1959) **19,** 402.
120. Kanematsu, S., Sawyer, C. H., *Endocrinology* (1963) **72,** 243.
121. Ramirez, V. D., McCann, S. M., *Endocrinology* (1964) **75,** 206.
122. Bates, R. W., Milkovic, S., Garrison, M. M., *Endocrinology* (1962) **71,** 943.
123. Grindeland, R. E., Harrison, E., Wherry, F. E., *Fed. Proc. Fed. Amer. Soc. Exper. Biol.* (1961) **20,** 183.
124. Takemoto, H., Yokoro, K., Furth, J., Cohen, A. I., *Cancer Res.* (1962) **22,** 917.
125. Dunning, W. F., Curtis, M. R., Segaloff, A., *Cancer Res.* (1953) **13,** 147.
126. Noble, R. L., *Proc. Am. Ass. Cancer Res.* (1967) **8,** 51.
127. Richards, J. F., Garland, M., Ng, T., *Cancer Res.* (1971) **31,** 1348.
128. Richards, J. F., Thomson, M., Garland, M., *Cancer Res.* (1973) **33,** 220.
129. Furtado-Dias, T., *C.R. Soc. Biol.* (1951) **145,** 1733.
130. Andervont, H. B., Shimkin, M. B., Canter, H. Y., *Natl. Cancer Inst. J.* (1957) **18,** 1.
131. Bonser, G. M., Robson, J. M., *J. Pathol. Bacteriol.* (1940) **51,** 9.
132. Hooker, C. W., Gardner, W. U., Pfeiffer, C. A., *J. Am. Med. Ass.* (1940) **115,** 443.
133. Shimkin, M. B., Grady, H. G., Andervont, H. B., *Natl. Cancer Inst. J.* (1941) **2,** 65.
134. Bonser, G. M., *J. Pathol. Bacteriol.* (1944) **56,** 15.
135. Gardner, W. U., *Cancer Res.* (1943) **3,** 757.
136. Hooker, C. W., Pfeiffer, C. A., *Cancer Res.* (1942) **2,** 759.
137. Huseby, R. A., *Ciba Found. Colloq. on Endocrinol.* (1958) **12,** 216.
138. Dominguez, O. V., Samuels, L. T., Huseby, R. A., *Ciba Found. Colloq. on Endocrinol.* (1958) **12,** 231.
139. Lucis, O. J., Lucis, R., *Cancer Res.* (1969) **29,** 1647.
140. Jacobs, B. B., Huseby, R. A., *Natl. Cancer Inst. J.* (1968) **41,** 1141.
141. Horning, E. S., *Br. J. Cancer* (1954) **8,** 627.
142. *Ibid.* (1956) **10,** 678.
143. Horning, E. S., Whittick, J. W., *Br. J. Cancer* (1954) **8,** 451.
144. Jolles, B., *Br. J. Cancer* (1962) **16,** 209.
145. Kirkman, H., *Cancer* (1957) **10,** 757.
146. Kirkman, H., *Natl. Cancer Inst. Monogr.* (1959) **1,** 1.
147. Kirkman, H., Bacon, R. L., *Cancer Res.* (1950) **10,** 122.
148. Kirkman, H., Bacon, R. L., *Natl. Cancer Inst. J.* (1952) **13,** 757.
149. *Ibid.,* 745.
150. Matthews, V. S., Kirkman, H., Bacon, R. L., *Proc. Soc. Exp. Biol. Med.* (1947) **66,** 195.
151. Lipschutz, A., Vargas, L., *Cancer Res.* (1941) **1,** 236.
152. Podilcak, M. D., *Neoplasia* (1959) **6,** 305.
153. Barbieri, G., Olivi, M., Sacco, O., *Lav. 1st Anat. Istol. Patol. Perugia* (1958) **18,** 165.
154. Gardner, W. U., Ferrigno, M., *Natl. Cancer Inst. J.* (1956) **17,** 601.
155. Baba, N., von Haam, E., *Progr. Exp. Tumor Res.* (1967) **9,** 192.
156. Gardner, W. U., Allen, E., *Yale J. Biol. Med.* (1939) **12,** 213.
157. Gardner, W. U., Allen, E., *Cancer Res.* (1941) **1,** 359.
158. Pan, S. C., Gardner, W. U., *Cancer Res.* (1948) **8,** 337.
159. Gardner, W. U., *Ann. N.Y. Acad. Sci.* (1959) **75,** 543.
160. Herbst, A. L., Scully, R. E., *Cancer* (1968) **25,** 745.
161. Herbst, A. L., Ulfelder, H., Poskanzer, D. C., *New Eng. J. Med.* (1971) **284,** 878.

162. Benedetti, E. L., van Nie, R., *Acta Unio Int. Contra Canc.* (1962) **18**, 197.
163. van Nie, R., Benedetti, E. L., Mühlbock, O., *Nature* (1961) **192**, 1303.
164. van Nie, R., Smit, G. M., Mühlbock, O., *Acta Unio. Int. Contra Canc.* (1962) **18**, 194.
165. Lipschutz, A., Iglesias, R., Salinas, S., *Endocrinology* (1963) **6**, 99.
166. Lipschutz, A., Iglesias, R., Pasanevich, V. I., Socorro, S., *Brit. J. Cancer* (1967) **21**, 153.
167. *Ibid.*, 144.
168. Jull, J. W., unpublished data.
169. Bern, H. A., Nandi, S., *Progr. Exp. Tumor Res.* (1961) **2**, 90.
170. Bonser, G. M., Dossett, J. A., Jull, J. W., "Human and Experimental Breast Cancer," Pitman Medical, London, 1961.
171. Nicoll, C. A., *Natl. Cancer Inst. J.* (1965) **34**, 131.
172. Dao, T. L., *Progr. Exp. Tumor Res.* (1964) **5**, 157.
173. Mühlbock, O., *Adv. Cancer Res.* (1956) **4**, 371.
174. Bittner, J. J., *Science* (1936) **84**, 162.
175. Bittner, J. J., *Natl. Cancer Inst. J.* (1940) **1**, 155.
176. Dmochowski, L., *Adv. Cancer Res.* (1953) **1**, 103.
177. Bittner, J. J., *Ann. N.Y. Acad. Sci.* (1958) **71**, 943.
178. Smith, F. W., Bittner, J. J., *Cancer Res.* (1945) **5**, 588.
179. Taylor, J. C., Waltmann, C. L., *Arch. Surg.* (1940) **40**, 733.
180. van der Lee, S., Boot, L. M., *Acta Physiol. Pharmacol. Neer.* (1956) **5**, 213.
181. Jull, J. W., *J. Pathol. Bacteriol.* (1954) **68**, 547.
182. Nandi, S., Bern, H. A., *Natl. Cancer Inst. J.* (1960) **24**, 907.
183. Nandi, S., *Proc. Soc. Exp. Biol. Med.* (1961) **108**, 26826.
184. Rivera, E. M., *Nature* (1966) **209**, 1151.
185. Bern, H. A., *Science* (1960) **131**, 1039.
186. DeOme, K. B., *Cancer Res.* (1965) **25**, 1348.
187. DeOme, K. B., Nandi, S., "Viruses Inducing Cancer," W. J. Burdette, Ed., p. 127, University of Utah, Salt Lake City, 1966.
188. Haaland, M., *Sci. Report, Imperial Cancer Res. Fund* (1911) **4**, 1.
189. Gardner, W. U., *Arch. Pathol.* (1939) **27**, 138.
190. Nandi, S., *Proc. Canad. Cancer Conf. Res.* (1966) **6**, 69.
191. Medina, D., DeOme, K. B., *Natl. Cancer Inst. J.* (1968) **40**, 1303.
192. *Ibid.* (1969) **42**, 303.
193. Armstrong, E. C., Bonser, G. M., *J. Pathol. Bacteriol.* (1947) **59**, 19.
194. Cantarow, A., Stasney, J., Paschkis, K. E., *Cancer Res.* (1948) **8**, 412.
195. Orr, J. W., *J. Pathol. Bacteriol.* (1943) **55**, 483.
196. Bonser, G. M., Orr, J. W., *J. Pathol. Bacteriol.* (1939) **49**, 171.
197. Bonser, G. M., *J. Pathol. Bacteriol.* (1954) **68**, 531.
198. Orr, J. W., *Br. Emp. Cancer Campaign Report* (1955) **33**, 235.
199. Huggins, C., Briziarelli, G., Sutton, H., *J. Exp. Med.* (1959) **109**, 25.
200. Huggins, C., Grand, L. C., Brillantes, F. P., *Nature* (1961) **189**, 204.
201. Dao, T. L., Tanaka, Y., Gawlak, D., *Natl. Cancer Inst. J.* (1964) **32**, 1259.
202. Marchant, J., *Br. J. Cancer* (1958) **12**, 62.
203. Dao, T. L., Tanaka, Y., Gawlak, D., *Cancer Res.* (1962) **22**, 973.
204. Marchant, J., *Br. J. Cancer* (1961) **15**, 568.
205. *Ibid.* (1958) **12**, 55.
206. Biancifiori, C., Caschera, F., *Br. J. Cancer* (1962) **16**, 721.
207. Marchant, J., *Nature* (1959) **183**, 629.
208. Sydnor, K. L., Cockrell, B., *Endocrinology* (1963) **73**, 427.
209. Jull, J. W., Huggins, C., *Nature* (1960) **188**, 73.
210. Helfenstein, J. E., Young, S., Currie, A. R., *Nature* (1962) **196**, 1108.
211. Haran-Ghera, N., *Cancer Res.* (1961) **21**, 790.
212. Cronkite, E. P., Shellabarger, C. J., Bond, V. P., Lippincott, S. W., *Radiat. Res.* (1960) **12**, 81.

213. Shellabarger, C. J., Cronkite, E. P., Bond, V. P., Lippincott, S. W., *Radiat. Res.* (1957) **6**, 501.
214. Silberberg, M., Silberberg, R., *Arch. Pathol.* (1950) **49**, 733.
215. Bond, V. P., Cronkite, E. P., Lippincott, S. W., Shellabarger, C. J., *Radiat. Res.* (1960) **12**, 276.
216. Pullinger, B. D., *Br. J. Cancer* (1954) **8**, 445.
217. Lacassagne, A., *C.R. Acad. Sci.* (1932) **195**, 630.
218. Bonser, G. M., *J. Pathol. Bacteriol.* (1936) **42**, 169.
219. Lacassagne, A., *Bull. Ass. Franc. Etude Cancer* (1939) **28**, 951.
220. Boot, L. M., Mühlbock, O., *Acta Unio Int. Contra Cancrum.* (1956) **12**, 569.
221. Heston, W. E., Deringer, M. K., *Proc. Soc. Exp. Biol. Med.* (1953) **82**, 731.
222. Cutts, J. H., *Proc. Can. Cancer Conf. Res.* (1966) **6**, 50.
223. Eisen, M. J., *Cancer Res.* (1941) **1**, 457.
224. Geschickter, C. F., *Arch. Pathol.* (1942) **33**, 334.
225. Geschickter, C. F., *Science* (1939) **89**, 35.
226. Mark, J., Biskind, G. R., *Endocrinology* (1941) **28**, 465.
227. Nelson, W. O., *Yale J. Biol. Med.* (1944) **17**, 217.
228. Noble, R. L., McEuen, C. S., Collip, J. B., *Can. Med. Ass. J.* (1940) **42**, 413.
229. Cutts, J. H., Noble, R. L., *Cancer Res.* (1964) **24**, 1116.
230. Noble, R. L., Collip, J. B., *Can. Med. Ass. J.* (1941) **44**, 1.
231. Boot, L. M., Mühlbock, O., Röpcke, G., Tengbergen, W. V. E., *Cancer Res.* (1962) **22**, 713.
232. Liebelt, A. G., Liebelt, R. A., *Cancer Res.* (1961) **21**, 86.
233. Silberberg, R., Silberberg, M., *Proc. Soc. Exp. Biol. Med.* (1949) **70**, 510.
234. Metcalf, D., *Adv. Cancer Res.* (1971) **14**, 181.
235. Hollander, V. P., Takakura, K., Yamada, H., *Recent Progr. Horm. Res.* (1968) **24**, 81.
236. Bertram, J. S., Craig, A. W., *Eur. J. Cancer* (1972) **8**, 587.
237. Weisburger, J. H., *N.Z. Med. J.* (1968) **67**, 44.

Work supported by National Cancer Institute of Canada.

Chapter

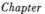

Carcinogenesis by Alkylating Agents

P. D. Lawley, Chester Beatty Research Institute, Institute of Cancer Research, Royal Cancer Hospital, Pollards Wood Research Station, Chalfont St. Giles, Buckinghamshire, HP8 4SP England

Introduction and General Considerations

The Roles of Direct Action and Metabolism for Biological Alkylating Agents. Chemical carcinogens act on cellular material of target organs by three principal mechanisms: the physical interaction of the carcinogen with cellular receptors, chemical reaction of the carcinogen with these receptors, or either type of metabolite–receptor interaction following metabolism of the carcinogen within the target organ or elsewhere.

In this survey, the essential feature of alkylation carcinogenesis that is stressed derives from the second alternative. Of course, the remaining processes occur with this group of carcinogens as with others. The first, purely physical, interactions may influence principally the penetration of the agents into target cells. In general, alkylating agents adsorb readily to cell surfaces. When suspensions of mammalian cells in aqueous media are treated with alkylating agents, the apparent half-life for the alkylation of cellular macromolecules is sometimes greater in the cells than for the same reactions in aqueous solution. Concomitantly, rapid uptake of the agent into whole cells occurs . A simple interpretation of the phenomena is that the agent, still in potentially reactive form, is rapidly sequestered within cells in a lipid or lipoprotein phase.It is then released relatively slowly by diffusion into the aqueous phase of the cell where alkylation occurs. This is documented for mustard gas [di(2-chloroethyl) sulfide] (**1**) in Ehrlich ascites cells (*1*), for several methylating agents and cultured hamster or human cells (*2*), and for chlorambucil (4-(4-di(2-chloroethyl)aminophenyl)butyric acid (**2**), and Yoshida ascites sarcoma (*3, 4, 5*).

Linford (*6*) and Hopwood and Stock (*7*) investigated the effects of proteins and molecules with extensive hydrophobic areas in slowing down the hydrolysis of aromatic nitrogen mustards such as chlorambucil and have concluded that this factor may be significant for transport of these agents

$Cl\ CH_2\ CH_2\ S\ CH_2\ CH_2\ Cl$ Mustard gas   1

$HO_2C\ (CH_2)_3$⟨benzene ring⟩$N(CH_2CH_2Cl)_2$ Chlorambucil   2

$Cl\ CH_2\ CH_2\ N(CH_3)\ CH_2\ CH_2\ Cl$ HN2   3

$(CH_3)_3N^+CH_2CH_2OH$ Choline   4

$Cl\ CH_2\ CH_2\ S\ CH_2\ CH_2\ OH$ Hemi-sulfur mustard   5

$CH_3O\ SO_2\ CH_3$ Methyl methanesulfonate   6

in the body. However, Hopwood and Stock (7) did not find any significant effect of administering chlorambucil as a complex with albumin or detergent on its cytotoxic activity against the Walker carcinosarcoma in the rat.

Goldenberg et al. (8, 9) showed that active transport of the aliphatic nitrogen mustard, HN2, [di(2-chloroethyl)methylamine] (3) occurs in L5178Y mouse lymphoma cells and that the same mechanism acts on the non-alkylating diol derived from it. The primary function of this carrier is to transport choline (4) which is structurally related to the mustard.

In general, then, penetration of alkylating agents into mammalian cells is facile. It is generally accepted that the alkylation of cellular constituents, particularly of functional macromolecules, is crucial in determining bio-logical response to these agents. It appears therefore that their chemical reactivity may be the predominant factor to be considered in this regard. The cellular constituents alkylated apparently present a fairly evenly dis-tributed array of nucleophilic centers reactive towards alkylating agents, since the main feature to emerge from relevant data is the general relative uniformity of alkylated macromolecular cellular constituents. Proteins and nucleic acids are generally alkylated about equally—expressed as alkylations per unit mass—both in the nucleus and the cytoplasm.

These findings are perhaps not surprising in view of the short distances within cells that chemical agents must diffuse before reacting. Even agents such as mustard gas and its monofunctional analog, 2-chloroethyl 2-hy-droxyethyl sulfide (5) which is generally regarded as highly reactive chemically with a half-life in water of about 1 min, can apparently diffuse rapidly both within cells and also presumably via the circulatory system in the animal. For example, following intraperitoneal injection in the mouse, the half sulfur mustard reacted extensively with constituents of liver, trans-planted hepatoma, and spleen (10).

However, alkylating agents are generally eliminated from the animal circulatory system at a greater rate than their hydrolysis in neutral aqueous solution (11). For example, methyl methanesulfonate (6) which hydrolyzes or alkylates bacterial cells in suspension with a half-life of about 5 hr (*12*) was eliminated from the blood of rats within 1.5 hr of its intravenous injection (*13*). Nevertheless, distribution of the agent in mice was rapid, and proteins and nucleic acids in a variety of organs were fairly evenly alkylated.

Evidently observations of this type reflect partial detoxification of the alkylating agent, mediated probably predominantly be reactions with gluta-thione which may be enzymatically catalyzed (*15*). The major excreted metabolites of various alkylating agents are derived from reactions with thiols (*16, 17*).

Another detoxification mechanism found with nitrogen mustard, HN2 (**3**), in mice, rats, and humans is N-dealkylation (*18*). Evidence suggests that the drug is largely converted to an inactive form by passage through rat liver (*19*).

It remains possible that in some cases enzymatic conversions *in vivo* may activate alkylating agents. However, little has been reported yet on the role of such activation in carcinogenesis because most studies relate to cytotoxic action.

Metabolic oxidation was implicated for aniline mustard, N,N-di(2-chloro-ethyl) aniline (**7**), converted to the *p*-hydroxy derivative (*20*). For cyclo-phosphamide [N,N-di(2-chloroethyl)-$N'O$-propylenephosphoric acid ester diamide] (**8**) the precise activation mechanism is uncertain (*21, 22, 23, 24, 25*). However, recently phosphoramide mustard (**9**) was implicated as the principal cytotoxic metabolite of cyclophosphamide (*26, 27*). (For studies of the carcinogenic action of cyclophosphamide *see* Refs. *28* and *29*). The role of metabolic activation in carcinogenesis for chlorambucil, a known carcinogen (*30, 31*), is uncertain, but some evidence suggests that such activation is involved in cytotoxic action (*4, 5*).

$\text{N(CH}_2\text{CH}_2\text{Cl)}_2$ Aniline mustard   **7**

ClCH$_2$CH$_2$ NH — CH$_2$
   N — P = O   CH$_2$ Cyclophosphamide   **8**
ClCH$_2$CH$_2$ O —— CH$_2$ (Endoxan, Cytoxan)

ClCH$_2$CH$_2$ O ⧵O$^-$
   N — P   Phosphoramide mustard   **9**
ClCH$_2$CH$_2$ NH$_2$

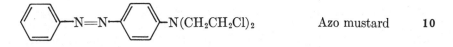

—N=N— $\text{—N(CH}_2\text{CH}_2\text{Cl)}_2$ Azo mustard   **10**

$$CH_2 \cdot X$$
$$HO \cdot C \cdot H$$
$$HO \cdot C \cdot H$$
$$H \cdot C \cdot OH$$
$$H \cdot C \cdot OH$$
$$CH_2 \cdot X$$

Mannitol myleran, X = $-OSO_2CH_3$;   **11**
Dibromomannitol, X = $-Br$;
Mannomustine, "Degranol",
   X = $-NH \cdot CH_2 \cdot CH_2 \cdot Cl$

Chlornaphazin (Erysan),   **12**
2-Naphthylamine mustard

Metabolic reduction of the azo linkage (*32*) activates the azo mustard *N,N*-di(2-chloroethyl)*p*-aminoazobenzene (**10**) and its derivatives in the rat, but this type of agent was not studied in carcinogenesis.

In some cases, a non-metabolic conversion *in vivo* was implicated, as for 1,6-disubstituted D-mannitols, mannitol myleran (**11**) and dibromo-mannitol (**11**), and related hexitol derivatives. Spontaneous epoxidation *in vivo* (*33, 34*) activated these agents. Mannitol myleran caused lung tumors in mice (*31*).

The cancer chemotherapeutic agent chlornaphazin [Erysan, *N,N*-di(2-chloroethyl)naphthylamine] (**12**) is another aromatic mustard which was carcinogenic in the test system of Shimkin *et al.* (*31*). It was suspected to cause bladder tumors in some treated patients, possibly following its meta-bolic conversion to the known carcinogen, 2-naphthylamine (*35, 36*).

If alkylating carcinogens undergo metabolic or other conversions before their reactions *in vivo*, this could presumably be detected by comparing the *in vitro* and *in vivo* reaction products. However, no studies of this type have been made yet with the compounds deduced to require metabolic activation.

Another aspect of the role of metabolism in carcinogenesis is that the alkylating drugs cyclophosphamide and HN2 inhibited the development of hepatic microsomal enzymes in livers of young rats and decreased the activity of these enzymes in adult rats (*37, 38*) at sublethal doses. Much higher dose levels were required to inhibit the enzymes *in vitro*. Further studies by Donelli and Garattini (*39*) showed that certain pretreatments with cytotoxic agents could stimulate, rather than inhibit, drug metabolism in adult rats.

Aspects of Chemical Reactivity of Alkylating Agents Relevant to Correlations with Biological Activity. With the proviso mentioned, that some alkylating agents may be activated by metabolism, it remains that many agents react *in vivo* mainly as *in vitro* in aqueous media. This simple concept led to several studies to correlate chemical reactivity with biological action of compounds of this type. Earlier correlations were devoted to cyto-toxic action of these agents (*40*), but recently mutagenic effectiveness has been correlated (*41*). Both factors are relevant to carcinogenic action, and the long-standing hypothesis equating somatic mutation and the initiation stage of carcinogenesis suggests that structure–activity relationships might be parallel for mutagenic and carcinogenic activity. The correlations between cytotoxicity and carcinogenesis might be more complex. These matters are discussed later.

Reactivity of alkylating agents may be discussed according to the classical concepts first developed by Ingold and his school (*42*). (For relevant reviews *see* Refs. *43* and *44*.) Aspects more particularly relevant to biological action have been reviewed (*17, 40, 45–48*). The process of alkylation has been discussed in terms of the S_N1 and S_N2 mechanisms, and the classification of typical alkylating agents is presented in Table I. These mechanisms may be regarded as limiting cases of a common mechanism in which alkylating agents are regarded as reacting through ion pairs (*63*) (*see* Scheme 1). Agents classified as reacting through the S_N1 mechanism

Scheme 1.

S_N1 and S_N2 mechanism (*42*):—

$$S_N1 \quad \text{R-X} \xrightarrow{k_1} \text{R}^+ + \text{X}^-; \ \text{R}^+ + \text{Y}^- \xrightarrow{k_2[\text{Y}]} \text{RY}$$

$$k_1 \ll k_2[\text{Y}]; \text{ unimolecular kinetics}$$

$$S_N2 \quad \text{Y}^- + \text{R-X} \rightarrow [\text{Y}^{\delta-} \ldots \text{R}^{\delta+} \ldots \text{X}^{\delta-}] \rightarrow \text{Y-R} + \text{X}^-$$

$$\text{Rate} = k_2 [\text{RX}] [\text{Y}^-]; \text{ bimolecular kinetics}$$

Unified mechanism (*63*):

$$\text{RX} \underset{k_{-1}}{\overset{k_1}{\rightleftharpoons}} \text{R}^+\text{X}^- \overset{k_\text{S}}{\underset{k_\text{Y}[\text{Y}]}{\Big\langle}} \begin{matrix} \text{ROH} \\ \text{RY} \end{matrix}$$

Limiting cases:

$$k_{-1}/k_\text{S} \rightarrow 0; \text{ resembles } S_N1$$
$$k_{-1}/k_\text{S} \rightarrow \infty; \text{ resembles } S_N2$$

will generally show lower sensitivity to the nucleophilicity of the attacking agents because of the high reactivity of the postulated carbonium ion intermediates (*42*). These properties of the alkylating agent (considered as the substrate) and of the attacking nucleophiles can be expressed quantitatively by Swain and Scott's (*49*) parameters s and n, respectively. Values of nucleophilicity for some representative groups are given in Table II. An alternative measure of the nucleophilicity parameter was used for reactions of nucleic acids and derivatives with the *N,N*-diethyleneimmonium ion (**13**) (derived from the nitrogen mustard (**14**) (*46*), *viz.*, the competition factor, *F*. This is related to n by the expression (bottom, p. 90):

Table I.   Representative Alkylating Agents Classified According Scott (49) and Their

Alkylating Agent	Formula	k'_o (h^{-1})
2-Oxopropyl methanesulfonate	$CH_3CO\ CH_2 \cdot OSO_2CH_3$	0.3
Iodoacetate	$^-OOC \cdot CH_2 \cdot I$	
Methyl iodide	$CH_3 \cdot I$	
Methyl bromide	$CH_3 \cdot Br$	0.0059
Glycidol	$HOCH_2\ CH\text{—}CH_2$ $\qquad\qquad O$	0.0068
Mustard gas	$S \cdot (CH_2CH_2Cl)_2$	ca. 33[f]
Mustard gas cation	CH_2 $\|\qquad S \cdot {}^+CH_2 \cdot CH_2 \cdot Cl$ CH_2	
Trimethyl phosphate	$(CH_3O)_3 \cdot PO$	
β-Propiolactone	$H_2C \text{ — } CH_2$ $\quad \| \;\cdot\cdot\; \| \;\cdot\cdot$ $\quad CO\text{—}O$	0.68[h]
Methyl methanesulfonate	$CH_3 \cdot OSO_2CH_3$	0.072[i]
n-Butyl methanesulfonate	$C_4H_9 \cdot OSO_2CH_3$	0.05[i]
Ethyl methanesulfonate	$C_2H_5 \cdot OSO_2H_3$	0.06[i]
Isopropyl methanesulfonate	$(CH_3)_2CH \cdot OSO_2CH_3$	3.1
N-Methyl-N-nitrosourea	$CH_3 \cdot N(NO) \cdot CONH_2$	2.74[j]
N-Ethyl-N-nitrosourea	$C_2H_5 \cdot N(NO) \cdot CONH_2$	2.36[j]

[a] Also given are the first order rate constants for reaction with water at 37°C (k_o'), and the half-life of hydrolysis ($t_{1/2}$). The value of $s = 1.00$ for methyl bromide is the reference standard, in the relationship $\log (k_y/k_o) = s \cdot n_y$, where k_y denotes the second order rate constants for reaction of a nucleophile of nucleophilic constant n with the alkylating agent and k_o the corresponding constant for water; $k'_o = k_o [H_2O] = 55.5\ k_o$.

[b] Osterman-Golkar et al. (41).

[c] Hawthorne et al. (50).

[d] Swain and Scott (49).

to Their Values of the Substrate Constant (s) of Swain and Suggested Reaction Mechanism

$t_{1/2}$ (h)	s	Mechanism	Remarks
2.3	1.9^b	S_N2	For a discussion of the effect of
	1.33^c	S_N2	β-carbonyl substituents, leading to relatively high s values, *see* Ref 58.
	1.15^c	S_N2	Ethyl also reacts mainly by S_N2
116	1.00^d	S_N2	mechanism; reactivity of RX increases in order $X = F \ll Cl < Br < I$ (40).
102	$0.96^{d,e}$	S_N2	Ring-opening reaction; $R \cdot \underset{\underset{O}{\textstyle\vert}}{CH} \cdot CH_2 + Y^- \rightarrow$ $R \cdot CHOH \cdot CH_2Y$ by S_N2 mechanism (59).
ca. 0.02			Shows S_N1-type kinetics (60)
	0.95^d	?	but may react through S_N2 mechanism; for discussion of $S,-$ N-mustards, *see* the text.
	0.8^e	S_N2	Only one methyl group reacts under pseudo-physiological conditions (40).
1.0	0.77^d	S_N2	Nucleophilic attack on β-C-atom.
9.5	0.83^b	S_N2	Dimethyl sulfate closely similar, one methyl group reacting
13.8	0.68^b	S_N2	under pseudo-physiological conditions (40).
11.5	0.67^b	mainly S_N2	"S_N1/S_N2 borderline" mechanism (61).
0.22	0.29^b	mainly S_N1	
0.25	0.42^k	mainly S_N1	Reacts *via* $CH_3N_2^+ \rightarrow CH_3^+$
0.29	0.26^k	mainly S_N1	Reacts *via* $C_2H_5N_2^+ \rightarrow C_2H_5^+$; the alkylnitrosourea decompositions are alkali-catalyzed; "exact mechanisms are in doubt" (62).

^{e} Petty and Nichols (51).
^{f} Banks *et al.* (extrapolated value), quoted by Ross (52).
^{g} Hudson (53).
^{h} Van Duuren and Goldschmidt (54).
^{i} Barnard and Robertson (55) (interpolated values), quoted by Ross (40).
^{j} Garrett, *et al.* (56) values refer to pH 7.18, 37°C.
^{k} Veleminsky *et al.* (57).

Table II. Nucleophilic Constants, Competition Factors, and Hard and Soft Character of Bases[a]

Nucleophile (Y)	n_y	Class	$\log F_y$
H_2O	0.00	hard	
CH_3COO^-	2.72	hard	
Cl^-	3.04	borderline	
Pyridine	3.6	borderline	
OH^-	4.2	hard	
Aniline	4.49	borderline	
I^-	5.04	soft	
HS^- (or cysteine)	5.1	soft	
$S_2O_3^{2-}$	6.36	soft	
$H_2PO_4^-$	2.8		
DNA (per P atom)	2.5–3.0		
Adenine, N-1			3.34
Adenine, N-3			3.88
Adenine, N-9			3.21
Adenosine, N-1			2.93
5'-Adenylic acid, N-1			2.91
5'-Adenylic acid, phosphate			4.06
Poly (A), N-1			3.29
Poly (A), phosphodiester			4.10
Guanosine, N-7			3.54
Guanylic acid, N-7			3.45
Guanylic acid, phosphate			3.97
Deoxycytidine, N-3			ca. 2.70
Thymidine, N-3			1.6
DNA, N-7 of guanine			5.18

[a] The nucleophilic constant n_y is defined by Swain and Scott (49) according to the equation $\log (k_y/k_o) = s \cdot n_y$ (cf. Table I), with the value n for H_2O assigned as 0.00. The competition factor F_y is related to n_y by the relationship $\log F_y = s \cdot n_y - 1.74$. The values reported refer to alkylation by the N,N-diethylethyleneimmonium ion at pH 7, 37° (46). The values of n_y are from Swain and Scott (49) except for $H_2PO_4^-$ and DNA (per P atom) which are from Osterman–Golkar et al. (41). The classification of nucleophiles as hard or soft Lewis bases is from Pearson and Songstad (64).

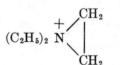

Immonium ion (derived from 14)   **13**

$(C_2H_5)_2 N \cdot CH_2CH_2Cl$ 2-Chloroethyl-diethylamine   **14**

$$\log F_y = \log (k_y/k_o) - \log [H_2O]$$

$$s \cdot n_y = \log (k_y/k_o)$$

$$\log F_y = s \cdot n_y - 1.74$$

Pearson and Songstad (64) classified nucleophiles as Lewis bases into "hard" and "soft" categories; these approximate the reagents of low and high n of Swain and Scott (49), (Table II). The electrophilic (acidic) components were classified in order of increasing hardness as $CH_3^+ < R_2CH^+ < R_3C^+$, $ROCH_2^+ < RCO^+$. Soft acids react rapidly with soft bases and hard acids with hard bases. In biological material, hydroxyl, phosphate, carboxylate, and aliphatic amino groups are "hard;" ring-nitrogen or aromatic amino groups are "borderline;" and thiol groups are "soft." Generally, the "harder" alkylating agents are those of lower s factor.

Alkylating agents of the "mustard" type present some special features in classification of their reaction mechanisms. This follows from the "neighboring group effect" $(43, 62, 65)$ which may be illustrated for the cases of mustard gas and nitrogen mustards (Scheme 2).

Scheme 2.   The neighboring group mechanism for sulfur and nitrogen mustards

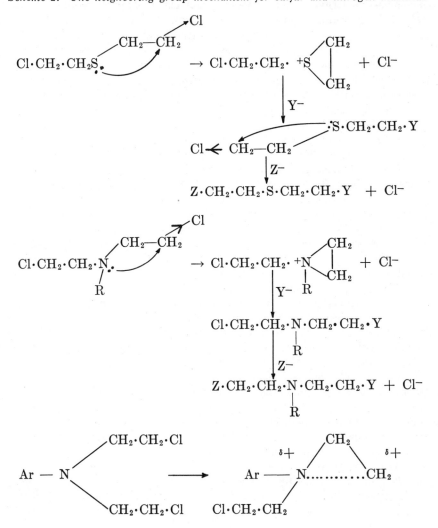

The mechanism is generally considered to consist of two successive S_N2 reactions (62, 65). However, Ross (40) regarded mustard gas as reacting by the S_N1 mechanism. This follows the opinion of Ogston (60), who showed that the kinetics of reactions of this mustard were consistent with ionization as the rate-controlling step, as required by the S_N1 mechanism. Streitweiser (43) stated that "the cyclic sulfonium intermediates have real carbonium-ion character." The reaction rate of mustard gas in aqueous media at 37°C is rapid, with $t_{\frac{1}{2}}$ about 2 min. On the other hand, the mustard cation has a fairly high Swain–Scott s factor (0.95) and was included by Swain and Scott (49) in a group of S_N2 agents (45). However, agents which react through the S_N1 mechanism can show a considerable range of competition factors which increase as the stability of the derived carbonium ion increases. Thus triphenylmethyl (trityl) halides give the relatively stable trityl cation, $(Ph)_3C^+$, which shows a quite high discrimination between nucleophiles (65a), corresponding to a s value of about 0.61. tert-Butyl chloride, which again reacts through the S_N1 mechanism but yields a less stable cation, shows a much lower range of competition factors (60) corresponding to s of the order of 0.4.

Aliphatic nitrogen mustards, typified by di(2-chloroethyl)methylamine, are generally thought to react mainly through the S_N2 mechanism, although Ludlum (66) obtained evidence suggesting S_N1 reaction with polynucleotide phosphodiester groups. Aromatic nitrogen mustards generally tend towards the S_N1 mechanism because of the lower basicity of the nitrogen atom (40, 52). Ross (52) showed that the effects of substituents in the aromatic moiety supported this concept; electron-releasing substituents ortho or para to the mustard group enhanced the hydrolysis rate while electron-withdrawing groups had the opposite effect. Bardos et al. (48) developed a method for comparing the relative abilities of aromatic mustards to alkylate the reagent 4-(p-nitrobenzyl)pyridine (S_N2 reaction) and to undergo solvolysis (S_N1). Their comparison between reactivities and antitumor activities agreed with Ross' previous deduction (82) that reaction by the S_N1 mechanism correlated positively with biological activity.

There are indications that this correlation may also apply to simple alkylating agents with respect to mutagenic action. Ehrenberg and his co-workers drew a parallel conclusion from their comparisons of mutagenic effectiveness of a series of alkyl methanesulfonates in barley (41). Also studies with a range of alkylating mutagens, including N-methyl- and N-ethyl-N-nitrosoureas which react through alkyldiazonium ions, in *Escherichia coli* (67, 68) and *Arabidopsis thaliana* (57) were consistent with this correlation. The more efficient mutagens had low values of the Swain–Scott constant s whereas alkylating agents with higher s values were either non-mutagenic or inefficient mutagens. Linear dose–response relationships could be shown with the agents of lower s, but those for agents of $s > 0.55$ were described as exponential (41, 68).

Osterman-Golkar et al. (41), pointed out that reagents of high s, typified by the β-carbonyl substituted alkylating agents such as 2-oxopropyl methanesulfonate or iodoacetamide, react more extensively *in vivo* with nucleophiles of high n, such as thiol groups, or with the more nucleophilic groups in

DNA. They concluded therefore that the groups in DNA of lower nucleophilicity were more specifically alkylated by the efficient mutagens. Alkylation of groups of higher n was indicated to be lethal.

Loveless (*69*) reached what appears to be essentially the same conclusion on different grounds. He deduced that O-alkylation, in particular the formation of O^6-alkylguanine, in DNA was a promutagenic reaction. In general ring-N atoms in the purines are the most nucleophilic centers. Evidently further work on the products of alkylation *in vivo* is again expected to clarify these questions, and the available information is reviewed in more detail below (pages 105–127).

Alkylating Agents Generated by the Metabolism of Other Chemical Carcinogens. As noted in the front section of this chapter, some alkylating agents may be activated by metabolism, although many can be biologically effective by direct reaction with target cellular material. Thus it is clear that alkylating agents can be regarded as simpler models for the action of the large class of indirectly acting carcinogens, *i.e.*, those whose biological action is mediated by reactive metabolites.

For directly acting alkylating agents, the ultimate carcinogen, *i.e.*, the molecular species that reacts with the essential target *in vivo*, is identical to the carcinogen itself if this reaction occurs by the S_N2 mechanism. If reaction involves the S_N1 mechanism, the ultimate carcinogen is a carbonium ion spontaneously generated in the cellular medium. Alternatively according to the unified mechanism discussed previously, an ion pair would fill this role.

For most chemical carcinogens, direct action of this type is impossible because of the extremely low, or almost nonexistent, reactivity of the compound under pseudo-physiological conditions. Furthermore, it is now accepted that physical interactions of such carcinogens with cellular receptors generally are unlikely to be the major cause of their carcinogenic action. However, in some cases, notably for acridine dyes, mutagenesis can result from such direct interaction with DNA in certain systems. Generally however, in organisms which cannot metabolize carcinogens of this type in appropriate ways, their mutagenic or carcinogenic action is not demonstrable.

The question then arises, which metabolic pathways can activate the pre-carcinogens? Miller and Miller (*70*) suggested an overall generalization that "the great majority, and perhaps all, of the chemical carcinogens are similar" in that "the reactive forms of chemical carcinogens all appear to be strong electrophiles." They qualify this statement by the further generalization that "S_N2 reactions or reactions of a type intermediate between S_N1 and S_N2 appear to predominate over pure S_N1 or free radical reactions with the reactive forms of chemical carcinogens" (referring to Price, *et al.* (*46*)). Evidently, a range of electrophilic reactivity characterizes the reactive forms of carcinogens. In DNA, an important target of carcinogens, the sites attacked by strong electrophilic reagents are pseudo-aromatic $\equiv$ CH groups at C-8 of purine residues and C-5 of pyrimidines whereas the most nucleophilic centers are ring N-atoms (*71, 72*). Thus the spectrum of electrophilicity covered by the reactive carcinogens or their metabolites also spans a range of probable receptor sites *in vivo*.

In justifying their emphasis on electrophilicity in this regard, Miller and Miller (73) (quoting Ref. 74) point out that tests of carcinogenic action of nucleophilic mutagens, such as hydroxylamine, were negative. Also, nucleic acid base analogs known to be mutagenic in microorganisms failed to yield tumors when tested in newborn mice (74, 75).

Since the metabolism of foreign compounds to water-soluble derivatives is directed presumably towards their detoxification (76), conversions to more toxic reactive metabolites seem unexpected a priori, and this relatively rare phenomenon can therefore be regarded as the key determinant of carcinogenic activity. A spectrum of such activity generally is found in various series of chemically related compounds. The metabolic pathways are generally the same, so that the reactivities of the metabolites may, in turn, become the significant parameter. If these are alkylating agents, then the relationships may resemble those for the directly acting compounds to some extent.

Some differences may be expected between directly acting and metabolically generated agents because of differences in physical pathways by which the reactive ultimate carcinogens reach the cellular targets. These differences may not be profound for proximate carcinogens. Thus, for the now-classical case of N-2-hydroxy-N-2-fluorenylacetamide (77) as proximate hepatocarcinogen derived from N-2-fluorenylacetamide (15), the active metabolite could be identified positively by its greater carcinogenic potency compared with the parent compound as shown using conventional methods of administration.

It appears, however, that, although this proximate carcinogen can arylate DNA in vitro (78) the ultimate carcinogen is almost certainly the derived N-sulfate. The proximate carcinogen is generated by a microsomal enzyme

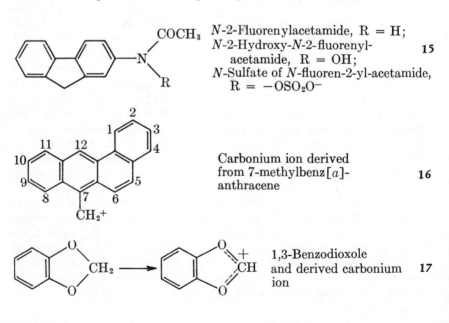

N-2-Fluorenylacetamide, R = H;
N-2-Hydroxy-N-2-fluorenyl-
    acetamide, R = OH;   **15**
N-Sulfate of N-fluoren-2-yl-acetamide,
    R = −OSO₂O⁻

Carbonium ion derived
from 7-methylbenz[a]-   **16**
anthracene

1,3-Benzodioxole
and derived carbonium   **17**
ion

Table III.   Suggested Alkylating Metabolites of Carcinogens

Carcinogen(s)	Suggested Metabolite(s)	References
Polynuclear aromatic hydrocarbons	epoxides	85,86,87,88,89
Methyl-substituted aromatic hydrocarbons	arylmethyl derivatives	82
	arylmethylcarbonium ions	83
Pyrrolizidine alkaloids	dihydropyrrolizine esters	90
Mitomycin C	reduction product(s)	91,92
Safrole	1'-acetoxysafrole	93,94
Aflatoxin B_1	2,3-epoxide	94
Penicillin	penicillenic acid	95
Alderlin	ethyleneimine derivative	96
N,N-Dimethyl-4-aminoazobenzene	protein-bound methionine derivative	97
Ethionine	S-adenosylethionine	98
N-Nitrosodimethylamine	N-nitrosomethylamine, methyldiazohydroxide	99
Vinyl chloride	choroethylene oxide	99a

system, the suspected ultimate carcinogen in the cytosol (*79*). The highly reactive ionic sulfate is not a carcinogen when administered to the animal. The essential cellular target is indicated to be nuclear DNA (*80*), and it is apparently still uncertain whether esterification must occur in the nucleus to permit arylation at this site (*81*).

Analogy with N-2-fluorenylacetamide suggests that reactive aralkylating agents might be generated *in vivo* from known hydroxyalkyl derivatives of polynuclear aromatic hydrocarbons (*82*), or direct generation of aralkyl carbonium ions, e.g., from 7-methylbenz[*a*]anthracene (**16**), could be envisaged (*83*) by analogy with a suggested metabolic activation of 1,3-benzodioxole (**17**) (*84*).

Alternatively, epoxides could be proximate, if not ultimate, carcinogens of the aralkylating type derived from aromatic hydrocarbons (*85, 86, 87*). The most recent evidence indicates that diol-epoxides are the important reactive metabolites for *in vivo* reactions of these hydrocarbons with DNA (*88, 89*). For both mechanisms, positive relationships were deduced between S_N1 character of the suggested metabolites and carcinogenic potency of hydrocarbons (*83*). Although these derivatives are alkylating agents in the strict sense, they are more properly dealt with in detail under the heading of aromatic hydrocarbons (*see* Chapter 5). Other cases where alkylating metabolites were suggested as proximate or ultimate carcinogens include those listed in Table III.

The hepatotoxic and carcinogenic (*100, 101, 102*) pyrrolizidine alkaloids, characterized by the general structure (**18**), have relatively weak alkylating ability *in vitro*. This is ascribed to the presence of the allylic ester grouping (*103*). For a review of substitution reactions of allylic compounds, *see* De Wolfe and Young (*104*). These alkaloids are oxidized by microsomal enzymes to dihydropyrrolizines, possibly *via* intermediate

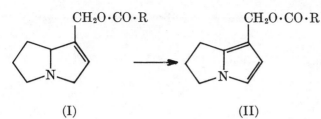

(I)   (II)

(I) Pyrrolizidine   (II) Derived condensed   **18**
alkaloid e.g. heliotrine,   pyrrole (dihydropyrrolizine)

$$R = -C \overset{CH(CH_3)_2}{\underset{OH}{\mid}} CH(CH_3)OMe$$

N-oxides. Those pyrrole derivatives with ester groups (as (**18**)) are highly reactive by the S_N1 mechanism (*90*), and certain of these derivatives can cross-link DNA *in vitro* (*105*).

An analogous metabolic conversion was proposed for Mitomycin C (**19**). Its reduced form contains an indole group embodying an allylic carbamate residue (*91*). This antibiotic is cytotoxic and carcinogenic (*106, 107*) but is inactive as a cytotoxic agent unless reduced chemically or metabolically.

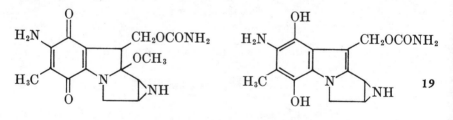

Mitomycin C   Suggested reduced form   **19**

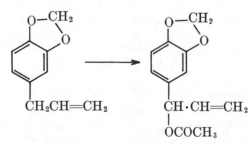

Safrole   1-Acetoxysafrole   **20**

It acts as a difunctional agent in cross-linking DNA (*91*). Safrole (**20**), a hepatocarcinogen from sassafras oil, was converted by metabolism to an allylic ester, 1-acetoxysafrole (*93*).

The potent hepatocarcinogenic fungal constituent aflatoxin B_1 (*108*), requires metabolic activation to yield its biological effects and is covalently bound to hepatic macromolecules in the rat (*109*). Mild acid hydrolysis of the *in vivo* reaction products with DNA and rRNA showed that the major part of these were derived from the 2,3-oxide of the aflatoxin (**21**) which is thus a probable ultimate carcinogenic metabolite (*94*).

Components of bracken fern showing radiomimetic properties in cattle yielded intestinal tumors in rats and mice (*102, 110,* Chapter 13). Van Duuren (quoted by Fishbein *et al.* (*25*)) ascribed the alkylating potential of bracken fern to dimethylsulfoniumpropionic acid (**22**). Further work by Evans and Osman (*99*) isolated a mutagen and carcinogen shikimic acid (**23**) from extracts of bracken, but this material also contains another more potent carcinogen (*111*).

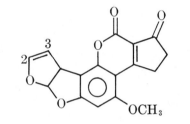

Aflatoxin B_1 21

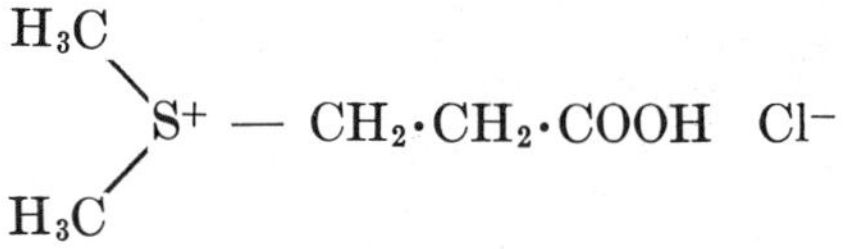

$$H_3C$$
$$\diagdown$$
$$S^+ - CH_2 \cdot CH_2 \cdot COOH \quad Cl^-$$
$$\diagup$$
$$H_3C$$

Dimethylsulfoniumpropionic acid hydrochloride   22

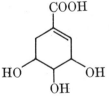

Shikimic acid   23

Penicillin (*see* Scheme 3), a relatively weak carcinogen (*112, 113*) at the site of injection in the rat, may be a relatively weak alkylating agent analogous to β-propiolactone (*113*). But Longridge and Timms (*95*) pointed out that in reactions with nucleophiles, penicillin acts as an acylating agent rather than an alkylating agent. Although acylation may be an *in vivo* reaction of certain cytotoxic agents, such as vinca alkaloids (*114*) and bisdioxopiperazines (*115*), it was thought more likely that a more powerful alkylating agent was generated *in vivo*, for which penicillenic acid (readily formed by oxidation of penicillin in aqueous media), was suggested as a model (*95*).

Scheme 3. *Possible reactions of penicillin and penicillenic acid* (95)

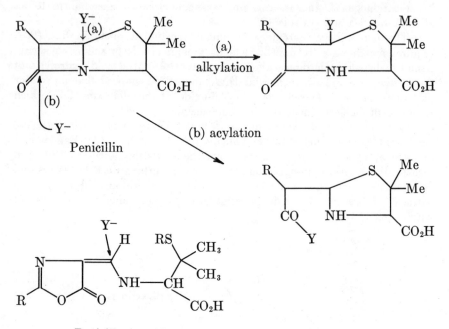

Penicillin

Penicillenic acid

Alderlin (**24**), a β-adrenergic blocking agent, yields thymic tumors in mice (*96*). Evidence implicated an ethyleneimine derivative as an aralkylating proximate carcinogen, and it was suggested further that abnormal metabolism of adrenalin (**25**) could give an analogous derivative, possibly an endogenous carcinogen (*96*).

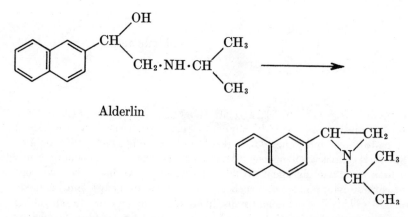

Alderlin   **24**

Metabolic intermediate

Myleran [Busulphan, 1,4-di(methanesulfonoxy)butane] (**26**), is a chemotherapeutic agent used in chronic myeloid leukemia. It is itself rather feebly reactive as an alkylating agent *in vitro* and *in vivo* (*116*) but is converted by metabolism in the rat (reacting with a cysteinyl moiety) to a cyclic sulfonium derivative (*117*). This is possibly also an *in vivo* alkylating agent, although it does not react with water or cysteine at pH 7, but yields *S*-dicysteinylbutane at pH 8. For a further discussion of the relevance of metabolic conversions of Myleran to its biological action, *see* "Difunctional Sulfonates," page 216.

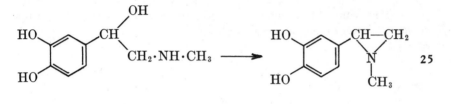

Adrenalin (Epinephrine)

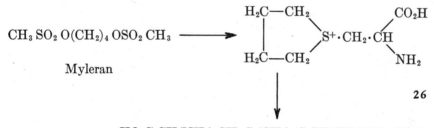

$$HO_2C\ CH(NH_2)\ CH_2\ S\ (CH_2)_4\ S\ CH_2CH(NH_2)\ CO_2H$$

1,4-Dicysteinylbutane

$$C_2H_5\ S\ CH_2\ CH\ CO\ NH\ CH_2\ CO_2H$$
$$|$$
$$NH\ CO\ CH_2\ CH_2\ CH(NH_2)CO_2H \qquad\qquad 27$$

S-Ethylglutathione

Urethane, a potent tumor initiator, yields *S*-ethylglutathione (**27**) as a metabolite in rat bile (*118*), but it is possible that this metabolite is not formed by direct ethylation, as occurs *in vivo* with ethyl methanesulfonate and thiols (*119*). A more likely mechanism suggests its formation by decarboxylation of the *S*-carbethoxy derivative (*118*). The principal mode of reaction of urethane with RNA after metabolic activation *in vivo* was claimed to involve introduction of the ethoxycarbonyl group (*120*), rather than ethylation. However, Lawson and Pound (*121*) reported recently that [^{14}C] ethyl-labeled urethane binds radioactivity to mouse liver DNA *in vivo* whereas [^{14}C] carbonyl-labeled urethane does not; thus, the bound metabolite was suggested to contain an ethyl group but not a carbonyl group.

The hepatocarcinogen *N,N*-dimethyl-4-aminoazobenzene yields 3-methyl-mercapto-*N*-methyl-4-aminoazobenzene (**28**) as a product from alkaline degradation of protein-bound dye in rat liver (*97*). The suggested precursor protein contains an "active" methionine residue which is possibly capable of abnormal methylation of cellular constituents. This protein thus would be a carrier for an alkylating group of possibly considerable specificity. A protein (ligandin) in liver and other organs that binds metabolites of azo-dye carcinogens with a high degree of affinity, appears to be identical with that acting as carrier of certain steroids (*122*).

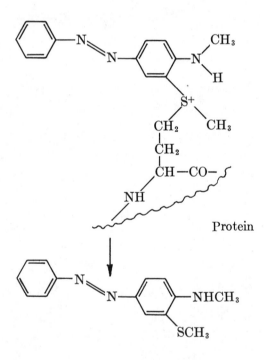

28

3-Methylmercapto-*N*-methyl-4-aminoazobenzene

Ethionine, a hepatocarcinogen, ethylated cellular constituents of liver including DNA on prolonged feeding to rats (*123, 124*). A suggested mechanism involves *S*-adenosyl-L-ethionine (**29**) as donor of ethyl groups (*98, 125*) since this is known to accumulate in liver of ethionine-treated rats, and the methyl analog is the source of methyl groups in minor bases of nucleic acids. However, as Craddock (*126*) points out, this analogy would lead to the expectation that 5-ethylcytosine would be formed in DNA of

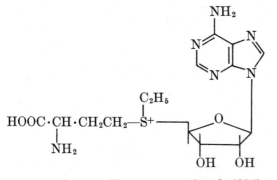

29

the treated rats. This was not found (*126*), as the only ethylated base detected was 7-ethylguanine (*124*).

The *N*-nitrosodialkylamines and related compounds are a large group of carcinogens that alkylate macromolecular constituents of target tissues (*127*, Chapter 11). The principal features of their metabolic conversions were established by Heath (*99*), who showed that methylating metabolites of *N*-nitrosodimethylamine were formed by N-demethylation to yield *N*-nitrosomethylamine which could tautomerize to methyldiazohydroxide, a source of methyldiazonium and methylcarbonium ions. The spontaneous chemical activations of *N*-methyl-*N*-nitrosourea (*56*) and *N*-methyl-*N'*-nitro-*N*-nitrosoguanidine (*128*) in neutral aqueous media are also postulated to yield the same group of methylating agents (Scheme 4). Reaction of *N*-methyl-*N'*-nitro-*N*-nitrosoguanidine with thiols also liberates the methylating species, and this is almost certainly a mode of activation *in vivo* (*128, 129*). However, *N*-methyl-*N*-nitrosourea is not activated in this way (*130*) so that thiol activation of alkylating nitroso compounds is not a general phenomenon.

The methyldiazonium ion can be considered as the conjugate acid of diazomethane base. The generation of alkali during reactions of diazomethane in non-buffered aqueous media shows that it is a fairly strong base. It is probable that in neutral solution it is ionized almost completely. The methylating species generated either metabolically from *N*-nitrosodimethylamine (*131*) or in chemical reactions, as with *N*-methyl-*N'*-nitro-*N*-nitrosoguanidine (*132, 133*), or with *N*-methyl-*N*-nitrosourea (*134*) transfers the methyl group of the precursors intact into the principal product in nucleic acid, 7-methylguanine. For consistency with these findings $CH_3 \cdot NH \cdot NO$, $CH_3 \cdot N{:}N \cdot OH$, $CH_3N_2^+$ or CH_3^+ could be considered as methylating intermediates, but CH_2N_2 is apparently not generated in appreciable amount before methylation occurs. The molecular species which diffuse *in vivo* from the metabolism sites of nitrosamines to the methylation sites are more likely to be those that are uncharged, but the migration of ion pairs of limited stability containing the methyldiazonium cation is perhaps possible. The latter, or the derived carbonium ions, are the ultimate reactive agents. March (*62*), referring to alkyldiazonium ions, stated that "no matter how produced, RN_2^+ are too unstable to be isolable, reacting presumably by the S_N1 or S_N2 mechanisms. Actually the exact mechanisms are in doubt . . ."

Scheme 4. Activation of N-nitrosodimethylamine (by metabolism) or of N-methyl-N-nitroso compounds (alkali- or thiol-catalyzed), to methylating agents [a]

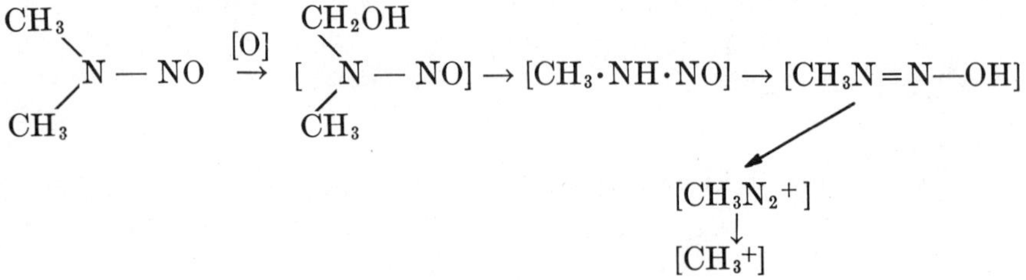

$$
\begin{array}{c}
CH_3 \\
\diagdown \\
\diagup \quad N - NO \quad \xrightarrow{[O]} \quad [\quad \diagdown N - NO] \to [CH_3 \cdot NH \cdot NO] \to [CH_3N = N-OH] \\
CH_3 \qquad\qquad\qquad CH_3
\end{array}
$$

$$[CH_3N_2^+]$$
$$\downarrow$$
$$[CH_3^+]$$

N-Nitrosodimethylamine

$$CH_3 N(NO)CONH_2 \xrightarrow{OH^-} [CH_3 \cdot NH \cdot NO] + NCO^- + H^+$$

N-Methyl-*N*-nitrosourea

$$CH_3N(NO)C(NH)NHNO_2 \xrightarrow{OH^-} [CH_3 \cdot NH \cdot NO] + NC \cdot \overline{N} \cdot NO_2 + H^+$$

N-Methyl-*N'*-nitro-*N*-nitrosoguanidine

$$CH_3N(NO)C(NH)NHNO_2 + HS \cdot CH_2 \cdot CH(NH_2)CO_2H$$

$$\to [CH_3 \cdot NH \cdot NO] + [HO_2C \cdot CH(NH_2) \cdot CH_2 \cdot S \cdot C(NH) \cdot NHNO_2]$$

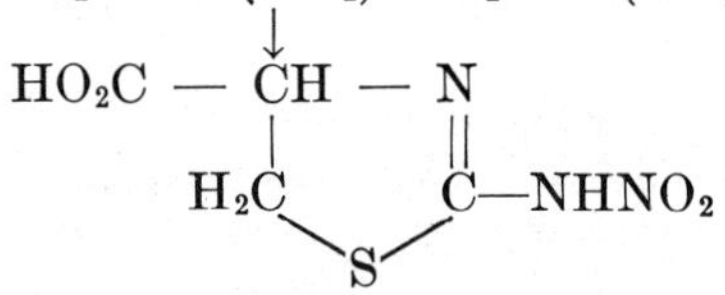

$$
\begin{array}{c}
HO_2C - CH - N \\
| \qquad\qquad \| \\
H_2C \qquad C-NHNO_2 \\
\diagdown S \diagup
\end{array}
$$

[a] *N*-Methyl-*N*-nitrosourea is not activated by thiols in neutral aqueous solution.

1-Aryl-3,3-dialkyltriazenes are another group of carcinogens that may be metabolized by a pathway analogous to that proposed for dialkylnitrosamines (*135*) (*see* Scheme 5). The analogous heterocyclic triazene, 4(5)-(3,3-dimethyltriazeno)imidazole-5(4)-carboxamide (DIC), is an *in vivo* methylating agent in the liver, kidney, lung, and brain of rats. The (^{14}C)methyl-labeled drug also produced 7-(^{14}C)methylguanine in urine of rats and humans (*136*) (Scheme 5).

Carcinogenic Action of Alkylating Agents in Relation to Mutagenic Action. SOMATIC MUTATION THEORY AND DOSE–RESPONSE RELATIONSHIPS FOR CARCINOGENESIS AND MUTAGENESIS. For historical reasons, the correlations between mutagenesis and carcinogenesis were stressed more for alkylating agents than for other chemical carcinogens, although recently this interest has spread increasingly to carcinogens in general. Heston (*138*) studied mustard gas as a carcinogen and showed its ability to induce tumors (mainly sarcomas) at the site of injection in mice, because of its known mutagenic action. The agent is generally quoted as the first discovered chemical mutagen (*139, 140*) although reports of mutation induction in *Aspergillus* by nitrous acid were made previously (*141*). *Drosophila melanogaster*, the test organism used by Auerbach, is used extensively in studies of the relationships between carcinogenicity and mutagenicity of chemicals (for recent work, *see* Refs. *142, 143*). The literature reporting mutagenic action of alkylating agents in a variety of organisms from bacteriophage to mammals is now prodigious (*25, 144, 145, 146*). Attention must be confined here to those studies more particularly relevant to correlations with carcinogenic action. Some generalities must first be dealt with concerning

Scheme 5.

(a) Enzymatic activation of 1-aryl-3,3-dialkyltriazenes (*135*) or of DIC (*136*) by oxidative *N*-demethylation

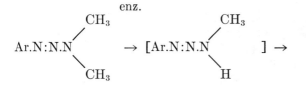

$$ArNH_2 + [CH_3NHNO] \rightarrow [CH_3N_2]^+$$

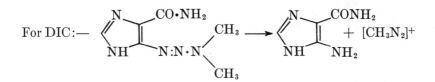

(b) Hydrolysis of 1-aryl-3,3-dialkyltriazenes (*137*)[a]

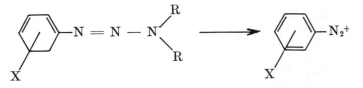

[a] This reaction, generating a diazo-coupling or arylating species, occurs at a rate which depends markedly on the nature and function of substitution of the group X, *e.g.*, electron-donating groups para to the azo linkage enhance the rate. A positive correlation between the Hammett constants (σ) and the hydrolysis rate at pH 7, 37° was found, and both were in turn positively correlated with ability to produce local tumors at the injection site. The alkylation mechanism which depends on metabolic oxidation correlates with the systemic action of more hydrolytically stable triazenes, which can induce tumors distant from the injection site.

dose–response relationships and their relevance to the multi-stage concept of carcinogenesis.

The type of relationship which emerges from data on tumor induction by chemicals can often be represented by equations of the form:

$$Y = aD^b \; \ldots \tag{1}$$

where Y denotes tumor yield, D denotes dose, and a and b are constants. (For examples of such derivations, see Refs. 31 and 147). Similar logarithmic equations fit the statistical data for human cancer incidence vs. age (148, 149). The exponent b (with values from somewhat over two to about seven depending on the tumor type) was considered a possible measure of the number of mutations or other discrete stages involved in carcinogenesis.

The latent period for tumor induction (L) by chemicals may also depend on the dose administered. Indices of carcinogenicity (I) for comparing a series of compounds of the type:

$$I = Y/D \cdot L \; \ldots \tag{2}$$

were proposed for aromatic hydrocarbons (150) and for alkylating agents (151).

The somatic mutation theory (152, 153, 154) and the multistage theory of carcinogenesis are both long standing. In the multistage concept (155) the most likely involvement of mutation is in the initiation stage (156). Initial mutation(s) possibly confer instability on the mitotic apparatus (157, 158) causing further mutations. Promotion involves proliferation of initiated cells and may be opposed by immunosurveillance (159, 160, 161).

The nature of the hypothetical cancer mutations remains speculative. Heritable change in cell surfaces (162, 163, 164, 165) or in transfer RNA (166, 167) were suggested as likely possibilities. However, experiments involving transplantation of tumor nuclei (168, 169) did not support the concept of somatic mutation, and the possibility remains that cancer is an epigenetic phenomenon. Genetic studies with somatic cells present obvious problems (170, 171) and so far the use of cell fusion techniques (172, 173, 174) seems most likely to resolve this question.

Some forms of cancer are inherited (175) e.g., retinoblastoma in man, for which the data on incidence vs. age suggest that two mutational events are required (176). This is a rather lower number than appears for most common cancers. It remains possible therefore that induced mutations caused by chemical agents could be added to inherited defects to produce cancer, (see Ref. 177 for radiation-induced cancer) but there is as yet no proof of this hypothesis.

It appears then that dose–response data for mutation induction are relevant to those for carcinogenesis if the somatic mutation hypothesis is followed. With alkylating agents a good measure of effective dose could be obtained if the extent of alkylation of the target genetic material were known. Few reports have appeared in which this measure of dosage has been determined. Verly *et al.* (*178*) studied induction of mutation in *E. coli* K-12 to streptomycin resistance, using ^{3}H-labeled ethyl methanesulfonate, and found a dose–response relationship of the type represented in Equation (1) (with Y as the mutation frequency per survivor and D as extent of alkylation of DNA guanine) having an exponent b of 2.3. Requirement for simultaneous alkylation of two or three sites in the appropriate locus was therefore indicated. With Myleran, which may be considered as the difunctional analog of ethyl methanesulfonate, analogous methods were applied (*179*) to study the induction of loss of resistance to streptomycin in *Chlamydomonas eugametos*. Here the exponent b was unity indicating that a single alkylation in a DNA target of 2700 nucleotides sufficed. This was interpreted as a deletion.

In other cases, dose–response data rely on concentration of the agent applied as a measure of dose, and although relative data can be obtained, this cannot be related to apparent target size. In some instances the nature of the target can reasonably be assumed. For example, Krieg (*180*) studied reversion of the phage T4rII mutant AP72 by ethyl methanesulfonate and found linear dose–response with a revertant frequency of about 10^{-3} per progeny phage per unit dose of 1-hr treatment with a $1M$ solution. These mutations were deduced to result from copy errors of an alkylated guanine base in DNA.

These isolated examples illustrate the problems facing attempts to deduce molecular mechanisms of mutagenesis from dose–response data since a fairly large deletion in molecular terms and a base-pairing error could apparently lead to the same type of linear dose–response. For a recent review of some chemical aspects of dose–response in mutagenesis, *see* Ref. *181*.

Empirically, differences in the form of dose–response curves dependent on locus studied and agents used can be taken as evidence for mutagen specificity. In the double auxotroph of *Neurospora*, first used for this purpose by Kølmark (*182*), interesting differences in the values of the exponent b were found when the alkylating carcinogens *N*-methyl-*N*-nitrosourea and butadiene dioxide were compared as inducers of reversions at the *ad* and *inos* loci (*183*). However, they did not help to assign molecular mechanisms. Malling and de Serres (*184*) compared some alkylating carcinogens as mutagens in the *Neurospora ad-3* system and similarly found different dose–response curves for *N*-methyl-*N'*-nitro-*N*-nitrosoguanidine and methyl methanesulfate. Molecular mechanisms were "tentatively" deduced from other data, such as comparison of spectra of complementation patterns (*see* the next section).

The most extensive series of dose–response data for a variety of alkylating agents, including epoxides, sultones, alkanesulfonates, and nitrogen mustards were tested as reversion inducers of three auxotrophs (arginine-, leucine-, or uracil-requiring) of *Schizosaccharomyces pombe* (*185*). Examples of approximately linear and markedly nonlinear responses were found, but no general conclusions emerged. Turtoczky and Ehrenberg (*67*) compared alkyl methanesulfonates as inducers of reversion of *E. coli* Sd-4 to streptomycin independence. They found a linear dose–response curve with isopropyl methanesulfonate, a possibly linear dose–response at low doses of ethyl methanesulfonate giving way to an exponential curve at higher doses, and a nonlinear response with methyl methanesulfonate.

Ehrenberg, *et al.* (*186*) introduced the terms "mutagenic effectiveness" as a measure of response per unit dose and "efficiency" in relation to toxicity or mutations per lethal hit. The latter concept is clearly useful when considering cases of nonlinear dose–response since this is often associated with "multi-hit" survival curves. These concepts were applied to compare relative mutagenicities of alkylating agents. Thus, Ehrenberg and Gustafsson (*187*) found butadiene dioxide a more effective mutagen in barley than ethylene oxide, but a less efficient one according to the the terms as defined. Kao and Puck (*188*), on this basis, found ethyl methanesulfonate a more efficient mutagen than the acridine mustard ICR–191 (**30**) for auxotrophy induction in cultural Chinese hamster CHO cells. Fahmy and Fahmy (*189*) found that induction of sex-linked recessive lethals in *Drosophila* sperm by four mesyloxy esters, including ethyl methanesulfonate and mannitol myleran, showed a linear dependence on dose administered by injection.

In summary, it appears from the limited amount of data available, that alkylating agents are unlikely to exhibit dose thresholds below which mutation cannot be induced. However, in some cases, nonlinear dose–response curves were found, and these might give an impression of a threshold, unless a dose range covering sufficiently low doses is studied. The interpretation of such data is apparently complex, and no obvious generalizations about structure, reactivity of mutagens, or correlations with molecular mechanisms have emerged. A probable reason for this complexity is the intervention of repair mechanisms, including those that can remove (excise) promutagenic lesions from alkylated DNA *in vivo* (*2, 12, 181, 190, 191, 192, 193*). Furthermore, by analogy with radiation-induced mutagenesis (*194, 195, 196*), some of these mechanisms may be more error-prone than others. These latter mechanisms are perhaps the recombinational or post-replicational type, rather than those involving excision (*197*).

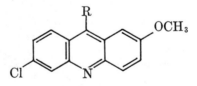

Acridine (quinacrine) mustards—
ICR-49, R $= -NH(CH_2)_3N(CH_2CH_2Cl)_2$;   **30**
ICR-50a, R $= -NH\ CH(CH_3)(CH_2)_3N(CH_2CH_2Cl)_2$;

ICR-170, R $= -NH\ (CH_2)_3N\begin{smallmatrix} C_2H_5 \\ \\ CH_2CH_2Cl \end{smallmatrix}$;

ICR-191, R $= -NH(CH_2)_3\ NH\ CH_2CH_2Cl$

Table IV. Correlation Between Mutagenicity (Induction of Small Chromosome Deletions, *Minutes*, in *Drosophila melanogaster*) and Carcinogenicity (Induction of Pulmonary Tumors in Strain A Mice)

Compound	Formula	Muta-genicity	Carcino-genicity
Triethylenemelamine (TEM)		92	560[b]
Uracil mustard		9	10420
Naphthylamine mustard		3.5	8.3
Melphalan (Sarcolysin)	$HO_2C \cdot CH(NH_2)$—〈 〉—M (L-)	1.5	2630
N,N-Di(2-chloroethyl)-2,3-dimethoxyaniline	MeO OMe	1.1	104
Butadiene dioxide	CH_2—CH—CH—CH_2	0.9	7.6
Mannitol myleran	$H_3C \cdot SO_2 \cdot O \cdot CH_2(CHOH)_4 \cdot CH_2 \cdot O \cdot SO_2 \cdot CH_3$	0.08	3.3

[a] Compounds were administered by injection into adult male flies. Mutagenicity (*142*) denotes induced mutation frequency per 10^3 divided by concentration of agent (mM) at a dose less than the LD_{30} of adult males. Carcinogenicity (*31*) denotes 10^4 divided by positive response dose, *i.e.*, dose (μmol/kg) at which one tumor per mouse was induced, as derived from a dose–response curve, log (no. of tumors per mouse) *vs.* log (dose). In formulae, M denotes the nitrogen mustard moiety, $-N(CH_2CH_2Cl)_2$.

[b] Calculated from data of Shimkin (*198*).

These various possibilities for dose–response relationships in muta-genesis obviously complicate the interpretation of dose–response for carcino-genesis if somatic mutations are involved. At present, comparisons of mutagenic and carcinogenic potencies based on such data might appear somewhat premature.

Nevertheless, this has been attempted. The most extensive studies were done by Fahmy and Fahmy (*142, 143*) referring in particular to 7 of the 29 alkylating agents assessed for carcinogenic potency by Shimkin *et al.* (*31*)

(Table IV). These comprised four compounds of the difunctional mustard type, a trifunctional triazene, a difunctional epoxide, and a difunctional alkanesulfonate. The Fahmys point out that for carcinogens in general, including alkylating agents, no positive correlations emerge between ability of compounds to induce point mutations (sex-linked recessive lethals) or gross deletions (including dominant lethals). A positive correlation was found between ability to induce small deletions, especially at the *Minute* and *bobbed* loci, i.e., those associated with RNA-forming genes (*199*).

However, an alternative correlation between carcinogenic and mutagenic potency was discerned for alkylating agents of simpler molecular structure (Table V). This suggests that, for tumor induction at certain sites—notably the kidney of the Albino rat or the lung of Swiss S mice—a greater response at a given dose results for alkylating agents that are able to induce transition mutations in T2 phage (*69, 206*) or are relatively more efficient mutagens for barley (induction of chlorophyll mutations) or for *E. coli* (reversions to streptomycin independence or from tryptophan requirement) (*41, 67, 68*). As previously mentioned, mutagenicity was positively correlated with ability to react by the S_N1 mechanism for this series of compounds.

Since it is likely that the two groups of alkylating carcinogens in Tables IV and V act through different mechanisms with respect to their effects on DNA templates, as discussed in the next section, the emergence of two apparently different correlations does not necessarily contradict any relationship between mutagenicity and carcinogenicity. It should also be noted in this connection that Malling and de Serres (*184*) concluded from studies of alkylation mutagenesis in *Neurospora* that "compounds that induce a high

Table V. Correlations Between Chemical Reactivity, Mutagenicity,

Compound	*Formula*	*Reactivity* s
2-Oxopropyl methanesulfonate	$CH_3COCH_2OSO_2CH_3$	1.9
Methyl methanesulfonate	$CH_3OSO_2CH_3$	0.83
n-Butyl methanesulfonate	$C_4H_9OSO_2CH_3$	0.65
Ethyl methanesulfonate	$C_2H_5OSO_2CH_3$	0.64
Isopropyl methanesulfonate	$(CH_3)_2CHOSO_2CH_3$	0.29
N-Methyl-N-nitrosourea	$CH_3N(NO)CONH_2$	0.42
N-Ethyl-N-nitrosourea	$C_2H_5N(NO)CONH_2$	0.26

[a] Chemical reactivity is expressed as the substrate constant s of Swain and Scott (*49*), cf. Table I, values generally referring to 37°C.   Mutagenicity for barley is expressed as percentage chlorophyll mutations per spike progeny per unit concentration (mM) from barley kernels treated with concentrations of agents leading to 50% survival, 24 hr, 20°C, or at a lower dose giving 2% mutations (s values for 20°C are closely similar to those for 37°C) (*41*).   For *E.coli*, mutations to streptomycin independence by reversion of mutant Sd-4 of strain B; mutants per 10^8 surviving cells per unit dose of 1 mM for 1 h 37°C (at the ID_{50} dose and at doses of less than 0.2 of that leading to 50% survival (*67*); for nitrosamides and *E.coli*, reversion of strain A58(try⁻) is expressed in the same units (*68*).   For *Drosophila*, "lethals" denotes sex-linked recessive lethals

percentage of mutants in which the specific gene product has an altered function are strong carcinogens, whereas compounds that induce a high percentage of mutants in which the specific gene product is nonfunctional have only a limited carcinogenic activity." Here again the compounds used were monofunctional alkylating agents.

DNA AS THE TARGET OF ALKYLATING CARCINOGENS, AND THE POSSIBLE ROLE OF DNA REPAIR IN ALKYLATION CARCINOGENESIS. Alkylation of DNA is thought to modify its template properties either by blocking DNA synthesis or by potentiating synthesis of a DNA with changed base sequence. Following the Watson and Crick model (207) for mutagenesis, the mis-pairing of anomalous induced tautomeric forms of bases in DNA became accepted as a general molecular mechanism for this process, which was termed "transition" by Freese (208). Later, Crick et al. (209) showed that an alternative mechanism, the "frameshift," was induced by acridine dyes. Both processes may occur in alkylation mutagenesis. The relevant evidence is principally the pattern of reversions induced by appropriate mutagens. Thus, hydroxylamine, at relatively high concentrations *in vitro*, reacts specifically with cytosine residues (210). It is generally regarded as diagnostic for transitions by causing those of the GC → AT type, *i.e.*, reverting those of the AT → GC type. Base analogs (211) also revert transitions, and acridines, but not base analogs, are diagnostic for frameshifts (25, 212, 213, 214, 215, 216).

The best known mechanism for inactivation of DNA templates by alkylation is the cross-linking action of di- and polyfunctional agents. Nitrogen mustard (217) was the first carcinogen shown to react with DNA

and Carcinogenicity of Monofunctional Alkylating Agents[a]

Mutagenicity							Carcinogenicity	
Barley		E.coli Sd-4		E.coli A58	Drosophila			
LD_{50}	Low Dose	LD_{50}	Low Dose	Low Dose	"Lethals"	Minutes	Mouse Lung	Rat Kidney
0	0	2	1.3					
6	4	45	11		26	2.7	0.04[b]	0.0
0.7	0.12	1	0.5		0.6			
1.5	0.25	74	6.5		7	0.5	0.30	0.08
0.3	0.14	150	150					
				67			0.58	0.52
				140			6.7	

from treated Oregon-K males (Muller-5 technique), mutations per 10^3/concentration (mM), compounds being injected in saline (189, 200); *Minutes*, as in Table IV (142) (the dose–response relationships were linear (189, 200). Carcinogenicity for mice (CFW/D inbred line of Swiss S) (lung adenomas) (201, 202), or for rats (Albino) (kidney tumors) (203, 204), is expressed as number of tumors per animal divided by dose (m mol/kg).

[b] Not significant; N.B. methyl methanesulfonate gave significant number of lung and other tumors in male RF mice on prolonged oral administration in water (30 mg/kg) (205).

(the purine fraction) *in vivo*. Subsequently, Brookes and Lawley(*1*) showed that mustard gas gave the same principal products in DNA *in vivo* as *in vitro*, *i.e.*, 7-alkylguanines. This difunctional mustard induces cross-links between guanine bases in opposite strands of DNA (*116, 218*) and within single strands of DNA (*219, 220, 221*) or RNA (*222*). Other carcinogens which cross-link DNA include triethylene melamine (*218, 223*) the nitrogen mustard HN2 (*224, 225, 226, 227*) (for *in vivo* studies, *see* Ref. *228*, ascites tumors in the mouse; Ref. *229*, chick embryos); thio-Tepa (**31**) [carcinogenesis, strain BR46 rats (*107*); cross-linking of DNA in chick embryos (*229*)]; butadiene dioxide (D- and L- forms cross-link DNA of T7 phage, but not the *meso* form (*230*); DL- and *meso* forms are carcinogenic (*54*); and mitomycin C (*231*). Monofunctional agents cannot cross-link by direct alkylation, but the subsequent hydrolytic depurination (*232, 233*) of DNA methylated by methyl methanesulfonate can cause cross-linkage to a relatively small extent (1 per 140 depurinations in T7 phage (*234*)), and this may therefore be general for agents inducing depurinations.

In addition to their ability to cross-link DNA, difunctional alkylating agents partially prevent DNA extraction by the phenol deproteinization procedures from alkylated Ehrlich ascites tumor cells (*235, 236*). Although this may in part be ascribed to formation of covalent alkylation cross-links between DNA and protein, it seems unlikely to account for all the observed effects since monofunctional alkylating agents and other cytotoxic agents, such as arsenate or arsenite, caused analogous decreased extractability of ascites cell DNA (*236*). It was also notable that the difunctional agent Trenimon (**33**), while effective in this respect in ascites and in newborn rat liver or kidney cells, was unable to prevent DNA extraction from liver or kidney of adult mice. This suggests that the effect was specific for proliferating tissues. Furthermore, the effect paralleled growth-inhibitory action on ascites cells, but it was not apparent with certain cytotoxic agents such as potassium cyanide or fluoroacetate. It was concluded that the significant

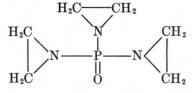

Tepa (in Thio-Tepa S replaces O)   **31**

$CH_3SO_2O(CH_2)_nOSO_2CH_3$ Methylene dimethanesulfonate, $n = 1$; Myleran (Busulphan), $n = 4$ **32**

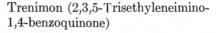

Trenimon (2,3,5-Trisethyleneimino-1,4-benzoquinone)   **33**

property of the effective agents was their ability to react with thiol groups of proteins.

In related studies on *in vitro* cross-linking, Nietert *et al.* (237) showed that the supposedly monofunctional alkylating carcinogen β-propiolactone can form DNA–protein complexes when the three components are incubated together for longer than 30 min. The nature of the protein–DNA bonds is not specified, but it was suggested that formation of such complexes *in vivo* could be significant by modifying the template function of DNA or by inhibiting repair of alkylated DNA.

Direct breakage of the sugar–phosphate chain of nucleic acids could result from alkylation of phosphodiester groups (238, 239). Phosphotriester groups are unstable in RNA at neutral pH (240). It is likely, therefore, that degradation of alkylated polyribonucleotides can be ascribed to their formation, as observed with HN2 (66), ethyl methanesulfonate (241), and N-methyl-N-nitrosourea (242). Sulfur mustards (243, 244) and dimethyl sulfate (245) did not degrade RNA, suggesting that phosphodiester alkylation occurs more with S_N1 than with S_N2 agents.

In alkylated DNA, phosphotriester groups were detected by chemical analysis only very recently. Bannon and Verly (246) found that about 20% of ethylation products from ethyl methanesulfonate and about 1% from methyl methanesulfonate were phosphotriesters which, at neutral pH, were stable to heating.

The cross-linking between strands of DNA molecules would prevent the separation of these strands necessary for DNA replication (247) and therefore induction of mutations by di- and polyfunctional alkylating agents would be expected to involve deletions of those units of DNA that are normally replicated. In view of the ability of difunctional agents to induce intramolecular, and possibly intermolecular, cross-links involving DNA, it seemed that these agents would induce a spectrum of mutations different from that given by monofunctional agents. The first detailed comparisons of the di- and monofunctional alkylating mutagens were made by Fahmy and Fahmy (200) using *Drosophila*. They found that difunctional mesyloxy esters, including mannitol myleran, induced more complete relative to mosaic mutants, a higher ratio of lethals to visibles, and more chromosome breaks than the monofunctional esters methyl and ethyl methanesulfonates. Watson (248, 249) compared the effects of di- monofunctional agents, butadiene dioxide and ethylene oxide or triethylenemelamine and ethylene imine on *Drosophila* sperm. He concluded that the greater efficiency of the difunctional agents in chromosome breakage was only revealed for alkylated sperm stored in the seminal receptacles of females for six days. As previously mentioned, Verly *et al.* (179) attributed mutations induced by myleran in *Chlamydomonas* to deletions of DNA molecules, but a subsequent study of the action of myleran and dimethyl myleran on phage T7 did not detect interstrand cross-linkage (227). Loveless (144) attributed the feeble mutagenic action of HN2 on T–even phages to the ability of this difunctional alkylating agent to inactivate the phage by cross-linkage (250). The relatively weak mutagenic activity detected with T4 (251, 252) was attributed to the monofunctional part of the reaction of HN2 with phage DNA.

However, DNA can be replicated after cross-linkage. This was clearly shown for *Bacillus subtilis* transforming DNA treated with HN2 (253). A resistant strain of *E. coli* (B/r) and a sensitive strain (B$_{S-1}$), after alkylation to equal extents with mustard gas, behaved quite differently on subsequent incubation (12, 244). The resistant strain, after a lag period depending on the mustard dose, resumed DNA synthesis apparently normally. In the sensitive strain DNA synthesis was blocked permanently by much lower doses. Following alkylation of DNA *in vivo*, the resistant strain removed the cross-linked bases from its DNA (12, 254) but not the principal monoalkylation product, 7-alkylguanine. Removal of interstrand cross-links *in vivo* can also be shown by physicochemical methods for HN2 and *E. coli* (255) and for mustard gas and *E. coli* (256).

These "excisions" of lesions in DNA induced by alkylating agents have been attributed therefore to "repair" endonuclease enzymes (12, 181, 190, 254). There is some analogy with the enzymic repair of the uv-induced thymine dimer lesion, and the processes of sequential excision of cross-links from DNA in *E. coli* and of the subsequent recombination process were elucidated in detail by Cole (257). Removal of an intrastrand cross-link, a known block to DNA synthesis in bacteriophage (219) formally resembles excision of the thymine dimer. However, removal of interstrand cross-linked bases involves excision at nearby points on both DNA strands, although the requisite information for repair of DNA could remain (190).

In mammalian cells, evidence for repair of the cross-link lesion was obtained, but the evidence from chemical analysis of the alkylated DNA did not show specific removal of cross-linked bases (192, 258, 259) but instead showed an overall loss of alkyl groups from DNA. According to McCann (229) "there is no known repair mechanism for covalent interstrand cross-links in DNA in higher cells."

It remains possible, however, that despite the apparent lack of evidence for specific removal of certain alkylated bases from DNA which would support the concept of excision repair, either "unhinging" of a cross-link could occur without complete removal of the alkylated bases involved, or "bypass" of the lesion with subsequent recombinational repair could occur by analogy with the scheme for uv repair in microorganisms (197).

One problem with mammalian cells in this respect is the lack of sensitive and resistant strains with defined differences in repair capability. Walker and Reid (260) recently isolated three substrains of mouse L-cells which exhibit a decreased sensitivity to mustard gas and also showed enhanced ability to excise alkylation products from their DNA when compared with the parental strains. On the other hand, Ball and Roberts (261) found no significant differences between alkylation of DNA by mustard gas or excision of alkylated bases from DNA on subsequent incubation in culture of a resistant sub-line of the Yoshida sarcoma compared with the original sensitive strain. Chun *et al.* (228) compared the alkylation and cross-linking of DNA by the nitrogen mustard, HN2, in sensitive and resistant lines of

Lettré–Ehrlich ascites tumors *in vivo* in Swiss S mice and found that the resistant strain showed about half the extent of alkylation and cross-linking of the sensitive line. Only a part of the observed acquired resistance could be ascribed to decreased permeability to the drug of the sub-line.

More recently Yin *et al.* (*262*) amplified these studies on HN2-sensitive and HN2-resistant Lettré–Ehrlich cells in the mouse. The principal conclusions were that both cell types rapidly opened HN2-induced DNA cross-links and removed alkylated bases from DNA. Preferential excision of diguaninyl products rather than of monoguaninyl products was found. The sensitivity of the more HN2-susceptible strain was ascribed to deficiencies in later stages of the repair process since this strain showed rapid strand-breakage of DNA which was not coordinated with subsequent rejoining of the broken ends by DNA ligase. This interpretation parallels that of Walker and Reid (*260*) for their strains of L-cells.

Another approach to the detection of DNA repair (*263, 264*) involves measuring non-semiconservative or unscheduled DNA synthesis as a response to induction of lesions into cellular DNA. This was fairly extensively investigated with alkylating carcinogens, and some of the reports are tabulated in Table VI.

The major interest in DNA repair as a factor in carcinogenesis stems from the work of Cleaver (*282*) and others (*283*) who showed that inherited diminished ability to repair uv-induced damage to DNA of skin cells was positively correlated with susceptibility to skin cancer in the condition xeroderma pigmentosum. So far, positive evidence of this kind relating defective repair and carcinogenesis for chemical carcinogens appears to be lacking, but the concept remains reasonable if somatic mutations are involved for agents which strongly inhibit DNA synthesis.

Cells from patients with xeroderma pigmentosum were used in studies with the alkylating carcinogens methyl methanesulfonate and *N*-methyl-*N'*-nitro-*N*-nitrosoguanidine (*267*) and led to the conclusion that their response with respect to repair replication following alkylation is the same as for normal cells. However, the results with the nitrogen mustard, HN2, were equivocal. The interpretation of the data was that excision of damage from DNA might be required for repair of HN2-induced lesions, but that it was not necessary for repair of damage caused by the methylating agents. This damage presumably consisted of single-strand breaks. This latter conclusion was previously drawn for microorganisms (*see* Refs. *273, 284;* for *B. subtilis, see* Ref. *274*) and implies that methylation damage, like that caused by x-irradiation, can be repaired by ligase action without the need for incision as a first step ⋅ enzymic repair. Recent evidence has indicated repair of single-strand breaks induced by alkylating carcinogens *in vivo* in DNA of rat liver. For example, breaks produced within 4 hr after administration of methyl methanesulfonate were repaired within 48 hr (*278, 279*).

This leaves unresolved the question whether the alkylation-induced breaks are produced by phosphotriester formation and subsequent hydrolysis (for which evidence was claimed using methyl or ethyl methanesulfonate as alkylating agents (*285*)) or by hydrolytic depurination (fission of the

Table VI.   Evidence for DNA Repair

Agent	Organism or Cell
Nitrogen mustard, HN2	*E.coli* murine mast cell tumour P-815 human lymphocytes in culture xeroderma pigmentosum cells in culture mouse ascites tumor *in vivo*
Mustard gas	*E.coli* *E.coli*
Mustard gas	cultured mammalian cells:- HeLa HeLa, Chinese hamster V79 mouse L-cells
Methyl methanesulfonate	*Bacillus subtilis* bacteriophage T4 *Haemophilus influenzae* bacteriophage λ in *E.coli* K12 HeLa, Chinese hamster V79 cells mouse L-cells rat myotubes rat liver *in vivo*
N-Methyl-N-nitrosourea	human lymphocytes HeLa, Chinese hamster V79 cells mouse L-cells rat liver *in vivo*
Ethyl methanesulfonate	bacteriophage λ in *E.coli* K 12 human lymphocytes HeLa, Chinese hamster V79 cells
β-Propiolactone	human lymphocytes
Mitomycin C	*E.coli* K-12 mouse L-cells

glycosidic alkylpurine linkages) and subsequent hydrolysis of the main chain (*238, 239, 286, 287*) or by action of an endonuclease different from that involved in excision of lesions induced by uv or by di- and polyfunctional alkylating agents. In this last connection, enzymes specific for methylated DNA are known in microorganisms, *e.g.*, *Micrococcus lysodeikticus* (*288*), and there is evidence for specific excision of certain methylated bases, *e.g.*, 3-methyladenine and O^6-methylguanine, from DNA of *E. coli* after treatment with N-methyl-N'-nitrosoguanidine (*191*). Recently, Kirtikar and Goldthwait (*289*) partially purified an enzyme, endonuclease II, which depurinates 3-methyladenine and O^6-methylguanine from DNA in *E. coli* treated with N-methyl-N-nitrosourea.

In summary, it is possible therefore that sublethal damage may remain in cellular DNA after incomplete or erroneous operation of enzymatic mechanisms that normally restore this template to its original functional condition—free of alkylation-induced damage. The question then arises, whether the state of the cell at the time of alkylation, either with regard to its functional status or stage of differentiation or with regard to its position

Following Alkylation; Representative Studies

Nature of Evidence	*References*
removal of cross-links	*255*
5-bromodeoxyuridine sensitivity	*265*
repair synthesis (unscheduled, insensitive to hydroxyurea)	*266*
non-semiconservative DNA synthesis	*267*
removal of cross-links, DNA strand breakage and rejoining	*262*
removal of mustard products	*268*
specific removal of cross-links	*12, 254,256*
removal of mustard products	*192, 258*
non-semiconservative DNA synthesis	*193,259,269*
caffeine sensitivity; removal of cross-links	*260,270*
repair synthesis; rejoining of single-strand breaks in DNA	*271,272,273*
ligase-defective mutant sensitive	*274*
recombinationless strains sensitive	*275*
Uvr⁻ and rec⁻ cells show impaired repair ability	*276*
non-semiconservative DNA synthesis	*269*
caffeine sensitivity	*270*
unscheduled DNA synthesis	*277*
DNA strand breakage and rejoining	*278*
repair replication	*266*
non-semiconservative DNA synthesis	*269*
caffeine sensitivity	*270*
DNA strand breakage and rejoining	*279*
Uvr⁻ and rec⁻ cells show impaired repair ability	*276*
repair replication	*266*
non-semiconservative DNA synthesis	*269*
repair replication	*266*
Uvr⁻ (excision-deficient) mutants sensitive	*280*
caffeine sensitivity	*281*

in the cycle of cell division, influences the repair response or the nature of the lesions induced in the first place. Clearly, significant effects of this type could account, at least in part, for some aspects of organotropism of alkylating carcinogens, *i.e.*, for lack of simple correlation between alkylation of cellular DNA and carcinogenic response.

Some evidence is already available that the action of chemical carcinogens in general depends on the status of the target cells. Thus, Warwick (*290*) reviewed evidence that proliferating cells are more vulnerable than resting cells. With regard to repair of DNA, this may imply that replicating DNA is more prone to errors in repair systems or that DNA near the "growing point" in DNA synthesis is replicated while still containing promutagenic alkylations. A similar conclusion may apply to DNA as an active template for RNA synthesis. Brock (*291*) found that the β-galactosidase locus of *E. coli* K-12 was more readily mutated by the carcinogen diethyl sulfate if alkylation occurred while the cells were induced to transcribe messenger RNA for β-galactosidase.

With regard to state of cellular differentiation, Hahn *et al.* (*277*) found that unscheduled DNA synthesis can be detected in nondifferentiated rat muscle (cultured myotube) cells following their alkylation by methyl methanesulfonate, but that as the cells progressed through the stages of differentiation in culture, they showed progressively less response of this type to methylation. The extent of cellular DNA alkylation did not depend on the stage of differentiation at which the agent was applied so that the conclusion followed that the more highly differentiated cells did not exhibit the repair response, at least not to as great an extent as the nondifferentiated cells.

The question then arises of the possible effects of promoting agents (Chapter 2) on carcinogen-damaged cells—whether an agent of this type that stimulated division of cells containing incompletely repaired DNA could thus increase the number of mutated cells. In this regard, Gaudin *et al.* (*292*) obtained evidence that typical promoting agents will inhibit the repair replication induced by uv irradiation of human lymphocytes (*293*). These cells respond also to alkylation by ethyl or methyl methanesulfonates, HN2, or β-propiolactone (*266*), but as yet no reports of the effects of promoting agents on this response have appeared. With regard to effects of known DNA repair inhibitors, caffeine breaks chromosomes in cultured mammalian cells at relatively high concentrations but was not mutagenic in a typical mammalian cell system (*188*) or in mice (*294*). It potentiated the lethal

Table VII. Mutagenic Activity of Alkylating Carcinogens

Compound	Formula	Phage Survival (%)	rII Mutants/10^4 Survivors
Ethyl methane-sulfonate	$C_2H_5OSO_2H_3$	100	*ca.* 1500
Diethyl sulfate	$(C_2H_5)_2SO_4$	60	*ca.* 125
β-Propiolactone	$\begin{array}{c} H_2C\text{---}CH_2 \\ \mid \quad\quad \mid \\ OC\text{---}O \end{array}$	0.1	50
1,3-Propanesultone	$\begin{array}{c} H_2C\text{---}CH_2 \\ \mid \quad\quad \mid \\ H_2C \quad\quad O \\ \diagdown\diagup \\ SO_2 \end{array}$	0.1	110
Glycidaldehyde	$\begin{array}{c} H_2C\text{---}CH\text{---}CHO \\ \diagdown\diagup \\ O \end{array}$	0.01	42
Nitrogen mustard, HN2	$CH_3N(CH_2CH_2Cl)_2$	0.1	17
Nitrogen mustard, HN2		1	10

[a] Bacteriophage was treated extracellularly. Number of mutants was greater than 10 times that of controls, except for HN2 (about five times greater). Types of mutation

action towards cultured mammalian cells of mitomycin C (*281*) and of several alkylating carcinogens, both difunctional (mustard gas) and mono-functional (methyl methanesulfonate, *N*-methyl-*N*-nitrosourea) (*270*). There is evidence that caffeine acts in mammalian cells by inhibiting repair of alkylated DNA, since it is ineffective if applied to the alkylated cells when the repair process is no longer operative as indicated from other evidence (*295*).

Whether sufficient concentrations of this repair inhibitor can exist in target cells of alkylating carcinogens *in vivo* is not yet known. Thayer and Kensler (*294*) reported that caffeine administered to mice in drinking water at concentrations up to 122 mg/kg/day (equivalent to 95 cups of coffee per day for humans) had no mutagenic effect, nor did it potentiate the induction of dominant lethal mutations by TEM or x-rays. On the other hand inhibition by caffeine of uv-induced induction of skin cancer in mice was reported (*296*).

It seems likely that some mechanisms for induced mutation may be caffeine-sensitive, but others are not. For example, Clarke (*297*) found that the frequency of reversions of *E. coli* B/r *try*-WWP2 induced by uv was enhanced by caffeine but that caused by the alkylating carcinogens, butadiene dioxide or *N*-methyl-*N*-nitrosourethane, was not. This may imply that the alkylating agents were acting by inducing directly miscoding promutagenic

in Bacteriophage T2 (*303*) or T4 (*180, 251, 252*) [a]

Predominant Type(s) of Mutation	References, Mutagenesis	References, Carcinogenesis
GC → AT transition	*180,303*	*204,304,305,306*
	180	*151*
GC → AT transition	*252*	*113,307,308,309,310*
GC → AT transition	*252*	*309,311*
Frameshift; AT → GC	*252*	*309*
Frameshift; large deletions	*252*	*31,312*
GC → AT, some frameshift	*251*	

were deduced from T4rII reversion studies. Data for ethyl methanesulfonate forward mutations are from Loveless (*303*), for reversions, from Krieg (*180*).

lesions and that repair was not involved in the mutagenic process in this system.

Another known inhibitor of DNA repair, 5-bromodeoxyuridine, increased the sensitivity of cultured mammalian cells (P-815-x2 murine mast cell tumor) to the lethal action of the alkylating agents HN2 and dimethylmyleran (265). 5-Bromodeoxyuridine is incorporated into cellular DNA and can induce mutations (to resistance to 8-azaguanine) in Chinese hamster cells (298) although it is generally regarded as noncarcinogenic.

Other effects associated with the repair response to DNA alkylation may be important in alkylation carcinogenesis apart from the possibility that mutations can be induced by errors in repair. Zimmermann (171) reviewed the possible significance of induced mitotic recombination and gene conversion as mechanisms which can lead to homozygosis of detrimental genes, the effects of which are only weak in the presence of wild-type alleles. A number of typical alkylating and other carcinogens can induce these effects. According to Zimmermann (171) the "general objection to the mutation hypothesis of cancer based on the apparent recessiveness of mutant vs. wild type alleles . . . should be considered with considerable reserve."

These remarks lead to a reiteration of what at first sight may seem to be contradictory evidence relevant to an assessment of the molecular mecha-

Table VIII. Suggested Molecular Mechanisms for Induction of T-even Bacteriophages

Compound(s)	Formula	Type of Mutation
Methyl methanesulfonate	$CH_3OSO_2CH_3$	Neurospora ad-3 locus Schizosaccharomyces pombe purple mutants (ad-6, ad-7)
Ethyl methanesulfonate	$C_2H_5OSO_2CH_3$	E.coli K12 lac⁻
		Phage S13, host range
		E.coli WWU (also called TAU⁻) reversion of arg locus Neurospora ad-3B
		S.pombe purple mutants
Diethyl sulfate	$(C_2H_5O)_2SO_2$	Salmonella typhimurium leu⁻ reversion
K-region epoxides of benz(a)anthracene and derivatives		Salmonella typhimurium his⁻ reversions

nisms indicated for cancer mutations. As previously noted, the work of the Fahmys drew attention to small deletions as a significant class of mutation associated with carcinogens. From knowledge of the mode of action of the di- and polyfunctional alkylating carcinogens, it seems possible that these deletions could result from errors in repair of cross-linked DNA. However, Malling and de Serres (*299*) and Zimmermann (*171*) have concluded that present knowledge indicates that carcinogens most frequently induce the missense type of mutation following from base substitution in DNA, such as the transitions or transversions in the nomenclature of Freese (*208, 215*). A third possibility, that alkylating agents with aromatic moieties act as frameshift mutagens, was recently suggested from studies of the mutagenic action of K-region epoxides of benz[*a*]anthracene derivatives in *Salmonella typhimurium* (*300*). The classical cases of alkylating agent mutagens acting by this mechanism are the acridine mustards (*216, 301, 302*), but of five such mustards tested for carcinogenesis by Shimkin *et al.* (*31*) only one was considered significantly positive, and one was classified as of borderline significance.

Alkylating carcinogens have been classified in terms of their molecular mechanisms of action as mutagens to show that all the various types of mechanisms are exhibited (Tables VII and VIII). Some agents act fairly

Mutations by Alkylating Carcinogens in Systems Other than and Mammalian Cells

Suggested Mechanism	Nature of Evidence	References
GC → AT transition	complementation spectra	*184*
transition (85%)	phenotypic, suppressor, and complementation analyses	*313*
transition, probably GC → AT	reversion by 2-aminopurine but not by ethyl methanesulfonate	*314*
transition, mainly G → A, C → T, some A → G, T → C	pattern of reversions induced by other mutagens	*315*
GC → AT transitions	induction of known suppressors	*316*
AT → GC (41%); GC → AT (17%); frameshift (9%); non-revertible, (deletions?) (7%)	pattern of reversions induced by other mutagens	*317*
transition (96%)	as for methyl methanesulfonate	*313*
GC → AT transition, AT → GC by depurination	comparison with action of other mutagens; time dependence	*318*
frameshift	strains known to be reverted only by frameshift inducing mutagens	*300*

specifically. For example ethyl methanesulfonate appears from the consensus to induce GC $\rightarrow$ AT transitions predominantly, but N-methyl-N'-nitro-N-nitrosoguanidine was tentatively classified mainly as an inducer of AT $\rightarrow$ GC transitions (184).

As previously discussed, since the alkylating agents can inactivate the DNA template by cross-linking or by depurination and chain-breakage, mutation resulting from errors in attempted repair of these lesions will be superimposed on those resulting from direct replication of promutagenic alkylated bases.

The question of which alkylation products are promutagenic by this direct mechanism remains unresolved. All four bases of DNA (Table VIII) and the phosphodiester groups (319) have been invoked as possible sites.

At present the most obvious choice in terms of the Watson–Crick mechanism for induction of transitions (see Scheme 6) is O^6-alkylguanine (69). This mechanism is strongly supported by the work of Gerchman and Ludlum (324) showing that poly(O^6-methylguanine) miscodes as a template by incorporating UTP and ATP in an in vitro polyribonucleotide synthesizing system. The O-6 atom of guanine is a site of relatively low reactivity to agents of the S_N2 type, but in agreement with theory it is more reactive towards S_N1 agents.

Alkylation of the most nucleophilic group in DNA, N-7 of guanine (238) by monofunctional agents appears to have little effect on the template properties and provokes little or no response from enzymes in E. coli that excise other products (191). The relatively feebly reactive N-3 atom of guanine could lead to miscoding on alkylation if the 3-alkylguanine retained the amino- as opposed to the imino-configuration (320).

Studies on miscoding in vitro of alkylated polynucleotides showed no positive evidence for miscoding directed by templates containing 7-methylguanine residues (325, 326). Positive evidence for miscoding was obtained with methylated polycytidylic acid or polydeoxycytidylic acid templates, which misincorporated uracil or adenine nucleotides in addition to the normal guanine (321). Since 3-methylcytosine is the only product detected from this methylated polynucleotide, it must be assumed that this residue is the miscoding base, although it would appear to block Watson–Crick hydrogen bonding.

Suggestions that 3- and 7-methyladenines can miscode are based on physicochemical theory (180, 322, 327, 328), but there is evidence from phage T4rII reversions that alkylated adenine can miscode (180).

Alkylated thymine can miscode, according to deductions from the pattern on induced reversions in phage containing single-stranded DNA (315). The most likely source of this miscoding would be alkylation of thymine at the O-4 atom. It may be noted that 1-methyluracil can be methylated at O-4 by diazomethane (329). Also a small extent of methylation of O-4 of thymine in DNA by N-methyl-N-nitrosourea was reported recently (323).

The general conclusion may be drawn, therefore, that S_N1 agents, by virtue of their ability to alkylate a wider spectrum of sites in DNA, including the O-atoms of bases and possibly of the sugar–phosphate chain (319) may

*Scheme 6. Watson–Crick base-pairs and suggested abnormal base-pairings of
alkylated bases in DNA*

Bases	*Formulae*	*References*
Cytosine: guanine (normal)		*207*
Thymine: ionized 7-alkylguanine		*232*
Thymine: O^6-alkylguanine		*69*
Thymine: 3-methylguanine (amino form)		*320*
3-Methylcytosine: adenine		*321*
Thymine: adenine (normal)		*207*
Cytosine: ionized 3-methyladenine		*322*
O^4-Methylthymine: guanine	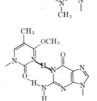	*323*

induce more promutagenic groups into DNA than S_N2 agents (*128, 330*). Conversely, the latter, by reacting relatively more at sites which potentiate depurination of DNA such as N-7 of guanine and N-3 of adenine (*232*), may induce relatively more inactivating lesions.

A possible exception to these generalizations is presented by the carcinogen β-propiolactone, which is generally classified as an S_N2 agent. This is known to alkylate N-7 of guanine in DNA of a target tissue, mouse skin (*307, 308*), and to induce *r* mutations in T4 phage (*252*) which are deduced to be of the GC → AT transition type (Table VII). It remains possible that the promutagenic groups induced by this compound are O-alkylated derivatives which have not yet been detected. It should also be noted that agents with more S_N2 character and higher Swain and Scott *s* factors *e.g.*, 3-chloro-, or 3-iodopropionic acids, or iodoacetic acid, reacted to lower extents with DNA of the target tissue at a given dose and were either not initiators of skin tumors (3-chloropropionic acid, iodoacetic acid) or were much weaker (3-iodopropionic acid) in this respect than β-propiolactone (*308*).

A general consideration relating to mispairing of bases as a cause of mutation concerns the relative acceptability of abnormal tautomeric forms of these bases to DNA polymerases. With mutagenic base analogs, such as 5-bromouracil, the polymerase may discriminate against the relatively rare tautomer that would pair with the abnormal base—in this case guanine instead of adenine. There is evidence that DNA polymerase of T4 phage can do this since mutants with discriminating ability, in this sense, markedly greater or less than that of the wild type can be isolated (*331*). The promutagenic group(s) induced by ethyl methanesulfonate were discriminated against only moderately by phage with the antimutator gene, and, in this respect, they resembled those induced by nitrous acid rather than by the antimetabolites. This finding suggests that the promutagenic ethylated base(s) exist(s) mainly in the tautomeric configuration that pairs abnormally in the Watson–Crick sense. O^6-Ethylguanine would fit this requirement, but not 7-ethylguanine. The tautomeric configuration of nucleosides of 3-alkylguanines is not known.

An action of certain alkylating carcinogens which may justifiably be discussed here, although its molecular mechanism is not known but may involve induced action of nuclease enzymes acting on damaged DNA, is that of latent virus induction. This was invoked as possibly involved in carcinogenesis since its discovery by Lwoff (*332*) as the phenomenon of induced lysogeny in *E. coli* (λ) strains, and it was recently reviewed, with respect to chemical inducers, by Heinemann (*333*). Loveless (*144*) concluded that di- and polyfunctional alkylating agents were better inducers of *E. coli* K12 (λ) than monofunctional agents. This conclusion is broadly supported by Heinemann's (*333*) data compilation, although the latter does not mention the report by Loveless and Shields (*334*) showing mustard gas as a effective inducing agent. Loveless (*144*) (*see also* Ref. *335*) concluded that the lethal properties of alkylating agents positively correlated with their inducing ability, possibly because of their ability to cause transient or permanent arrest of DNA synthesis.

A limited number of cases of release by chemical action of a tumor virus from a mammalian cell previously transformed by the virus have been reported (*336*). Mitomycin C induced certain SV-40-transformed clones of hamster kidney cells to produce infectious virus, but other SV-40- and adenovirus- or polyoma-transformed cells could not be induced.

Frei (*201, 202*) compared the carcinogenic action of low molecular weight alkylating agents in an inbred line of Swiss mice (strain CFW/D) with regard to induction of lung adenomas and lymphomas. These latter tumors may originate from induction of a latent virus containing RNA (*337*). Ethyl methanesulfonate was an effective inducer of adenomas, but not of lymphomas. *N*-Methyl- and *N*-ethyl-*N*-nitrosoureas induced either type of tumor. However, the induction of latent virus by these nitroso compounds has not been reported as yet.

A provisional conclusion may therefore be drawn from studies of the general mutagenic action of alkylating carcinogens so far available. The results of these studies are quite consistent with the somatic mutation hypothesis in so far as virtually all alkylating carcinogens tested induced mutations in almost all systems used. However, the comparisons between mutational spectra and carcinogenic potency have not yet clarified the molecular mechanism of carcinogenesis, at least with respect to the initiation stage. What has emerged from mutation studies with alkylating agents illustrates the diversity of possible mechanisms; so far, none of these stands out as particularly involved in cancer mutations. Direct mispairing of promutagenic alkylated bases in DNA is indicated to be the principal mode of action of certain monofunctional agents, typified by ethyl methanesulfonate and more particularly those that are classified as S_N1 agents; but these are not always outstandingly potent carcinogens. Small deletions, caused by induction of frameshifts or the result of errors in repair of alkylation lesions in DNA, may be more likely to cause cancer-initiating mutations than the simple transition mechanism, although this may not be the case for certain target organs. This conclusion would agree with the correlations between mutagenicity and carcinogenicity found by the Fahmys and would also agree with the apparent lack of carcinogenicity of base analog transition-inducing mutagens. Blocks to DNA synthesis leading to the repair response may be expected from cross-linking of DNA and from depurination or chain-breakage. Agents containing aromatic or heterocyclic moieties appear to be particularly effective as inducers of frameshifts. In addition to stimulating repair mechanisms, blocks to DNA synthesis may lead to induction of latent virus.

ALKYLATION-INDUCED MUTAGENESIS WITH MAMMALIAN SYSTEMS. According to Kao and Puck (*338*), "it would appear that the mammalian cell system may afford a valuable approach in exploring mutagenic action in a large variety of carcinogenic compounds. Since genetic changes are studied directly in mammalian somatic cells, the mutagenic response so obtained should be much more similar to those producing the carcinogenic response than is the case when microorganisms or *Drosophila* are used as the test system."

Table IX.   Mutagenesis by Alkylating

Compound	Cell
Methyl methanesulfonate	Chinese hamster V79
Ethyl methanesulfonate	Chinese hamster CHO/Pro⁻K1
	CHO/Pro⁻
	V79
	human lymphocytes
N-Methyl-N'-nitro-N-nitrosoguanidine	CHO/Pro⁻K1
	CHO/Pro⁻
	V79
	human lymphocytes
N-Methyl-N-nitrosourea	CHO/Pro⁻K1
N-Methyl-N-nitrosourethane	CHO/Pro⁻K1
ICR–170, Acridine mustard (30)	V79
ICR–191, Acridine mustard (30)	CHO/Pro⁻
K-region epoxides of 3-methylcholan-threne, benz(a)anthracene, 7-methyl-benz(a)anthracene, dibenz(a,b)-anthracene	V79–4C16

A further important feature of the mammalian cell systems is that they can be used for comparative mutation and transformation studies (*339*). It is not yet clear whether the phenomenon of transformation (sometimes denoted "*in vitro* carcinogenesis") involves mutation, although virtually all chemical transforming agents so far tested are also mutagens. According to Harris (H.) (*174, 340*) malignancy can be shown to constitute a recessive heritable characteristic of tumor cells by cell fusion techniques. It seems likely that the mutations involved, if in fact they are gene mutations, affect the cell surface (*164*).

However, in one much used test system for mammalian cell mutagenesis in which selection is based on induced resistance of Chinese hamster V79 cells to 8-azaguanine (*341*) the spontaneous mutation rate was reported to be relatively high compared with the known rates for germ cells in mice or man (*342*). Moreover, cells of different ploidy showed about the same mutation rates (*343*). According to Harris (M.) (*343*), the data suggest that "at least some variations may arise in somatic cells by stable shifts in phenotypic expression rather than by changes in genetic information." The molecular basis of such "shifts" is not known.

Table X.   Transformation or Morphological Conversion

Compound	Cell
N-Methyl-N-nitrosourea	Chinese hamster lung tissue cell line
N-Methyl-N'-nitro-N-nitrosoguanidine	secondary Syrian hamster cells
	hamster embryo cells
	mouse prostate clone C311-G23

Carcinogens in Mammalian Cell Systems

Type of Mutation Induced	*References*
resistance to 8-azaguanine	*344*
gly⁻ (mainly)	*345*
reversion to prototrophy	*345*
resistance to 8-azaguanine and its reversion	*344*
resistance to 6-thioguanine	*346*
gly⁻+*thy*⁻+*hypox*⁻ (mainly)	*345*
reversion to prototrophy	*345*
resistance to 8-azaguanine and its reversion	*344*
resistance to 6-thioguanine	*346*
thy⁻	*338*
gly⁻ (and other auxotrophs)	*338*
resistance to 8-azaguanine and its reversion	*347*
auxotrophy, *gly*⁻, *hypox*⁻	*188*
resistance to 8-azaguanine	*339*

The principal studies to date of mutation (irrespective of the provisos of the last paragraph) and transformation of mammalian cells by alkylating agents are summarized in Tables IX and X, respectively. These tables concern mainly nitroso compounds, and among simple aliphatic alkylating agents only ethyl and methyl methanesulfonates have been used so far. It was notable that the spectrum of mutations to auxotrophy in Chinese hamster ovary cells induced by the ethylating agent was different from that induced by the acridine mustard, ICR-191 (**30**), which is known to be mainly a frameshift-inducing mutagen. The ethylating agent induced mainly glycine requirement, the acridine mustard both glycine and hypoxanthine requirements. Also the ethylating agent caused chromosome breaks and chromatid exchanges to a greater extent than the acridine mustard at equal lethalities (*188, 338, 345*). Whereas while some mutations to 8-azaguanine resistance by ethyl methanesulfonate or by *N*-methyl-*N*'-nitro-*N*-nitrosoguanidine were reverted by either alkylating agent, those induced by the acridine mustard ICR-170 were not, but a few were reverted only by the acridine mustard (*347*). Most of the induced mutants, irrespective of the agent, were not revertible. It appears therefore that a minority of the mutations induced

of Mammalian Cells by Alkylating Carcinogens

Effects Observed	*References*
"morphological conversion"; converted cells induced tumors in Syrian hamsters	*348*
transformation ("criss-cross pattern of spindle cells"); transformed cells produced tumors in hamsters	*349*
transformation; tumors in hamsters	*87*
transformation; tumors in mice	*350*

in mammalian cells are single base-pair changes (347), some are frameshifts, and some are intragenic changes or deletions.

Several studies of induced mutations in mammals treated with carcinogens were done chiefly with mice (351) but these included few studies of visible mutation. In the early work of Auerbach et al. (352) treatment of the house mouse with the nitrogen mustard HN2 caused some sterility, as expected, but progeny of the treated mice included one visible mutant— "crinkled"—(353) possibly induced by the alkylating agent. With carcinogenic hydrocarbons, Strong (154) claimed to have induced coat color mutations in mice. Specific locus mutations (mainly of the coat color type) were induced in mice by triethylenemelamine (351) and by alkyl methanesulfonates (351, 355, 356). Most studies on mutagenesis in mammals with alkylating carcinogens involved detection of dominant lethals and translocations (357, 358). The principal studies are listed in Table XI.

Little appears to be known about the molecular aspects of either specific locus or dominant lethal mutations in mammals. It is generally assumed that induction of dominant lethals reflects reaction of mutagens with DNA, although, as in other systems, the process could be affected by alkylation of other cellular constituents. The relatively few studies of the alkylation of mammalian DNA in vivo by carcinogens (see the next section) support the view that alkylating carcinogens can react with DNA of target tissues, but virtually nothing is yet known about the repair response to such alkylation in the animal. It will be evident from Table XI that most alkylating agents act on spermatozoa of rodents at the postmeiotic stage, but some,

Table XI.   Induction of Dominant Lethal

Compound	Species
Methyl methanesulfonate	mouse
Ethyl methanesulfonate	mouse
	rat[a]
n-Propyl methanesulfonate	mouse
Isopropyl methanesulfonate	mouse
	rat[a]
Trimethyl phosphate	mouse
N-Methyl-N'-nitro-N-nitrosoguanidine	mouse
ICR-170 (30)	mouse
Butadiene dioxide	mouse
	mouse
Myleran (32)	mouse
TEM	mouse
	mouse
Tepa, thio Tepa (31)	mouse
Trenimon (33)	mouse
Cyclophosphamide (8)	mouse

[a] "Mutagenic" effects refer to measurements of preimplantation loss.

notably isopropyl methanesulfonate, Myleran, and triethylenemelamine (TEM), are active in meiotic and premeiotic sperm. Evidently further information will be required on metabolism of alkylating agents and other carcinogens and on the possible repair responses in the various phases of spermatogenesis before these differences can be interpreted at the molecular level (*146, 368*).

The host-mediated assay, a technique introduced fairly recently, enables mutagenic action of chemicals to be studied *in vivo* in mammals, by using microorganisms as test objects. This permits a useful correlation with mutations that were studied more intensively at the mechanistic level (*369, 370, 371*). So far, the principal test objects were histidine auxotrophs of *S. typhimurium*, a system developed mainly by Whitfield *et al.* (*372*), and conidia of *Neurospora crassa* (*373*). Using *S. typhimurium*, in the peritoneum of the mouse, Gabridge and Legator (*374*) found that *N*-methyl-*N'*-nitro-*N*-nitrosoguanidine was an active mutagen following intramuscular injection. However, this carcinogen did not give a positive result when *Neurospora* was used as indicator organism (*370*) although methyl and ethyl methanesulfonates were both active in this system.

ALKYLATION OF NUCLEIC ACIDS *In Vivo.* As previously noted, the first evidence for *in vivo* alkylation of nucleic acids was obtained by Wheeler and Skipper (*217*). They showed that the purine fraction of nucleic acid of liver and intestine of rats or mice treated with [^{14}C]methyl-labeled HN2 contained radioactivity, but the nature of the products was not determined. Subsequently several analogous studies using isotropically labeled antitumor

Mutations in Male Mammals by Alkylating Agents

Type of Cell Affected

Spermatozoa (weeks 1–2)	Spermatids (weeks 3–5)	Spermatocytes (weeks 6–8)	References
++	++	−	359, 360
++	++	−	359
++	++	−	361
++	++	−	354
+	+	++	354
+	+	++	361
++	++		362
−	−	−	359
−	−	−	359
−	−	−	363
++	+	+	364
++	−	++	364
++	++	+	365
++	++	+	364
+	+	−	363
+	+	−	366
+	+	−	367

agents were done, and in some cases nucleic acids were isolated and shown to have incorporated radioactivity. Relatively few attempts have been made so far to show that the bound products resulted from alkylation of nucleic acids *in vivo* at specific chemical sites. In view of the possibility that breakdown of the drugs and metabolic utilization of isotopic label (^{14}C or ^{3}H) could have occurred, resulting in the labeling of normal nucleic acid bases (*375, 376*), such studies must be regarded as incomplete with respect to establishing *in vivo* alkylation (*377*). Furthermore, the bound radioactivity might in some instances be present in non-nucleic acid impurities.

Isolation of radioactive bases in such *in vivo* studies and their identification with known alkylation products were first achieved by Brookes and Lawley (*1*) using ^{35}S-labeled mustard gas. The principal site of nucleic acid alkylation *in vitro* as *in vivo* was N-7 of guanine. This was confirmed using ^{14}C-labeled nitrogen mustard by Chun *et al.* (*228*). Other minor alkylation sites *in vitro* were subsequently found; in adenine, N-1, N-3, and N-7; in cytosine, N-3; and in guanine, N-3, and O-6 (*128, 232, 238, 320, 330, 378, 379*). Certain aralkylating agents can react directly with extranuclear N atoms in nucleic acids (*380*) but, with simple alkylating agents, N^6-alkyladenine production is more likely to result from the slow rearrangement of 1-alkyladenine residues.

Currently, there is interest in obtaining evidence that the minor alkylation sites are attacked *in vivo*. This may be significant with respect to mutagenesis and carcinogenesis, since some alkylated bases may be more promutagenic than others; *e.g.* induction of O^6-alkylguanines given by S_N1 reagents may cause transition mutations. At the time of writing, the formation of this base in nucleic acid of a target issue *in vivo* has been shown for N-[^{14}C]methyl-N-nitrosourea in DNA of various mouse organs (*202*) and for N-nitrosodi[^{14}C]methylamine in RNA or DNA of rat liver (*381, 382*).

A summary of results obtained, showing *in vivo* nucleic acid alkylation, or probable alkylation for those cases where products have yet to be

Table XII.   Alkylation of Nucleic Acids

Compound	Animal	Route	Tissue(s)
[^{35}S] Mustard gas	mouse	i.p.	ascites tumour
[^{35}S] Half mustard	mouse	i.p.	spleen, liver
N-Nitrosodi[^{14}C]methyl-amine[a]	rat	i.p.	liver

isolated· and identified, by various agents in whole animals is given in Table XII. In all cases so far studied where alkylation was found, it occurred in all types of cellular nucleic acid examined, e.g., ³H-labeled N-nitrosodimethylamine methylated rRNA, tRNA, and nuclear RNA (*395*) of mouse liver.

In cases where mitochondrial DNA and nuclear DNA were compared, the specific radioactivity of the mitochondrial DNA of rat or hamster livers and kidneys was somewhat higher (up to about sevenfold) with the carcinogens used [N-[^{14}C]-methyl-N-nitrosourethane (*387*), N-nitrosodi[^{14}C]methylamine (*396*)] than that of the nuclear DNA, as measured by the 7-[^{14}C]-methylguanine yields.

With regard to the possible incorporation of ^{14}C from alkylating agents into nucleic acids by metabolism through the "one-carbon pool," there is evidence that this does occur *in vivo*, giving radioactive "normal" bases (*375, 376, 381, 397*). However, the concept that 7-methylguanine formed in DNA *in vivo* could be derived from biomethylation (*398*), since it was claimed to be found in DNA isolated from cultured mammalian cells after growth in media containing ^{14}C-labeled methionine, was contraindicated by investigations of biomethylation of rat liver DNA *in vivo* (*399, 400*) and in cultured cells (*384*). Only 5-methylcytosine could be detected as a product of biomethylation in mammalian DNA, and this was never found as a product of methylation by mutagens or carcinogens.

A few studies of the stability of nucleic acids alkylated by carcinogens *in vivo* have been made. Rat liver rRNA, methylated either by N-nitrosodi-[^{14}C]methylamine or by [^{14}C]methyl methanesulfonate, had a half-life of three and a half days as measured by 7-methylguanine loss (*376*). This may be compared with the value found for this rRNA isotopically labeled with orotic acid as precursor of four to five days (*376*). Muramatsu *et al.* (*395*) considered that this difference reflected induced enhanced instability of RNA caused by methylation *in vivo*. McElhone *et al.* (*376*) considered that it

in Whole Animals—Sites of Alkylation

Nucleic Acid(s)	Site(s) of Alkylation[c]	References
RNA, DNA	N-7 of guanine	1
RNA, DNA	N-7 of guanine, N-3 of adenine	10
RNA, DNA	N-7 of guanine	126
DNA	N-7 of guanine, N-3 of adenine	383
RNA	N-7 of guanine, N-1 of adenine, N-3 of cytosine	383
rRNA	O-6, N-7 of guanine, N-1, N-3, N-7 of adenine, N-3 of cytosine	384

Table XII.

Compound	Animal	Route	Tissue(s)
N-[¹⁴C]Methyl-N-nitrosourethane	rat	intragastric i.p.	liver, stomach liver, intestines
N-[¹⁴C]Methyl-N-nitrosourea	rat	intragastric or i.v. i.p.	liver, kidney, lung, intestine, stomach, brain liver, kidney plus heart
N-Methyl-N-nitrosourea	mouse	i.p.	bone narrow, spleen thymus, kidney, liver, lung
Di[¹⁴C]methyl sulfate	rat	i.v.	liver, kidney, lung, brain
[¹⁴C]Methyl methane-sulfonate	rat rat	i.v. i.p.	liver, kidney, lung, testis, brain liver
N-Methyl-N'-nitro-N-nitrosoguanidine	rat	intragastric	stomach plus small intestine
[¹⁴C]Ethyl methane-sulfonate	rat	i.p.	kidney
N-[¹⁴C]Ethyl-N-nitrosourea	rat	i.v.	kidney
N-Nitrosodi[¹⁴C]ethyl-amine	rat	i.p.	kidney
[³H]-β-Propiolactone	mouse	skin	skin
Di(2-chloro[¹⁴C]ethyl)-methylamine (HN2)	rat	i.p.	ascites tumor
Di(2-chloroethyl)[¹⁴C]-methylamine (HN2)	rat, mouse	i.p.	liver, intestine
[¹⁴C]Myleran	mouse	i.p.	lymphoma, regenerating liver
[³H]Myleran	mouse	i.p.	liver, leukemic spleen
Tris[¹⁴C]ethyleneimino-s-triazene (TEM)	mouse	i.p.	lymphoma, regenerating liver
Di[¹⁴C]chloroethyl-p-aminophenylbutyric acid (Chlorambucil)	mouse	i.p.	lymphoma, regenerating liver
[¹⁴C]Thio Tepa	hamster	i.p.	liver, plasmacytoma
[¹⁴C]Cyclophosphamide	hamster	i.p.	plasmacytoma
[³H]Aniline mustard	mouse rat	i.p. s.c.	myeloma ascites tumor
[⁴H]Naphthylamine mustard	mouse	i.p.	myeloma

ᵃ Several other studies with nitrosamines have been reported; those selected here are for comparison with other alkylating carcinogens.

Continued

Nucleic Acid(s)	Site(s) of Alkylation[c]	References
RNA, DNA	N-7 of guanine	385
RNA, DNA	N-7 of guanine	386
RNA, DNA	N-7 of guanine	203
tRNA, rRNA nucDNA, mitDNA	N-7 of guanine	387
DNA	O-6, N-7 of guanine, N-3 of adenine	202
RNA, DNA	N-7 guanine	203
RNA, DNA	N-7 of guanine	203
RNA	N-7 of guanine, N-1 of adenine, N-3 of cytosine	388
rRNA	N-7 of guanine, (trace of O-6?) N-1, N-3, N-7 of adenine, N-3 of cytosine	381
DNA[b]	N-7 of guanine	389
DNA	N-7 of guanine	390
DNA	N-7 of guanine	390
DNA	N-7 of guanine	390
RNA, DNA	N-7 of guanine	307, 308
DNA	N-7 of guanine	228
NA purines	n.d.	217
RNA, DNA	n.d.	391
RNA, DNA	n.d.	10
RNA, DNA	n.d.	391
RNA, DNA	n.d.	391
DNA	n.d.	392
DNA	n.d.	392
RNA, DNA	n.d.	393
DNA	n.d.	394
RNA, DNA	n.d.	393

[b] DNA was prelabeled *in vivo* using [^{14}C] formate.
[c] n.d. = not determined; some radioactivity may have been incorporated metabolically.

reflected reutilization of labeled precursors from the orotic acid-labeled RNA and that the half-life as measured by the disappearance rate of the [^{14}C]methyl label from RNA was the true measure of its turnover rate.

Induced instability of polyribosomes of rat liver following *in vivo* treatment with *N*-nitrosodimethylamine was reported (*401, 402*), and it was suggested that degradation of methylated mRNA had occurred. This could in turn be ascribed to direct chemical action through phosphotriester formation; or to enzymatic action. Comparable studies with a carcinogen such as dimethyl sulfate, which does not appear to degrade RNA by direct chemical action, might help to elucidate this question.

Loss of 7-methylguanine from rat liver DNA methylated *in vivo* by *N*-nitrosodi[^{14}C]methylamine was somewhat more rapid than by hydrolysis from methylated DNA *in vitro*. Craddock (*403*) reported a half-life of about two to three days for the *in vivo* loss following administration of 1–2 mg/kg of the carcinogen, but noted that at higher dosage of 26 mg/kg the half-life was shorter, probably reflecting tissue necrosis.

Whether this loss reflects enzymatic excision of 7-methylguanine is thus not yet clear. Such a phenomenon would, however, be more convincingly indicated if specific excisions of alkylated bases could be shown, especially of those not lost by hydrolysis from alkylated DNA at neutral pH.

Recently, evidence for specific excision *in vivo* of certain methylation products was found for liver DNA of rats injected with *N*-nitrosodi[^{14}C]-methylamine (*382*). These findings parallel those reported for excision of products from DNA of *E. coli* treated with *N*-[^{14}C]methyl-*N'*-nitro-*N*-nitrosoguanadine (*191*). The order of ease of removal is: 3-methyladenine $> O^6$-methylguanine removed with a half-life of 13 hr $>$ material associated with pyrimidine nucleotides, including possibly phosphotriesters $>$ 7-methylguanine.

It now seems likely that these specific depurinations from DNA methylated *in vivo* by carcinogens are mediated by the enzyme endonuclease II which was partially purified from *E. coli* by Kirtikar and Goldthwait (*289*). It is also indicated to be present in rat liver (personal communication from D. A. Goldthwait).

Analogous removal of the ethylated purines 3-ethyladenine and O^6-ethylguanine occurred from DNA of various organs of rats treated with *N*-ethyl-*N*-nitrosourea. The removal rate of O^6-ethylguanine was significantly slower from DNA of a target organ—the brain of the 10-day-old rat—than from DNA of liver, an organ not susceptible to tumor induction by this agent (*404*).

Other cases of specific excisions from DNA of alkylated bacteria include 3-alkyladenine derived from half sulfur mustard (*405*) and extranuclear *N*-aralkyl derivatives derived from 7-bromomethylbenz[*a*]anthracene (*406*), N^2-aralkylguanine being lost more rapidly than N^6-aralkyladenine or N^4-aralkylcytosine. It is not yet known whether analogous excisions occur *in vivo* from animal DNA with these or other alkylating agents.

Using human lymphocytes *in vitro*, Lieberman and Dipple (*407*) found that N^6-benzanthranylmethyladenine was excised more rapidly than the amino-*N*-alkylated guanine or cytosine, which is a different specificity pattern from that found for the same alkylating agent in *E. coli* by Venitt and Tarmy (*406*).

Studies on the action of certain nucleases on methylated DNA (*408*) led to the conclusion that extensive methylation had little inhibitory effect on an alkaline deoxyribonuclease from rat liver or pancreatic deoxyribonuclease I, but the activity of an acid deoxyribonuclease was diminished. Methylated DNA was completely degraded by snake venom exonuclease. The effects of other alkylating agents in this respect have not been studied at all extensively, although the nitrogen mustard HN2, (again at high extents of alkylation of DNA), did protect to some extent against the action of deoxyribonuclease *in vitro* (*392*).

In view of the reports that alkylation stimulates DNA repair in mammalian cells and that specific excisions occur *in vivo*, it would appear that nucleases specific for alkylated DNA must exist, but these have evidently yet to be isolated, apart from the case of endonuclease II already mentioned (*289*).

With regard to extent and time course of nucleic acid alkylations *in vivo*, the data available refer mainly to methylated DNA and to the principal product 7-methylguanine. These data are summarized in Table XIII.

Some quantitative specificity of reaction between various classes of nucleic acid is evident, but, as previously noted, in no case so far reported has alkylation been confined to any one type of nucleic acid. It seems unlikely therefore that the distribution of monoalkyl groups chemically induced within any nucleic acid molecule should depart markedly from a random attack or that it should, for example, depend on base sequence in any marked fashion.

At the time of writing, no study of the detailed distribution of induced monoalkyl groups in the base sequence of DNA has been reported. Pegg (*409*) investigated the pattern of oligonucleotides derived from partial enzymatic digestion of tRNA methylated with *N*-methyl-*N*-nitrosourea and found all guanine sites equally susceptible to methylation at the N-7 atom. This atom is sterically available in the "wide groove" of a double helix of the Watson–Crick type, so that this finding is not unexpected. It remains possible that alkylation sites that are involved in Watson–Crick hydrogen bonding, such as N-3 of cytosine, N-1 of adenine, and O-6 of guanine, might show a reactivity dependence on base sequence, but no studies relevant to this possibility have been reported yet.

The situation with regard to difunctional alkylation is, of course, rather different. Whereas attachment of the first "arm" of a difunctional agent at the N-7 position of guanine in DNA might occur in random fashion, the possibility of completion of difunctional reaction with DNA, as opposed to hydrolysis of the second "arm," might seem likely to depend on base sequence. A simple hypothesis was proposed by Brookes and Lawley (*116*) based on consideration of the Watson–Crick model. This hypothesis predicted that interstrand cross-linkage would be favored by the sequence GpC on either DNA strand; intrastrand linkage would be favored by GpG in that strand. Chun *et al.* (*228*) analyzed DNA from mouse Ehrlich ascites tumor

Table XIII.   Extents of Alkylation of

Compound	Animal	Route	Dose mg/kg	µC₁/kg	Tissue
N-Nitrosodi[¹⁴C]methylamine[c]	rat	i.p.	1	33.2	liver
			2	11.7	liver
			26	8.0	liver
	rat	i.p.	31	325	liver
			31	325	kidney
	rat	i.p.	2	90	liver
	hamster	i.p.	31	325	liver
	hamster	i.p.	31	325	kidney
	rat	i.p.	27	86	liver
			27	86	kidney
N-[¹⁴C]Methyl-nitrosourea	rat	i.v.	90	39	liver
					kidney
	rat	i.p.	43.3	700	liver
[¹⁴C]Methyl-methanesulfonate	rat	i.v.	120	33	liver
					kidney
					liver
					kidney
					testis
	rat	i.p.	50	46	liver
	rat	i.p.	54	350	liver
N-Methyl-N'-nitro-N-nitrosoguanidine[f]	rat	intragastric	273[f]	—[f]	liver
					stomach +ileum
N-Nitrosodi[1-¹⁴C]ethylamine	rat	i.p.	250	1560	liver
					kidney
					lung

Nucleic Acids *in vivo* by Carcinogens

Time[a] (hr)	Extent of Alkylation (mmole/mole NA-P)[b]				References
	7-alkylguanine		Other		
	RNA	DNA	RNA	DNA	
5		0.07			*403*
50		0.04			
5		0.11			
50		0.06			
5		1.8			
50		0.3			
5		1.3 (nuc)[d]			*396*
		6.6 (mit)[d]			
5		0.17 (nuc)[d]			
		0.70 (mit)[d]			
5	0.27[e]	0.11	1-MeAde, 0.004	0.001	*381, 382*
			3-MeAde, 0.0008	0.003	
			7-MeAde, 0.004	0.001	
			3-MeCyt, 0.010	0.001	
			O^6-MeGua, 0.010	0.008	
5		2.0 (nuc)[d]			*396*
		7.6 (mit)[d]			
5		0.33 (nuc)[d]			
		2.0 (mit)[d]			
5	4.0	1.9			*203*
5	0.54	0.23			
4	0.51	0.26			*203*
4	0.44	0.24			
6		0.12 (nuc)[d]			*387*
		0.26 (mit)[d]			
4	0.37	0.45			*203*
4	0.34	0.50			
16	0.18	0.23			
16	0.17	0.24			
16	0.09	0.11			
4	0.10[e]	0.11	1-MeAde, 0.013	0.0015	*381, 382*
			3-MeAde, 0.002	0.018	
			7-MeAde, 0.001	0.0011	
			3-MeCyt, 0.0012	0.0006	
			3-MeGua, —	0.0008	
2	0.13				*388*
24	0.13				*389*
8		0.44			*389*
8		0.66			
24	0.085	0.075			*390*
24	0.022	0.018			
24	0.005	0.015			

Table XIII.

| | | | Dose | | |
Compound	Animal	Route	mg/kg	μC₁/kg	Tissue
N-[2-¹⁴C]Ethyl-N-nitrosourea	rat	i.v.	150	220	liver kidney lung brain
[1-¹⁴C]Ethyl-methanesulfonate	rat	i.p.	270	920	liver kidney lung ileum brain

ᵃ Time of isolation of NA (generally after administration of single dose of carcinogen). Generally maximal alkylation was achieved after about 2–5 hr. For details of time-course the original references should be consulted.

ᵇ Extents of alkylation are expressed per mole NA–P, or average nucleotide unit, of MW 337 for animal DNA. In some cases literature data are quoted as % guanine converted to 7-alkylguanine. Values of 0.22 for the molar proportion of guanine per DNA P and of 0.34 for rat liver rRNA have been assumed to convert these to mmoles 7-alkylguanine per mole DNA P. It should not be assumed that absence of entries for other bases in this table necessarily implies their absence in the nucleic acids analyzed.

alkylated *in vivo* by ¹⁴C-labeled HN2 and found that 25% of the products were of the diguaninyl type and 7–8% gave interstrand cross-links. They assumed that the nearest neighbor frequencies were the same as for calf-thymus DNA, *i.e.*, that the proportion of guanines in GpG sequences was 22.3% and in GpC 11.5%. The predicted ratio of inter- to intra-strand linkages is thus about 0.5 and in reasonable agreement with that found.

Differential staining of chromosomes of both plant and animal cells using fluorochromes, including several acridine mustards such as "quinacrine mustard" (ICR-50a), "propyl quinacrine mustard" (ICR-49), and "propyl quinacrine half mustard" (ICR-170) (for formulae, *see* 30), was reported by Caspersson *et al.* (410), and it is now a well established example of mutagen binding specificity. The reasons for this specificity are not yet clear, but it seems likely that the physical interaction of the quinoline moiety of the fluorochromes is the principal factor involved, since covalent binding by the mustard moiety is not essential for the effect. An approximate correlation between fluorescent bands and regions of maximal induced chromosome breakage was found in the M-chromosome of *Vicia*; these are the hetero-chromatic regions, which are also susceptible to alkylating agents in general.

It is thus possible that chromosome structure may determine regions of preferential chemical attack by alkylating agents, either in general or, more particularly, those containing aromatic or heterocyclic moieties. In this connection, the evidence obtained by the Fahmys, showing specific loci of induced small deletion mutations, might be consistent with such specificity of reaction, since the heterochromatin of the *Drosophila* chromosome studied was involved and since the compounds studied contained aromatic or hetero-

Continued

Extent of Alkylation $(mmole/mole\ NA\text{-}P)^b$

$Time^a$ (hr)	7-alkylguanine		Other		References
	RNA	DNA	RNA	DNA	
2	0.006	0.009			390
2	0.006	0.007			
2	0.005	0.007			
2	0.006	0.007			
17	0.08	0.10			390
17	0.10	0.09			
17	0.09	0.10			
17	0.08	0.11			
17	0.13	0.08			

[c] This compilation of data for N-nitrosodimethylamine is not exhaustive but is included for comparison with other alkylating carcinogens.

[d] (nuc) denotes nuclear DNA, total MW of the order of 10^{10} nucleotide units; (mit) mitochondrial DNA, 1.4×10^4 nucleotides, 0.194 guanines per DNA-P.

[e] Refers to ribosomal RNA, MW about 7×10^3 nucleotide units. In other cases, where rRNA was not isolated, a value of 0.34 for the molar proportion of guanine, *i.e.*, equal to that of rRNA, has been assumed.

[f] The carcinogen was administered in five doses of 55 mg/kg at intervals during 8 hr prior to killing. The DNA of the animals was prelabeled using [^{14}C] formate.

cyclic moieties. However, the acridine mustards were not particularly potent carcinogens in the test system of Shimkin *et al.* (*31*), so that a superficial correlation between chromosome binding in certain test systems and carcinogenesis is not warranted. This does not, of course, rule out the possibility of specificity of alkylation of certain chromosomal regions in the animal cells in which tumors can be induced, and further studies in this area are desirable.

With regard to the reported preferential methylation of mitochondrial, as opposed to nuclear, DNA by the carcinogens N-nitrosodimethylamine and N-methyl-N-nitrosourea (*387, 396*), the relative extents of reaction per nucleotide unit of DNA were around fivefold greater for mitochondrial DNA. After a relatively high dose of N-nitrosodimethylamine (31mg/kg) the extent of the reaction of this DNA in rat liver was of the order of 100 molecules 7-methylguanine per molecule of mitochondrial DNA and of the order of 10 molecules in rat kidney mitochondrial DNA. It is not clear at present how general this preferential attack is for other carcinogens. Also there does not appear to be evidence for the concept that chemical agents specific for their effects on mitochondrial DNA, such as ethidium (*34*) (*411*), are carcinogenic. However, the methylating carcinogen, N-methyl-N'-nitro-N-nitrosoguanidine, was noted early as a potent inducer of cytoplasmic mutation involving deletion of DNA-containing organelles such as chloroplasts of *Euglena* (*412*).

With regard to the somatic mutation hypothesis in its original form, it is clear from Table XIII that multiple alkylations of nuclear DNA in target organs can result from the *in vivo* action of carcinogens. Assessment of the likelihood that these will cause somatic mutations might be derived from data relating mutational frequency extent and mode of DNA alkylation in mammalian cell systems. This has yet to be achieved, although as previously mentioned, the rather scanty dose-response data available suggest that "no-effect thresholds" are unlikely for cultured cells, although they cannot be ruled out. If they exist, they would presumably reflect complete "repair" of promutational lesions in DNA. Such a repair mechanism would be "error-free," and available evidence suggests that "excision repair" is more likely than other mechanisms to approximate to this requirement.

The question of "promotion" of initiated (mutated ?) cells then remains. As previously mentioned, this might involve stimulation of cell division, possibly with inhibition of repair mechanisms as a contributory factor. For example, if cells were to replicate their DNA prior to excision of promutational groups, this might lead to deleterious fixation of altered DNA base sequences.

This raises a further question concerning the relevance of studies of the action of carcinogens on cultured mammalian cells to their *in vivo* effects. The pattern of initial alkylation of DNA in cultured cells appears to be closely similar to that for *in vivo* alkylation. However, evidence for specific excision of certain methylation products, such as O^6-methylguanine, from DNA methylated by N-methyl-N'-nitro-N-nitrosoguanidine or by methyl methanesulfonate was not found for the HeLa S3 or V79-379a cell lines (413). On the other hand, specific removal of 3-methyladenine from DNA of N-methyl-N-nitrosourea-treated HeLa cells (but not from mouse L cells) was recently reported by Walker and Ewart (414). If such specific excisions play a part in preventing mutation fixation by removing induced promutational groups prior to DNA replication, their absence in certain cultured cell systems might result in a relatively high rate of induced mutation at a given extent of alkylation of cellular DNA. It might then be misleading to assume that a similar somatic mutation rate would arise *in vivo* at the same extent of DNA alkylation, if mammalian cells in their natural milieu possessed more effective mechanisms for removing promutational groups.

With regard to the promutational effectiveness of various induced alkylated groups in DNA, the relationship between the structure of these groups and the Watson–Crick hydrogen-bonding scheme has already been discussed. As shown by Table XIII, few studies of the minor products derived from DNA alkylation *in vivo* have been reported yet, either with regard to their extent of formation or their possible enzymatic removal. The influence of the nature of the chemical structure of the alkylating carcinogens on the nature and distribution of alkylation products *in vivo* as so far revealed is that these reflect the chemical reactivities of the carcinogens or ultimate carcinogens *in vitro*. Thus the relative proportions of O^6-alkylguanine in the nucleic acid alkylation products *in vivo* are greater for N-nitrosodimethylamine which is thought to act through the methyldiazonium ion, than for methyl methanesulfonate (384, 397). Clearly further studies of minor alkylation products induced *in vivo* by other alkylating carcinogens are desirable.

With regard to minor alkylation products induced in RNA *in vivo*, these might affect the function of the various molecular species of RNA in certain cases. The type of RNA most likely to be affected is messenger RNA. However, there is no direct evidence for its alkylation because of the difficulties in isolating this material in sufficient quantity. On the reasonable assumption that it is alkylated to the same extent as the bulk of cellular RNA, Venitt *et al.* (*415*) deduced that mRNA for β-galactosidase in *E. coli* was inactivated by a few alkylations per molecule by mustard gas or the corresponding half mustard. Shooter *et al.* (*244*) found that of the few alkylations per molecule of viral RNA necessary to inactivate bacteriophage μ2, those that prevented Watson–Crick hydrogen bonding were probably effective, *i.e.*, formation of 7-alkylguanine was not a lethal event, unless cross-linkage was involved. These data can, therefore, accord with the concept that the template function of a single-stranded RNA of the mRNA type is particularly vulnerable to alkylation since virtually all alkylations, apart from mono-alkylation at N-7 of guanine, appear to cause inactivation. This result may be contrasted with the observations that bacteriophage containing double-stranded DNA is relatively resistant to mono-alkylation, although a few depurinations subsequent to alkylation can inactivate (*219, 416*). The possible role of mRNA inactivation *in vivo* by carcinogens would clearly involve inhibition of protein synthesis (*402*) although the significance of this with regard to tumor induction remains unknown.

Biomethylation of RNA is of course a well established phenomenon, and several investigators, following Borek (*166, 167, 417*), proposed that abnormal methylations or other alkylations of RNA caused by carcinogens may play a significant part in the induction of tumors in which enhancement of tRNA methylase activity appears to be a common feature. This effect was also positively associated with morphological conversion of cultured cells by *N*-methyl-*N*-nitrosourea *in vitro* (*418*). No obvious mechanism by which such enhancement could be related to *in vivo* RNA methylation, or alkylation in general by carcinogens has been revealed yet. The base sequence in RNA could be altered in heritable fashion by induced somatic mutations in RNA-coding genes.

It is also conceivable that chemically modified cellular RNA could be "mutated" to a form that stimulated its activity as a template for RNA-directed DNA polymerase, the type of enzyme associated with RNA tumor viruses (*419*), but this is speculative. Presumably mRNA would be the most likely type of cellular template to be involved.

Studies of the effects of chemical methylation by dimethyl sulfate on the *in vitro* functional activity of transfer RNA's from *E. coli* were made by Pillinger *et al.* (*420*) and by Hay *et al.* (*421*). About 10 methylations of various tRNA molecules inactivated their abilities to accept amino acids and to function in an *in vitro* polypeptide synthesizing system. Such alkylation levels are statistically unlikely to occur as a result of alkylation by carcinogens *in vivo* since *t*RNA is a relatively small target of about 85 nucleotide units and is not specifically susceptible to alkylation. In a study of the methylation of mouse liver RNA *in vivo* by *N*-nitrosodi[³H]methylamine, *e.g.* Muramatsu *et al.* (*395*) reported ratios of methylation at N-7 of guanine of 1.2 : 1.0 : 1.8 for 28s, 18s, and 4s RNA respectively. However, since the spectrum of alkylated chemical sites depends on the nature of the agent, it remains possible that other chemical carcinogens could be more effective as inactivators of RNA.

A further conceivable effect of tRNA alkylation could be the ultimate generation of alkylated nucleosides with some sort of growth stimulatory activity, analogous to that of cytokinins (422). In this respect, N^6-substituted adenosines are the most potent structural types. As already noted, extra-nuclear N-atoms of nucleic acid bases are directly attacked by certain aralkylating agents (380). Otherwise, the slow rearrangement of 1-alkyl-adenosine residues (232) could result in the formation of such N^6-alkyladeno-sines in RNA. Although it is an intriguing possibility, involvement of pseudo-cytokinins in carcinogenesis is a highly speculative mechanism about which little is known for mammalian as opposed to plant cells.

In summary, regarding possible effects of nucleic acid alkylation *in vivo* in target tissues of carcinogens, the older hypothesis of somatic mutation must receive some support from quantitative measurements of such alkyla-tion. So far, in every substantiated case alkylation of DNA in a target tissue has been shown to occur. This conclusion may not apply to N-nitrosodi-methylamine, which is claimed to cause tumors in the liver of rainbow trout without ability to methylate either nucleic acid or protein in this organ (423). However, the number of quantitative estimates of the extent of such alkylation is still small, and questions can cogently be raised with regard to the relationships between extent and mode of DNA alkylation and tumor induction in specific tissues.

In view of the relatively small amount of data available, the relative lack of knowledge of DNA repair *in vivo*, and the dose–relationships for induced mutagenesis in mamalian systems (which, as noted, may not be the same for cells *in vivo* as for cultured cells *in vitro*), it seems premature at this time to assess this problem in too much detail. Some authors have already, apparently, discounted any relationship between DNA or RNA alkylation and carcinogenesis, at least for alkylnitrosamides and dialkyl-nitrosamides. For example, Schoental (386) stated that "the finding that N-methyl-N-nitrosourethane, a carcinogen that does not induce liver tumors, yet methylates guanine at the 7-position in DNA and RNA of rat liver, indicates that this reaction cannot be significant for the initiation of carcinogenesis." Similar conclusions were reached by Krüger *et al.* (424) who used N-methyl-N-nitrosourea and by Lijinsky and Ross (425) and Lijinsky *et al.* (426) who used various nitrosamines.

This type of argument may be regarded as inconclusive, however, by analogy with other biological actions of alkylating agents in which the molecular mechanisms are more clearly defined than for the carcinogenic process. Such an action is mutagenesis, in which few would doubt that DNA alkylation plays an essential role. It is plausible to assume that inhibi-tion of some key cellular protein, such as a repair enzyme or polymerase enzyme, might enhance mutation rate, but here again alkylation of a macromolecular cellular constituent would have to be invoked. For induction of mutations in extracellularly treated bacteriophage, alkylation of DNA seems the only reasonable causative process. As mentioned before, the available data suggest that no simple relationship need exist between extent or mode of alkylation of target DNA and the presumed-consequent induced mutation rate, when various test systems are compared for their response to various alkylating agents. For example, methylation or ethylation of T-even bacteriophages to about the same extents as measured by lethal effects can yield widely different mutation frequencies in progeny of phage alkylated by various agents (*206*). If the interpretation of dose–response in such an apparently relatively simple system is admitted to be complex, it is perhaps sanguine to expect simple relationships to hold for tumor induction.

Among obvious deviations from a simple positive correlation between extent of DNA alkylation and carcinogenic activity may be quoted those found for various methylating and ethylating agents by Swann and Magee (*204, 370*) (see Table XIV). These may be summarized as follows:

1. Methylation of DNA does not necessarily lead to carcinogenesis, *e.g.*, for various agents in rat liver or for methyl methanesulfonate in any organ of the rat except brain.

2. Comparisons of extents of ethylation, as opposed to methylation, at the doses giving comparable tumor yields show that ethylation is generally more effective. However, only ethylation at N-7 of guanine has been estimated so far; extents of alkylation at other chemical sites in DNA are not yet known.

3. Among ethylating carcinogens, the nitrosamides or nitrosamines tested were effective carcinogens at much lower extents of DNA ethylation of rat kidney than was ethyl methanesulfonate. Here also differences in the spectra of reaction products are expected in view of the probable involvement of the ethyldiazonium ion for the nitroso compounds. In agreement with this view, Goth and Rajewsky (*404*) recently found that the ratio of ethylation by *N*-ethyl-*N*-nitrosourea at O-6 of guanine in DNA to that at N-7 is higher (about 0.6) than that found for corresponding methylations by *N*-methyl-*N*-nitrosourea (about 0.1) (*134*).

The distribution of the alkyl groups—*e.g.*, relative extents of reaction of mitochondrial as opposed to nuclear DNA (except for the cases noted in Table XIII), or in certain types of cells in a tissue as opposed to others, or at the level of distribution within the various chromosomal regions—are also not known.

The balance of this type of evidence, however, incomplete though it may be, makes it improbable that any simple positive correlation will emerge between tumor induction in a given tissue and overall alkylation of even a specific chemical site in DNA, such as the supposedly promutational O-6 atom of guanine. This provisional conclusion is not perhaps surprising in view of the multistage hypotheses of carcinogenesis. The initiation phase could still be positively correlated with extent of induction of promutational DNA alkylations, but the separation of the process of carcinogenesis into the proposed stages is difficult, especially for internal tissues.

From another viewpoint, the question may be posed whether alkylation of DNA *in vivo* indicates a carcinogenic hazard. With regard to the com-

Table XIV.   Extents of Alkylation of Nucleic Acid in Tissues of the Same or Nearly the Same Dose and Mutagenic Activity (for Alkylating

Compound	Dose (mg/kg)	Route	Tissue
Methyl methanesulfonate	120	i.v.	liver
			kidney
			brain
Dimethyl sulfate	80	i.v.	liver
			kidney
			brain
N-Nitrosodimethylamine	27	i.p.	liver
			kidney
N-Methyl-N-nitrosourea	90	i.v.	liver
			kidney
			intestine
			brain
Ethyl methanesulfonate	270	i.p.	liver
			kidney
			brain
N-Nitrosodiethylamine	250	i.p.	liver
			kidney
N-Ethyl-N-nitrosourea	152	i.v.	liver
			kidney

[a] From Refs. 203 and 390 for alkylation and carcinogenesis data; from Ref. 206 for mutagenesis data.

[b] Weak mutagenic activity for T-even phage was claimed by Bautz and Freese (427) and confirmed by J. W. Drake (personal communication); Loveless (303) classified methyl methanesulfonate as non-mutagenic in this type of test; the compound is certainly markedly less active than the ethyl analog or the N-alkyl-N-nitrosoureas considered here.

pounds so far examined in detail, evidently no clear-cut positive answer can be given. However, the ability of a compound to alkylate DNA *in vivo* certainly should stimulate investigation of its carcinogenic potency. The greater effectiveness in certain cases (*e.g.*, N-nitrosodimethylamine in liver and ethyl methanesulfonate in kidney) of continuous or multiple dosages should be remembered in this regard. Possibly maintenance of a certain low level of alkylation *in vivo* for a prolonged period might be a greater carcinogenic hazard in some cases than an equivalent single large dose; but only the latter treatment might lead to an easily detectable extent of DNA alkylation.

Alkylating Agents and Cancer in Humans

Since, in general, the alkylating agents are obviously toxic compounds, few examples of human exposure to any specific compound in doses sufficient to cause significant biological effects would be expected. The principal areas in which such exposure could occur are those of industrial or labora-

**Rat Compared with Carcinogenic Activity in Those Tissues, at the
Extracellularly Treated Bacteriophage) of Various
Carcinogens**[a]

Extent of Alkylation (% Guanine at N-7)		Yield of Tumors (No. of Tumors/	Mutagenic Action
RNA	DNA	No. of Rats)	Bacteriophage T2
0.053	0.09	0/16	—[b]
0.051	0.096	0/16	—
n.d.	0.105	3/20	—
0.007	0.008	0/9	n.d.
0.010	0.014	0/9	n.d.
n.d.	0.046	0/9	n.d.
1.16	0.87	0/15[d]	n.d.[c]
0.16	0.106	3/15	n.d.
0.15	0.12	0/16	+
0.13	0.11	7/16	+
0.12	0.095	5/16	+
n.d.	0.085	1/16	+
0.024	0.045	0/22	+
0.031	0.041	0/22[e]	+
		(12/24)[e]	
0.038	0.038	1/22	+
0.025	0.034	0/14	n.d.[c]
0.007	0.008	6/14[f]	n.d.
0.002	0.004	0/17[g]	+
0.002	0.0034	7/17[g]	+

[c] Mutagenic action of N-nitrosodialkylamines would not be expected in microorganisms incapable of generating alkylating agents therefrom by oxidative metabolism.

[d] Carcinogenic for rat liver when administered by continuous feeding in water.

[e] Not carcinogenic when administered as single dose. Tumor yield in brackets refers to three successive doses. Mesenchymal tumors.

[f] Epithelial cell tumors.

[g] Data from Druckrey *et al.* (*428*). Dosage, 80 mg/kg (oral) to 30-day old rats. Mesenchymal tumors.

tory usage of alkylating agents and the administration of such agents in chemotherapy, particularly as antineoplastic drugs. A third possibility must be considered, that pesticides or other environmental chemicals may have alkylating potential or that they could be converted to alkylating agents in the environment or by metabolism. Prolonged exposures to small dose levels of weakly active compounds, although difficult to detect and assess, might be the most likely source of alkylating compounds to the total carcinogenic hazard of the environment. For these reasons, sufficient reliable dose–response data should be amassed for alkylating, as for other, carcinogens, to reasonably extrapolate to environmental exposure levels.

Relatively weak carcinogenic activity for individual alkylating agents does not necessarily indicate that their status as a carcinogenic hazard in totality is negligible. Evidence was presented (*429, 430, 431*) that sub-carcinogenic doses of chemical agents given together may produce at least an additive effect. This "syncarcinogenesis" did appear, however, to apply only to carcinogens which act on the same tissues. For example, the known hepatocarcinogens N-nitrosodiethylamine and N,N-dimethyl-4-phenylazoaniline (4-dimethylaminoazobenzene) were syncarcinogens for rat liver (431). The nitrosamine and 4-stilbenamine gave an additive effect on liver, for which both are effective carcinogens, but not on the auditory canal, a tissue in which only the stilbenamine induced tumors (430). The additive effects observed also correlate with the known reaction sites of the carcinogens, mediated by their appropriate metabolites, with DNA of the respective tissues, e.g., nitrosamines (203, 390) and the azo-dye (117, 432, 433). It is possible, therefore, that syncarcinogenesis reflects the additive effect of the totality of unrepaired lesions in the appropriate DNA targets, irrespective of their chemical nature.

It is generally impracticable to determine whether chemical carcinogens react in vivo with human DNA, although, for the reasons already discussed, this seems certain to occur with directly acting compounds such as alkylating agents. The hepatocarcinogen, 2-fluorenylacetamide, which requires metabolic activation through N-hydroxylation to potentiate its in vivo reaction with DNA of rat liver (434), also undergoes this key metabolic step in man (435). The antitumor drug DIC [4(5)-(3,3-dimethyl-1-triazeneimidazole 5(4)-carboxamide] similarly yielded isotopically labeled 7-methylguanine in urine after administration of the [^{14}C]methyl-labeled compound to humans (136). Again this indicates by analogy with animal experiments, that the appropriate metabolic activation through oxidative N-demethylation (see Schemes 4 and 5) had occurred to yield an in vivo-alkylating intermediate.

It may be concluded tentatively, therefore, that additivity of effects of small subcarcinogenic doses of chemical carcinogens, whether directly acting or metabolically activated, would be anticipated in humans as in experimental animals. Clearly, research to detect early effects of carcinogens in man requires further attention if progress is to be made in assessing this possibility quantitatively.

The question now arises, whether the lesions induced by the initiating action of chemical carcinogens and not relatively rapidly repaired by appropriate early defense mechanisms such as the DNA repair systems already mentioned will remain as a permanent potential source of initiated tissues, perhaps to be subject to the subsequent phases of carcinogenesis including promotion and progression. As previously pointed out, the irreversibility of the initiation phase which is possibly consistent with its nature as involving potential somatic mutation, has been accepted as one of the principal features distinguishing this phase from promotion, which is generally found to have some degree of reversibility (436, 437, Chapter 2).

However, recent evidence from experiments using the mouse skin system, for which the two-stage scheme of carcinogenesis in its classical form (438) was developed, showed that some degree of reversibility of tumor initiation can be detected (439). In this work, 7,12-dimethylbenz[a]anthracene was used as initiator and a phorbol ester as promoting agent. Generalization from these findings was subject to the proviso that the papillomas obtained are subject to regression.

In summary, it may be speculated that alkylating agents could induce potential tumor-initiating chemical lesions in human tissues and that these may be subject to repair processes, both relatively rapidly after their initial induction (such as action of DNA repair enzymes) and subsequently by as yet less defined mechanisms.

The available evidence for carcinogenesis and allied effects in humans by alkylating agents must now be discussed and currently suspected environmental hazards attributable to such compounds assessed.

Industrial Exposure to Alkylating Agents. The classical case of cancer caused by an industrial alkylating chemical is the induction of neoplasia of the respiratory tract by mustard gas, the agent commonly regarded as the first established chemical mutagen. The use of this compound as a war gas during 1914–1918 led to numerous exposures, but statistical analysis of data relating these exposures to cancer deaths did not establish causality conclusively (*440, 441*). The more prolonged exposures suffered by workers in a mustard gas plant in Okuno-jima, Japan, during 1929–1945 were associated with a significant incidence of respiratory neoplasia. Among 322 males who had worked with mustard gas, 33 deaths from such neoplasms (30 of which were histologically confirmed) were traced for 1948–1966 (*442*). The expected number based on mortality rates for males with the same age distribution is 0.9. Neoplasms of the squamous or undifferentiated cell type occurred along the main airways of the respiratory tract, tongue, pharynx, sphenoidal sinus, larynx, trachea, and bronchi. No adenocarcinomas were found. There was a similarity between the fiindings for mustard gas and those for induced neoplasia in uranium miners, which is consistent with the known "radiomimetic" character of the alkylating agent.

The epidemiology of lung cancer was reviewed by Berg (*443*) who concluded that adenocarcinoma predominates in nonsmokers, and this may therefore be taken as the typical "spontaneous" type of tumor at this site. In cases attributed to industrial exposure, asbestos appeared to cause this type of tumor. This may support the concept that this agent is a promoting rather than an initiating agent. Otherwise, industrial exposure was associated with increased incidence of squamous cell and oat cell carcinoma, which is compatible with the observations for tumor induction by mustard gas.

Druckrey *et al.* (*444*) reported that one. case of human cancer could plausibly be attributed to industrial exposure to another alkylating agent, dimethyl sulfate. The latent period was 11 years, and the age at death in this case was 47 years. The carcinoma was characterized histologically as being of the oat cell type and was sited in the upper respiratory tract. Dimethyl sulfate has also proved carcinogenic in model experiments using an inhalation technique in the rat (*151*), where squamous nasal carcinoma was induced.

In the chemical industry, as in the research laboratory, many compounds are in common use that present possible carcinogenic hazards. In fact, any alkylating agent should be used under carefully controlled conditions where contact or ingestion is effectively ruled out. Alkyl halides and sulfates; diazomethane and its precursors, including N-methylnitrosamides; ethyleneimines; and reactive lactones, including β-propiolactone, are obvious examples. Extensive relevant surveys of the industrial usages of alkylating agents are available, notably in the recent publications of Fishbein *et al.* (25) and Fishbein (445).

Less obviously reactive esters, such as trimethyl phosphate, may also be regarded as a potential hazard. This quite widely used industrial chemical induced dominant lethal mutations in mice (362) and alkylated and degraded DNA *in vitro* (446). It has not been tested for carcinogenic potency, but some alkyl phosphates have been claimed to be positively carcinogenic (*see* Table XIX).

Carcinogenesis tests of groups of compounds have appeared which reflect particularly the recognition of the possible hazards of their industrial use. Weil *et al.* (447) studied an extensive series of epoxides, and more detailed investigations of selected compounds of this type were carried out by Van Duren *et al.* (448). Walpole (449) reviewed early work on ethyleneimines with some reference to epoxides. The reviews of carcinogenesis by lactones compiled by Dickens (108, 113, 450) and Van Duuren (448) are relevant in part to their industrial use. It seems likely that more tests will involve oral administration (451) or inhalation techniques, since they are more relevant to assessment of environmental hazards than the classical tests using skin painting or injections, which at present constitute almost all the available data for alkylating carcinogens.

Much early work in this area was devoted to the study of the simpler halogenated alkanes, which include widely used industrial solvents. For the choloromethanes, toxicity to mice was positively correlated with ease of hydrolysis in the order $CH_3Cl > CHCl_3 > CCl_4 > CH_2Cl_2$ (452) and might reflect the involvement of *in vivo* alkylation. Chloroform and carbon tetrachloride are hepatocarcinogenic to rodents by intragastric administration of relatively large doses (*see* Table XV, and the I.A.R.C. Monograph "Evaluation of Carcinogenic Risk of Chemicals to Man," Vol. 1, 1972). Carbon tetrachloride also gave tumors on inhalation. The mode of action of carbon tetrachloride was suggested to involve oxidative conversion to either a free radical or to the carbonium ion, CCl_3^+ (472, 473, 474).

Methyl bromide was reported early to hydrolyze to some extent *in vivo* (477), but it was not tested as a possible carcinogen. Methyl iodide yielded sarcomas at the injection site and a few tumors at other sites when administered by subcutaneous injection to rats (151).

Chloral hydrate, $(Cl_3C \cdot CH(OH)_2)$ was tested for initiating activity in the mouse skin system (476). A few tumors were obtained, but the incidence was not significantly greater than for the controls.

Ethylene dibromide was tested in a variety of animal species by oral and skin contact administration, but no tumors were reported (466). Recently this compound was found to be carcinogenic to rats and mice on administration by oral intubation (467).

Evidently the carcinogenic activity of the simpler haloalkanes generally is relatively weak, but the number of tests reported must be regarded as not very extensive. A striking demonstration of carcinogenic potency of an industrially used alkyl halide is the work of Viola *et al.* (*471*). It shows that inhalation of vinyl chloride, the monomer of the plastic polyvinyl chloride, caused a variety of tumors in rats, including a high yield of epidermoid carcinoma and bone and skin tumors. Very recently, exposure to vinyl chloride was considered a possible industrial hazard, since five cases of the normally rare angiosarcoma of the liver were reported among workers in polyvinyl chloride plants in the U.S. and Britain (*477*).

In summary, therefore, evidence relating industrial exposure to specific alkylating agents (apart from vinyl chloride, which is not a reactive alkylating agent) with cancer in humans appears to be limited to cases involving probably relatively high levels of mustard gas and dimethyl sulfate, but its positive nature in these cases appears to be established. Representative animal tests showed that some members of virtually all classes of alkylating agent can be carcinogenic. The doses involved are generally high, and extrapolation from animals (nearly always rats or mice) to man on a simple dose relationship would suggest that the contribution of alkylation carcinogenesis to the sum total of human cancer caused by the industrial uses of alkylating agents would be small. Adequate means for measuring alkylation damage in man are not yet available. The question whether low levels of exposure to alkylating agents would be completely negated by the body's defenses remains unresolved. In reviewing cancer epidemiology, Higginson (*478*) stated that although some studies with animals did indicate minimal tumorigenic doses for chemical carcinogens, this might not be true generally.

Possible Ingestion of Alkylating Agents and Related Compounds Used in Chemotherapy or as Pesticides etc. Certain alkylating agents were used in cancer chemotherapy, and several are currently available (as listed for example in "Martindale": The Extra Pharmacopoeia, 26th ed., 1972). These have been quite extensively investigated for their ability to induce tumors in animal tests. In particular, Schmähl and Osswald (*107*) used dose schedules in rats which were designed to mimic the chemotherapeutic usage of such agents. Tumors were obtained in significantly greater yield than in controls for six alkylating drugs: the nitrogen mustards HN2 (**3**) and its *N*-oxide, "mannomustine" "Degranol") (**11**), cyclophosphamide (Endoxan, Cytoxan) (**8**), and the tris(ethyleneimine) compounds Trenimon (**33**) and Thio TEPA (**31**). The results with the bis-alkanesulfonate, myleran (Busulphan) (**32**) were not conclusive. These results may indicate a possible carcinogenic hazard of such drugs to man.

As previously mentioned, 2-naphthylamine mustard (**12**) was indicated to be a bladder carcinogen in man. It seems likely that this action was mediated by metabolism to the parent carcinogenic amine, 2-naphthylamine, rather than by direct alkylation (*479, 480*). The ability of the compound to induce sarcomas at the injection site in rodents (*481*) may, on the other hand, be ascribed to direct reaction, since chromosomal damage characteristic of alkylating agents in general was found.

Furthermore, there is evidence that effects in man related to the mutagenic action of alkylating agents can occur. Hobbs (*482*) drew attention to the possibility that myeloma cells in patients treated with alkylating drugs may undergo induced mutation. This might account for the development of clones of cells which resist the growth inhibitory effect of the drug.

Multiple myeloma patients treated with melphalan or cyclophosphamide showed increases in acute leukemia (483), but "it was not clear whether the drugs caused the neoplasm or whether prolonged survival had allowed time for development of a cancer that is part of the underlying disease for which they were used" (484).

The mutagenic properties of Myleran were suggested to cause side effects, following its use in therapy of chronic granulocytic leukemia. These effects include diffuse interstitial pulmonary fibrosis, atypical alveolar cell hyperplasia, bronchiolar cell carcinoma in a lung with diffuse atypical alveolar cell changes (485), dysplastic epithelial changes in many tissues, and possibly carcinoma of the breast (486). Miller (487) found that aspermia can result in patients treated with chlorambucil and cyclophosphamide. This may parallel some of the known antifertility effects of alkylating agents in animals.

These observations may indicate that the antineoplastic alkylating agents can react with DNA and other cellular constituents in the human body, as expected from animal experiments and that these reactions, especially those inactivating template DNA, inhibit cell division, as deduced for other systems.

With regard to the carcinogenic hazard involved in the chemotherapeutic use of such agents, Shimkin (31, 488) gave the opinion that their use in fatal diseases—such as the lymphomas, for which they have palliative value—should not be restricted. However, he expressed caution with regard to the use of known carcinogens to treat chronic diseases.

Certain alkylating agents notably HN2 and cyclophosphamide, have been used as immuno-suppressants. This action is positively correlated with cytotoxicity or the ability to cause "so-called reproductive cell death" (489).

As noted elsewhere, penicillin and related compounds may be classified as alkylating agents and were carcinogenic at high dose levels. No human cancer attributable to the use of this antibiotic has been detected (108).

The use of certain compounds of this type as insect chemosterilants is related to the general cytotoxic action of the alkylating agents (490). Triethylenemelamine (TEM), a known carcinogen (see Table XXXVII), was proposed for such use. This led to assessment of the possible genetic and presumably carcinogenic hazard to man (491, 492). From their work on induction of mutations in Drosophila, Fahmy and Fahmy (491) considered that a dose level of 3 mg/kg of TEM would be mutagenically equivalent to exposure to 1000 R of ionizing radiation. In addition to their potential value in insect control, the use of certain alkanesulfonates as male contraceptives by oral administration has been considered. Hrushesky et al. (306) found "high" carcinogenicity of ethyl methanesulfonate in the rat which "may preclude such use, pending further evaluation."

In a preliminary report of pesticide bioassays for tumorigenicity in mice using oral administration of maximal tolerated doses, the insecticide bis(2-chloroethyl)ether, a potential alkylating agent, induced a significantly elevated incidence of tumors *(451)*. Other tests showed this compound to be a carcinogen (*see* Table XXIX).

Maleic hydrazide (**36**), a herbicide, although not known to act as an alkylating agent, was included by Dickens and Jones *(493)* in tests of a series of reactive lactones and their structural analogs and was a carcinogen for the rat and mouse. In subsequent tests, showing that this compound is a hepatocarcinogen by injection into infant mice, Epstein *et al.* *(494)* assessed the possible carcinogenic hazard to man. They concluded that a carcinogenic dose could be ingested in four and a half years by humans from vegetables containing the maximum tolerance level of 50 ppm. The basis of their calculation could in principle be extended to other carcinogens, including those classified as directly acting alkylating agents.

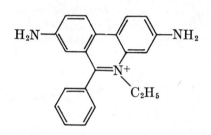

Ethidium   **34**

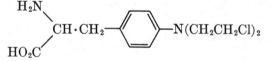

Melphalan, (*p*-Di(2-chloroethylamino)-L-phenylalanine)   **35**

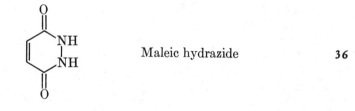

Maleic hydrazide   **36**

The extrapolation from mouse to man rested essentially on the assumption that the effective carcinogenic dose to mice, expressed as mg/kg body weight, should be divided by a factor of about 10 to 15 to give a corresponding effective dose to man. This factor was derived from a survey of relative toxicities of several drugs to the two species. The range of compounds considered included several alkylating drugs *(495)*. The conclusion reached from these data was that, for the various compounds, the maximum tolerated doses to either species were consistently approximately equal if dose was expressed as mg/m^2 of body surface area. This finding was remarkable in that the range of dosages covered was about 1000-fold. The predicted effective

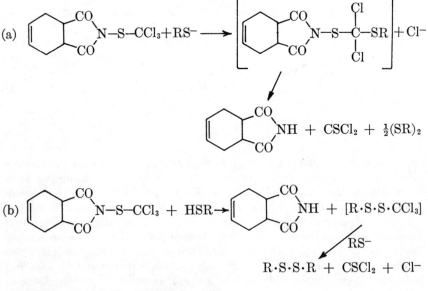

$$\text{(structure)} \quad N - S - CCl_3 \qquad \text{Captan} \qquad \mathbf{37}$$

carcinogenic doses were thus derived on the assumption that the same relationship would apply to this parameter as to toxicity.

Among other pesticides, the fungicide Captan (**37**) and the insecticide DDT (**38**) are currently under intensive investigation as potential hazards. Both compounds embody the -CCl₃ group and might possibly act in part through an alkylation mechanism *in vivo*, by analogy with carbon tetrachloride. Captan reacted with reduced glutathione *in vitro*, yielding oxidized glutathione suggesting an alkylation reaction as a first stage (*496*) (*see* Scheme 7a). However, the alternative exchange mechanism (b) was considered at least equally likely. The thiophosgene formed evidently reacted less rapidly with an excess of glutathione than did Captan itself. Occurrence of this reaction (c) also apparently yielded oxidized glutathione *via* thiocarbonate decomposition. Captan is mutagenic to *E. coli* (*497*), but its mode of action is not yet defined with respect to the chemical reaction involved. In the preliminary report by Innes *et al.* (*451*), Captan did not cause a significant increase in tumors on oral administration to mice, but DDT did cause an elevated tumor incidence. Aramite (**39**), an acaricide, proved to be carcinogenic in animal tests (*see* Table XXIX) and by virtue of the -CH₂CH₂Cl group in the molecule was classified as an alkylating agent.

Scheme 7.   Reaction of Captan with thiols (496)

(a) ... N–S–CCl₃+RS⁻ ⟶ [... N–S–C–SR]+Cl⁻

... NH + CSCl₂ + ½(SR)₂

(b) ... N–S–CCl₃ + HSR→ ... NH + [R·S·S·CCl₃]

R·S·S·R + CSCl₂ + Cl⁻

(c)   CSCl₂ + 2RS⁻ → CS(SR)₂ + 2Cl⁻

The benzylidenemalononitriles, of which the riot control agent "CS gas" is a well known exampl⸱, are reactive compounds capable of forming adducts with amines and thiols, and a zwitterionic resonance form embodying a benzylidene carbonium ion moiety contributes to their structure (**40**). Very recently, a rapid bioassay system in mouse skin, which has been claimed to indicate potential carcinogens by histological methods, showed a positive response to "CS gas" (*498*). This procedure demonstrates *in vivo* suppression of nonspecific esterase activity, possible caused by *in vivo* reactions with thiol groups. Barry *et al.* (*498*) proposed on the basis of their work that CS should now be investigated fully for carcinogenic activity.

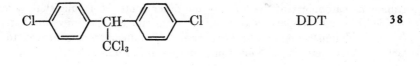

DDT   **38**

(CH$_3$)$_3$C—⬡—OCH$_2$CH(CH$_3$)—O—$\overset{\text{O}}{\underset{}{\overset{\|}{\text{S}}}}$—OCH$_2CH_2$Cl   Aramite   **39**

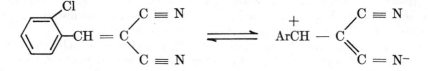

"CS gas", *o*-chlorobenzylidenemalononitrile   **40**

$$O\begin{cases} \text{CH — COOEt} \\ \text{CH — COOEt} \end{cases}$$

Diethyl epoxysuccinate   **41**

An interesting example of possible ingestion of an alkylating agent is presented by the occurrence of diethyl succinate in wine (*499*). Boyland and Down (*500*) think that distillation to produce spirits could yield diethyl *cis*- or *trans*-epoxysuccinates (**41**) which they showed to be alkylating agents *in vitro*. They further discussed the possibility that formation of alkylating compounds in spirits could be a causal factor in the etiology of cancer of the esophagus in spirit drinkers.

With regard to the association between betel-nut chewing and cancer of the oropharynx, Boyland and Nery (*501*) pointed out that the betel-nut alkaloid, arecoline (**42**), is a biological alkylating agent because of its ability to undergo addition reactions across the reactive △ ^{3}-ethylenic bond.

The carcinogenic properties of the naturally occurring lactones were reviewed by Dickens (*108, 113, 450*). Dickens *et al.* (*502*) reported on tests

CO·O·CH₃

Arecoline   42

N
|
CH₃

of certain compounds of this type using intratracheal administration, with relevance to the possibility that lactones may be involved in lung cancer induction by cigarette smoke. Several lactones shown to be active carcinogens by subcutaneous injection in the rat (*see* Tables XXIV–XXVI) were negative when given by intratracheal intubation, but β-propiolactone gave one squamous carcinoma of the lung by the latter route. The fungistatic agents sorbic acid and dehydroacetic acid were carcinogens by injection but not by oral administration in drinking water. Certain aflatoxins proved to be potent carcinogens given both orally and by injection.

Representative Oncogenesis Tests with Alkylating Agents

In this section, data on animal tests are summarized in Tables XV–XXXVII for compounds classified according to chemical type. Sufficient detail has been given to enable fairly rapid comparisons to be made without reference to original literature, although the latter must generally be consulted for details such as precise methods of dosimetry and administration, sex and age of animals, and any statistical evaluation of data.

The diversity of the chemical nature of the compounds and also of the type of test system used are obvious features of any attempted survey of this kind. This prevents any overall quantitative comparison of carcinogenic potency of compounds. However, such comparisons can be valid when a single well defined test system is used. It may be noted, for example, that Shimkin *et al.* (*31*) (*see also,* Ref. *503*) assigned numerical values for carcinogenic potency to 29 alkylating agents tested over a range of dose levels administered by intraperitoneal injection for ability to induce lung tumors in strain A/J mice. Druckrey *et al.* (*151*) assigned numerical tumorigenicity indices to 12 alkylating agents administered by subcutaneous injection to BD rats.

Shimkin *et al.* (*31*) compared their data with that obtained in strain A mice for other chemical types of carcinogens. They deduced the dose at which one lung tumor per mouse would be induced from data relating logarithm of the number of tumors found at 39 weeks and logarithm of the dose, expressed as μmoles/kg. These data gave straight-line plots of almost equal slopes but with different intercepts. The value of the dose at the one-tumor-per-mouse level was taken as a measure of carcinogenic potency, expressed as 10,000/this dose.

Among the alkylating agents tested, uracil mustard, HN2, Melphalan, and TEM were the most potent, with values over 500, and were of the same order of potency as 3-methylcholanthrene, dibenz[*a,h*]anthracene, and 4-nitroquinoline-*N*-oxide. Cyclophosphamide (Cytoxan), 2-naphthylamine mustard, diepoxybutane, and mannitol myleran were weakly positive in this test with potencies of about 10; *i.e.*, of the same order of potency as ethyl carbamate (urethane). Several nitrogen mustards were classified as inactive (*see* Tables XXX–XXXVII).

The index derived by Druckrey *et al.* (*151*) was of the form:

$$I = A/t.D. \times 10^3$$

where A denotes tumor yield, t average induction time, and D the total dose administered in mg/kg. Of the compounds tested, veratryl chloride and *n*-butyl-*p*-toluenesulfonate were inactive; di-*n*-butyl sulfate, ethyl *p*-toluenesulfonate, ethylene sulfide, and trimethylene oxide gave I values of about 10; methyl iodide, benzyl chloride, dimethyl sulfate, and methyl methanesulfonate, 30–40; methyl-*p*-toluenesulfonate, 49; and diethyl sulfate, 63. 1,3-Propanesultone was a more potent carcinogen, giving I values of 130–210 by multiple injection and 470–800 by single injection (*311*). For the other compounds, single injections of about half the LD_{50} dose generally gave higher I values than multiple smaller doses. For comparison, values of 200 for *N*-methyl-*N'*-nitro-*N*-nitrosoguanidine (MNNG), 500 for β-propiolactone, and about 2,000 for TEM were derived.

It appears, therefore, that alkylating agents are not generally potent carcinogens when compared with polynuclear aromatic hydrocarbons. However, among monofunctional agents diethyl sulfate, β-propiolactone, and 1,3-propanesultone appear to be fairly potent. The trifunctional ethyleneimine derivative, TEM, emerges as probably the most potent polyfunctional alkylating agent taking all tests into consideration, although uracil mustard and certain other nitrogen mustards gave higher potency indexes in strain A mice.

Clayson (*504*) considered that "with few exceptions, it is difficult to accept that the carcinogenic activity of the biological alkylating agents has been firmly established, because so much of the evidence is concerned with the induction of subcutaneous sarcomas in the rat." He called for further tests using subcutaneous injection or skin painting in mice. The early tests with β-propiolactone (*112, 505*) appeared vulnerable to this criticism, although their results did show that in control animals multiple injections of the vehicles used gave either no tumors during the test period or gave tumors after longer induction times than the tested compound. The use of subcutaneous injection tests was reviewed by Carter (*506*).

McDonald (*507*) found that nitrogen mustard, HN2, enhanced the rate of tumor appearance in female rats of the Holtzman strain, but tumors appeared in about the same numbers and of the same types in control animals kept for more than one year after the injections were started. It was therefore concluded that HN2 "was not in itself the carcinogenic agent," and "might have acted as a co-carcinogen in these groups of animals."

The concept of alkylating agents as co-carcinogens may appear to be at variance with the more generally accepted classification of these agents as initiators rather than promoting agents. In the classical two-stage carcinogenesis test using the mouse skin system, several alkylating agents were classi-

fied as initiating agents. Roe and Salaman (476) found TEM and β-propiolactone to be initiators in this system, and Salaman and Roe (30) found
chlorambucil positive in this sense, but HN2, Myleran, and Melphalan were
inactive.

Colburn and Boutwell (307, 308) used alkylation of DNA, RNA, or
protein of mouse skin as an index of potency of several alkylating agents
in this regard. They found a positive correlation between *in vivo* alkylation
of DNA and initiating ability increasing in the order: iodoacetic acid,
3-chloropropionic acid (non-initiators), 3-iodopropionic acid (weak initiator), and β-propiolactone (active initiator). With regard to promoting
activity, they stated that "the binding data for β-propiolactone and iodoacetic
acid are compatible with the theory that protein binding is important in
promotion of skin tumorigenesis."

The situation may be envisaged as of some complexity *a priori*, since
in vivo alkylation of DNA, as discussed previously can lead both to mutagenesis and to "reproductive cell death." The ability to initiate may
be reasonably associated positively with mutagenic action. On the other
hand, the cytotoxic action may be considered as "anti-promotional" since
promotion is associated with stimulation of target cell division. It is not
surprising therefore that alkylating agents can be initiating agents on the
one hand and "anti-carcinogenic" on the other. This latter finding was
reported for mustard gas (508) and for butadiene dioxide (437, 448)
which were found to inhibit tumor initiation in mouse skin by aromatic
hydrocarbons. Furthermore, since alkylating agents are not specific reagents
for DNA *in vivo*, but also react with proteins, the concept that alkylation of
protein can play a role in promotion could accord with the activity of alkylating agents as complete carcinogens in some cases. These considerations are
still reasonable hypotheses, not established mechanisms; the mutations involved in initiation have not been specified, and the protein receptors involved
in promotion have yet to be defined. The reactions of both DNA and proteins
with alkylating agents *in vivo* seem most likely *a priori* to be of a random
nature, and this might explain why alkylating agents are generally weak
carcinogens. Nevertheless, some specificity of mutagenic action correlated
with carcinogenic potency has been discerned for certain agents.

The most comprehensive series of investigations of some alkylating
agents of relatively simple structural types by several administration routes
are those by Van Duuren et al. (448). β-Propiolactone and β-butyrolactone
were classified as positive because they gave malignant tumors in long-term
tests by four routes; application to skin of mice, subcutaneous injections in
mice and rats, and gastric feeding to rats. The epoxides glycidaldehyde,
d,l-1,2,3,4-diepoxybutane, and 1,2,5,6-diepoxyhexane gave tumors by the first
three routes, but gastric tumors could not be induced. This was ascribed to
rapid acid-catalyzed hydrolysis of epoxides. At the estimated stomach pH of
1, β-lactones are not hydrolyzed.

It is evident from the tables that mice or rats were used in nearly all the
tests recorded. In view of the supposition that alkylating agents act by direct
reaction with target tissues, species-dependent differences reflecting different

modes of metabolism should therefore not be expected to be very important. Parish and Searle (*509, 510*) confirmed this assumption by showing that β-propiolactone can induce skin tumors in the guinea pig and golden hamster. The susceptibility of the latter species to melanotic tumor induction, noted for 7,12-dimethylbenz[*a*]anthracene and 4-nitroquinoline *N*-oxide, was also found with this alkylating agent.

In the overall assessment of alkylating agents as weak carcinogens, it was often necessary to use either relatively high doses, with the resulting complication of decreased survival of tested animals relative to controls, or multiple doses throughout a major part of the life span of the animals. In the search for more sensitive testing techniques, injection of neonatal animals has been a notable introduction. Walters *et al.* (*305*) used this method with ethyl methanesulfonate and two strains of mice. They found that five daily subcutaneous injections during the first five days of life was a more effective administration method than a single injection within one day of birth. Five injections of 200 μg ethyl methanesulfonate in 3% aqueous gelatine induced lung adenomas in all surviving Balb/c mice at 50 weeks, compared with 8.3% in the controls. However the same procedure with arachis oil as the vehicle was ineffective, although a positive response was obtained in C57Bl mice.

Chernozemski and Warwick (*511*) found that β-propiolactone was a potent hepatocarcinogen for male suckling mice, (C57Bl/6 x A)F_1, whereas treated baby females gave few hepatomas but enhanced incidence of malignant lymphomas. Adult mice were not susceptible to hepatocarcinogenesis by this agent.

Transplacental administration of alkylating agents was used, notably by Druckrey *et al.* (*151, 311*), by injection of single doses into pregnant rats at the 15th day of gestation. Dimethyl and diethyl sulfates and 1,3-propanesultone gave malignant tumors in the offspring, mainly in tissues of the nervous system.

Although tumors generally have been induced by alkylating agents at the application site, as expected from their ability to alkylate tissues in that vicinity, (as shown, for example, in Colburn and Boutwell's (*307, 308*) *in vivo* alkylation studies) many examples show tumor induction at distant sites. In some cases (*see* Table XII) alkylation of cellular constituents was demonstrated at such sites. The apparent lack of simple positive correlation between extent of the *in vivo* alkylation reactions and the tumor yields has been noted already.

In view of the general assessment that alkylating carcinogens are initiators rather than promoters, the inability of alkylation to cause tumorigenesis in particular organs might be ascribed in part to lack of appropriate promotional stimulus. The applicability of the classical two-stage scheme of carcinogenesis to organs other than skin remains a problem for further study. The findings of Chernozemski and Warwick (*511*) for hepatocarcinogenic action of β-propiolactone illustrate the possible importance of hormonal status of the animal; male baby mice were much more susceptible than female.

Whether some form of activation of latent virus is involved in oncogenesis by alkylating agents is at present unresolved. However, it does seem a definite possibility in some cases where inbred strains of animals were used, as for example in Frei's (*201, 202*) work on lymphoma induction in CFW/D mice. This type of mechanism cuts across the generalized scheme of two-stage carcinogenesis in terms of initiation and promotion. Perhaps the presence of the provirus associated with the genome of the particular strain of animal should be considered as the primary oncogenic stimulus. The alkylating agents should then be classified as acting as co-carcinogens. As already mentioned, this latter action may be associated with the induced stimulus to DNA repair mechanisms, which are as yet little understood in the whole animal.

Oncogenesis Tests with Alkylating Agents in Relation to their Chemical Structure and Reactivity. SIMPLER ALKYL HALIDES (Table XV). Extensive tests with methyl iodide, chloroform, and carbon tetrachloride, showed positive results. Of these, methyl iodide almost certainly acts by direct alkylation at the injection site. Hepatocarcinogenesis by chloroform and carbon tetrachloride appears to require activation of the carcinogens to free radicals or, perhaps less likely, to carbonium ions.

Vinyl chloride is remarkable in showing a measure of carcinogenic potency in the rat and in man while possessing negligible reactivity as an alkylating agent. Further studies related to its mode of action are clearly desirable.

Possibly the remaining compounds of this group are essentially unreactive towards tissue constituents *in vivo* and may be effectively eliminated either unchanged or by detoxificative metabolism. In view of possible ingestion of some of these compounds in industrial use, more intensive studies might be advisable.

β-CARBONYL-SUBSTITUTED ALKYL HALIDES (Table XVI). These compounds are classical S_N2 reagents and react principally with groups of high nucleophilicity, such as thiols. Although evidently feeble initiators, perhaps

Table XV. Representative Oncogenesis Tests with Alkylating Agents

Compound	Formula	Animal	Strain or Type	Route
Methyl bromide	CH_3Br	rat	white	inhal.
Methyl iodide	CH_3I	rat	BD	s.c.
		mouse	—	inhal.
		rat	white	p.o.

reflecting their lack of reactivity towards DNA, they may act as promoting agents by virtue of their ability to react with proteins *in vivo* (*307, 308*).

ARALKYL HALIDES (Table XVII). Evidently this group contains some significantly potent carcinogens, possibly reflecting the ability to react through the S_N1 mechanism.

The studies with halomethylbenz[a]anthracene derivatives were stimulated to some extent by their possible relationship to reactive metabolites of the parent hydrocarbons (*83*). The relationship between carcinogenic and mutagenic action and reactions with DNA are currently under investigation.

MONOFUNCTIONAL ALKYL SULFATES AND SULFONATES (Table XVIII). As already mentioned, this group includes chemically highly reactive compounds. The methyl and ethyl esters of methanesulfonic acid, being more soluble in aqueous media than the sulfates, were extensively studied as *in vivo* alkylating agents. This led to the hypothesis, already discussed, that the relatively greater tendency of the ethyl esters to react by the S_N1 mechanism may correlate with their higher mutagenic and carcinogenic activity. It may be speculated further that the relatively high activity of allyl methanesulfonate should be ascribed to the same cause since allylic mesomerism would stabilize the derived carbonium ion:

$$CH_2{=}CH{-}\overset{+}{C}H_2 \rightleftharpoons \overset{+}{C}H_2{-}CH{=}CH_2.$$

Notable features of the action of the methanesulfonates include their ability to induce tumors in tissues remote from the site of injection. Although alkylation has been found in these tissues, the relationship between this factor and tumor induction remains largely obscure. Lymphoma induction may involve some form of viral activation.

ALKYL PHOSPHATES, THIOPHOSPHONATES, AND PHOSPHONATES (Table XIX). Weak activity has been claimed for two compounds of this group. Trichlorphon gave liver carcinomas and papillomas of the forestomach, and di-isopropyl fluorophosphate gave pituitary tumors.

(and Some Related Compounds)[a]—Alkyl Halides (Haloalkanes)

Dose (mg/kg)	Duration (Days)	Tumors	Remarks	References
0.28-0.42[b]	176	none	probably inconclusive	458
10, wkly × 50	580[c]	9/12 local sarcomas	a few tumors at other sites	151
20, wkly × 45	620[c]	6/20 local sarcomas		
50, single	610[c]	4/14 local sarcomas		
0.5[b] × 20	30	none	probably inconclusive	459
100-500, daily	71	none		

Table XV.

Compound	Formula	Animal	Strain or Type	Route
Methylene dichloride[d]	CH_2Cl_2	mouse	NMRI, F_1, 2-3 months old	skin
Chloroform	$CHCl_3$	mouse	A	p.o. (intra-gastric)
		mouse	C3H	inhal.
		mouse	(C57 $\times$ DBA/2) F_1, new-born	a.c.
Carbon tetrachloride[f]	CCl_4	mouse	A	p.o. (intra-gastric)
Ethylene chlorohydrin	$CH_2Cl \cdot CH_2OH$	rat	—	p.o.
Ethylene dibromide	$CH_2Br \cdot CH_2Br$	rat	—	inhal.
		rat	Osborne–Mendel	p.o. (intub-ation)
Ethylene dichloride	$CH_2Cl \cdot CH_2Cl$	rat	Wistar	inhal.
Freon 112 (1,1,2,2-Tetra-chloro-1,2-difluoroethane)	$CFCl_2 \cdot CFCl_2$	mouse	Swiss S, newborn	s.c.
Freon 113 (1,1,2-Tri-chloro-1,2,2-trifluoroethane)	$CFCl_2 \cdot CF_2Cl$	rat	Wistar albino	inhal.
Vinyl chloride	$CH_2 {:} CHCl$	rat	Wistar Ar/IRE (m)	inhal.

[a] Alkylnitroso compounds and dialkylnitrosamines or other carcinogens known to be metabolized to yield alkylating agents are not included in this compilation of data; but certain compounds generally classified as alkylating agents, although they are almost certainly converted to more reactive molecular species *in vivo*, such as cyclophosphamide are included. Urethane and analogs (alkyl carbamates) are not included. For reasons of space, details about administration and histopathology are not given, and the original references should be consulted for this information. Generally only the principal types of tumor induced are listed. Tumor yields are expressed as no. of tumors/no. of animals used. For survival data, see original references.

[b] Inhalation dose, mg/l. of air; 8 hr/day, 5 days/week.

Continued

Dose (mg/kg)	Duration (Days)	Tumors	Remarks	References
0.2ml[d] × 25, (twice weekly)	675	2/50 tumors	one skin tumor	460
590 × 30		3/5 hepatomas	tumors in females only; males died	461
1180 × 30		4/5 hepatomas	from renal necrosis	
5[b]	540	0/72		462
200 μg[e] 200 μg × 8	519	not sig. greater than controls		463
160-2600	150	136/300 hepatomas	dose–response study	464
0.01-0.24%[e] in diet	up to 403	0/35		465
25 ppm[g] 7 hr. daily	213	0/40		466
[h]	378	31/31 gastric squamous carcinoma		467
200 ppm[g] 157 × 7 hr. exposures	212	0/30		468
not stated	365	1% s.c. sarcomas 5% hepatomas		469
12000 ppm[g] 2 hr/day 5 days/week	730	1/6 fibrangio-sarcoma	1/6 s.c. and 1/6 lung tumors in controls	470
3%[g] 4 hr 5 days weekly	380	15/26 skin (mostly epi-dermold ca.) 6/26 lung 3/26 osteo-chondroma		471

[c] Average time of death.
[d] Inhalation tests over 6 months with various animal species have been reported (453), but no tumors were found.
[e] Amount given per dose, not mg/kg.
[f] Several other studies have been made; generally, inhalation or s.c. injection did not give tumors; see Hartwell (454), p. 30; Shubik and Hartwell (455), p. 29; Shubik and Hartwell (456), p. 40; Shubik and Hartwell (457), p. 38, for relevant references.
[g] Inhalation dose, ppm of air.
[h] Maximum tolerated dose; *see* ref. for details.   Also active in $(C57B1 \times C3H)F_1$ mice by same route.   Also active at half the maximum tolerated dose.

Table XVI. Representative Oncogenesis

Compound	Formula	Animal	Strain or Type	Route
Chloracetic acid	$Cl \cdot CH_2 \cdot CO_2H$	mouse	(C57B1/6 × C3H/Anf)F_1	p.o.
Chloracetone	CH_3COCH_2Cl	mouse	stock	skin
		mouse	albino	skin
Iodoacetic acid[b]	$I \cdot CH_2CO_2H$	rat	hybrid	s.c.
		mouse	Swiss	p.o.
		mouse		skin
3-Bromopropionic acid	$BrCH_3CH_2\text{-}CO_2H$	mouse	albino	skin
3-Iodopropionic acid	$I \cdot CH_2CH_2\text{-}CO_2H$	mouse		skin

[a] Promotion with croton oil, 0.2 ml, 0.3% in acetone, 20 weeks. For details of time-course and survival *see* original reference.

Table XVII. Representative

Compound	Formula	Animal	Strain or Type	Route
Benzyl chloride	⟨benzene⟩—CH₂Cl	rat	BD	s.c.
Veratryl chloride (3,4-Bis(methoxy)-benzyl chloride)	MeO—, MeO—⟨benzene⟩—CH₂Cl	rat	BD	s.c.

Tests—β-Carbonyl-substituted Alkyl Halides

Dose	Duration (Days)	Tumors	Remarks	References
46.4 mg/kg	540	none		*451*
—	183	none		*514*
0.2 ml, 0.3% in acetone × 24[a]	365	44/19 papillomas	10/20 papillomas in controls	*515*
multiple, total, 960 mg	596	1 inj. site fibroma, 1 inj. site fibrosarcoma, 1 plasma cell sarcoma		*516*
45 doses, total, 36 mg	315	2/40 papillomas of forestomach	3/42 papillomas of forestomach in controls	*517*
10 mcmole × 6	210	none	with or without promotion by croton oil; alkylation of RNA, DNA, and protein studied	*307, 308*
0.2 ml, 0.3% in acetone × 24[a]	365	78/20 papillomas	10/20 papillomas in controls	*515*
120 mcmole × 6	210	none	with or without croton oil	*307, 308*

[b] Iodoacetic acid is a co-carcinogen in the mouse skin test system (*512*) and is a mitotic stimulator in this tissue (*513*).

Oncogenesis Tests—Aralkyl Halides

Dose (mg/kg) (or as Stated)	Duration (Days)	Tumors	Remarks	Refercnees
40, wkly × 52	500	3/14 local sarcomas		*151*
80, wkly × 46	500	6/8 local sarcomas		
10, wkly × 36		0/12	Tumors (local	*151*
20, wkly × 37		0/12	sarcomas)	
50, wkly × 12		0/14	obtained in	
100, wkly × 12		0/6	Sprague– Dawley rats (Schmähl *et al.* quoted by reference	*151*

Table XVII.

Compound	Formula	Animal	Strain or Type	Route
1,1,1-Trichloro-2,2-bis(p-chloro-phenyl) ethane (DDT)	$\left(Cl\text{—}\bigcirc\right)_2 CH\cdot CCl_3$	mouse	(C57B1/6 × C3H/Anf)-F_1 (C57B1/6 × AKR)F_1	p.o. (diet)
7-Bromo-methylbenz-(a)anthracene	CH_2Br	rat	CB–hooded (f)	s.c.
		mouse	Swiss S (f)	skin[a]
		mouse	Swiss S (f, new-born)	s.c. (i.s.)[d]
			Swiss S (m, new-born)	s.c. (i.s.)[d]
4-Bromo-7-bromomethylbenz-(a)anthracene	Br, CH_2Br	mouse	Swiss S (f)	skin[a]
4-Chloro-7-bromomethylbenz-(a)anthracene	Cl, CH_2Br	mouse	Swiss S (f)	skin[a]
		mouse	Swiss S (f, new-born)	s.c. (i.s.)[d]
		mouse	Swiss S (m, new-born)	s.c. (i.s.)[d]
1-Methyl-7-bromomethylbenz-(a)anthracene	Me, CH_2Br	mouse	Swiss S (f)	skin[a]
7-Bromomethyl-12-methylbenz-(a)anthracene	Me, CH_2Br	rat	CB–hooded (f)	s.c.
		mouse	Swiss S (f)	skin[a]
		mouse	Swiss S (f, new-born)	s.c. (i.s.)[d]
			Swiss S (m, new-born)	s.c. (i.s.)[d]
		rat	Sprague–Dawley (f)	s.c.

Continued

Dose (mg/kg) (or as Stated)	Duration (Days)	Tumors	Remarks	References
140 ppm	567	hepatomas	sig. > controls	*451*
		hepatomas	sig. > controls	
		lymphomas	sig. > controls	
12.5, single	365	0/10		*518*
1 μmole[b] (321 μg)	112	4/25 papillomas[c]	1.2 papillomas/ mouse	*518*
266 μg × 3	up to 431	15/26 lung[c] 1/26 liver[c]		*519*
266 μg × 3	up to 431	33/43 lung[c] 35/43 liver[c]	2 malignant lymphoma, 1 i.site sarcoma	
1 μmole[b]	112	2/25 papillomas		*520*
1 μmole[b]	112	1/25 papillomas		*520*
294 μg × 3	up to 431	1/38 lung		*519*
294 μg × 3	up to 431	1/32 lung 8/32 liver[c]		
1 μmole[b]	112	5/25 papillomas[c]	1.2 papillomas/ mouse	*519*
12.5, single	365	10/10 i.site sarcomas		*518*
1 μmole[b]	112	22/25 papillomas[c]	4.1 papillomas/ mouse	*520*
277 μg × 3	up to 431	16/17 lung[c] 3/17 liver		*519*
277 μg × 3	up to 431	24/26 lung[c] 23/26 liver[c]		
0.1 mg × 20	200	6/12 i.site sarcomas	no mammary cancer	*521*
1 mg × 20	200	3/5 i.site sarcomas		

Table XVII.

Compound	Formula	Animal	Strain or Type	Route
7-Chloromethyl-12-methylbenz-(a)anthracene	Me ... CH_2Cl	rat	Sprague–Dawley (f)	s.c.
7-Iodomethyl-12-methylbenz-(a)anthracene	Me ... CH_2I	rat	Sprague–Dawley (f)	s.c.

[a] Promoted with Hecker's croton oil fraction A, (10 μg, twice weekly, ×25).
[b] Single dose, as initiator.

Table XVIII.   Representative Oncogenesis Tests—

Compound	Formula	Animal	Strain or Type	Route
Dimethyl sulfate	$(CH_3)_2SO_4$	rat	BD	s.c.
				i.v. inhala- tion
				trans- pla- cental i.v.
Diethyl sulfate	$(C_2H_5)_2SO_4$	rat	BD	s.c.
Di-n-butyl sulfate	$(CH_3(CH_2)_3)_2SO_4$	rat	BD	s.c.

Continued

Dose (mg/kg) (or as Stated)	Duration (Days)	Tumors	Remarks	References
1 mg × 20	200	9/9 i.site sarcomas	no mammary cancer	*521*
0.1 mg × 20	200	5/5 i.site sarcomas	no mammary cancer	*521*
1 mg × 20	200	4/11 i.site sarcomas		

[c] Refers to number of tumor-bearing animals; some had multiple tumors.
[d] Injection near root of tail to deliver to interscapular region.

Alkyl Sulfates and Sulfonates (Monofunctional)

Dose (mg/kg) (or as Stated)	Duration (Days)	Tumors or Tumors-bearing Animals	Remarks	References
8 wkly × 58	500[b]	7/12 local sarcoma 1/12 hepatocellular ca.		*151*
16 wkly × 49	330[b]	4/6 local sarcoma		
50 single		7/15 local sarcoma		
2–4, wkly		negative tumors		
3–10 ppm 1 hr, 5 × wkly		8/27 tumors, squamous ca. of nasal cavity, and others		
20		7/59 mostly of nervous system		
25 wkly × 32	415[b]	6/12 local sarcoma	also active by transplacental route	*151*
50 wkly × 32	350[b]	11/11 local sarcoma 1/11 adenocarcinoma		
500 wkly × 19	675[b]	2/7 local sarcoma		*151*

Table XVIII.

Compound	Formula	Animal	Strain or Type	Route[a]
Methyl meth-anesulfonate	$CH_3OSO_2CH_3$	rat	BD	s.c.
		rat	Wistar albino	i.v.
		mouse	RF/Un (m, 1wk old)	p.o.
		mouse	CFW/D inbred	i.p.
Ethyl meth-anesulfonate	$C_2H_5OSO_2CH_3$	mouse	CBA	i.p.
		mouse	Balb/C (new-born)	s.c.
				s.c.
		mouse	C57B1 (new-born)	s.c.

Continued

Dose (mg/kg) (or as Stated)	Duration (Days)	Tumors or Tumor-bearing Animals	Remarks	References
4 wkly × 46	635[b]	3/12 local sarcoma 1/12 nephro-blastoma		*151*
8 wkly × 46	490[b]	3/8 local sarcoma		
72	—	1/20 spinal cord meningioma 2/20 brain astrocytoma		*203, 204*
96	—	1/20 neurofibroma 1/20 brain oligo-dendroglioma		
120	—	0/16		
20 mg/100 ml in drinking water, approx. 30 mg/kg/ day	550	2.1% stomach 4.2% liver 14.9% thymic lymphoma 70.2% lung adenoma 44.7% other (mainly retic. cell sarcoma) (% of 47 animals)	in controls, 0 3.7% 3.7% 38.9% 60.5% (% of 162 animals)	*205*
660	365	2/35 lymphoma 8/35 lung adenoma	not statistically sig. greater than controls	*201, 202*
200 × 3[f]	693[b]	5% kidney, carcinoma 28% kidney, cystic papillary adenoma 89% lung, solid adenoma 11% lymphoma	3% kidney, 20% lung, 5% lymphoma in controls	*304*
200 μg[c]	280	9/45 lung adenoma	not sig. greater than controls	*305*
200 μg × 5[c]		8/51 lung adenoma		
200 μg × 5[d]	280	31/31 lung adenoma	13.6 adenomas per survivor	
200 μg × 5[c]	420	5/39 lung adenoma	no tumors in controls	

Table XVIII.

Compound	Formula	Animal	Strain or Type	Route[a]
Ethyl meth- anesulfonate (*continued*)		mouse	CFW/D inbred	i.p.
		rat	Wistar albino	i.p.
		rat	Sprague– Daw- ley	i.p.
n-Butyl meth- anesulfonate	$CH_3(CH_2)_3OSO_2CH_3$	mouse	Albino "S"	skin
Methyl *p*-tolu- enesulfonate	$CH_3OSO_2\langle\ \rangle CH_3$	rat	BD	s.c.
Ethyl *p*-tolu- enesulfonate	$C_2H_5OSO_2\langle\ \rangle CH_3$	rat	BD	s.c.
n-Butyl *p*-tolu- enesulfonate	$C_4H_9OSO_2\langle\ \rangle CH_3$	rat	BD	s.c.
Allyl meth- anesulfonate	$HC_2{:}CH \cdot CH_2OSO_2CH_3$	mouse	Albino "S"	skin
Propargyl meth- anesulfonate	$HC{\equiv}C \cdot CH_2OSO_2CH_3$	mouse	Albino "S"	skin

[a] In s.c. injections, compounds were administered in arachis oil unless otherwise stated.
[b] Mean survival time.
[c] Vehicle, arachis oil.

Table XIX.   Representative Oncogenesis Tests—

Compound	Formula	Animal	Strain or Type	Route
Dimethyl- 2,2-chlorovinyl phosphate (DDVP, Dichlorvos)	$(CH_3O)_2PO \cdot OCH{:}CCl_2$	rat	White– Sher- man	p.o. (diet)
		rat	albino	p.o.

Continued

Dose (mg/kg) (or as Stated)	Duration (Days)	Tumors or Tumor-bearing Animals	Remarks	References
675	210	1/22 lymphoma	not sig.	*201, 202*
		20/22 lung adenoma	sig.	
275 × 3	—	12/24 kidney mesenchymal		*204, 390*
350	—	1/22 brain ependymoma		
3 × 33 mg	365	Various, 74%(f) 53%(m) 0% in controls	mainly anaplastic carcinoma of lung and especially in (f) adeno-carcinoma of abdominal wall	*306*
10 × 0.8 mg[e]	140	0/10		*522*
10 × 8 mg[e]	140	0/10		
15 wkly × 53	470	7/10 local sarcoma 1 bronchial ca. 1 mammary ca. 1 ovarial ca.		*151*
50 wkly × 65	600	3/11 local sarcoma		*151*
250 wkly × 34	up to 828	0/15		*151*
10 × 1.35 mg[e]	140	12/20 papillomas	total of 42 papillomas	*522*
10 × 1.3 mg[e]	140	4/19 papillomas	1/20 papillomas in controls; not sig. (*t* test)	*522*

[d] Vehicle, 3% aqueous gelatine.
[e] Promotion with 18 weekly applications of 0.5% croton oil.
[f] At intervals of three weeks.

Alkyl Phosphates, Thiophosphates, and Phosphonates

Dose (mg/kg) (or as Stated)	Duration (Days)	Tumors	Remarks	References
0.4–69.9	90	0/10		*523*
10	42	0/?		*524*

Table XIX.

Compound	Formula	Animal	Strain or Type	Route
Dimethyl 1-hydroxy-2,2,2-trichloroethyl phosphonate (Dipterex, Trichlorphon)	$(CH_3O)_2PO \cdot CH(OH)$ CCl_3	rat	Sprague–Dawley	i.p.
		rat	BD	s.c.
		rat	Wistar	
		rat	Wistar	s.c.
		mouse	AB	skin
		mouse	AB	skin[a]
Diethyl 2-chlorovinyl phosphate	$(C_2H_5O)_2 \cdot PO \cdot OCH:$ $CHCl$	rat	Long–Evans	p.o. (diet)
Dimethyl dithiophosphate of diethyl mercaptosuccinate (Malathion)	$(CH_3O)_2 \cdot PS \cdot S \cdot$ $\underset{\overset{\mid}{CH_2CO_2C_2H_5}}{CH \cdot CO_2C_2H_5}$	rat	—	p.o. (diet)
Diethyl p-nitrophenyl thiophosphate	$(C_2H_5O)_2 \cdot PS\langle\bigcirc\rangle NO_2$	rat	albino	p.o. (diet)
Diethyl S-ethylmercaptoethanol thiophosphate (Systox)	$(C_2H_5O)_2 \cdot PS \cdot OCH_2-$ $CH_2 \cdot S \cdot C_2H_5$	rat	albino	p.o. (diet)
Diethyl S-[2-ethylthio)-ethyl] phosphorodithioate (Di-Syston)	$(C_2H_5O)_2 \cdot PS \cdot SCH_2-$ $CH_2SC_2H_5$	rat	Sprague–Dawley	i.p.
Diisopropyl fluorophosphate	$((CH_3)_2CHO)_2 \cdot PO \cdot F$	rat	Wistar	i.m.
2-Ethylhexyl-diphenyl-phosphate	$(C_6H_5O)_2 \cdot PO \cdot OCH_2-$ $CH(C_2H_5)(CH_2)_3CH_3$	rat	Carworth albino	p.o. (diet)

[a]Promotion with croton oil, weekly.

Continued

Dose (mg/kg) or as Stated)	Duration (Days)	Tumors	Remarks	References
50–150, daily	60	0/15		*525*
50	800	2/24 i.site sarcoma		*526*
30, 3 × wkly	up to 705	3/52 papilloma, forestomach		*527*
30, 3 × wkly	up to 720	7/61 papilloma, forestomach		
30, 3 × wkly	up to 790	1/16 liver carcinoma 1/16 papilloma, forestomach		
30, 3 × wkly	up to 781	1/19 liver carcinoma 2/19 papilloma, forestomach 1/19 local sarcoma		
6.3–100 ppm	60	0/24		*528*
100–5000 ppm	730	0/?		*529*
10–50 ppm	365	1 sarcoma, mediastinum	considered not sig.	*530*
1–50 ppm	112	0/90		*531*
0.25–1.5	60	0/25		*532*
0.5 (every 72 hr)	730	16/100 pituitary tumors (chromophobe adenoma)	spont. incidence "rare"	*222*
0.625–5%	730	24/160 various	not sig. (9/40 in controls)	*533*

Table XX. Representative Oncogenesis Tests—

Compound	Formula	Animal	Strain or Type	Route
Ethyl formate	$C_2H_5O \cdot CHO$	mouse	albino "S"	skin[a]
Diethyl carbonate	$(C_2H_5O)_2 \cdot CO$	mouse	albino "S"	skin[a]
Tricaprylin	$[CH_3(CH_2)_6COO]_3C_3H_5$	rat	albino	s.c.
		mouse	albino	s.c.
Tributyrin	$(CH_3CH_2CH_2COO)_3C_3H_5$	rat	AES	p.o. (diet)
n-Butyl stearate	$CH_3(CH_2)_{16}COO(CH_2)_3CH_3$	rat	Sprague–Dawley	p.o. (diet)

Table XXI. Representative Oncogenesis

Compound	Formula	Animal	Strain or Type	Route
Ethylene oxide		rat	albino	s.c.[a]
Propylene oxide		rat	albino	s.c.[a]
Glycidaldehyde[b]		mouse	ICR/Ha Swiss	skin
				s.c.

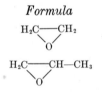

Miscellaneous Esters, Alkyl Formates, Carbonates, etc.

Dose	Duration (Days)	Tumors	Remarks	References
10 × 276 mg wkly	133	0/20		*476*
10 × 290 mg	210	2/25 papillomas	4/20 papillomas in controls	*30*
0.1 ml	480	0/20	often used as a	*539*
0.1 ml	400	0/57	vehicle for carcinogens	
15–25%	245	papillomatosis of forestomach		*540*
0.01–6.25%	730	0/90		*541*

a Promotion with 18 weekly applications of croton oil (0.3 ml. in acetone).

Tests—Epoxides (Monofunctional)

Dose (mg/kg)	Duration (Days)	Tumors	Remarks	References
100[b]	—	0/12		*449*
150[b]	739	8/12 local sarcomas	9/67 local sarcomas and 14/67 other neoplasms in analogous controls (*505*)	*449*
150[c]	737	3/12 local sarcomas		
10 mg, 3 × wkly in acetone	598	6/41 papillomas 3/41 squamous ca.		*542*
3 mg, 3 × wkly in benzene		16/30 papillomas 8/30 squamous ca.		
0.1 mg, wkly	595	2/50 fibro-sarcomas 1/50 squamous ca.		*543*
3.3 mg, wkly	536	3/30 fibro-sarcomas 2 squamous ca. 1 undiff. sarcoma		

Table XXI.

Compound	Formula	Animal	Strain or Type	Route
Glycidal-dehyde (*continued*)		rat	Sprague–Daw-ley	p.o. (in-tragas-tric)
		rat	Sprague–Daw-ley	s.c.
Glycidol	H_2C——CH—CH_2OH , O	mouse	ICR/Ha Swiss	skin
1,2-Epoxy-butene	H_2C——CH—$CH_2 \cdot CH_3$, O	mouse	ICR/Ha Swiss	skin
1,2-Epoxy-butene-3	H_2C——CH—CH=CH_2 , O	mouse	Swiss–Miller-ton	skin
1,2-Epoxy-hexadecane	H_2C——$CH \cdot (CH_2)_3 CH_3$, O	mouse	ICR/Ha Swiss	skin
Styrene oxide	H_2C——CH—⬡ , O	mouse	Swiss–Miller-ton	skin
Epichloro-hydrin	H_2C——$CHCH_2Cl$, O	mouse	C$_3$H	?
Glycidyl ester of: hexanoic acid	H_2C——$CH \cdot CH_2 \cdot CO_2(CH_2)_4 CH_3$, O	rat	albino	s.c.[a]
dodecanoic acid	H_2C——$CH \cdot CH_2 \cdot CO_2(CH_2)_{11} CH_3$, O	rat	albino	s.c.[a]
octadecanoic (stearic acid)	H_2C——$CH \cdot CH_2 \cdot CO_2(CH_2)_{16} CH_3$, O	rat	albino	s.c.[a]

[a] Generally twice weekly.
[b] Total dose in arachis oil.
[c] Total dose in water.

Continued

Dose (mg/kg)	Duration (Days)	Tumors	Remarks	References
33 mg, wkly	492	0/5		*543*
1 mg, wkly	558	1/50 fibro-sarcoma		*543*
33 mg, wkly	539	5/20 local sarcomas		*544*
5 mg, 3 × wkly in acetone	520	0/20		*542*
10 mg, 3 × wkly in acetone	540	0/30		
100 mg, 3 × wkly no solvent	237[e]	3/30 papillomas 1/30 squamous ca.	considered active	*545*
10 mg, 3 × wkly in acetone	427	2/41 papillomas 1/41 squamous	considered active; 1,2-epoxydo-decane inactive	*542*
10 mg, 3 × wkly in benzene	431[e]	3/30 papillomas 1/30 squamous ca.	considered active; sat. analog, ethyleneoxy-cyclohexane inactive; styrene oxide reported in-active (*447*)	*545*
5 μmoles	?	3% skin 10% malignant lymphomas 3% pulmonary adenomas		*546*
200[b]	658	7/12 local sarcoma		*449*
440[b]	626	6/12 local sarcoma		*449*
550[b]	608	4/12 local sarcoma		*449*

[d] May be effectively difunctional since both the aldehyde and epoxide groups react with guanosine (*542*).

[e] Median survival time.

The use of compounds of this type as pesticides stimulated interest in their alkylating ability. For example, the anticholinesterase Dichlorvos (DDVP, dichlorovinyl dimethyl phosphate), the active constituent of an insecticidal strip, can methylate DNA *in vitro*, but the reaction is slow (534). This compound is weakly mutagenic to *E. coli* and several other bacterial species, but, in the opinion of one group of investigators (534a), the mutagenic potency is "insufficient for the compound to be regarded as dangerously mutagenic to man." Methylation of DNA in *E. coli* by dichlorvos was detected (535), and mice treated with [^{14}C]methyl-dichlorvos excreted 7-[^{14}C]methylguanine in urine (536). The metabolism of ^{32}P- and ^{14}C-labeled dichlorvos in the pig and rat are under investigation, and relevant preliminary reports have appeared (537, 538). Further relevant studies on the cytotoxicity and potential mutagenicity of dichlorvos were reported recently by workers at Shell Research Ltd. (538a). No mutagenic action was found in the mammalian systems studied.

MISCELLANEOUS ESTERS (Table XX). Esters of fatty acids appear generally to be inactive. This conclusion is possibly consistent with their hydrolysis at the acyl–oxygen rather than at the alkyl–oxygen linkage, in contrast to the alkylating abilities of sulfate and phosphate esters.

MONOFUNCTIONAL EPOXIDES (Tables XXI and XXII). The parent compound, ethylene oxide, typifies the reactivity conferred by the strained 3-membered ring. However, as a potential carcinogen, it is generally considered to be inactive, although it might be considered as not exhaustively tested in view of the relatively weak activity found for propylene oxide (449). Van Duuren et al. (542, 543, 544) found other simple aliphatic epoxides generally to be inactive. It appears necessary to elongate the aliphatic chain of the molecule to enhance activity or to include other relatively hydrophobic groups conferring greater lipid solubility, but not all such modifications are effective in this respect (Table XXII).

An apparent exception to this generalization is glycidaldehyde. However, as shown by Van Duuren et al. (542) this can act as a difunctional agent in its reaction with guanosine, and difunctional epoxides are in general more potent carcinogens than monofunctional (448). It has been

Table XXII. Representative Oncogenesis Tests— Epoxides (Monofunctional) Reported to be Inactive

Compound	Formula	Test System	References
Ethylene oxide	H$_2$C——CH$_2$ \\ O /	mouse skin rat, s.c.	309, 449
Glycidol	H$_2$C——CH CH$_2$OH \\ O /	mouse skin	309
Epichlorhydrin[a]	H$_2$C——CH CH$_2$Cl \\ O /	mouse skin	447

Table XXII. Continued

Compound	Formula	Test System	References
Epibromohydrin	H₂C——CH CH₂Br (epoxide O)	mouse skin	309
1,2-Epoxybutane	H₂C——CH CH₂CH₃ (epoxide O)	mouse skin	309
2,3-Epoxy-2-methyl-propyl acrylate	CH_3 / H₂C——C—CH₂OCOCH:CH₂ (epoxide O)	mouse skin	447
9,10-Epoxystearic acid	CH₃(CH₂)₇—CH—CH—(CH₂)₇CO₂H (epoxide O)	mouse skin mouse, rat, s.c.	309
Glycidyl ester of stearic acid	H₂C——CH·CH₂·CO₂(CH₂)₇CH: CH(CH₂)₇CH₃ (epoxide O)	rat s.c.	449
1,2-Epoxydodecane	H₂C——CH·(CH₂)₉CH₃ (epoxide O)	mouse skin	309
Epoxycyclohexane	(cyclohexene oxide)	mouse skin rat, s.c.	309
1-Vinyl-3,4-epoxycyclohexane	CH:CH₂ (epoxycyclohexane)	mouse skin	309
Epoxycyclooctane	(cyclooctene oxide)	mouse skin	309
Indan epoxide	(indan oxide)	mouse skin	309
Limonene monoxide	CH_3 ... C=CH₂ / CH₃	mouse skin	309
Ethyleneoxycy-clohexane	(ethyleneoxy cyclohexane)	mouse skin	309
Dieldrin[b]	Cl Cl / O CH₂ CCl₂ Cl / Cl	rat, dog, p.o. rabbit skin	547
Endrin[c]		rat, p.o. rabbit skin rat, p.o.	548 547 549

[a] Reported positive by Kotin and Falk (*546*); *see* Table XXI.
[b] Endo, exo isomer.
[c] Endo, endo isomer of dieldrin.

suggested further that monofunctional agents with adjacent centers of unsaturation may be converted *in vivo* to difunctional agents (*542*).

Thus, while epoxides can act as alkylating agents in neutral aqueous media and were shown to be mutagenic in numerous instances (*25, 144*), it may be concluded that either the simpler monofunctional epoxides alkylate to insufficient extent *in vivo* to cause carcinogenesis, or the types of reaction undergone do not lead to this effect. Propylene oxide reacts slowly with DNA in aqueous solution (*550*) introducing the -$CH_2CH(OH)CH_3$ group by the S_N2 mechanism.

No studies of *in vivo* alkylation by epoxides appear to have been reported. However, active monofunctional epoxides such as styrene oxide and 1,2-epoxybut-3-ene (Table XXI) might react in part by the S_N1 mechanism, the derived carbonium ion being stabilized mesomerically. This in turn might correlate with enhanced mutagenic, and therefore possibly tumor

Table XXIII. Representative Oncogenesis

Compound	Formula	Animal	Strain or Type	Route
Ethyleneimine	$HN{<}^{CH_2}_{CH_2}$	rat	albino (m) albino (f)	s.c.
			albino (m)	s.c.
			albino (f)	
N-Acetylethyl-eneimine	$CH_3CON{<}^{CH_2}_{CH_2}$	rat	albino	s.c.
			albino (m) albino (f)	s.c.
		mouse	C(m)	s.c.
			C3Hf(f)	s.c.

initiating, activity according to the arguments discussed previously. Epoxides derived from polynuclear aromatic hydrocarbons are of interest as potential reactive metabolites and are discussed by Dipple (Chapter 5).

MONOFUNCTIONAL ETHYLENEIMINES (Table XXIII). Apart from recent work by Van Duuren *et al.* (*551*) the relatively early work of Walpole's group (reviewed by Ref. *449*) remains the principal contribution for this type of agent. The parent compound, ethyleneimine, is a more potent inducer of sarcoma at the injection site than the analogous heterocycle ethylene oxide. The other active monofunctional ethyleneimines reflect the interest of Walpole's group in the effectiveness conferred by substitution of long-chain alkyl groups into the ethyleneimine (aziridine) nucleus. This, no doubt, enhances the retention of this potentially reactive group in the tissues near the injection site. However, studies of *in vivo* alkylation by these compounds have not been made yet.

Tests—Ethyleneimines (Monofunctional)

Dose (mg/kg)	Duration (Days)	Tumors	Remarks	References
20[a]	546	5/6 local sarcoma 1/6 local sarcoma	1/19 local sarcoma, 1/19 local fibroma, 4/19 other tumors in controls, but latent period generally longer in controls	505
12[b]	540	0/6 local sarcoma 1/6 kidney carcinoma 2/6 local sarcoma		
up to 210[a]	515	13/30 local sarcoma 3/30 other		
160[b]	449	3/6 local sarcoma		
80[b]		1/6 local sarcoma		
200[a]	371	6/20 local sarcoma		
180[a]		5/20 local sarcoma		

Table XXIII.

Compound	Formula	Animal	Strain or Type	Route
N-Butyrylethyl-eneimine	$CH_3CH_2CH_2CON\begin{smallmatrix}CH_2\\|\\CH_2\end{smallmatrix}$	rat	albino	s.c.
				s.c.
		mouse	C3Hf	s.c.
N-Diethylace-tylethylene-imine	$(C_2H_5)_2CHCON\begin{smallmatrix}CH_2\\|\\CH_2\end{smallmatrix}$	rat	albino	s.c.
		mouse	C3Hf(f)	s.c.
N-Caproylethyl-eneimine	$CH_3(CH_2)_4CON\begin{smallmatrix}CH_2\\|\\CH_2\end{smallmatrix}$	rat	albino	s.c.
		mouse	C3Hf(m)	s.c.
			C3Hf(f)	s.c.
N-Nonanoyl-ethyleneimine	$CH_3(CH_2)_7CON\begin{smallmatrix}CH_2\\|\\CH_2\end{smallmatrix}$	rat	albino	s.c.
				s.c.
		mouse	C3Hf(m)	s.c.
N-Laurylethyl-eneimine	$CH_3(CH_2)_{10}CON\begin{smallmatrix}CH_2\\|\\CH_2\end{smallmatrix}$	rat	albino	s.c.
N-Myristoyl-ethyleneimine	$CH_3(CH_2)_{12}CON\begin{smallmatrix}CH_2\\|\\CH_2\end{smallmatrix}$	rat	albino	s.c.
		mouse	C3Hf(m)	s.c.
N-Oleylethyl-eneimine	$CH_3(CH_2)_7CH{:}CH(CH_2)_7CON\begin{smallmatrix}CH_2\\|\\CH_2\end{smallmatrix}$	rat	albino	s.c.

Continued

Dose (mg/kg)	Duration (Days)	Tumors	Remarks	References
220[a]	489	11/12 local sarcoma 4/12 other		*505*
225[b]	428	10/12 local sarcoma 1/12 other		
488[a]	504	3/20 local sarcoma		
420–440[a]	314	9/12 local sarcoma 3/6 mammary ca. in (f) 2/6 other in (f)		
225[b]	428	10/12 local sarcoma 1/12 other		
400–460[c]	346	11/12 local sarcoma 5/6 mammary ca. in (f)		
488[a]	443	10/16 local sarcoma		
49.5–51[a]	314	12/12 local sarcoma		
52.5[c]	450	8/12 local sarcoma		
765[a]	385	5/16 local sarcoma		
360[a]		2/20 local sarcoma		
760–860[a]	296	11/12 local sarcoma 3/12 other		
720–740[c]	324	9/12 local sarcoma 5/12 other		
500[a]	504	4/20 local sarcoma		
1000[a]	up to 741	1/12 local sarcoma 4/12 other		
3325[a]	229	8/12 local sarcoma		
1600[a]	395	13/20 local sarcoma		
17[a]	178	11/12 local sarcoma		

Table XXIII.

Compound	Formula	Animal	Strain or Type	Route
N-Stearoyl-ethyleneimine	$CH_3(CH_2)_{16}CON{<}^{CH_2}_{CH_2}$	rat	albino	s.c.
Ethyleneimino-sulfonylpropane	$CH_3(CH_2)_2SO_2N{<}^{CH_2}_{CH_2}$	rat	albino	s.c.
Ethyleneimino-sulfonylpentane	$CH_3(CH_2)_4SO_2N{<}^{CH_2}_{CH_2}$	rat	albino	s.c.
Ethyleneimino-sulfonylheptane	$CH_3(CH_2)_6SO_2N{<}^{CH_2}_{CH_2}$	rat	albino	s.c.
4-Chloro-6-ethyleneimino-2-phenylpyrimidine		rat	albino	s.c.
N-Cycloethyleneureidoazobenzene		rat	albino	s.c.
Aziridine ethanol (3-Hydroxy-1-ethylaziridine)	$HOCH_2CH_2N{<}^{CH_2}_{CH_2}$	mouse	ICR/Ha Swiss	s.c.
Propyleneimine	$CH_3CH_2CH_2N{<}^{CH_2}_{CH_2}$	rat	Charles River CD	i.g.

a Total dose; twice-weekly injection in arachis oil.
b Total dose; twice-weekly injection in water.
c Total dose; twice-weekly injection in Carbowax 300.

OXETANES, LACTONES, AND RELATED COMPOUNDS (FOUR-MEMBERED RINGS) (Table XXIV). Compounds of this group, like the epoxides and ethyleneimines, embody strained-ring structures conferring reactivity towards nucleophiles (reviewed by Ref. 113) with cleavage of the CH_2-O bond.

The parent compound, oxetane (trimethylene oxide), and its β,β-dimethyl derivative are active but not very potent sarcomagens at the injection site. Druckrey et al. (151) derived a value of their carcinogenic index of 19 for trimethylene oxide.

Continued

Dose (mg/kg)	Duration (Days)	Tumors	Remarks	References
27.5[a]	441	7/12 local sarcoma 2/12 other		505
1250[a]	601	0/12		
900[a]	601	0/12		
1500[a]	601	0/12		
960[a]	154	11/12 local sarcoma		
1110–1140[a]	570	7/12 local sarcoma 1/12 other	Corresponding N-dimethyl analog gave no local sarcomas, but did give 7/12 tumors at other sites	
0.3 mg × 75[d]	525	10/30 local sarcoma		551
10 × 120[e]	420	20/26 breast 8/26 other in females 4/26 leukemia 4/26 glioma 9/26 other in males		563

[d] Weekly injection in tricaprylin.
[e] Twice weekly, administration, by gavage, in water.

The oxetanones, β-propiolactone and 4-membered-ring lactones, are fairly generally, but not always (Table XXVII), active carcinogens. The extensively investigated β-propiolactone is a "potent, though slow-acting carcinogen" (*113, 151*) with carcinogenic index of 500. Substitution in the β-propiolactone ring weakens its activity.

Some progress towards correlation of *in vivo* reactions and carcinogenic activity, with regard to the classical two-stage mechanism, for β-propio-lactone and related alkylating agents containing carbonyl substituents has

Table XXIV. Representative Oncogenesis Tests—Oxetanes,

Compound	Formula	Animal	Strain or Type	Route
Trimethylene oxide (Oxetane)	H_2C—CH_2 O—CH_2	rat	BD	s.c.
β,β-Dimethyltrimethylene oxide	H_2C—$C(CH_3)_2$ O—CH_2	rat	Wistar	s.c.
β-Propiolactone (2-Oxetanone, 3-Hydroxypropionic acid lactone)	H_2C—CH_2 O—CO	rat	albino	s.c.
		mouse	albino "S"	skin
				skin
				i.v., tail
		rat	Wistar	s.c.
		mouse	albino	skin
		mouse	Swiss	skin
		mouse	Swiss ICR/Ha	s.c.
		guinea-pig	—	skin

Lactones and Related Compounds (Four-Membered Rings)

Dose (mg/kg) (or as Stated)	Duration (Days)	Tumors	Remarks	References
40 × 56, wkly	550[a]	6/14 local sarcomas		*151*
80 × 56, wkly	550	5/6 local sarcomas 1/6 vaginal carcinoma		
1 mg × 102[e]	742	2/4 local sarcomas		*552*
440–480[b]	508	9/12 local sarcomas		*449*
155 mg[c]	133	160/19 papillomas		*476*
7.5 mg, wkly × 52	385	5/10 papillomas	2 malignant ca.	*553*
1–10 mg[d]	183	inj. site papillomas	no lung tumors	
0.1 mg × 68[c]	238	4/4 local sarcomas	1/11 thoracic tumor in controls	*112*
1.0 mg × 88[d]	308	10/10 local sarcomas		
2.0 mg × 66[f]	385	2/4 local sarcomas		
7.5 mg × 70[g]	322	1/25 squamous carcinoma	weak response attributed to hydrolysis in impure acetone	*554*
7.5 mg × 120[g]	420	20/45 squamous ca. and others		
5 mg, 3 × wkly[g]	ca. 250	21/30 papillomas 11/30 cancers	dose–response study, *see* original ref.	*555*
0.73 mg, wkly[h]	503	9/30 fibrosarcomas 3/30 adenoca. 6/30 squamous cell ca.		*543*
12.5 mg, 2 × wkly[g]	up to 1176	3/9 kerato-acanthomas 1/9 melanoma 1/9 hepatoma 1/9 lacrimal gland tumor	also pigmented naevi	*509*

Table XXIV.

Compound	Formula	Animal	Strain or Type	Route
β-Propiolactone (2-Oxetanone, 3-Hydroxypropionic acid lactone) (*continued*)		golden hamster	—	skin
		mouse	"Susceptible" (f)	
		mouse	B6AF₁, neonates (m)	i.p.
			neonates (f)	i.p.
			neonates (m)	skin
			neonates (f)	skin
			adults (m)	i.p.
			adults (f)	i.p.
β-Butyrolactone	CH_3CH-CH_2 $\mid$ $\quad$ $\mid$ $O-CO$	mouse	Swiss ICR/Ha	skin
		mouse	Swiss ICR/Ha	skin

Continued

Dose (mg/kg) (or as Stated)	Duration (Days)	Tumors	Remarks	References
12.5 mg, 2 × wkly[g]	up to 700	8/17 keratoacan-thomas 4/17 melanomas 5/17 papillomas 2/17 squamous cell ca.		510
120 μmoles × 6[c]	210	97% papillomas 11% carcinomas	binding to DNA, RNA, and protein studied	307, 308
0.5 mg (ca. 100 mg i/kg)	476	65% hepatomas 47% lung tumors 9% lymphomas	controls 4% hepatomas, 49% lung tumors, nil lymphomas	511
0.5 mg[i]		nil hepatomas 27% lung tumors 20% lymphomas	controls nil hepatomas, 24% lung tumors, nil lymphomas	
3 mg[j]	476	19% hepatomas 44% lung tumors nil lymphomas		
3 mg[j]	476	3% hepatomas 55% lung tumors 3% lymphomas		
80 mg/kg[i]	546	9% hepatomas 55% lung tumors 14% lymphomas	controls, 6.7% hepatomas, 44% lung tumors, nil lymphomas	
80 mg/kg[i]	546	nil hepatomas 40% lung tumors 17% lymphomas	controls, 1% hepatomas, 34% lung tumors, 5% lymphomas	
10 mg, 3 × wkly[j]	466	4/30 papillomas 21/30 carcinomas		556
1 mg, single	468	0/20 papillomas 0/20 carcinomas		
1 mg, single, then croton resin promotion	468	3/20 papillomas 1/20 carcinomas		
10 mg, 3 × wkly[j]	598	1/40 papillomas 1/40 cancer		542
10 mg, 3 × wkly[k]	467	20/30 papillomas 16/30 cancers		

Table XXIV.

Compound	Formula	Animal	Strain or Type	Route
4,5-Epoxy-3-hydroxyvaleric acid β-lactone	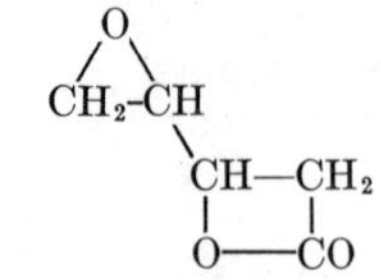 (see structure)	mouse	Swiss ICR/ Ha	skin
α-Carboxy-β-phenyl-β-propiolactone	Ph.CH—CH.COOH | | O——CO	rat	Wistar	s.c.
α,α-Diphenyl-β-propiolactone	H_2C—CPh_2 | | O—CO	rat	Wistar	s.c.
Penicillin G	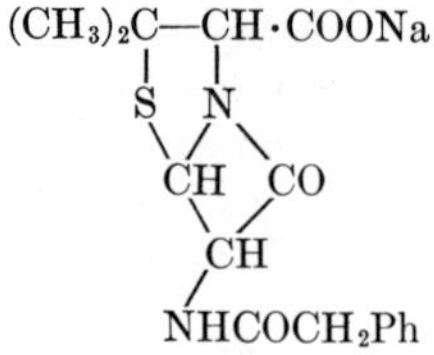 $(CH_3)_2C$—CH·COONa (see structure)	rat	Wistar	s.c.

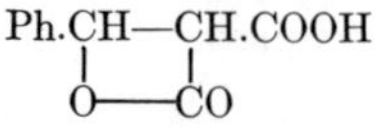

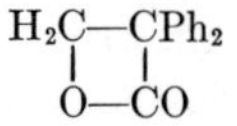

Structure for 4,5-Epoxy-3-hydroxyvaleric acid β-lactone:

$$CH_2-CH \overset{O}{\diagup\diagdown}$$
$$CH-CH_2$$
$$\underset{O-CO}{|\quad|}$$

Structure for Penicillin G:

$$(CH_3)_2C-CH\cdot COONa$$
$$S\quad N$$
$$CH\quad CO$$
$$CH$$
$$NHCOCH_2Ph$$

[a] Mean time of death of tumor-bearing animals.
[b] Twice weekly injection in arachis oil, total dose stated.
[c] Multiple doses in acetone, total dose stated, promotion with croton oil.
[d] Multiple doses in Ringer solution, total dose stated.
[e] Twice weekly, injection in arachis oil.
[f] Twice weekly injection in water.

emerged from the work of Boutwell *et al.* (*557*). Van Duuren (*448*) has also reviewed structure–activity relationships and has raised the question whether the principal reaction of β-propiolactone with DNA *in vivo* to yield 7-(2-carboxyethyl)guanine (*557*) is important for carcinogenic action or whether other, as yet apparently undefined, reaction sites could be involved.

Penicillin, although originally included by Dickens and Jones (*112*) as a reactive lactone, may convert to more reactive derivatives (page 95). The relationship between the reactions of penicillenic acid and those of five-membered ring lactones will be evident from the subsequent discussion of these compounds.

LACTONES AND RELATED COMPOUNDS (FIVE-MEMBERED RINGS) (Table XXV). Unlike the β-lactones, γ-lactones are not inherently reactive because of ring strain. This lack of reactivity of γ-butyrolactone, therefore, is in accord with its inactivity as a carcinogen (*113, 448*).

However, certain modifications of the five-membered ring structure,

Continued

Dose (mg/kg) (or as Stated)	Duration (Days)	Tumors	Remarks	References
10 mg, 3 × wkly[k]	514	5/30 papillomas	benign tumors only; considered negative as carcinogen	556
2 mg × 128[e]	735	1/4 local sarcoma		112
1 mg × 38[e]	735	1/3 local sarcoma		
2 mg × 92[e]	700	1/4 local sarcoma 1/4 remote fibroma 1/4 thyroid alveolar carcinoma		112
2 mg × 104[e]	735	1/4 local sarcoma		552
2 mg × 130[e]	742	2/4 local fibro-sarcoma		

[g] Applied in acetone solution (generally twice weekly).
[h] In tricaprylin (octanoin).
[i] In arachis oil.
[j] In acetone.
[k] In benzene.

notably the presence of ethylenic bonds, can enhance both chemical reactivity (which has so far been studied principally with regard to reactions with thiols) and sometimes carcinogenicity. The relationship between reactivity towards thiols and carcinogenic potency is not a simple positive correlation (*558*). For example, the α,β-unsaturated γ-lactones (*e.g.*, 4-hydroxypent-2-enoic acid lactone, Scheme 8) react with thiols in neutral aqueous solution, with the β-carbon atom as the electrophilic center, to give alkylation products. Several lactones of this type are carcinogenic (*113*). Thiols also react with the noncarcinogen, 4-hydroxypent-3-enoic acid lactone, but the products are derived by S-acylation rather than by S-alkylation and are unstable; the product with cysteine rearranges rapidly to yield an N-acylated cysteine. Jones and Young (*558*) point out that this latter reaction *in vivo* would be reparable by proteolytic enzymes whereas alkylation would be irreversible. The alkylation products can also undergo further nucleophilic attack at the carbonyl group, thus introducing the possibility of *in vivo* cross-linking

Table XXV. Representative Oncogenesis Tests—

Compound	Formula	Animal	Strain or Type	Route
γ-Butyrolactone (3-Hydroxybutyric acid lactone, 4-Hydroxybutanoic acid lactone)	H$_2$C—CH$_2$ CH$_2$ CO O	rat mouse	Wistar ICR/Ha	s.c. skin
Maleic anhydride	HC=CH CO CO O	rat	Wistar	s.c.
α, β-Dimethyl maleic anhydride	CH$_3$·C=C·CH$_3$ CO CO O	rat	Wistar	s.c.
Succinic anhydride	H$_2$C—CH$_2$ CO CO O	rat	Wistar	s.c.
4-Hydroxyhex-2-enoic acid lactone	HC=CH C$_2$H$_5$·CH CO O	rat	Wistar	s.c.
Methyl protoanemonin (4-Hydroxyhexo-2,4-dienoic acid lactone)	HC=CH CH$_3$CH=C CO O	rat	Wistar	s.c.
4-Hydroxyhex-4-enoic acid lactone	H$_2$C—CH$_2$ CH$_3$·CH=C CO O	rat	Wistar	s.c.
Patulin (Clavacin)	CHOH O C=CH CH$_2$ C CO CH O	rat	Wistar	s.c.
Penicillic acid	CH$_3$O—C=CH CH$_3$ C CO C O CH$_2$ OH	rat mouse	Wistar	s.c.
Bovolide	CH$_3$C=CCH$_3$ CH$_3$(CH$_2$)$_3$CH=C CO O	rat	Wistar	s.c.

Lactones and Related Compounds (Five-Membered Rings)

Dose	Duration (Days)	Tumors	Remarks	References
2 mg × 122[a]	700	0/5		*112*
10 mg, 3 × wkly[b]	292	2/30 papillomas	Considered negative	*545*
		1/30 cancer		
1 mg × 122[a]	742	2/3 local fibro-sarcomas		*552*
2 mg × 130[a]	728	3/5 local sarcomas		*493*
2 mg × 130[a]	742	3/3 local sarcomas		*493*
2 mg × 128[a]	714	2/4 local fibro-sarcomas	isomeric-3-enoic lactone inactive	*112*
2 mg × 128[a]	735	3/5 local fibro-sarcomas		*112*
1 mg × 116[a]	693	3/5 local sarcomas		*112*
0.2 mg × 122[a]	483	4/4 local sarcomas		*112*
1 mg × 128[a]	469	4/4 local sarcomas		*112*
0.1 mg × 122[a]	742	1/4 local sarcomas		
2 mg × 104[c]	723	4/5 local sarcomas		*552*
0.2 mg × 76[a]	588	6/19 local sarcomas		*493*
2 mg × 130[a]	742	5/5 local sarcomas		*493*

Table XXV.

Compound	Formula	Animal	Strain or Type	Route
α-Methyltetronic acid	HO·C=C·CH₃ CH₂ CO O	rat	Wistar	s.c.
Vinylene carbonate	HC=CH O O CO	rat	Wistar	
Sarkomycin	NaOOC·CH—C=CH₂ CH₂ CO O	rat	Wistar	s.c.

^a In arachis oil.
^b In benzene.
^c In water.

reactions. Although studies of *in vivo* reactions of the unsaturated γ-lactones have not been made, they might thus prove to be of considerable interest.

Dickens (*113*) has shown further that inclusion of an external double bond at the 4-position of the γ-lactones, as in methylprotoanemonin, conferred carcinogenic activity and also enhanced that of the α,β-unsaturated lactones.

Scheme 8. Reactions of unsaturated γ-lactones with cysteine (RSH; R = ·CH₂CH(NH₂)CO₂H) at pH 7 (558)

(a) α,β-unsaturated γ-lactones, *e.g.* 4-hydroxypent-2-enoic acid lactone

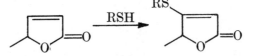

(b) β,γ-unsaturated γ-lactones, *e.g.* 4-hydroxypent-3-enoic acid lactone

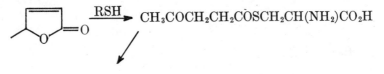

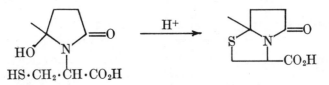

Continued

Dose	Duration (Days)	Tumors	Remarks	References
2 mg × 130[a]	693	2/4 local sarcomas	not trans-plantable	
2 mg × 130[a]	588	6/6 local sarcomas		
2 mg × 84[a]	742	1/6 local myxo-sarcoma		

With regard to vinylene carbonate, Jones and Young (*558*) found no cysteine reaction products and suggested that an *in vivo* hydrolysis product was probably the ultimate carcinogen. Dickens (*113*) noted that several natural products embody the structural features of the reactive γ-lactones and suggested that compounds of this type might occur as endogenous carcinogens.

LACTONES AND RELATED COMPOUNDS (SIX-MEMBERED RINGS) (Table XXVI). With respect to chemical reactivity, this group of compounds may be considered analogous to the five-membered ring lactones, *i.e.*, the presence of α,β-ethylenic bonds is necessary for activity, and the results of onco-genesis tests are generally also parallel (*113*). Sorbic acid, an open-chain analog of α,β-unsaturated lactones, also proved active in one test, but this was not confirmed subsequently (*502a*).

The aflatoxins (Chapter 12) fall into the structural class of six-membered ring lactones, but their carcinogenic potency can be both quantitatively higher and qualitatively different from typical lactones, *e.g.*, they are highly active by oral and intratracheal administration. The question of their possibly acting through reactive metabolites was first discussed by Lijinsky, and the time course of binding of ^{3}H-labeled aflatoxins B_1 and G_1 to macro-molecules of liver and other organs of rats was reported by Lijinsky *et al.* (*109*). Recently, Swenson *et al.* (*94*) showed that *in vivo* reactions of aflatoxin B_1 are largely mediated by the 2,3-epoxide. Maleic hydrazide is also unlikely to act by direct *in vivo* alkylation, and its mode of action is as yet uncertain.

The chromene and isochromene derivatives studied by Lacassagne *et al.* (*561, 562*) embody six-membered lactone rings. More detailed discussion of these compounds is given by Dipple (Chapter 5).

Table XXVI. Representative Oncogenesis Tests—

Compound	Formula	Animal	Strain or Type	Route
(+) Parasorbic acid		rat	Wistar	s.c.
Maleic hydrazide		rat	Wistar	s.c.
		mouse	Swiss (infant male)	s.c.
Aflatoxin B₁ᶜ		rat	Wistar	s.c.
Aflatoxin G₁ᶜ		rat	Wistar	s.c.
Sterigmatocystin		rat	Wistar	s.c.
Gedunin		rat	Wistar	s.c.
Sorbic acid		rat	Wistar	s.c.
Dehydroacetic acid				

Lactones and Related Compounds (Six-Membered Rings)

Dose	Duration (Days)	Tumors	Remarks	References
0.2 mg × 64[a]	665	4/6 local sarcomas		*552*
2 mg × 64[a]	742	4/5 local sarcomas		
2 mg × 130[a]	742	3/6 local sarcomas 1/6 hepatoma		*493*
55 mg[b]	343	65% hepatomas	8% in controls	*559*
20 μg, 2 × wkly	259	6/6 local sarcomas		*493*
20 μg, 2 × wkly	350	4/6 local sarcomas		*493*
0.5 mg × 48[a]	455	3/6 local sarcomas 1/6 hepatoma 1/6 cholangioma		*502*
2 mg × 130[a]	721	1/1 local sarcoma		
2 mg × 130[a]	679	5/6 local sarcomas	reactive open-chain analog of lactones; reported inactive by *502a*	*502*
2 mg × 130[a]	595	5/6 local sarcomas		

Table XXVI.

Compound	Formula	Animal	Strain or Type	Route
N^6-(3,4-Benzo-coumarinyl)-acetamide	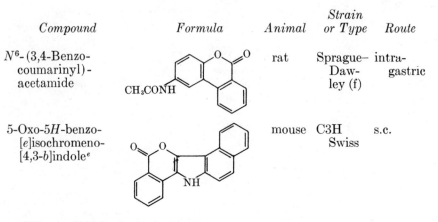	rat	Sprague–Daw-ley (f)	intra-gastric
5-Oxo-5H-benzo-[e]isochromeno-[4,3-b]indole[e]	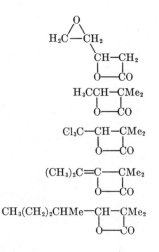	mouse	C3H Swiss	s.c.

[a] Twice weekly injection in arachis oil.
[b] During first three weeks of life; in water or tricaprylin.

Table XXVII.   Representative Oncogenesis Tests—

Compound	Formula
Four-Membered Rings Diketene	H_2C——C=CH_2 $\quad\quad\ \ CO$—O
4,5-Epoxy-3-hydroxyvaleric acid β-lactone	
3-Hydroxy-2,2-dimethylbutyric acid β-lactone	H_3CCH—CMe_2 $\quad\ O$——CO
3-Hydroxy-2,2-dimethyl-4,4,4-trichlorobutyric acid β-lactone	Cl_3C—CH—CMe_2 $\quad\quad\ \ O$——CO
2,2,4-Trimethyl-3-hydroxy-3-pentenoic acid β-lactone[a]	$(CH_3)_2C$=C——CMe_2 $\quad\quad\quad\ O$——CO
3-Hydroxy-2,2,4-trimethyl-heptanoic acid β-lactone	$CH_3(CH_2)_2CHMe$—CH—CMe_2 $\quad\quad\quad\quad\quad\ O$——$CO$

Continued

Dose	Duration (Days)	Tumors	Remarks	References
1000 mg[d]	270	6/19 mammary ca. and other tumors	6-acetamidocou- marin inactive	560
0.6 mg × 3	450 183	26/28 sarcomas 26/26 sarcomas	rapidly acting potent car- cinogen	561

Ref. *457*.
  [d] Total dose.

Lactones and Related Compounds Reported Inactive

Species	Route	References
mouse	skin	*309, 545*
mouse	s.c.	
rat	s.c.	
mouse	skin	
mouse	skin	*309*
mouse	skin	*309*
mouse	skin	*309*
mouse	s.c.	
mouse	skin	*309*

Table XXVII.

Compound	*Formula*
Five-Membered Rings γ-Butyrolactone	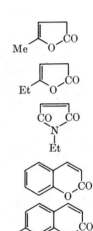
β-Angelicalactone	
α-Angelicalactone	
4-Hydroxyhex-3-enoic acid lactone	
N-Ethylmaleimide	
Six-Membered Rings Coumarin	
6-Acetamidocoumarin	

ᵃ Reported positive for rat, s.c. by Van Duuren *et al.* (*543*).

CYCLIC SULFIDES AND SULTONES (Table XXVIII). Ethylene sulfide, the analog of ethylene oxide, is a sarcomagen at the injection site in the rat, although not of high potency. The value of the carcinogenic index derived by Druckrey *et al.* (*151*) was 9, compared with 500 for β-propiolactone.

1,3-Propanesultone is "highly reactive" and "a potent carcinogen" with an index of 130–210 by multiple injection and 470–800 by single injection (*311*). The next higher homolog, 1,4-butanesultone, was much less carcinogenic. The reactivity towards nucleophiles presumably involves fission of the CH₂-O bond, as with β-propiolactone, the enhanced reactivity relative to that of saturated γ-lactones being ascribed to the greater electron withdrawing power of the —O—SO₂-group compared with that of the —O—CO-group. No studies of *in vivo* alkylation by sultones have been reported as yet.

HALOALKYL ETHERS (Table XXIX). This group of compounds has found wide industrial use and exhibits cytotoxic and irritant properties associated with chemical reactivity of alkylating type (*448*). The α-chloroethyl ethers, chloromethyl ether and α,α-dichloromethyl methyl ether, were inactive as complete carcinogens on mouse skin or by subcutaneous injection in rats

Continued

Species	Route	References
mouse	skin	*545*
rat	s.c.	*112*
mouse	skin	*112, 309, 544*
rat	s.c.	
mouse	skin	*542*
rat	s.c.	*112*
rat	s.c.	*112*
rat	s.c.	*493*
rat	s.c.	*493*
rat	i.g.	*560*

but were initiating agents in two-stage carcinogenesis. Bis(chloromethyl) ether is a potent carcinogen and tumor initiator. Although it is evidently a difunctional alkylating agent, reaction with DNA did not yield any isolable base-alkylation products (*309*).

NITROGEN MUSTARDS (MONOFUNCTIONAL AND 2-CHLOROETHYLSULFONIC ACID DERIVATIVES) (Table XXX). Few monofunctional nitrogen mustards, have been tested, and no simple compound of this type has been reported as active. *N*-(2-Chloroethyl)-*N*-nitrosourethane may owe its carcinogenic potency to its structure as a "mixed difunctional" compound, embodying both the mustard and alkylnitroso groups (*567*) although its mode of reaction has apparently yet to be defined. Aramite has also been classified as an alkylating carcinogen although again the *in vivo* reactions are not known.

Monofunctional aliphatic 2-chloroethylamines yield relatively stable cyclic imonium ions in aqueous solution. Detailed studies with 2-chloroethyldiethylamine suggested that reaction of these ions with nucleophiles proceeds by the S_N2 mechanism (*46*). As previously discussed, this may not be true for 2-chloroethylarylamines, which may react in part through the S_N1

Table XXVIII. Representative Oncogenesis

Compound	Formula	Animal	Strain or Type	Route
Ethylene sulfide	H_2C—CH_2 $\diagdown$S$\diagup$	rat	BD	s.c.
1,3-Propanesultone (1,2-Oxathialone 2,2-dioxide)	H_2C—CH_2 H_2C SO_2 $\diagdown$O$\diagup$	rat	BD	s.c.
				p.o.
				i.v.
				i.v.
				trans-pla-cental
	rat	Charles River CD	i.g.	
	mouse	ICR/Ha Swiss	s.c.	

Tests—Cyclic Sulfides and Sultones

Dose (mg/kg)	Duration (Days)	Tumors	Remarks	References
8 × 50[a]	500[b]	1/15 local sarcomas		*151*
16 × 50		4/12 local sarcomas		
15 × 14[a]	295[b]	7/12 local sarcomas 1/12 tumor of nervous tissue 1/12 other		*151*
30 × 13[a]	270[b]	11/11 local sarcomas		
15 × 15[c]	280[b]	18/18 local sarcomas		
10[d]	500[b]	4/15 local sarcomas		
30[d]	400[b]	12/18 local sarcomas		
100[d]	285[b]	18/18 local sarcomas		
30[e]	340[b]	2/10 nervous tissue 2/10 other		
10–40, wkly[c]	492	5/29 nervous tissue 4/29 other		
150[c]	350[b]	3/32 nervous tissue 6/32 other		
20		3/25 nervous tissue		
60		2/25 nervous tissue 2/25 other		
28 × 120[f]	420	in males, 12/26 glioma, 11/26 other in females, 7/26 breast, 15/26 glioma, 10/26 other	similar results using 56 mg/kg for 32 wks	*563*
0.3 mg × 63	371[g]	12/30 local sarcomas 9/30 other		*551*

Table XXVIII.

Compound	Formula	Animal	Strain or Type	Route
1,4-Butanesultone		rat	BD	s.c.
				i.v.
				p.o.

$$\begin{array}{c} CH_2 \\ H_2C \diagup \quad \diagdown CH_2 \\ H_2C \diagdown \quad \diagup SO_2 \\ O \end{array}$$

a Weekly injection in arachis oil.
b Mean induction time.
c Injection in aqueous buffer solution.
d Single injection in oil.

Table XXIX.   Representative Oncogenesis

Compound	Formula	Animal	Strain or Type	Route
Chloromethyl methyl ether	$ClCH_2 \cdot OCH_3$	mouse	ICR/Ha Swiss	skin
		rat	Sprague–Dawley	s.c.
		mouse	ICR Swiss (newborn)	s.c.
Bis(chloromethyl) ether	$ClCH_2 \cdot OCH_2Cl$	mouse	ICR/Ha	skin
				skin
		rat	Sprague–Dawley	s.c.
		mouse	ICR Swiss (newborn)	s.c.
		mouse	A/Heston	inhalation

Continued

Dose (mg/kg)	Duration (Days)	Tumors	Remarks	References
30 × 76[e]	610[b]	1/12 local sarcoma		*151*
30 × 84		0/16		
30[e]	708	2/16 adeno ca. 6/16 other		

[e] Weekly injection or fed in aqueous solution.
[f] Twice weekly, by gavage in water.
[g] Weekly injection in tricaprylin.

Tests—Haloalkyl Ethers

Dose	Duration (Days)[a]	Tumors	Remarks	References
0.1–1 mg[b]	540	0/60	active as initiator	*309*
0.1 mg[c]	496	7/20 papillomas 4/20 carcinomas		
1 mg[b]	488	5/20 papillomas 1/20 carcinoma		
3 mg × 45[d]	515	1/20 fibro-sarcoma	considered inactive	
125 μl/kg[e]	183	17/99 adenomas	7/50 in controls	*565*
2 mg × 129[b]	313	13/20 papillomas 12/20 carcinomas	active carcinogen	*309*
1 mg[b]	474	5/20 papillomas 2/20 carcinomas	active as initiator	
3 mg × 16 then 1 mg wkly		5/20 fibro-sarcoma		
12.5 μl/kg[e]	183	45/100 ade-nomas	7/50 in controls	*565*
1 ppm, 6th/day, 82 days	196	55% lung tumors	statistically sig. rel. to controls; analogous expt. with chloro-methyl methyl ether not sig. positive	*564*

Table XXIX.

Compound	Formula	Animal	Strain or Type	Route
Octachlorodi-n-propyl ether	$(ClC \cdot CHCl \cdot CH_2)_2O$	mouse	ICR/Ha Swiss	skin
α,α-Dichloromethyl ether	$Cl_2CH \cdot O \cdot CH_3$	mouse	ICR/Ha Swiss	skin
Monochloro-acetaldehyde diethyl acetal	$ClCH_2 \cdot CH(OC_2H_5)$ $\cdot O \cdot CH_2CH_3$	mouse	ICR/Ha Swiss	skin

[a] Median survival time.
[b] In benzene.
[c] Promotion with phorbol ester.

Table XXX.   Representative Oncogenesis Tests—Nitrogen 2-Chloroethylsulfonic

Compound	Formula	Animal	Strain or Type	Route
(2-Chloroethyl)-trimethylammonium chloride	$ClCH_2CH_2{}^+N(CH_3)_3Cl^-$	mouse	(C57-BL/6 × C3H/Anf) F_1	i.g. p.o.
N-(2-Chloro-ethyl)amino-azobenzene	ClCH₂CH₂NH⟨⟩N:N⟨⟩	rat	Wistar	p.o.
N-(2-Chloro-ethyl)-N-nitro-sourethane	$ClCH_2CH_2N(NO)$ COOEt	rat	White, Porton	intra-gastric
"Quinacrine ethyl half mustard," "ICR-125," 9-(2-(2-Chloro-ethyl)amino)-ethylamino)-6-chloro-2-meth-oxyacridine	HN·CH₂CH₂NHCH₂CH₂Cl, —OCH₃, Cl	mouse	A/J	i.p.
"ICR-170," 9-(3-(Ethyl-2-chlo-roethyl)amino)-ethylamino)-6-chloro-2-meth-oxyacridine	HN·CH₂CH₂N(Et)(CH₂CH₂Cl), —OCH₃, Cl	mouse	A/J	i.p.

Continued

Dose	Duration (Days)[a]	Tumors	Remarks	References
1 mg[e]	450	3/20 papillomas	active as initiator	309
		1/20 carcinoma		
1 mg[e]	450	3/20 papillomas	active as initiator	
		1/20 carcinoma		
1 mg[e]	450	1/20 papillomas	considered inactive	

[d] In nujol.
[e] In arachis oil.

Mustards (Monofunctional) (2-Chloroethylamines) and Acid Derivatives

Dose	Duration (Days)	Tumors	Remarks	References
21.5 mg/kg × 21 then 65 ppm in diet	540	Lymphomas, pulmonary and liver tumors	in "uncertain range" statistically	451
0.07% in diet	240	0/14		566
6–100 mg/kg	up to 400	4/10 stomach carcinomas 2/10 other carcinomas	"Mixed difunctional" agent- mustard and nitroso compound	567
1280 μmol/kg[a]	273	pulmonary, rel. potency[b] 7.8	"borderline activity"	31
			inactive	31

Table XXX.

Compound	Formula	Animal	Strain or Type	Route
Methanesulfonic acid 2-chloro-ethyl ester, "CB 1506"	$ClCH_2CH_2O \cdot SO_2CH_3$	mouse	A/J	i.p.
"Aramite,"2-(4-*t*-Butylphenoxy) isopropyl-2-chloroethyl sulfite	$ClCH_2CH_2O \cdot SO \cdot OCH_2\overset{\underset{\displaystyle O-\!\!\langle\bigcirc\rangle\!\!-C(CH_3)_3}{\mid}}{\overset{CH_3}{\mid}}CH$	rat	Wistar	p.o.
		dog	mongrel	p.o.
		mouse	(C57-BL/6 × C3H/Anf) F_1	i.g. then p.o.

[a] Range of dose levels used; "positive response dose," giving 1 tumor/mouse shown, was deduced from data.
   [b] Denotes (10,000/positive response dose), see [a].

mechanism. No studies of *in vivo* alkylation by monofunctional nitrogen mustards have been made. The sulfur mustard analog, 2-chloroethyl 2-hydroxyethyl sulfide, alkylated tissue constituents *in vivo*, including DNA, but has not been tested as a carcinogen.

The monofunctional acridine mustard, ICR-170, was used as a fluorochrome (*410*). Its binding specificity to certain chromosomal regions does not apparently confer carcinogenic potency with respect to induction of pulmonary tumors in the test system of Shimkin *et al.* (*31*) although some difunctional acridine mustards were moderately active in this system.

DI- AND POLYFUNCTIONAL NITROGEN AND SULFUR MUSTARDS (Tables XXXI, XXXII, and XXXIII). Mustard gas, although a carcinogen in man was relatively difficult to establish as a carcinogen by testing in animals (Table XXXI). Somewhat similarly, only the more recent tests with the nitrogen mustard HN2 have been entirely convincing. Both these compounds and the potentially trifunctional HN3 are potent cytotoxic agents. The difunctional agents have been extensively studied with regard to the concept that their cytotoxic action arises principally from their ability to inactivate template DNA by cross-linking. Considerable attention has also been devoted to their related effects in stimulating DNA repair mechanisms.

In two-stage carcinogenesis, HN2 was only of borderline activity as an initiating agent (*30*), whereas the mustards Chlorambucil and Melphalan, like TEM and β-propiolactone, were unequivocally active. The most conclusive evidence for carcinogenic potency of HN2, as with several analogous difunctional mustards, has been obtained by Shimkin *et al.* (*31*) for induc-

Continued

Dose	Duration (Days)	Tumors	Remarks	References
380 μmoles/kg[a]	273	pulmonary, rel. potency[b] 26	"borderline activity"	*31*
400 ppm in diet	730	2/100 hepatic carcinomas 5/100 cholangeal adenomas		*568*
500–1429 ppm in diet	1280	20/19 adenocarcinomas and other tumors		*569*
1112 ppm in diet	567	sig. yield of lymphomas, hepatomas, and pulmonary tumors		*451*

[c] Range of dose levels used; highest level did not give "positive response" of statistical significance relative to controls.

tion of lung tumors in strain A mice. These authors further noted hepatotoxic action with some mustards suggesting that in longer term experiments hepatomas would be expected. In addition, statistically significant yields of tumors at various sites were obtained by Schmähl and Osswald (*107*) using intravenous administration in rats according to a dose schedule designed to mimic the use of the mustard as a chemotherapeutic agent. The *N*-oxide of HN2 appears to be more carcinogenic than HN2 itself.

The extensive series of mustards used by Shimkin *et al.* (*31*) showed no clear correlation between carcinogenicity and tumor growth inhibitory properties, but, as already discussed, Fahmy and Fahmy (*142*) found correlations with mutagenicity for certain mustards. Specifically, ability to induce mutations at certain loci (RNA-forming genes) in *Drosophila* was positively correlated with carcinogenicity, not overall mutagenicity.

Evidently, until more details are known about the *in vivo* reactions of the mustards with chromosomes and other possibly significant cellular receptors, interpretation of these correlations in molecular terms must be largely speculative. As noted for the monofunctional mustards, the likely influence of reaction mechanism on biological action remains largely unexplored.

Another doubtless important factor concerns the transport of the mustards to the essential sites of their various biological actions *in vivo*, as discussed, for example, by Shimkin *et al.* (*31*). The high relative potency of "uracil mustard" may, for example, be caused by the presence in the molecule of a modified RNA base residue, perhaps favoring active transport

**Table XXXI.   Representative Oncogenesis Tests—Sulfur
Di(2-chloroethyl)methylamine,**

Compound	Formula	Animal	Strain or Type	Route
Mustard gas, Di-(2-chloroethyl)-sulfide, "H"	$(ClCH_2CH_2)_2S$	mouse	A	i.v.
		mouse	A	s.c.
			C3H	s.c.
			A	inhalation
Di-(2-chloroethyl)methylamine, "HN2," "Nitrogen mustard," "Dichloren," "Mustine"	$(ClCH_2CH_2)_2NCH_3$ (as hydrochloride)	mouse	—	s.c.
		mouse	C3H	s.c.
		mouse	Swiss	i.v., i.p., s.c.
		mouse	albino	s.c.
		mouse	albino	skin
		mouse	albino	s.c., i.p.
		mouse	RF	i.v.
		mouse	A/J	i.p.

and Nitrogen Mustards (Di(2-chloroethyl)sulfide, and Tri(2-chloroethyl)amine

Dose	Duration (days)	Tumors	Remarks	Ref.
0.25 ml of sat. aq. soln. (0.065% × 4	112	93% lung adenomas	61% in controls	*312*
	112	68% lung adenomas	13% in controls	*138*
0.05 ml of 0.05% soln. in olive oil × 5	450	13/26 lung adenomas 3/26 other	15/30 lung adenomas 7/30 other in controls	
as above × 6	600	8/16 mammary 5/16 other	7/16 mammary in controls 10/16 other	
15 min. exposure to vapor	520	44% lung adenomas	27% in controls	*570*
1 mg/kg wkly × 50	580	3/20 lung carcinoma 2/20 lung adenoma 2/20 other		*571*
0.025 mg × 6	*ca.* 360	21/37 pulmonary 17/37 hepatoma and some other	6/39 pulmonary 18/39 hepatoma in controls	*138*
0.5 mg/kg wkly	up to 270	15-20% sarcomas and adeno-carcinoma	no tumors in controls	*572*
0.3-0.4 mg/kg wkly × 64	448	1/138 lymphoma	strain with no spont. lung adenoma	*573*
0.1 mg × 15[a]	133	4/10 skin tumors		*476*
0.4 mg/kg monthly × 9	600	15.6% tumors mostly sar-comas	13.2% in controls, but mustard inj. animals showed tumors earlier	*507*
0.4 mg/kg single	600	13.3% tumors		
1 mg/kg × 9,	600	17.2% tumors		
1 mg/kg single	600	13.3% tumors		
2.4 mg/kg × 4	554	21% thymic lymphoma	8% in controls	*574, 575*
3 μmol/kg[b]	273	lung tumors rel. potency[c] of mustard—3300	"highly potent" inj. in water, "barely active" in tricaprylin	*31*

Table XXXI.

Compound	Formula	Animal	Strain or Type	Route
Di(2-chloro-ethyl)methyl-amine, "HN2," "Nitrogen mustard," "Dichloren," "Mustine" (*continued*)		mouse	A/J	i.v.
		rat	BR46	i.v.
Tri(2-chloro-ethyl)amine, "HN3"	$(ClCH_2CH_2)_3N$ (as hydrochloride)	mouse	—	s.c.

a In acetone; promotion with croton oil.
b Injection in water, 3 × weekly; range of dose levels, "positive response dose," shown, giving 1 lung tumor/mouse.

**Table XXXII. Representative Oncogenesis Tests—
Di-(2-chloroethyl)amine), Excluding**

Compound	Formula*a*	Animal	Strain or Type	Route
Nitrogen mustard N-oxide, "Mitomen," Di(2-chloro-ethyl)methyl-amine N-oxide	O $\uparrow$ $(ClCH_2CH_2)_2NCH_3$	rat	BD	s.c.
		mouse	dd/I (7-day old)	s.c.
		rat	BR46	i.v.
"Chlorambucil," N,N-Di-(2-chloroethyl)-p-aminophenyl-butyric acid	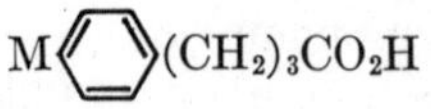 M⟨⟩$(CH_2)_3CO_2H$	mouse	albino S	skin
		mouse	A/J	i.p.

Continued

Dose	Duration (Days)	Tumors	Remarks	Ref.
0.5 μmole/kg[b]	294	lung tumors rel. potency[c]— 20,000		31
0.11 mg/kg, total 5.72 mg/kg	480[d]	26% malignant tumors 18% benign[e]	dose of 7% of LD$_{50}$ to simulate chemotherapy; 6% malignant tumors in controls, 5% benign; statistically sig. positive	107
1 mg/kg wkly × 10	567	2/4 lung carcinoma 1/4 local sarcoma 1/4 lung adenoma		571

[c] Denotes (10,000/positive response dose), see [b].
[d] Average induction time.
[e] Variety of tumor types, *see* original reference for histopathology.

Nitrogen Mustards (Difunctional) (Derivatives of Derivatives of Heterocyclic Amines

Dose	Duration (Days)	Tumors	Remarks	References
15 mg/kg × 16	730	2/36 sarcomas 1/36 carcinoma	a few tumors also by i.v. or i.p.	576
650 mg/kg × 4	180	57% thymic lymphomas 43% lung adenomas 21% lung cancer 16% Harderian gland adenomas	22% lung adenomas, no other tumors in controls	577
4.2 mg/kg, multiple, total 218 mg/kg	480[b]	27% malignant, 7% benign tumors[c]	statiscally sig. positive; dose simulates chemotherapy	107
0.27 mg × 10[d]	224	30/25 papillomas		30
60 μmol/kg[e]	273	rel. potency[f] 170		31

Table XXXII.

Compound	Formula[a]	Animal	Strain or Type	Route
"Melphalan,"3-p-(Di(2-chloro-ethyl)amino)-phenyl-L-alanine, L-sarcolysin	M◯CH₂CH(NH₂)CO₂H	mouse	albino S	skin
		mouse	A/J	i.p.
"Aniline mustard" N,N-Di-(2-chloroethyl)-aniline	M◯	mouse	A/J	i.p.
		rat	—	s.c.
		mouse	—	s.c.
"p-Toluidine mus-tard," N-N-Di-(2-chloroethyl)-p-toluidine	M◯CH₃	rat	—	s.c.
		mouse	—	s.c.
"α-Naphthylamine mustard,"N,N-Di-(2-chloroethyl)-l-naphthylamine	M naphthalene	rat	—	s.c.
		mouse	—	s.c.
"β-Naphthylamine mustard,"N,N-Di-(2-chloroethyl)-2-naphthylamine	naphthalene M	rat	—	s.c.
		mouse	—	s.c.
		mouse	A/J	i.p.
"Mannomustine," "Degranol," "Mannitol mustard," 1,6-Di-(2-chloroethyl-amino)-1,6-deoxy-d-mannitol	ClCH₂CH₂·NH·CH₂(CHOH)₄·CH₂·NH·CH₂CH₂Cl	mouse	A/J	i.p.
		rat	BR46	i.v.
"Hydroquinone mustard," 2,5-Bis(bis-(2-chloroethyl) aminomethyl) hydroquinone	hydroquinone structure with CH₂M and MCH₂ groups, OH	mouse	A/J	i.p.

[a] M = mustard group, -N(CH₂CH₂Cl)₂; generally hydrochlorides were used, not free bases.

[b] Mean induction time.

[c] Various types, *see* original reference for histopathology.

[d] Applied in acetone; promotion with croton oil.

Continued

Dose	Duration (Days)	Tumors	Remarks	References
0.144 mg $\times$ 10[d]	224	7/25 papillomas	D-enantiomer of equal activity	*30*
3.8 μmoles/kg[e]	273	rel. potency[f] 2630		*31*
96 μmoles/kg[e]	273	rel. potency[f] 104		*31*
2 mg/kg, wkly $\times$ 20	400[g]	5/12[h]	mitotic ab- normalities	*481*
1 mg/kg, wkly $\times$ 20	400[g]	1/12[h]	observed in primary tumors	
2 mg/kg, wkly $\times$ 20	365[g]	5/12[h]		*481*
1 mg/kg, wkly $\times$ 20	330[g]	2/12[h]		
2 mg/kg, wkly $\times$ 20	270[g]	6/12[h]		*481*
1 mg/kg, wkly $\times$ 20	400[g]	2/12[h]		
2 mg/kg, wkly $\times$ 20	240[g]	12/12[h]		*481*
1 mg/kg, wkly $\times$ 20	300[g]	2/12[h]		
1200 μmoles/kg[e]	273	rel. potency[f] 8.3		*31*
60 μmoles/kg[e]	273	rel. potency[f] 280		*31*
4 mg/kg, multiple, total 208 mg/kg	450[b]	11% malignant, 5% benign tumors[c]	statiscally sig. positive; dose simulates chemotherapy	*107*
66 μmoles/kg[e]	273	rel. potency[f] 150		*31*

[e] Twelve 3 $\times$ weekly injection in water over a range of dose levels; "positive response dose" quoted gave 1 lung tumor/mouse.

[f] Relative potency denotes (10,000/positive response dose), see [e].

[g] Latent period.

[h] "Mostly sarcomas at site of injection".

Table XXXIII.   Representative Oncogenesis Tests—

Compound	Formula[a]	Animal	Strain or Type	Route
"Uracil mustard," 5-(Di-2-chloroethyl) aminouracil	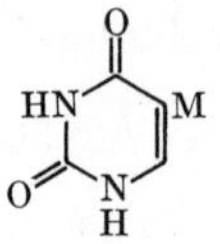	mouse	A/J	i.p.
"Chloroquine mustard," 4-(4-(Di-(2-chloroethyl)-amino)-1-methyl-butylamino)-7-chloroquinoline	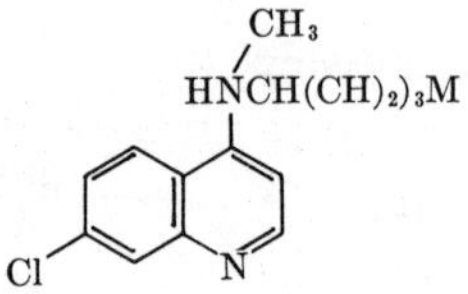	mouse	A/J	i.p.
"Quinacrine ethyl mustard,"9-(2-(Di-(2-chloroethyl) amino)ethylamino)-6-chloro-2-methoxy-acridine	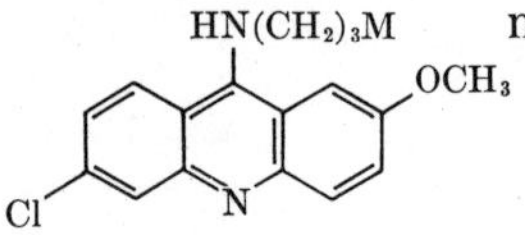	mouse	A/J	i.p.
"Benzimidazole mustard," 2-(Di-2-chloroethyl) aminomethyl-5,6-dimethylbenzimidazole	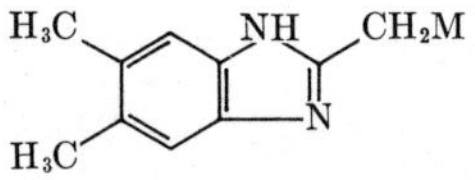	mouse	A/J	i.p.
"Cytoxan," "Cyclophosphamide," "Endoxana," 2-H-1,3,2-Oxazaphosphorinane, 2-(Di(2-chloroethyl)amino)2-oxide, N,N-di(2-chloroethyl)-N,O-propylenephosphoric acid ester diamide	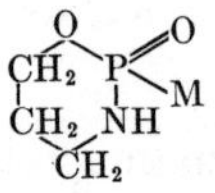	mouse	A/J	i.p.
		mouse	A	i.p.
		mouse	A	i.p.
		mouse	dd	i.p.
		rat	BR46	i.v.
"Quinacrinepropyl mustard,"9-(3-(Ethyl-2-chloroethyl)amino) propylamino-6-chloro-2-methoxy-acridine	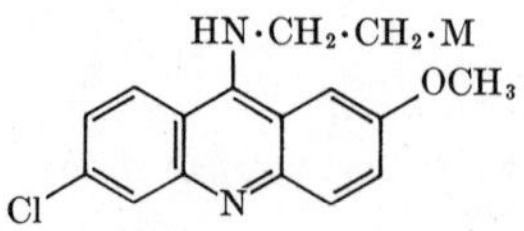	mouse	A/J	i.p.

The formula structures shown in the table:

- Uracil mustard: uracil ring with HN, O, M substituent
- Chloroquine mustard: CH_3, $HNCH(CH_2)_3M$, chloroquinoline with Cl and N
- Quinacrine ethyl mustard: $HN(CH_2)_3M$, OCH_3, acridine with Cl and N
- Benzimidazole mustard: H_3C, NH, CH_2M, H_3C, benzimidazole with N
- Cyclophosphamide: O, O, CH_2, P, M, CH_2, NH, CH_2
- Quinacrinepropyl mustard: $HN\cdot CH_2\cdot CH_2\cdot M$, OCH_3, acridine with Cl and N

Nitrogen Mustards Derived from Heterocyclic Compounds

Dose	Duration (Days)	Tumors	Remarks	References
0.96 μmole/kg[b]	273	lung, rel. potency[c] 10,420		31
18 μmoles/kg[b]	273	lung, rel. potency[c] 560	active as hydro-chloride, inactive as pamoate (salt of $CH_2(C_{10}$-$H_5OHCO_2H)_2$)	31
30 μmoles/kg[b]	273	lung, rel. potency[c] 330		31
36 μmoles/kg[b]	273	lung, rel. potency[c] 280		31
360 μmoles/kg[b]	273	lung, rel. potency[c] 28		31
0.02 mg $\times$ 5		pulmonary adenomas		578
5 mg/kg $\times$ 30	294	37.5% various[d]	18% in controls, p = 0.263	28
5 mg/kg $\times$ 30	336	55% various	30% in controls, p = 0.183	
13 mg/kg, multiple, 676 mg/kg, total		11% benign, 17% malignant[d]	statistically sig. positive	107
16.5 μmoles/kg[e]	273	rel. potency nil		31

Table XXXIII.

Compound	Formula[a]	Animal	Strain or Type	Route
"5-Chloroquine mustard," 4-(4-(Di-(2-chloroethyl)amino)-1-methylbutylamino)-5-chloroquinoline		mouse	A/J	i.p.
"Benzalpurine mustard," p-(Di(2-chloroethyl)amino) benzaldehyde, purin-6-ylhydrazone		mouse	A/J	i.p.

[a] M denotes di-(2-chloroethyl)amino-.
[b] Range of dose levels used; "positive response dose" giving 1 lung tumor/mouse quoted.

to a critical site. Such considerations were, of course, in addition to those relating to chemical reactivity, important determinants in the design of these agents for cancer chemotherapy.

As already noted, yet another factor is significant from these various aspects, that of the role of mustard metabolism. For example, Cytoxan (Cyclophosphamide) was designed as a compound of latent activity, to be selectively metabolized in tumor tissues to a reactive alkylating agent. Evidently, some form of metabolic activation can confer carcinogenic potency as well as growth inhibitory activity in this case.

The possible role of metabolic detoxification of mustards in relation to their carcinogenic activity has been discussed in some detail by Shimkin et al. (31), who noted the need for further studies.

DIFUNCTIONAL SULFONATES (Table XXXIV). The carcinogenicity of compounds falling into this category has not been very extensively studied, in contrast to their cytotoxicity. The straight chain dimethanesulfonoxyalkanes of the type $CH_3SO_2O(CH_2)_nOSO_2CH_3$ have been of considerable interest as cytotoxic agents, particularly in chronic myeloid leukemia (579). The specific action as depressants of circulating neutrophils of a homologous series ($n = 2$–10) showed that activity was maximal at $n = 4$, i.e., with Myleran (Busulfan). Chemical reactivity as measured by solvolysis increased from $n = 2 - 4$, but for $n = 4$–10 it was approximately the same. Introduction of methyl substituents to the terminal C-atoms of the alkyl chain was expected to change the mechanism of alkylation from "largely S_N2 to an S_N1 type" (580), (cf. the change in mechanisms through methyl, ethyl, and isopropyl halides). In the resulting series, $CH_3SO_2OCH(CH_3)$-$(CH_2)_{n-2}CH(CH_3)OSO_2CH_3$, the cytotoxic action was again maximal at $n = 4$ but was overall lower.

Continued

Dose	Duration (Days)	Tumors	Remarks	References
25 μmoles/kg[e]	273	rel. potency nil		*31*
36 μmoles/kg[e]	273	rel. potency nil		*31*

[c] Relative potency denotes 10,000/"positive response dose," *see* [b].
[d] For details of histopathology, *see* original reference.
[e] Highest dose, negative response relative to controls.

Various suggestions have been made to explain the rather specific cytotoxic action of Myleran and its homologs, but as yet none appear to be convincing. Although too few studies of carcinogenicity have yet been made to enable any useful assessment of the relevance of these hypotheses in this area, it may be useful to mention some of these briefly, with regard to any future work.

The principal *in vivo* reactions of Myleran and its monofunctional analog ethyl methanesulfonate are with thiol groups. The ability of Myleran to form cyclic sulfonium ions (derivatives of tetrahydrothiophene, *see* Scheme 9) was demonstrated by Roberts and Warwick (*581*) as already discussed. Clearly this type of reaction could account for the dependence of cytotoxicity on chain length, since cycloalkylation would be favored at around $n = 4$ or 5, as previously noted by Timmis and Hudson (*580*). As already noted, the products of cycloalkylation are unstable and decompose *in vivo* to yield tetrahydrothiophene derivatives, *i.e.*, "dethiolation" of cysteinyl groups results (*582*).

The possible importance of cycloalkylation for cytotoxicity has been questioned, notably recently by Jones and co-workers (*583*) who found that the homolog 1,3-bis(methanesulfonyloxy)propane ($n = 3$) resembles Myleran in its effects on hemopoiesis and spermatogenesis but does not cycloalkylate *in vitro* or *in vivo* (*584*). Furthermore, studies with dimethanesulfonates of cyclohexane showed that noncycloalkylating isomers (1,3- and 1,4-derivatives, Scheme 9) are cytotoxic, but the 1,2-derivative is inactive, although able to dethiolate cysteine ethyl ester (*583*).

The 1,3- and 1,4-dimethanesulfonates undergo S_N1-elimination reactions with this cysteine derivative, and elimination reaction products were found

Table XXXIV.   Representative Oncogenesis

Compound	Formula	Animal	Strain or Type	Route
"Myleran," "Busulfan," 1,4-Dimethane-sulfonoxy-butane	$H_3CSO_2O(CH_2)_4$ OSO_2CH_3	mouse	albino	skin
		mouse	RF	i.v.
		rat	BR46	p.o.
		rat	—	s.c.
		mouse	—	s.c.
1,6-Dimethane-sulfonoxyhexane	$H_3CSO_2O(CH_2)_6$ OSO_2CH_3	rat	—	s.c.
		mouse	—	s.c.
1,8-Dimethane-sulfonoxyoctane	$H_3CSO_2O(CH_2)_8$ OSO_2CH_3	rat	—	s.c.
		mouse	—	s.c.
"Mannitol myleran," 1,6-Dimethane-sulfonoxy-d-mannitol	$H_3CSO_2OCH_2$ $(CHOH)_4\cdot$ $CH_2OSO_2CH_3$	mouse	A/J	i.p.

[a] Multiple application in acetone; promotion with croton oil.
[b] Average induction time.
[c] For details of histopathology, see original reference.

in rat urine after administration of ^{35}S-labeled trans-1,4-dimethanesulfonate. It was therefore suggested that cycloalkylation and dethiolation represent detoxification processes whereas the significant cytotoxic action of the methanesulfonates may involve cleavage of the methanesulfonyloxy group to yield sulfene ($CH_2 = SO_2$), a highly reactive electrophile, which Jones and Campbell (583) suggest may be liberated in vivo by a base-activated reaction.

Further evidence contraindicating a conventional alkylation mechanism for Myleran was obtained by Addison and Berenbaum (585), who found that exogenous cysteine potentiated rather than diminished the immunosuppressive action of Myleran in mice.

As these authors also point out, whereas Myleran can react with DNA, albeit to a small extent even in vitro, it inactivates phage T7 in the manner characteristic of a monofunctional agent, and interstrand cross-linkage could not be detected (227).

Whatever molecular mechanisms contribute to the biological action of Myleran, they evidently do not confer marked carcinogenic potency, since

Tests—Alkanesulfonates (Difunctional)

Dose	Duration (Days)	Tumors	Remarks	References
2–6 mg total[a]	154	1/33	inactive as initiator at highest tolerated dose	476
12 mg/kg × 4	614	35% thymic lymphomas	8% in controls	574, 575
0.13 mg/kg multiple, 6.76 mg/kg total	670[b]	6% benign,[c] 11% malignant	statistical sig. in doubt	107
2 mg/kg × 20	240[b]	5/10 local sarcomas		481
1 mg/kg × 20	450[b]	1/10		
2 mg/kg × 20	365[b]	4/10		481
1 mg/kg × 20	300[b]	2/10		
2 mg/kg × 20	365[b]	4/10		481
1 mg/kg × 20	430[b]	1/10		
3000 μmol/kg[d]	273	rel. potency[e] 3.3		31

[d] Range of doses used; "positive response dose" giving 1 lung tumor/mouse quoted.
[e] Denotes (10,000/"positive response dose").

most investigators using this agent found no significantly positive results (Table XXXIV). Koller (*481*) briefly reported the induction of sarcomas at the injection site in mice and rats by Myleran and two homologs. Shimkin *et al.* (*31*) found Mannitol Myleran a relatively weak inducer of lung adenomas in strain A/J mice (relative potency of 3.3, compared with 280 for the analogous mannitol mustard) and expected that Myleran (not tested) would behave similarly. Evidently further studies of the carcinogenicity of alkanesulfonates, especially directed towards structure–activity relationships, appear to be warranted.

DIFUNCTIONAL EPOXIDES (Table XXXV). The relationship between structure and activity for this group of compounds has been discussed in some detail by Van Duuren (*448*). As mentioned in the discussion of mono-epoxides, he considered that three of the monoepoxides found to be active might be converted *in vivo* to difunctional agents.

The importance of the ability of carcinogenic epoxides to react with two nucleophilic centers was stressed, although it should be noted that not all difunctional epoxides are active (Table XXXVI). Van Duuren (*448*)

Scheme 9.   Reactions and metabolism of Myleran and cyclohexane dimethane-
sulfonates

Reactions with cysteine or derivatives–"dethiolation"; (a) (*582*) ; (b) (*583*)

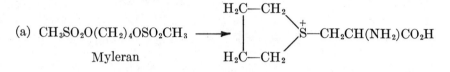

(a) CH₃SO₂O(CH₂)₄OSO₂CH₃   ⟶

Myleran

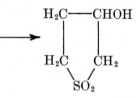

Urinary metabolite

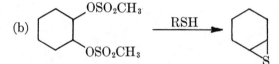

(b)

Cyclohexane *cis*-1,2-
dimethanesulfonate

Dethiolation product from
reaction with cysteine ethyl ester

Elimination reaction (*583*)

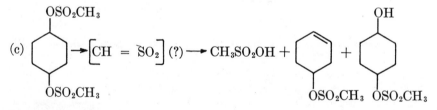

(c)

Cyclohexane *trans*-1,4-
dimethanesulfonate

Urinary metabolites

pointed out that the distance between the reactive groups in the difunctional
epoxides could range from about 0.4 nm (diepoxybutane) to about 1.0 nm.
It was considered that cross-linking between nucleic acid molecules or between
DNA and nucleohistones was more likely to be important for carcinogenicity
than cross-linking between the strands of the DNA double helix. This last
reaction, if it occurred between the most reactive nucleophilic sites in DNA
at N-7 atoms of guanine residues would be required to span a distance of
about 0.8 nm.

The ability of D- and L- forms of diepoxybutane to induce interstrand cross-linking in DNA of T7 phage has been demonstrated (*230*), but cross-linking by the meso-form was not detected, and it was the least efficient isomer in the inactivation of the phage. It may be noted that *d,l*-diepoxy-butane was a somewhat more effective initiator than the meso-form in two-stage carcinogenesis in mouse skin (*448*). The alkylation sites in DNA which are involved in interstrand cross-linking by diepoxybutane do not appear to have been specified as yet.

DI- AND POLYFUNCTIONAL ETHYLENEIMINES (Table XXXVII). All the compounds tested have been classed as positive, except the chemosterilant Apholate; they are all mutagens and chromosome-breaking agents (for a comprehensive review, *see* Ref. *25*).

TEM (*223*) and Mitomycin C (*231*) are powerful cross-linking agents for DNA, although the latter requires metabolic or chemical reduction for activation. The induction of lymphoma in mice by TEM may involve some form of activation of a tumor virus (*575*).

Summary and Conclusions

The alkylating agents include carcinogens of particular chemical interest. Their reactions *in vivo* will often, but not always, be the same as *in vitro* since in some cases metabolic activation may intervene. This stimulates interest in their mode of action, not only in their own right, but as models for reactive metabolites of other carcinogens.

As previously noted (*588*), the initial hopes that the relative simplicity of *in vivo* alkylation reactions would enable specification of the essential cellular receptors of chemical carcinogens were not fulfilled. First, alkylating agents do not appear to react specifically with any cellular target; in fact the major type of reaction which generally appears to occur *in vivo* with thiols is now regarded fairly widely as mainly detoxificative in nature. It should not, however, be assumed that protein alkylation plays no part in carcinogenesis, since as Colburn and Boutwell (*307, 308*) have pointed out, this is particularly likely to be a significant process in the promotion stage of the two-stage mechanism of carcinogenesis.

Historically, the alkylating agents emerged as the classical carcinogenic mutagens. With aromatic hydrocarbons and amines, demonstration of carcinogenicity preceded that of mutagenicity. With the alkylating agents, the reverse has often been true. This, of course, is understandable since many test organisms in chemical mutagenesis do not metabolize many carcinogens at all or inappropriately to yield the ultimate reactive forms. Generally, there are no effective barriers to reactions of alkylating agents with DNA *in vivo*.

It is not surprising therefore that considerable attention has been devoted to this group of compounds in the area of the detection of chemical modifications of DNA as an index of potential mutagenic action (*377*). The question remains whether this approach is relevant for assessment of a carcinogenic hazard. Probably few would now doubt the equation of the initiation stage in carcinogenesis with some type of somatic mutation.

Table XXXV.   Representative Oncogenesis

Compound	Formula	Animal	Strain or Type	Route[a]
Butadiene dioxide, 1,2,3,4-Diepoxy-butane	 $H_2C-CH-CH-CH_2$ (*d,l*-form)	rat	albino	i.p.
		mouse	ICR/Ha Swiss	skin
				skin
		rat	Sprague–Daw-ley	s.c.
				s.c.
	$H_2C-CH-CH-CH_2$ (meso-form)	mouse	ICR/Ha Swiss	skin
				skin
		mouse	C3H	skin
	L-form	mouse	A	i.p.
1,2,4,5-Diepoxy-pentane	$H_2C-CH \cdot CH_2 \cdot CH-CH_2$	mouse	ICR/Ha Swiss	skin
1,2,5,6-Diepoxy-hexane	$H_2C-CH(CH_2)_2CH-CH_2$	mouse	ICR/Ha	skin
				s.c.
		rat	Sprague–Daw-ley	s.c.
1,2,6,7-Diepoxy-heptane	$H_2C-CH(CH_2)_3CH-CH_2$	mouse	ICR/Ha	skin
1,2,7,8-Diepoxy-octane	$H_2C-CH(CH_2)_4CH-CH_2$	mouse	ICR/Ha	skin
1-Ethyleneoxy-3,4-epoxycyclohexane, "Vinylcyclohexene dioxide"		mouse	Swiss	skin
		mouse	C3H	skin

Test—Epoxides (Difunctional)

Dose	Duration (Days)	Tumors	Remarks	References
1–2 mg/kg × 12	540	1/14 sarcoma	reported inactive on mouse skin	586
3 mg, 3 × wkly	475[a]	6/30 carcinomas	weakly active	556
1 mg, single[b]	137[c]	7/20 papillomas 2/20 carcinomas	active as initiator, in promotion tests an active inhibitor	309, 310
1.1 mg, wkly[d]	589	5/30 local malignant sarcomas	inactive by gastric feeding	543
1 mg, wkly[d]	550	9/50 local malignant sarcomas 1/50 adeno-carcinoma		
10 mg, 3 × wkly	357[a]	4/30 carcinomas		556
1 mg, single[b]	163[c]	4/20 papillomas 0/20 carcinomas	less active as initiator than d,l-	309
continuous painting	450	1/4 cancer 2/4 papillomas		447
1320 μmoles/kg[e]	273	lung, rel. potency[f] 7.6		31
10 mg, 3 × wkly	490[a]	10/30 papillomas 3/30 carcinomas		556
2 mg, 3 × wkly	427[a]	13/30 papillomas 10/30 carcinomas		542
1 mg, wkly[d]	533	2/30 fibro-sarcomas 1/30 adeno-carcinoma		543
1 mg, wkly[d]	552	1/50 fibro-sarcoma		
1 mg, 3 × wkly	464[a]	9/30 papillomas 1/30 carcinomas		556
1 mg, 3 × wkly	385[c]	7/30 kerato-acanthomas 4/30 carcinomas		542
10 mg, 3 × wkly	326[a]	14/30 papillomas 9/30 carcinomas	first studied by Ref. 586	545
continuous painting	520	3/17 papillomas 1/17 cancer	weakly positive in rats	447

Table XXXV.

Compound	Formula	Animal	Strain or Type	Route[a]
3,4-Epoxy-6-methyl-cyclohexylmethyl-3,4-epoxy-6-methylcyclo-hexanecarboxy-late		mouse	ICR/Ha	skin
Modified bis-phenol diglycidyl ethers	"indefinite"	mouse	C3H	skin
Triethylene glycol, diglycidyl ether, "Epodyl"		mouse	A	i.p.

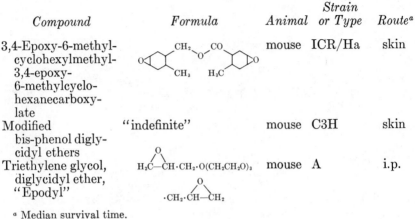

[a] Median survival time.
[b] Promotion with phorbol esters.
[c] Appearance of first papilloma, duration generally about 550 days.
[d] About 65 mg total dose.

Table XXXVI.   Representative Oncogenesis Tests—

Compound	Formula
Bis(2,3-epoxy-2-methylpropyl) ether	
Ethylene glycol bis(2,3-epoxy-2-methylpropyl) ether	
Bis(3,4-epoxy-6-methyl-cyclohexyl-methyl)adipate	
Limonene dioxide	
1,2,3,4-Diepoxy-cyclohexane	
1,2,5,6-Diepoxy-cyclooctane	

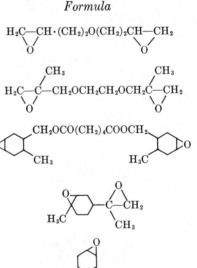

Continued

Dose	Duration (Days)	Tumors	Remarks	References
1 mg, 3 × wkly	392[c]	11/30 kerato-acanthomas 11/30 carcinomas	first studied by Ref. 447 and reported positive	542
continuous painting	700	6/28 papillomas 3/28 cancers		447
14,400 μmoles/ kg[e]	273	lung, rel. potency 0.7		31

[e] Range of doses; "positive response dose" giving 1 lung tumor/mouse quoted.
[f] Relative potency denotes (10,000/positive response dose).
[g] In skin painting applications, acetone was generally used as solvent.

Epoxides (Difunctional) Reported Inactive[a]

Animal	Route	References
mouse	skin	447
mouse	skin	447
mouse	skin	447
mouse	skin	447
mouse	skin	448
mouse	skin	

Table XXXVI.

Compound	*Formula*
9,10,12,13-Diepoxy- stearic acid	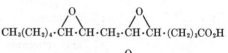 $CH_3(CH_2)_4 \cdot CH \cdot CH \cdot CH_2 \cdot CH \cdot CH \cdot (CH_2)_3CO_2H$
Resorcinoldi- glycidyl ether	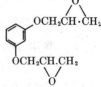
Hexaepoxysqualene	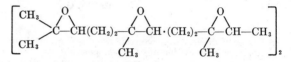
1,4-Bis(2,3- epoxypropyl) piperazine 1,1′-Bis(2,3- epoxypropyl)- 4-4′-bipiperidine	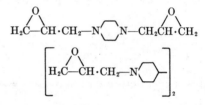

a Ref. *447* also reported 10 other compounds of this type inactive.

Table XXXVII.   Representative Oncogenesis

Compound	*Formula*	*Animal*	*Strain* *or Type*	*Route*
Triethylene melamine, "TEM"	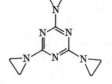	mouse	A	i.p.
		mouse	A	i.p.
		mouse	albino S	skin
		mouse	RF	i.p.
		rat	—	s.c.
		Wistar		s.c.

Continued

Animal	Route	References
mouse	skin	*448*
mouse	skin	
mouse	skin	
mouse	i.p.	*31*
mouse	i.p.	

Tests—Ethyleneimines (Di- and Polyfunctional)

Dose	Duration (Days)	Tumors	Remarks	References
7.5 µg × 10	100	8/10 pulmonary adenomas	2/15 in controls	*587*
50 µg × 2	126	24/30 animals with pulmonary tumors	2.64 tumors/ mouse	*488*
240 µg	154	0/10		*476*
240 µg[a]	154	18/10	active initiator	
1.5 mg/kg × 4	563	33% thymic lymphoma	8% in controls; myeloid leukemia incidence accelerated but no overall increase	*574, 575*
10 mg/kg[b] total	450	11/12 local sarcomas		*449, 505*
10 mg/kg[b], total	506	5/12 local sarcomas		

Table XXXVII.

Compound	Formula	Animal	Strain or Type	Route
1,3-Bis(ethyl-eneiminosul-fonyl)propane	$N\cdot SO_2\cdot(CH_2)_3SO_2\cdot N$	rat	Wistar	s.c.
"Trenimon," 2,3,5-Tri-(1-aziridinyl) p-benzoquinone	(structure)	rat	BR46	i.v.
Tris(1-aziridinyl) phosphine oxide, "Tepa," "Aphoxide"	(structure)	rat	Fischer	p.o.
2,2,4,4,6,6-Hexakis (1-aziridinyl)-2,2,4,4,6,6-hexa-hydro-1,3,5,2,4,-6-triazatri-phosphorine, "Apholate"	(structure)	rat	Fischer	p.o.
Bis(1-aziridinyl) morpholino-phosphine sulfide, "OPSPA"	(structure)	mouse	A/J	i.p.
Tris(1-aziridinyl) phosphine sulfide, "Thio Tepa," "TESPA"	(structure)	mouse	A/J	i.p.
		rat	BR46	i.v.
Mitomycin C[f]	(structure)	rat	BR46	i.v.

[a] Applied in acetone; followed by promotion with croton oil.
[b] Repeated injection in arachis oil of 1 mg/kg.
[c] For details see original reference.
[d] Range of doses used; "positive response dose" giving 1 lung tumor/mouse quoted.

As yet, demonstration of the nature of the required mutation(s) has not been achieved, although several suggestions have been made including mutations causing instability of the structure of chromosomes or of the cell surface or deletions of RNA-forming genes. The key problems in this area are doubtless those concerned with the control of cell division.

Continued

Dose	Duration (Days)	Tumors	Remarks	References
8 mg/kg[b], total		6/12 local sarcomas		*449*
0.03 mg/kg, total 1.56 mg/kg	450	11% benign[e], 24% malignant	considered positive	*107*
1–300 µg per day × 260	up to 565	33/58 neo-plastic[e] lesions	part of detailed methodological study; classed as weakly carcinogenic	*75*
3–300 µg per day × 260	up to 565	18/60 neo-plastic[e] lesions	detailed study; tumor distribution similar to that of controls	*75*
120 µmol/kg[d]	273	lung, rel. potency[e] 83		*31*
60 µmol/kg[d]	273	lung, rel. potency[e] 170		*31*
1 mg/kg, total 52 mg/kg	450	17% benign[e] 30% malignant	considered positive	*107*
0.52 mg/kg × 5	540	4% benign 34% malignant,	5% benign, 6% malignant in controls	*107*

[e] Denotes (10,000/positive response dose).
[f] Although strictly a monofunctional ethyleneimine, behaves as difunctional agent *in vivo*.

   The ability of alkylating agents to induce significant chemical lesions in cellular DNA, and thus to cause appropriate DNA repair mechanisms to operate, has been demonstrated with mammalian cells both *in vitro* and to some extent *in vivo*. Three principal mechanisms by which tumor initiation could result have thus been suggested—mutation induction by the replication of DNA containing promutagenic alkylated bases or phosphotriesters, mutation induction by replication of mis-repaired alkylated DNA, and tumor virus activation by derepression of provirus. In addition, the ability of alkylating agents to react with cellular RNA may also be significant in carcinogenesis. *In vivo* reactions with ribosomal and transfer RNA have been demonstrated, and it is reasonable to speculate that messenger RNA might also be susceptible.

Some attention has been devoted to the question whether certain types of alkylation damage may be more effective than others in causing various biological effects. The cross-linking action of difunctional alkylating agents appears to be reasonably well established as conferring cytotoxicity by interference with replication of DNA. With respect to mutagenesis, current interest concerns the indication that alkylating agents reacting through the S_N1 mechanism may be more powerful mutagens since they are able to attack a wider range of nucleophiles than S_N2 reagents, including, in nucleic acids, O-atoms, and in some cases amino groups, in addition to the ring N-atoms that are generally the most nucleophilic centers. Specific suggestions have been made concerning the nature of the induced promutagenic groups, notably the O^6-alkylguanines (69).

It may therefore become possible to relate carcinogenic hazard of chemicals in a rather broad sense with the ability of compounds with or without activating metabolism, to react with nucleic acids *in vivo* at certain sites and to certain extents. The question whether repair mechanisms, which may include those operating at the level of damage to DNA or at subsequent stages, can be regarded as virtually completely effective up to certain levels of reaction leading to no-effect thresholds in dose–response relationships may prove to be particularly difficult to answer. Even if dose–response relationships for chemical carcinogens are established from animal studies, their extrapolation to man would then be required.

Literature Cited

1. Brookes, P., Lawley, P. D., *Biochem. J.* (1960) **77**, 478.
2. Roberts, J. J., Pascoe, J. M., Plant, J. E., Sturrock, J. E., Crathorn, A. R., *Chem. Biol. Interact.* (1971) **3**, 29.
3. Hill, B. T., Jarman, M., Harrap, K. R., *J. Med. Chem.* (1971) **14**, 614.
4. Hill, B. T., *Biochem. J.* (1972) **129**, 44P.
5. Hill, B. T., *Biochem. Pharmacol.* (1972) **21**, 495.
6. Linford, J. H., *Can. J. Biochem.* (1963) **41**, 931.
7. Hopwood, W. J., Stock, J. A., *Chem. Biol. Interact.* (1971/72) **4**, 31.
8. Goldenberg, G. J., Vanstone, C. L., Bihler, I., *Science* (1971) **172**, 1148.
9. Goldenberg, G. J., Vanstone, C. L., Israels, L. G., Ilse, D., Bihler, I., *Cancer Res.* (1970) **30**, 2285.
10. Brookes, P., Lawley, P. D., "Isotopes in Experimental Pharmacology," L. J. Roth, Ed., p. 403, University of Chicago, Chicago, 1965.
11. Ulfohn, A., Kramer, S. P., Dorfman, H., Witten, B., Williamson, C., Sass, S., Miller, J. I., Seligman, A. M., *Cancer Res.* (1964) **24**, 1659.
12. Lawley, P. D., Brookes, P., *Biochem. J.* (1968) **109**, 433.
13. Swann, P. F., *Biochem. J.* (1968) **110**, 49.
14. Cumming, R. B., Walton, M. F., *Mutat. Res.* (1970) **10**, 365.

15. Boyland, E., Chasseaud, L. F., *Adv. Enzymol.* (1969) **32**, 173.
16. Roberts, J. J., Warwick, G. P., *Nature* (1957) **179**, 1181.
17. Warwick, G. P., *Cancer Res.* (1963) **23**, 315.
18. Trams, E. G., Nadkarni, M. V., *Cancer Res.* (1956) **16**, 1069.
19. Cobb, L. M., *Int. J. Cancer* (1966) **1**, 329.
20. Connors, T. A., *Cancer Res.* (1969) **29**, 2443.
21. Arnold, H., Bourseaux, F., *Angew. Chemie* (1958) **70**, 539.
22. Connors, T. A., Grover, P. L., McLoughlin, A. M., *Biochem. Pharmacol.* (1970) **19**, 1533.
23. Alarcon, R. A., Meienhofer, J., *Nature New Biol.* (1971) **233**, 250.
24. Connors, T. A., Foster, A. B., Gilsenan, A. M., Jarman, M., Tisdale, M. J., *Biochem. Pharmacol.* (1972) **21**, 1373.
25. Fishbein, L., Flamm, W. G., Falk, H. L., "Chemical Mutagens, Environmental Effects on Biological Systems," Chap. 7 and 8, Academic, New York, 1970.
26. Colvin, M., Padgett, C. A., Fenselav, C., *Cancer Res.* (1973) **33**, 915.
27. Connors, T. A., Cox, P. J., Farmer, P. B., Foster, A. B., Jarman, M., *Biochem. Pharmacol.* (1974) **23**, 115.
28. Tokuoka, S., *Gann* (1965) **56**, 537.
29. Schmähl, D., *Dtsch. Med. Wochenschr.* (1967) **92**, 1150.
30. Salaman, M. H., Roe, F. J. C., *Br. J. Cancer* (1956) **10**, 363.
31. Shimkin, M. B., Weisburger, J. H., Weisburger, E. K., Gubareff, N., Suntzeff, V., *J. Natl. Cancer Inst.* (1966) **36**, 915.
32. Ross, W. C. J., Warwick, G. P., *J. Chem. Soc.* (1956) 1364, 1724.
33. Elson, L. A., Jarman, M., Ross, W. C. J., *Eur. J. Cancer* (1968) **4**, 617.
34. Horvath, I. P., Sellei, C., Eckhardt, S., Kralovanszky, J., *Int. Cancer Congr. Abstr., 10th* (1970) 415.
35. Videbaek, A., *Acta Med. Scand.* (1964) **176**, 45.
36. Thiede, T., Chievitz, E., Christensen, B. C., *Acta Med. Scand.* (1964) **175**, 721.
37. Tardiff, R. G., Dubois, K. P., *Arch. Int. Pharmacodyn.* (1969) **177**, 445.
38. Donelli, M. G., Franchi, G., Rosso, R., *Eur. J. Cancer* (1970) **6**, 125.
39. Donelli, M. G., Garattini, S., *Eur. J. Cancer* (1971) **7**, 361.
40. Ross, W. C. J., "Biological Alkylating Agents," Butterworths, London, 1962.
41. Osterman-Golkar, Ehrenberg, L., Wachtmeister, C. A., *Radiat. Bot.* (1970) **10**, 303.
42. Ingold, C. K., "Structure and Mechanism in Organic Chemistry," 2nd ed., Chap. VII, Cornell University, New York, G. Bell and Sons Ltd., London, 1969.
43. Streitweiser, A., *Chem. Rev.* (1956) **56**, 571.
44. Wells, P. R., *Chem. Rev.* (1963) **63**, 171.
45. Price, C. C., *Ann. N.Y. Acad. Sci.* (1958) **68**, 663.
46. Price, C. C., Gaucher, G. M., Koneru, P., Shibakawa, R., Sowa, J. R., Yamaguchi, M., *Ann. N.Y. Acad. Sci.* (1969) **163**, 593.
47. Bardos, R. J., Datta-Gupta, N., Hebborn, P., Triggle, D. J., *J. Med. Chem.* (1965) **8**, 167.
48. Bardos, T. J., Chmielewicz, Z. F., Hebborn, P., *Ann. N.Y. Acad. Sci.* (1969) **163**, 1006.
49. Swain, C. G., Scott, C. B., *J. Am. Chem. Soc.* (1953) **75**, 141.
50. Hawthorne, M. F., Hammond, G. S., Graybill, B. M., *J. Am. Chem. Soc.* (1955) **77**, 486.
51. Petty, W. L., Nichols, P. L., Jr., *J. Am. Chem. Soc.* (1954) **76**, 4385.
52. Ross, W. C. J., *Adv. Cancer Res.* (1953) **1**, 397.
53. Hudson, R. F., "Structure and Mechanism in Organo-Phosphorus Chemistry," p. 110, Academic, London, 1965.
54. Van Duuren, B. L., Goldschmidt, B. M., *J. Med. Chem.* (1966) **9**, 77.
55. Barnard, P. W. C., Robertson, R. E., *Can. J. Chem.* (1961) **39**, 881.

56. Garrett, E. R., Goto, S., Stubbins, J. F., *J. Pharm. Sci.* (1965) **54,** 119.
57. Veleminsky, J., Osterman-Golkar, S., Ehrenberg, L., *Mutat. Res.* (1970) **10,** 169.
58. Pearson, R. G., Langer, S. H., Williams, R. V., McGuire, W. J., *J. Am. Chem. Soc.* (1952) **74,** 5130.
59. Parker, R. E., Isaacs, N. S., *Chem. Rev.* (1959) **59,** 737.
60. Ogston, A. G., *Trans. Faraday Soc.* (1948) **44,** 45.
61. Hudson, R. F., Withey, R. J., *J. Chem. Soc.* (1964) 3513.
62. March, J., "Advanced Organic Chemistry: Reactions, Mechanisms and Structure," Chap. 10, McGraw-Hill, New York, 1968.
63. Sneen, R. A., Larsen, J. W., *J. Am. Chem. Soc.* (1969) **91,** 362.
64. Pearson, R. G., Songstad, J., *J. Am. Chem. Soc.* (1967) **89,** 1827.
65. Sykes, P., "Guidebook to Mechanism in Organic Chemistry," Chap. 3, Longmans, London, 1961.
65a. Swain, G. C., Scott, C. B., Lohmann, K. H., *J. Am. Chem. Soc.* (1953) **75,** 136.
66. Ludlum, D. B., *Biochim. Biophys. Acta* (1967) **142,** 282.
67. Turtoczky, I., Ehrenberg, L., *Mutat. Res.* (1969) **8,** 229.
68. Neale, S., *Mutat. Res.* (1972) **14,** 155.
69. Loveless, A., *Nature* (1969) **223,** 206.
70. Miller, J. A., Miller, E. C., *J. Natl. Cancer Inst.* (1971) **47,** v.
71. Pullman, B., *Biopolym. Symp.* (1964) **1,** 141.
72. Pullman, B., *J. Chem. Phys.* (1965) **43,** S233.
73. Miller, E. C., Miller, J. A., "Chemical Mutagens, Principles and Methods for Their Detection," A. Hollaender, Ed., Vol. 1, Chap. 3, Plenum, New York, London, 1971.
74. Poirier, L. A., Thesis, University of Wisconsin (1965).
75. Hadidian, Z., Fredrickson, T. N., Weisburger, E. K., Weisburger, J. H., Glass, R. M., Mantel, N., *J. Natl. Cancer Inst.* (1968) **41,** 985.
76. Brodie, B. B., Maickel, R. P., "Metabolic Factors Controlling Duration of Drug Action," B. B. Brodie, E. G. Erdös, Eds., p. 299, Pergamon, Oxford, 1962.
77. Miller, J. A., Miller, E. C., *Prog. Exp. Tumor Res.* (1969) **11,** 273.
78. Kriek, E., *Biochem. Biophys. Res. Commun.* (1965) **20,** 793.
79. De Baun, J. R., Miller, E. C., Miller, J. A., *Cancer Res.* (1970) **30,** 577.
80. Matsushima, T., Weisburger, J. H., *Chem. Biol. Interact.* (1970) **1,** 211.
81. Weisburger, J. H., Yamamoto, R. S., Williams, G. M., Grantham, P. H., Matsushima, T., Weisburger, E. K., *Cancer Res.* (1972) **32,** 491.
82. Flesher, J. W., Sydnor, K., *Int. J. Cancer* (1970) **5,** 253.
83. Dipple, A., Lawley, P. D., Brookes, P., *Eur. J. Cancer* (1968) **4,** 493.
84. Hennessy, D. J., *J. Agri. Food Chem.* (1965) **13,** 218.
85. Boyland, E., *Symp. Biochem. Soc.* (1950) **5,** 40.
86. Grover, P. L., Forrester, J. A., Sims, P., *Biochem. Pharmacol.* (1971) **20,** 1297.
87. Grover, P. L., Sims, P., Huberman, E., Marquardt, H., Kuroki, T., Heidelberger, C., *Proc. Natl. Acad. Sci.* (1971) **68,** 1098.
88. Sims, P., Grover, P. L., Swaisland, A., Pal, K., Hewer, A., *Nature* (1974) **252,** 326.
89. Swaisland, A. J., Hewer, A., Pal, K., Keysell, G. R., Booth, J., Grover, P. L., Sims, P., *FEBS Lett.* (1974) **47,** 34.
90. Mattocks, A. R., *J. Chem. Soc. (C)* (1969) 1155.
91. Szybalski, W., Iyer, V. N., *Fed. Proc.* (1964) **23,** 946.
92. Murakami, H., *J. Theor. Biol.* (1966) **10,** 236.
93. Borchert, P., Wislocki, P. G., Miller, J. A., Miller, E. C., *Cancer Res.* (1973) **33,** 575.
94. Swenson, D. H., Miller, E. C., Miller, J. A., *Biochem. Biophys. Res. Commun.* (1974) **60,** 1036.

95. Longridge, J. L., Timms, D., *J. Chem. Soc. (B)* (1971) 848.
96. Howe, R., *Nature* (1965) **207**, 594.
97. Scribner, J. D., Miller, J. A., Miller, E. C., *Biochem. Biophys. Res. Commun.* (1965) **20**, 560.
98. Stekol, J. A., Mody, U., Perry, J., *J. Biol. Chem.* (1960) **235**, PC59.
99. Heath, D. F., *Biochem. J.* (1962) **85**, 72.
99a. Malaveille, C., Bartsch, H., Barbin, A., Camus, A. M., Montesano, R., Croisy, A., Jacquignon, P., *Biochem. Biophys. Res. Comm.* (1975) **63**, 363.
100. Schoental, R., *Cancer Res.* (1968) **28**, 2237.
101. Schoental, R., Hard, G. C., Gibbard, S., *J. Natl. Cancer Inst.* (1971) **47**, 1037.
102. Wogan, G. N., *Prog. Exp. Tumor Res.* (1969) **11**, 134.
103. Culvenor, C. C. J., Dann, A. T., Dick, A. T., *Nature* (1962) **195**, 570.
104. De Wolfe, R. H., Young, W. G., *Chem. Rev.* (1956) **56**, 753.
105 White, I. N. H., Mattocks, A. R., *Biochem. J.* (1972) **128**, 291.
106. Ikegami, R., Akamatsu, Y., Haruta, M., *Acta Pathol. Jpn.* (1967) **17**, 495.
107. Schmähl, D., Osswald, H., *Arzneimittelforsch.* (1970) **20**, 1461.
108. Dickens, F., "U.I.C.C. Monograph, No. 7," R. Truhaut, Ed., p. 144, Springer, Berlin, 1967.
109. Lijinsky, W., Lee, K. W., Gallagher, C. H., *Cancer Res.* (1970) **30**, 2280.
110. Evans, I. A., Mason, J., *Nature* (1965) **208**, 913.
111. Evans, I. A., Osman, M. A., *Nature* (1974) **250**, 348.
112. Dickens, F., Jones, H. E. H., *Br. J. Cancer* (1961) **15**, 85.
113. Dickens, F., *Br. Med. Bull.* (1964) **20**, 96.
114. Moncrief, J. W., Heller, K. S., *Cancer Res.* (1967) **27**, 1500.
115. Creighton, A. M., Birnie, G. D., *Int. J. Cancer* (1970) **5**, 47.
116. Brookes, P., Lawley, P. D., *Biochem. J.* (1961) **80**, 496.
117. Roberts, J. J., Warwick, G. P., *Int. J. Cancer* (1966) **1**, 179, 573.
118. Boyland, E., Nery, R., *Biochem. J.* (1965) **94**, 198.
119. Roberts, J. J., Warwick, G. P., *Biochem. Pharmacol.* (1958) **1**, 60.
120. Williams, K., Kunz, W., Petersen, K., Schneiders, B., *Z. Krebsforsch.* (1971) **76**, 69.
121. Lawson, T. A., Pound, A. W., *Chem. Biol. Interact.* (1973) **6**, 99.
122. Litwack, G., Ketterer, B., Arias, M., *Nature* (1971) **234**, 466.
123. Farber, E., *Adv. Cancer Res.* (1963) **7**, 383.
124. Swann, P. F., Pegg, A. E., Hawks, A., Farber, E., Magee, P. N., *Biochem. J.* (1971) **123**, 175.
125. Farber, E., McConomy, J., Franzen, B., Marroquin, F., Stewart, G. A., Magee, P. N., *Cancer Res.* (1967) **27**, 1761.
126. Craddock, V. M., *Chem. Biol. Interact.* (1971) **4**, 149.
127. Magee, P. N., Barnes, J. M., *Adv. Cancer Res.* (1967) **10**, 163.
128. Lawley, P. D., Thatcher, C. J., *Biochem. J.* (1970) **116**, 693.
129. Schulz, U., McCalla, D. R., *Can. J. Chem.* (1969) **47**, 2021.
130. Wheeler, G. P., Bowdon, B. J., *Biochem. Pharmacol.* (1972) **21**, 265.
131. Lijinsky, W., Loo, J., Ross, A. E., *Nature* (1971) **218**, 1174.
132. Lingens, F., Haerlin, R., Süssmuth, R., *FEBS Lett.* (1971) **13**, 241.
133. Süssmuth, R., Haerlin, R., Lingens, F., *Biochim. Biophys. Acta* (1972) **269**, 276.
134. Lawley, P. D., Shah, S. A., *Chem. Biol. Interact.* (1973) **7**, 115.
135. Preussmann, R., Von Hodenberg, A., Hengy, H., *Biochem. Pharmacol.* (1969) **18**, 1.
136. Skibba, J. L., Bryan, G. T., *Toxicol. Appl. Pharmacol.* (1971) **18**, 707.
137. Kolar, G. F., Preussmann, R., *Z. Naturforsch.* (1971) **26b**, 950.
138. Heston, W. E., *J. Natl. Cancer Inst.* (1953) **14**, 131.
139. Auerbach, C., Robson, J. M., *Nature* (1946) **157**, 302.

140. Auerbach, C., *Hereditas Suppl. Proc. 8th Int. Congr. Genet. (1949)* 128.
141. Thom, C., Steinberg, T. A., *Proc. Natl. Acad. Sci.* (1939) **25,** 329.
142. Fahmy, O. G., Fahmy, M. J., *Cancer Res.* (1970) **30,** 195.
143. *Ibid.* (1972) **32,** 550.
144. Loveless, A., "Genetic and Allied Effects of Alkylating Agents," Butterworths, London, 1966.
145. Barthelmess, A., "Chemical Mutagenesis in Mammals and Man," F. Vogel and G. Röhrborn, Eds., Chap. 3, Springer-Verlag, Berlin-Heidelberg-New York, 1970.
146. Auerbach, C., Kilbey, B. J., *Annu. Rev. Genet.* (1971) **5,** 163.
147. Bryan, W. R., Shimkin, M. B., *J. Natl. Cancer Inst.* (1943) **3,** 503.
148. Ashley, D. J. B., *Br. J. Cancer* (1969) **23,** 313.
149. Cook, P. J., Doll, R., Fellingham, S. A., *Int. J. Cancer* (1969) **4,** 93.
150. Iball, J., *Am. J. Cancer* (1939) **35,** 188.
151. Druckrey, H., Kruse, H., Preussmann, R., Ivankovic, S., Landschütz, C., *Z. Krebsforsch.* (1970) **74,** 241.
152. Murray, J. A., *Sci. Rep. Imperial Cancer Res. Fund* (1908) 69.
153. Boveri, T., "Origin of Malignant Tumours" (translated by M. Boveri), p. 111, Williams and Wilkins Co., Baltimore, 1929.
154. Strong, L. C., *Br. J. Cancer* (1949) **3,** 97.
155. Berenblum, I., *Cancer Res.* (1954) **14,** 471.
156. Ryser, H. J. P., *New England J. Med.* (1971) **285,** 721.
157. Nicholls, W. W., *Hereditas* (1963) **50,** 53.
158. Cole, L. J., Nowell, P. C., *Science* (1965) **150,** 1782.
159. Thomas, L., "Cellular and Humoral Aspects of Hypersensitive States," H. W. Lawrence, Ed., p. 529, Hoeber-Harper, New York, 1961.
160. Burnet, F. M., *Transplant. Rev.* (1971) **7,** 3.
161. Good, R. A., *Proc. Natl. Acad. Sci.* (1972) **69,** 1026.
162. Coman, D. R., *Cancer Res.* (1944) **4,** 625.
163. Carter, S. B., *Nature* (1968) **220,** 970.
164. Burger, M. M., *Curr. Top. Cell. Regul.* (1971) **3,** 135.
165. Warren, L., Critchley, D., Macpherson, I., *Nature* (1972) **235,** 275.
166. Borek, E., *Cancer Res.* (1971) **31,** 596.
167. Craddock, V. M., *Nature* (1970) **228,** 1264.
168. King, T., McKinnell, R. G., "Cell Physiology of Neoplasia," p. 591, Univ. of Texas, Austin, 1960.
169. McKinnell, R. G., Deggins, B. A., Labat, D. D., *Science* (1969) **165,** 394.
170. Ruddle, F. H., "Control Mechanisms in the Expression of Cellular Phenotypes," H. A. Padykula, Ed., p. 233, Academic, New York, London, 1970.
171. Zimmermann, F. K., *Biochem. Pharmacol.* (1971) **20,** 985.
172. Barski, G., Cornefert, F., *J. Natl. Cancer Inst.* (1962) **28,** 801.
173. Harris, H., Watkins, J. F., *Nature* (1965) **205,** 640.
174. Harris, H., *Proc. Roy. Soc. Lond.* (1971) **B179,** 1.
175. Knudson, A. G., Jr., *Adv. Cancer Res.* (1973) **17,** 317.
176. Knudson, A. G., Jr., *Proc. Natl. Acad. Sci.* (1971) **68,** 820.
177. Burch, P. R. J., *Proc. Roy. Soc.* (1965) **B162,** 223.
178. Verly, W. G., Barbason, H., Dusart, J., Petitpas-Dewandre, A., *Biochim. Biophys. Acta* (1967) **145,** 752.
179. Verly, W. G., Dewandre, J., Moutschen-Damen, J., Moutschen-Damen, M., *J. Mol. Biol.* (1963) **6,** 175.
180. Krieg, D. R., *Genetics* (1963) **48,** 561.
181. Lawley, P. D., *Mutat. Res.* (1974) **23,** 283.
182. Kølmark, G., *Hereditas* (1953) **39,** 270.
183. Auerbach, C., Ramsay, D., *Mol. Gen. Genet.* (1968) **103,** 72, 384.
184. Malling, H. V., De Serres, F. J., *Ann. N.Y. Acad. Sci.* (1969) **163,** 788.
185. Heslot, H., *Abh. Dtsch. Akad. Wiss. Berlin Kl. Med.* (1962) **II,** 193.
186. Ehrenberg, L., Lundqvist, U., Strom, G., *Hereditas* (1958) **44,** 330.

187. Ehrenberg, L., Gustafsson, A., *Hereditas* (1957) **43,** 595.
188. Kao, F. T., Puck, T. T., *J. Cell. Physiol.* (1969) **74,** 245.
189. Fahmy, O. G., Fahmy, M. J., *Genetics* (1961) **46,** 1111.
190. Lawley, P. D., "Molekulare Biologie des Malignen Wachstums," H. Holzer and A. W. Holldorf, Eds., p. 126, Springer-Verlag, Berlin-Heidelberg-New York, 1966.
191. Lawley, P. D., Orr, D. J., *Chem. Biol. Interact.* (1970) **2,** 154.
192. Roberts, J. J., Brent, T. P., Crathorn, A. R., *Eur. J. Cancer* (1971) **7,** 515.
193. Roberts, J. J., Crathorn, A. R. Brent, T. P., *Nature* (1968) **218,** 970.
194. Witkin, E. M., *Brookhaven Symp. Biol.* (1968) **20,** 17.
195. Witkin, E. M., *Mutat. Res.* (1969) **8,** 9.
196. Witkin, E. M., *Ann. Rev. Microbiol.* (1969) **23,** 487.
197. Rupp, W. D., Howard-Flanders, P., *J. Mol. Biol.* (1968) **31,** 291.
198. Shimkin, M. B., *Adv. Cancer Res.* (1955) **3,** 223.
199. Ritossa, F. M., Atwood, K. C., Spiegelman, S., *Genetics* (1966) **54,** 663, 819.
200. Fahmy, O. G., Fahmy, M. J., *Genetics* (1961) **46,** 447.
201. Frei, J. V., *Chem. Biol. Interact.* (1971) **3,** 117.
202. Frei, J. V., *Int. J. Cancer* (1971) **7,** 436.
203. Swann, P. F., Magee, P. N., *Biochem. J.* (1968) **110,** 39.
204. Swann, P. F., Magee, P. N., *Nature* (1969) **223,** 947.
205. Clapp, N. K., Craig, A. W., Toya, R. E., Sr., *Science* (1968) **161,** 913.
206. Loveless, A., Hampton, C. L., *Mutat. Res.* (1969) **7,** 1.
207. Watson, J. D., Crick, F. H. C., *Nature* (1953) **171,** 737, 964.
208. Freese, E., *Brookhaven Symp. Biol.* (1959) **12,** 63.
209. Crick, F. H. C., Barnett, L., Brenner, S., Watts-Tobin, R. J., *Nature* (1961) **192,** 1227.
210. Phillips, J. H., Brown, D. M., *Prog. Nucleic Acid Res. Mol. Biol.* (1967) **7,** 349.
211. Freese, E., *Proc. Nat. Acad. Sci.* (1961) **47,** 540.
212. Drake, J. W., "Molecular Basis of Mutation," Holden-Day, San Francisco, 1970.
213. Loprieno, N., *Scientia* (1971) **25,** 408.
214. Banks, G. R., *Sci. Prog., Oxford* (1971) **59,** 475.
215. Freese, E., "Chemical Mutagens, Principles and Methods for their Detection," A. Hollaender, Ed., Vol. 1, Chap. 1, Plenum, New York-London, 1971.
216. Ames, B. N., "Chemical Mutagens, Principles and Methods for Their Detection," A. Hollaender, **1,** p. 267, Plenum, London and New York, 1971.
217. Wheeler, G. P., Skipper, H. E., *Arch. Biochem. Biophys.* (1957) **72,** 465.
218. Lawley, P. D., Brookes, P., *J. Mol. Biol.* (1967) **25,** 143.
219. Lawley, P. D., Lethbridge, J. H., Edwards, P. A., Shooter, K. V., *J. Mol. Biol.* (1969) **39,** 181.
220. Walker, I. G., *Can. J. Biochem.* (1971) **49,** 332.
221. Edwards, P. A., Shooter, K. V., *Biopolymers* (1971) **10,** 2079.
222. Glow, P. H., *Nature* (1969) **221,** 1265.
223. Doskočil, J., *Collect. Czech. Chem. Commun.* (1965) **30,** 479.
224. Geiduschek, E. P., *Proc. Natl. Acad. Sci.* (1961) **47,** 950.
225. Doskočil, J., Šormova, Z., *Collect. Czech. Chem. Commun.* (1965) **30,** 481.
226. Kohn, K. W., Spears, C. L., Doty, P., *J. Mol. Biol.* (1966) **19,** 266.
227. Verly, W. G., Brakier, L., *Biochim. Biophys. Acta* (1969) **174,** 674.
228. Chun, E. H. L., Gonzales, L., Lewis, F. S., Jones, J., Rutman, R. J., *Cancer Res.* (1969) **29,** 1184.
229. McCann, J. J., Lo, T. M., Webster, D. A., *Cancer Res.* (1971) **31,** 1573.
230. Verly, W. G., Brakier, L., Feit, P. W., *Biochim. Biophys. Acta* (1971) **228,** 400.
231. Iyer, V. N., Szybalski, W., *Science* (1964) **145,** 55.
232. Lawley, P. D., Brookes, P., *Biochem. J.* (1963) **89,** 127.
233. Margison, G. P., O'Connor, P. J., *Biochim. Biophys. Acta* (1973) **331,** 343.

234. Burnotte, J., Verly, W. G., *Biochim. Biophys. Acta* (1972) **262**, 449.
235. Steele, W. J., *Proc. Am. Assoc. Cancer Res.* (1962) **3**, 364.
236. Grunicke, H., Bock, K. W., Becher, H., Gäng, V., Schnierda, J., Puschendorf, B., *Cancer Res.* (1973) **33**, 1048.
237. Nietert, W. C., Kellicutt, L. M., Kubinski, H., *Cancer Res.* (1974) **34**, 859.
238. Lawley, P. D., *Prog. Nucleic Acid Res. Mol. Biol.* (1966) **5**, 89.
239. Strauss, B. S., "Chemical Mutagens, Principles and Methods for their Detection," A. Hollaender, Ed., Vol. 1, Chap. 5, Plenum, New York, London, 1971.
240. Brown, D. M., Todd, A. R., *J. Chem. Soc.* (1953) 2040.
241. Ludlum, D. B., *Biochim. Biophys. Acta* (1969) **174**, 773.
242. Shooter, K. V., *Jerusalem Symp. Quantum Chem. Biochem.* (1972) **4**, 509.
243. Abell, C. W., Rosini, L. A., Ramseur, M. R., *Proc. Natl. Acad. Sci.* (1965) **54**, 608.
244. Shooter, K. V., Edwards, P. A., Lawley, P. D., *Biochem. J.* (1971) **125**, 829.
245. Smith, K. D., Armstrong, J. L., McCarthy, B. J., *Biochim. Biophys. Acta* (1967) **142**, 323.
246. Bannon, P., Verly, W. G., *Eur. J. Biochem.* (1972) **31**, 103.
247. Meselson, M., Stahl, F. W., *Proc. Natl. Acad. Sci.* (1958) **44**, 671.
248. Watson, W. A. F., *Z. Vererbungsl.* (1964) **95**, 374.
249. Watson, W. A. F., *Mutat. Res.* (1966) **3**, 455.
250. Loveless, A., Stock, J. C., *Proc. Roy. Soc.* (1959) **B150**, 486.
251. Löbbecke, A. E., *Genetics* (1963) **48**, 691.
252. Corbett, T. H., Heidelberger, C., Dove, W. F., *Mol. Pharmacol.* (1970) **6**, 667.
253. Kohn, K. W., Green, D. M., *J. Mol. Biol.* (1966) **19**, 289.
254. Lawley, P. D., Brookes, P., *Nature* (1965) **206**, 480.
255. Kohn, K. W., Steigbigel, N. H., Spears, C. L., *Proc. Natl. Acad. Sci.* (1965) **53**, 1154.
256. Venitt, S., *Biochem. Biophys. Res. Commun.* (1968) **31**, 355.
257. Cole, R. S., *Proc. Natl. Acad. Sci.* (1973) **70**, 1064.
258. Crathorn, A. R., Roberts, J. J., *Nature* (1966) **211**, 150.
259. Roberts, J. J., Brent, T. P., Crathorn, A. R., "Interaction of Drugs and Subcellular Components," P. N. Campbell, Ed., p. 5, Churchill, London, 1968.
260. Walker, I. G., Reid, B. D., *Cancer Res.* (1971) **31**, 510.
261. Ball, C. R., Roberts, J. J., *Chem. Biol. Interact.* (1970) **2**, 321.
262. Yin, L., Chun, E. H. L., Rutman, R. J., *Biochim. Biophys. Acta* (1973) **324**, 472.
263. Painter, R. B., "Genetics Concepts and Neoplasia," p. 593, Williams and Wilkins, Baltimore, 1970.
264. Painter, R. B., Cleaver, J. E., *Radiation Res.* (1969) **37**, 451.
265. Schindler, R., Ramseier, L., Grieder, A., *Biochem. Pharmacol.* (1966) **15**, 2013.
266. Lieberman, M. W., Baney, R. N., Lee, R. E., Sell, S., Farber, E., *Cancer Res.* (1971) **31**, 1297.
267. Cleaver, J. E., *Mutat. Res.* (1971) **12**, 453.
268. Papirmeister, B., Davison, C. L., *Biochem. Biophys. Res. Commun.* (1964) **17**, 608.
269. Roberts, J. J., Pascoe, J. M., Smith, B. A., Crathorn, A. R., *Chem. Biol. Interact.* (1971) **3**, 49.
270. Walker, I. G., Reid, B. D., *Mutat. Res.* (1971) **12**, 101.
271. Reiter, H., Strauss, B. S., *J. Mol. Biol.* (1965) **14**, 179.
272. Strauss, B. S., Coyle, M., Robbins, M., *Trans. N.Y. Acad. Sci.* (1969) **163**, 765.
273. Prakash, L., Strauss, B. S., *J. Bacteriol.* (1970) **102**, 760.
274. Baldy, M. W., Strom, B., Bernstein, H., *J. Virol.* (1971) **7**, 407.
275. Kimball, R. F., Setlow, J. K., Liu, M., *Mutat. Res.* (1971) **12**, 21.
276. Ronen, A., Atidia, J., *Mutat. Res.* (1971) **11**, 175.

277. Hahn, G. M., King, D., Yang, S. J., *Nature New Biol.* (1971) **230**, 242.
278. Cox, R., Damjanov, I., Abanobi, S. E., Sarma, D. S. R., *Cancer Res.* (1973) **33**, 2114.
279. Damjanov, I., Cox, R., Sarma, D. S. R., Farber, E., *Cancer Res.* (1973) **33**, 2122.
280. Boyce, R. P., Howard-Flanders, P., *Z. Vererbungsl.* (1964) **95**, 345.
281. Rauth, A. M., Barton, B., Lee, C. P. Y., *Cancer Res.* (1970) **30**, 2724.
282. Cleaver, J. E., *Nature* (1968) **218**, 652.
283. Bootsma, D., Mulder, M. P., Pot, F., Cohen, J. A., *Mutat. Res.* (1970) **9**, 507.
284. Searashi, T., Strauss, B. S., *Biochem. Biophys. Res. Commun.* (1965) **20**, 680.
285. Rhaese, H. J., Freese, E., *Biochim. Biophys. Acta* (1969) **190**, 418.
286. Strauss, B. S., Hill, T., *Biochim. Biophys. Acta* (1970) **213**, 14.
287. Uhlenhopp, E. L., Krasna, A. I., *Biochemistry* (1971) **10**, 3290.
288. Strauss, B. S., Robbins, M., *Biochim. Biophys. Acta* (1968) **161**, 68.
289. Kirtikar, D. M., Goldthwait, D. A., *Proc. Natl. Acad. Sci.* (1974) **71**, 2022.
290. Warwick, G. P., *Fed. Proc.* (1971) **30**, 1760.
291. Brock, R. D., *Mutat. Res.* (1971) **11**, 181.
292. Gaudin, D., Gregg, R. S., Yielding, K. L., *Biochem. Biophys. Res. Commun.* (1971) **45**, 630.
293. Evans, R. G., Norman, A., *Radiat. Res.* (1968) **36**, 287.
294. Thayer, P. S., Kensler, C. J., *Toxicol. Appl. Pharmacol.* (1973) **25**, 157.
295. Roberts, J. J., 5th Miles Symposium, Molecular and Cellular Repair Processes, Baltimore, *Johns Hopkins Med. J. Suppl.* (1972) **1**, 226.
296. Zajdela, F., Latarjet, R., *C.R. Acad. Sci.* (1973) **277D**, 1073.
297. Clarke, C. H., *Mutat. Res.* (1969) **8**, 35.
298. Huberman, E., Heidelberger, C., *Mutat. Res.* (1972) **14**, 130.
299. Malling, H. V., DeSerres, F. J., *Mol. Gen. Genet.* (1970) **106**, 195.
300. Ames, B. N., Sims, P., Grover, P. L., *Science* (1972) **176**, 47.
301. Ames, B. N., Whitfield, H. J., Jr., *Cold Spring Harbor Symp. Quant. Biol.* (1966) **31**, 22.
302. Brusick, D. J., *Mutat. Res.* (1969) **8**, 247.
303. Loveless, A., *Proc. Roy. Soc. B.* (1959) **150**, 497.
304. Alexander, P., Connell. D. I., "Cellular Basis and Etiology of Late Somatic Effects of Ionizing Radiation," R. J. C. Harris, Ed., p. 259, Academic, London, 1962.
305. Walters, M. A., Roe, F. J. C., Mitchley, B. C. V., Walsh, A., *Br. J. Cancer* (1967) **21**, 367.
306. Hrushesky, W., Sampson, D., Murphy, G. P., *J. Natl. Cancer Inst.* (1972) **49**, 1077.
307. Colburn, N. H., Boutwell, R. K., *Cancer Res.* (1966) **26**, 1701.
308. *Ibid.* (1968) **28**, 642, 653.
309. Van Duuren, B. L., Sivak, A., Goldschmidt, B. M., Katz, C., Melchionne, S., *J. Natl. Cancer Inst.* (1969) **43**, 481.
310. Van Duuren, B. L., Sivak, A., Katz, C., Melchionne, S., *Cancer Res.* (1969) **29**, 947.
311. Druckrey, H., Kruse, H., Preussmann, R., Ivankovic, S., Landschütz, C., Gimmy, J., *Z. Krebsforsch.* (1970) **75**, 69.
312. Heston, W. E., *J. Natl. Cancer Inst.* (1950) **11**, 415.
313. Loprieno, N., Guglielminetti, R., Bonatti, S., Abbondandolo, A., *Mutat. Res.* (1969) **8**, 65.
314. Schwartz, N. M., *Genetics* (1963) **48**, 1357.
315. Tessman, I., Poddar, R. K., Kumar, S., *J. Mol. Biol.* (1964) **9**, 352.
316. Osborn, M., Person, S., Phillips, S., Funk, F., *J. Mol. Biol.* (1967) **26**, 437.
317. Malling, H. V., De Serres, F. J., *Mutat. Res.* (1968) **6**, 181.
318. Ronen, A., *J. Gen. Microbiol.* (1964) **37**, 49.
319. Olson, A. O., Baird, K. M., *Biochim. Biophys. Acta* (1969) **179**, 513.
320. Lawley, P. D., Orr, D. J., Shah, S. A., *Chem. Biol. Interact.* (1972) **4**, 389.

321. Ludlum, D. B., *Biochim. Biophys. Acta* (1971) **247**, 412.
322. Krieg, D. R., *Prog. Nucleic Acid Res. Mol. Biol.* (1963) **2**, 125.
323. Lawley, P. D., Orr, D. J., Shah, S. A., Farmer, P. B., Jarman, M., *Biochem. J.* (1973) **135**, 193.
324. Gerchman, L., Ludlum, D. B., *Biochim. Biophys. Acta* (1973) **308**, 310.
325. Hendler, S., Fürer, E., Srinivasan, P. R., *Biochemistry* (1970) **9**, 4141.
326. Ludlum, D. B., *J. Biol. Chem.* (1970) **245**, 477.
327. Nagata, C., Imamura, A., Saito, H., Fukui, K., *Gann* (1963) **54**, 109.
328. Brookes, P., Lawley, P. D., *J. Cell Comp. Physiol. Suppl. 1* (1964) **64**, 111.
329. Wong, J. L., Fuchs, D. S., *J. Org. Chem.* (1971) **36**, 848.
330. Lawley, P. D., Shah, S. A., *Biochem. J.* (1972) **128**, 117.
331. Drake, J. W., Greening, E. O., *Proc. Natl. Acad. Sci.* (1970) **66**, 823.
332. Lwoff, A., *Bacteriol. Rev.* (1953) **17**, 269.
333. Heinemann, B., "Chemical Mutagens, Principles and Methods for their Detection," Vol. 1, Chap. 8, Plenum, New York, London, 1971.
334. Loveless, A., Shields, G., *Virology* (1964) **24**, 668.
335. Kondo, S., *Proc. Int. Congr. Genet., 12th, Tokyo* (1968) **2**, 126.
336. Burns, W. H., Black, P. H., *Virology* (1969) **39**, 625.
337. Igel, H. J., Huebner, R. J., Turner, H. C., Kotin, P., Falk, H. L., *Science* (1969) **166**, 1624.
338. Kao, F. T., Puck, T. T., *J. Cell. Physiol.* (1971) **78**, 139.
339. Huberman, E., Aspiras, L., Heidelberger, C., Grover, P. L., Sims, P., *Proc. Natl. Acad. Sci.* (1971) **68**, 3195.
340. Harris, H., Miller, O. J., Klein, G., Worst, P., Tachibana, T., *Nature* (1969) **223**, 363.
341. Chu, E. H. Y., Brimer, P., Jacobson, K. B., Merriam, E. V., *Genetics* (1969) **62**, 359.
342. Shapiro, N. I., Khalizev, A. E., Luss, E. V., Marshak, M. I., Petrova, O. N., Varshaver, N. B., *Mutat. Res.* (1972) **15**, 203.
343. Harris, M., *J. Cell. Physiol.* (1971) **78**, 177.
344. Chu, E. H. Y., Malling, H. V., *Proc. Natl. Acad. Sci.* (1968) **61**, 1306.
345. Kao, F. T., Puck, T. T., *Proc. Natl. Acad. Sci.* (1968) **60**, 1275.
346. Sato, K., Slesinski, R. S., Littlefield, J. W., *Proc. Natl. Acad. Sci.* (1972) **69**, 1244.
347. Chu, E. H. Y., "Chemical Mutagens, Principles and Methods for their Detection," A. Hollaender, Ed., Vol. 2, Chap. 15, Plenum, New York, London, 1971.
348. Sanders, F. K., Burford, B. O., *Nature* (1967) **213**, 1171.
349. DiPaolo, J. A., Nelson, R. L., Donovan, P. J., *Nature* (1972) **235**, 278.
350. Marquardt, H., Kuroki, T., Huberman, E., Selkirk, J. E., Heidelberger, C., Grover, P. L., Sims, P., *Cancer Res.* (1972) **32**, 716.
351. Cattanach, B. M., *Mutat. Res.* (1966) **3**, 346.
352. Auerbach, C., Falconer, D. S., *Nature* (1949) **163**, 678.
353. Falconer, D. S., Slizynski, B. M., Auerbach, C., *J. Genet.* (1952) **51**, 81.
354. Ehling, U. H., "Chemical Mutagenesis in Mammals and Man," F. Vogel, G. Rohrborn, Eds., Chap. 5, Springer-Verlag, Berlin, 1970.
355. Ehling, U. H., Russell, W. L., *Genetics* (1969) **61**, s14.
356. Cattanach, B. M., "Chemical Mutagens, Principles and Methods for their Detection," A. Hollaender, Ed., Vol. 2, Chap. 20, Plenum, New York-London, 1971.
357. Röhrborn, G., "Chemical Mutagenesis in Mammals and Man," F. Vogel and G. Röhrborn, Eds., Chap. 19, Springer-Verlag, Berlin, 1970.
358. Bateman, A. J., Epstein, S. S., "Chemical Mutagens, Principles and Methods for their Detection," A. Hollaender, Ed., Vol. 2, Chap. 21, Plenum, New York-London, 1971.
359. Ehling, U. H., Cumming, R. B., Malling, H. V., *Mutat. Res.* (1968) **5**, 417.
360. Partington, M., Bateman, A. J., *Heredity* (1964) **19**, 191.

361. Partington, M., Jackson, H., *Genet. Res.* (1963) **4**, 333.
362. Epstein, S. S., Bass, W., Arnold, E., Bishop, Y., *Science* (1970) **168**, 584.
363. Epstein, S. S., Shafner, H., *Nature* (1968) **219**, 385.
364. Moutschen, J., *Genetics* (1961) **46**, 291.
365. Cattanach, B. M., *Z. Vererbungsl.* (1959) **90**, 1.
366. Röhrborn, G., *Humangenetik* (1965) **1**, 576.
367. Brittinger, D., *Humangenetik* (1966) **3**, 156.
368. Dubinin, N. P., Soyfer, V. N., *Mutat. Res.* (1969) **8**, 353.
369. Legator, M. S., "Chemical Mutagenesis in Mammals and Man," F. Vogel, G. Röhrborn, Eds., Chap. 15, Springer-Verlag, Berlin, 1970.
370. Malling, H. V., Cosgrove, G. E., "Chemical Mutagenesis in Mammals and Man," F. Vogel and G. Röhrborn, Eds., Chap. 16, Springer-Verlag, Berlin, 1970.
371. Legator, M. S., Malling, H. V., "Chemical Mutagens, Principles and Methods for their Detection," A. Hollaender, Ed., Vol. 2, Chap. 22, Plenum, New York, London, 1971.
372. Whitfield, H. J., Martin, R., Ames, B. N., *J. Mol. Biol.* (1966) **21**, 335.
373. De Serres, F. J., Kølmark, G., *Nature* (1958) **182**, 1249.
374. Gabridge, M. G., Legator, M. S., *Proc. Soc. Exp. Biol. Med.* (1969) **130**, 831.
375. Lee, K. Y., Lijinsky, W., Magee, P. N., *J. Natl. Cancer Inst.* (1964) **32**, 65.
376. McElhone, M. J., O'Connor, P. J., Craig, A. W., *Biochem. J.* (1971) **125**, 821.
377. Brookes, P., Lawley, P. D., "Chemical Mutagens, Principles and Methods for their Detection," A. Hollaender, Ed., Vol. 1, Chap. 4, Plenum, New York, London, 1971.
378. Lawley, P. D., Brookes, P., *Exp. Cell Res.*, *Suppl.* (1963) **9**, 512.
379. Lawley, P. D., Brookes, P., *Biochem. J.* (1964) **92**, 19c.
380. Dipple, A., Brookes, P., Mackintosh, D. S., Rayman, M., *Biochemistry* (1971) **10**, 4323.
381. O'Connor, P. J., Capps, M. J., Craig, A. W., Lawley, P. D., Shah, S. A., *Biochem. J.* (1972) **129**, 519.
382. O'Connor, P. J., Capps, M. J., Craig, A. W., *Br. J. Cancer* (1973) **27**, 153.
383. Lawley, P. D., Brookes, P., Magee, P. N., Craddock, V. M., Swann, P. F., *Biochim. Biophys. Acta* (1968) **157**, 646.
384. Lawley, P. D., Crathorn, A. R., Shah, S. A., Smith, B. A., *Biochem. J.* (1972) **128**, 133.
385. Schoental, R., *Biochem. J.* (1967) **102**, 5c.
386. *Ibid.* (1969) **114**, 55P.
387. Wunderlich, V., Schutt, M., Bottger, M., Graffi, A., *Biochem. J.* (1970) **118**, 99.
388. Whittle, E. D., *Biochim. Biophys. Acta* (1969) **195**, 381.
389. Craddock, V. M., *Chem. Biol. Interact.* (1969) **1**, 234.
390. Swann, P. F., Magee, P. N., *Biochem. J.* (1971) **125**, 841.
391. Trams, E. G., Nadkarni, M. V., Smith, P. K., *Cancer Res.* (1961) **21**, 560.
392. Wheeler, G. P., Alexander, J. A., *Arch. Biochem. Biophys.* (1957) **72**, 476.
393. Connors, T. A., Jeney, A., Warwick, G. P., Whisson, M. E., "Isotopes in Experimental Pharmacology," L. J. Roth, Ed., p. 433, University of Chicago, Chicago, 1965.
394. Poynter, R. W., *Biochem. Pharmacol.* (1970) **19**, 1387.
395. Muramatsu, M., Azama, Y., Takayama, S., *Cancer Res.* (1972) **32**, 702.
396. Wunderlich, V., Tetzlaff, I., Graffi, A., *Chem. Biol. Interact.* (1971) **4**, 81.
397. Craddock, V. M., *Biochem. Biophys. Acta* (1973) **312**, 202.
398. Culp, L. A., Dore, E., Brown, G. M., *Arch. Biochem. Biophys.* (1970) **136**, 73.
399. Craddock, V. M., Villa-Treviño, S., Magee, P. N., *Biochem. J.* (1968) **107**, 179.
400. Craddock, V. M., *Biochim. Biophys. Acta* (1971) **240**, 376.
401. Mizrahi, I. J., Emmelot, P., *Biochim. Biophys. Acta* (1964) **91**, 362.

402. Villa-Treviño, S., *Biochem. J.* (1967) **105**, 625.
403. Craddock, V. M., *Biochem. J.* (1969) **111**, 497.
404. Goth, R., Rajewsky, M. F., *Z. Krebsforsch.* (1974) **82**, 37.
405. Papirmeister, B., Dorsey, J. K., Davison, C. L., Gross, C. L., *Fed. Proc.* (1970) **29**, Abstract No. 2716.
406. Venitt, S., Tarmy, E. M., *Biochim. Biophys. Acta* (1972) **287**, 38.
407. Lieberman, M. W., Dipple, A., *Cancer Res.* (1972) **32**, 1855.
408. Margison, G. P., O'Connor, P. J., *Biochem. J.* (1972) **128**, 138P.
409. Pegg, A. E., *Chem. Biol. Interact.* (1973) **6**, 393.
410. Caspersson, T., Zech, L., Modest, E. J., Foley, G. E., Wagh, U., Simonsson, E., *Exp. Cell. Res.* (1969) **58**, 128.
411. Bauer, W., Vinograd, J., *J. Mol. Biol.* (1970) **33**, 141.
412. McCalla, D. R., *J. Protozool.* (1967) **14**, 480.
413. Pascoe, J. M., Thesis, London (1972).
414. Walker, I. G., Ewart, D. F., *Can. J. Biochem.* (1973) **51**, 148.
415. Venitt, S., Brookes, P., Lawley, P. D., *Biochim. Biophys. Acta* (1968) **155**, 521.
416. Brakier, L., Verly, W. G., *Biochim. Biophys. Acta* (1970) **213**, 296.
417. Borek, E., Kerr, S. J., *Adv. Cancer Res.* (1972) **15**, 163.
418. Wilkinson, R., Pillinger, D. J., *Int. J. Cancer* (1971) **8**, 401.
419. Temin, H. M., Mizutani, S., *Nature* (1970) **227**, 887.
420. Pillinger, D. J., Hay, J., Borek, E., *Biochem. J.* (1969) **114**, 429.
421. Hay, J., Pillinger, D. J., Borek, E., *Biochem. J.* (1970) **119**, 587.
422. Hall, R. H., *Prog. Nucleic Acid Res. Mol. Biol.* (1970) **10**, 57.
423. Krüger, F. W., Walker, G., Wiessler, M., *Experientia* (1970) **26**, 520.
424. Krüger, F. W., Ballweg, H., Maier-Borst, W., *Experientia* (1968) **24**, 592.
425. Lijinsky, W., Ross, A. E., *Proc. Am. Assoc. Cancer Res.* (1969) **10**, 51.
426. Lijinsky, W., Tomatis, L., Wenyon, C. E. M., *Proc. Soc. Exp. Biol.* (1969) **130**, 945.
427. Bautz, E., Freese, E., *Proc. Natl. Acad. Sci.* (1960) **46**, 1585.
428. Druckrey, H., Schagen, B., Ivankovic, S., *Z. Krebsforsch.* (1970) **74**, 141.
429. Schmähl, D., *Z. Krebsforsch.* (1970) **74**, 457.
430. Schmähl, D., Thomas, C., *Z. Krebsforsch.* (1965) **67**, 135.
431. Schmähl, D., Thomas, C., König, K., *Z. Krebsforsch.* (1963) **65**, 342.
432. Roberts, J. J., *Jerusalem Symp. Quantum Chem. Biochem.* (1969) **1**, 229.
433. Dingman, W. C., Sporn, M. B., *Cancer Res.* (1967) **27**, 938.
434. Sporn, M. B., Dingman, C. W., *Nature* (1966) **210**, 531.
435. Weisburger, J. H., Grantham, P. H., Vanhorn, E., Steigbigel, N. H., Rall, D. P., Weisburger, E. K., *Cancer Res.* (1964) **24**, 475.
436. Boutwell, R. K., *Prog. Exp. Tumor Res.* (1964) **4**, 207.
437. Van Duuren, B. L., *Prog. Exp. Tumor Res.* (1969) **11**, 31.
438. Berenblum, I., *Cancer Res.* (1941) **1**, 807.
439. Roe, F. J. C., Carter, R. L., Mitchley, B. C. V., Peto, R., Hecker, E., *Int. J. Cancer* (1972) **9**, 264.
440. Case, R. A. M., Lea, A. J., *Br. J. Prev. Soc. Med.* (1955) **9**, 62.
441. Beebe, G. W., *J. Natl. Cancer Inst.* (1960) **25**, 1231.
442. Wada, S., Miyanishi, M., Nishimoto, Y., Kambe, S., Miller, R. W., *Lancet* (1968) **i**, 1611.
443. Berg, J. W., "Morphology of Experimental Respiratory Carcinogenesis," P. Netterheim, M. G. Hanna, Jr., J. W. Deatherage, Jr., Eds., p. 93, U.S. Atomic Energy Commission, Division of Technical Information, 1970.
444. Druckrey, H., Preussmann, R., Nashed, N., Ivankovic, S., *Z, Krebsforsch.* (1966) **68**, 103.
445. Fishbein, L., "Chromatography of Environmental Hazards, Carcinogens, Mutagens and Teratogens," Vol. 1, Elsevier, Amsterdam, 1972.
446. Rosenkranz, H. S., Rosenkranz, S., *Experientia* (1972) **28**, 386.

447. Weil, C. S., Condra, N., Haun, C., Striegel, J. A., *Am. Ind. Hyg. Assoc. J.* (1963) **24,** 305.
448. Van Duuren, B. L., *Ann. N.Y. Acad. Sci.* (1969) **163,** 633.
449. Walpole, A. L., *Ann. N.Y. Acad. Sci.* (1958) **68,** 750.
450. Dickens, F., *Carcinog. Collect. Pap. Annu. Symp. Fundmen. Cancer Res. 20th* (1967), 447.
451. Innes, J. R. M., Ulland, B. M., Valerio, M. G., Petrucelli, L., Fishbein, L., Hart, E. R., Pallotta, A. J., Bates, R. R., Falk, H. L., Gart, J. J., Klein, M., Mitchell, I., Peters, J., *J. Natl. Cancer Inst.* (1969) **42,** 1101.
452. Williams, R. T., "Detoxication Mechanisms," Chap. 2 and 8, Chapman and Hall, London, 1959.
453. Heppel, L. A., Neal, P. A., Perrin, T. L., Orr, M. L., Porterfield, V. T., *J. Ind. Hyg. Toxicol.* (1944) **26,** 8.
454. Hartwell, J. L., "Survey of Compounds which have been tested for Carcinogenic Activity," 2nd ed., National Cancer Institute, National Institute of Health, Bethesda, Maryland, 1951.
455. Shubik, P., Hartwell, J. L., "Survey of Compounds which have been tested for Carcinogenic Activity, Suppl. **1,**" U.S. Dept. of Health, Education and Welfare, Public Health Service (Publication No. 149), Washington, D.C., 1957.
456. *Ibid.,* Suppl. **2,** 1969.
457. Shubik, P., Hartwell, J. L., (successors to) For National Cancer Inst., Public Health Service (Publication No. **149**), J. I Thompson and Co., Rockville, Md., 1968–1969.
458. Irish, D. D., Adams, E. M., Spencer, H. C., Rowe, V. K., *J. Ind. Hyg. Toxicol.* (1940) **22,** 218.
459. Buckell, M., *Br. J. Ind. Med.* (1950) **7,** 122.
460. Muller, E., *Arch. Hyg. Bakt.* (1968) **152,** 23.
461. Eschenbrenner, A. B., Miller, E., *J. Natl. Cancer Inst.* (1945) **5,** 251.
462. Deringer, M. K., Dunn, T. B., Heston, W. E., *Proc. Soc. Exp. Biol. Med.* (1953) **83,** 474.
463. Roe, F. J. C., Carter, R. L., Mitchley, B. C. V., *Annu. Rep. Br. Empire Cancer Campaign* (1968) **46,** 13.
464. Eschenbrenner, A. B., *J. Natl. Cancer Inst.* (1944) **4,** 385.
465. Ambrose, A. M., *Arch. Ind. Hyg.* (1950) **2,** 591.
466. Rowe, V. K., Spencer, H. C., McCollister, D. D., Hollingsworth, R. L., Adams, E. M., *Arch. Ind. Hyg.* (1952) **6,** 158.
467. Olson, W. A., Habermann, R. T., Weisburger, E. K., Ward, J. M., Weisburger, J. H., *J. Natl. Cancer Inst.* (1973) **51,** 1993.
468. Spencer, H. C., Rowe, V. K., Adams, E. M., McCollister, D. D., Irish, D. D., *Arch. Ind. Hyg.* (1951) **4,** 482.
469. Fujii, K., Epstein, S. S., *Toxicol. Appl. Pharmacol.* (1969) **14,** 613.
470. Desoille, H., Truffert, L., Bourguignon, A., Delavierre, P., Philbert, M., Girard-Wallon, C., *Arch. Mal. Prof.* (1968) **29,** 381.
471. Viola, P. L., Bigotti, A., Caputo, A., *Cancer Res.* (1971) **31,** 516.
472. Slater, T. F., *Nature* (1966) **209,** 36.
473. Reynolds, S. E., *J. Pharmacol. Exp. Therap.* (1967) **155,** 117.
474. Miller, J. A., *Cancer Res.* (1970) **30,** 559.
475. Miller, D. P., Haggard, H. W., *J. Ind. Hyg.* (1943) **25,** 423.
476. Roe, F. J. C., Salaman, M. H., *Br. J. Cancer* (1955) **9,** 177.
477. *Br. Med. J.* (1974) **i,** 590.
478. Higginson, J., "Proceedings of the 8th Canadian Cancer Conference," J. F. Morgan, Ed., p. 40, Pergamon, Oxford, 1969.
479. Boyland, E., "UICC Monographs, Vol. 7," R. Truhaut, Ed., p. 204, Springer-Verlag, Berlin, 1967.
480. Boyland, E., *Prog. Exp. Tumor Res.* (1969) **11,** 222.
481. Koller, P. C., *Mutat. Res.* (1969) **8,** 207.

482. Hobbs, J. R., *Br. Med. J.* (1971) **2**, 67.
483. Kyle, R. A., Pierre, R. V., Bayrd, E. D., *N. Engl. J. Med.* (1970) **283**, 1121.
484. Fraumeni, J. F., Jr., Miller, R. W., *J. Natl. Cancer Inst.* (1972) **48**, 1267.
485. Min, K.-W., Györkey, F., *Cancer* (1968) **22**, 1027.
486. Nelson, B. M., Andrews, G. A., *Am. J. Clin. Pathol.* (1964) **42**, 37.
487. Miller, D. G., *J. Am. Med. Assoc.* (1971) **217**, 1662.
488. Shimkin, M. B., *Cancer* (1954) **7**, 410.
489. Berenbaum, M. C., *Antiobiot. Chemother.* (1969) **15**, 155.
490. Borkovec, A. B., *Ann. N. Y. Acad. Sci.* (1969) **163**, 860.
491. Fahmy, O. G., Fahmy, M. J., *Ann. N.Y. Acad. Sci.* (1969) **160**, 228.
492. Obe, G., Sperling, K., Belitz, H. J., *Angew. Chem. (Int. Ed.)* (1971) **10**, 302.
493. Dickens, F., Jones, H. E. H., *Br. J. Cancer* (1965) **19**, 392.
494. Epstein, S. S., Andrea, J., Jaffe, H., Joshi, S., Falk, H., Mantel, N., *Nature* (1967) **215**, 1388.
495. Rall, D. P., *Environ. Res.* (1969) **2**, 360.
496. Owens, R. G., Blaak, G., *Contrib. Boyce Thompson Inst.* (1960) **20**, 475.
497. Bridges, B. A., Mottershead, R. P., Rothwell, M. A., Green, M. H. L., *Chem. Biol. Interact.* (1972) **5**, 77.
498. Barry, D. H., Chasseaud, L. F., Hunter, B., Robinson, W. E., *Nature* (1972) **240**, 560.
499. Sapis, J. C., Ribéreau-Gayor, P., *Ann. Technol. Agric.* (1969) **18**, 207. 1244.
500. Boyland, E., Down, W. H., *Eur. J. Cancer* (1971) **7**, 495.
501. Boyland, E., Nery, R., *Biochem. J.* (1969) **113**, 123.
502. Dickens, F., Jones, H. E. H., Waynforth, H. B., *Br. J. Cancer* (1966) **20**, 134.
502a. *Ibid.* (1968) **22**, 762.
503. Zweifel, J. R., *J. Natl. Cancer Inst.* (1966) **36**, 937.
504. Clayson, D. B., "Chemical Carcinogenesis," J. and A. Churchill Ltd., London, 1962.
505. Walpole, A. L., Roberts, D. C., Rose, F. L., Hendry, J. A., Homer, R. F., *Br. J. Pharmacol.* (1954) **9**, 306.
506. Carter, R. L., "Metabolic Aspects of Food Safety," F. J. C. Roe, Ed., p. 569, Blackwells, Oxford, 1970.
507. McDonald, G. O., "Dissemination of Cancer, Prevention and Therapy," W. H. Cole, G. O. McDonald, S. S. Roberts, H. W. Southwick, Eds., Appleton-Century-Crofts, Inc., New York, 1961.
508. Berenblum, I., *J. Pathol. Bacteriol.* (1931) **34**, 731.
509. Parish, D. J., Searle, C. E., *Br. J. Cancer* (1966) **20**, 200.
510. *Ibid.*, 206.
511. Chernozemski, I. N., Warwick, G. P., *J. Natl. Cancer Inst.* (1970) **45**, 709.
512. Gwynn, R. H., Salaman, M. H., *Br. J. Cancer* (1953) **7**, 482.
513. Rusch, H. P., Bosch, D., Boutwell, R. K., *Acta Unio Int. Cancrum* (1955) **11**, 699.
514. Crabtree, H. G., *J. Pathol. Bacteriol.* (1940) **51**, 303.
515. Searle, C. E., *Cancer Res.* (1966) **26**, 12.
516. Tagashira, Y., *Gann* (1954) **45**, 601.
517. Berenblum, I., Haran-Ghera, N., *Cancer Res.* (1957) **17**, 329.
518. Dipple, A., Slade, T. A., *Eur. J. Cancer* (1970) **6**, 417.
519. Roe, F. J. C., Dipple, A., Mitchley, B. C. V., *Br. J. Cancer* (1972) **26**, 461.
520. Dipple, A., Slade, T. A., *Eur. J. Cancer* (1971) **7**, 473.
521. Flesher, J. W., Sydnor, K. L., *Cancer Res.* (1971) **31**, 1951.
522. Roe, F. J. C., *Cancer Res.* (1957) **17**, 64.
523. Durham, W. F., Gaines, T. B., McCanley, R. H., Sedlak, B. S., Mattson, A. M., Hayes, W. J., *Arch. Ind. Health* (1957) **15**, 340.
524. Klotsche, C., *Z. Angew. Zool.* (1956) 87.
525. Du Bois, K. P., Cotter, G. J., *Arch. Ind. Health* (1955) **11**, 53.

526. Preussmann, R., *Food Cosmet. Toxicol.* (1968) **6,** 576.
527. Gibel, W., Lohs, K., Wildner, G. P., Ziebarth, D., *Arch. Geschwulstforsch.* (1971) **37,** 303.
528. Kodama, J. K., Morse, M. S., Anderson, H. H., Dunlap, M. K., Hine, C. H., *Arch. Ind. Hyg.* (1954) **9,** 45.
529. Hazleton, L. W., Holland, E. G., *Arch. Ind. Hyg.* (1953) **8,** 399.
530. Barnes, J. M., Denz, F. A., *J. Hyg.* (1951) **49,** 430.
531. Barnes, J. M., Denz, F. A., *Br. J. Ind. Med.* (1954) **11,** 11.
532. Bombinski, T. J., du Bois, K. P., *Arch. Ind. Health* (1958) **17,** 192.
533. Treon, J. E., Dutra, F. M., Cleveland, F. P., *Arch. Ind. Hyg.* (1953) **8,** 170.
534. Löfroth, G., *Naturwissenschaften* (1970) **57,** 393.
534a. Voogd, C. E., Jacobs, J. J. J. A. A., Van der Stel, J. J., *Mutat, Res.* (1972) **16,** 413.
535. Lawley, P. D., Shah, S. A., Orr, D. J., *Chem. Biol. Interact.* (1974) **8,** 171.
536. Wennerberg, R., Löfroth, G., *Chem. Biol. Interact.* (1974) **8,** 339.
537. Hutson, D. H., Blair, D., Hoadley, E. C., Pickering, B. A., *Toxicol. Appl. Pharmacol.* (1971) **19,** 378.
538. Loeffler, J. E., De Vries, D. M., Young, R., Page, A. C., *Toxicol. Appl. Pharmacol.* (1971) **19,** 378.
538a. *Arch. Toxicol.* (1972) **30,** 1.
539. Miller, E. C., Miller, J. A., *Cancer Res.* (1960) **20,** 133.
540. Salmon, W. D., Copeland, D. H., *J. Natl. Cancer Inst.* (1949) **10,** 361.
541. Smith, C. C., *Arch. Ind. Hyg.* (1953) **7,** 310.
542. Van Duuren, B. L., Langseth, L., Goldschmidt, B. M., Orris, L., *J. Natl. Cancer Inst.* (1967) **39,** 1217.
543. Van Duuren, B. L., Langseth, L., Orris, L., Teebor, G., Nelson, N., Kuschner, M., *J. Natl. Cancer Inst.* (1966) **37,** 825.
544. Van Duuren, B. L., Langseth, L., Orris, L., Baden, M., Kuschner, M., *J. Natl. Cancer Inst.* (1967) **39,** 1213.
545. Van Duuren, B. L., Nelson, N., Orris, L., Palmes, E. D., Schmitt, F. L., *J. Natl. Cancer Inst.* (1963) **31,** 41.
546. Kotin, P., Falk, H. L., *Radiat. Res. Suppl. 3* (1963) 193.
547. Treon, J. F., Cleveland, F. P., *J. Agr. Food Chem.* (1955) **3,** 402.
548. Ortega, P., Wayland, J. H., Durham, W. F., *Arch. Pathol.* (1957) **64,** 614.
549. Speck, L. B., Maaske, C. A., *Arch. Ind. Health* (1958) **18,** 268.
550. Lawley, P. D., Jarman, M., *Biochem. J.* (1972) **126,** 893.
551. Van Duuren, B. L., Melchionne, S., Blair, R., Goldschmidt, B. M., Katz, C., *J. Natl. Cancer Inst.* (1971) **46,** 143.
552. Dickens, F., Jones, H. E. H., *Br. J. Cancer* (1963) **17,** 100.
553. Roe, F. J. C., Glendenning, O. M., *Br. J. Cancer* (1956) **10,** 357.
554. Searle, C. E., *Br. J. Cancer* (1961) **15,** 804.
555. Palmes, E. D., Orris, L., Nelson, N., *Am. Ind. Hyg. Assoc. J.* (1962) **23,** 257.
556. Van Duuren, B. L., Orris, L., Nelson, N., *J. Natl. Cancer Inst.* (1965) **35,** 707.
557. Boutwell, R. K., Colburn, N. H., Muckerman, C., *Ann. N.Y. Acad. Sci.* (1969) **163,** 751.
558. Jones, J. B., Young, J. M., *J. Med. Chem.* (1968) **11,** 1176.
559. Epstein, S. S., Mantel, N., *Int. J. Cancer* (1968) **3,** 325.
560. Griswold, D. P., Jr., Casey, A. E., Weisburger, E. K., Weisburger, J. H., *Cancer Res.* (1968) **28,** 924.
561. Lacassagne, A., Buu-Hoi, N. P., Zajdela, F., Jacquignon, P., Mangane, M., *Science* (1967) **158,** 387.
562. Lacassagne, A., Buu-Hoi, N. P., Zajdela, F., Stora, C., Mangane, M., Jacquignon, P., *C.R. Acad. Sci. Paris, ser. D.* (1971) **272,** 3102.
563. Ulland, B., Finkelstein, M., Weisburger, E. K., Rice, J. M., Weisburger, J. H., *Nature* (1971) **230,** 460.
564. Leong, B. K. J., Macfarland, H. N., Reese, W. H., Jr., *Arch. Environ. Health*

(1971) **22,** 663.
565. Gargus, J. L., Reese, W. H., Jr., Rutter, H. A., *Toxicol. Appl. Pharmacol.*
     (1969) **15,** 92.
566. Kensler, (?), (1957) quoted by Shubik, P. and Hartwell, J. L. in "PHS
     Publication No. 149, Suppl. 1," Washington, U.S. Dept. of Health, Educa-
     tion and Welfare, 1957.
567. Schoental, R., Bensted, J. P. M., *Cancer Res.* (1971) **31,** 573.
568. Popper, H., Sternberg, S. S., Oser, B. L., Oser, M., *Cancer* (1960) **13,** 1035.
569. Sternberg, S. S., Popper, H., Oser, B. L., Oser, M., *Cancer* (1960) **13,** 780.
570. Heston, W. E., Levallain, W. D., *Proc. Soc. Exp. Biol. Med.* (1953) **82,** 457.
571. Boyland, E., Horning, E. S., *Br. J. Cancer* (1949) **3,** 118.
572. Griffin, A. C., Brandt, E. L., Tatum, E. L., *J. Am. Med. Assoc.* (1950) **144,**
     571.
573. Narpozzi, A., *Boll. Soc. Ital. Biol. Sper.* (1954) **29,** 1168.
574. Conklin, J. W., Upton, A. C., Christenberry, K. W., *Cancer Res.* (1965) **25,**
     20.
575. Upton, A. C., Jenkins, V. K., Walburg, H. E., Jr., Tyndall, R. L., Conklin,
     W. L., Wald, N., *Natl. Cancer Inst. Monogr.* (1966) **22,** 329.
576. Steinhoff, D., Kuk, B. T., *Z. Krebsforsch.* (1957) **62,** 112.
577. Matsuyama, M., Suzuki, H., Nakamura, T., *Br. J. Cancer* (1969) **23,** 167.
578. Duhig, J. T., *Arch. Pathol.* (1965) **79,** 177.
579. Haddow, A., Timmis, G. M., *Lancet* (1953) **i,** 207.
580. Timmis, G. M., Hudson, R. F., *Ann. N.Y. Acad. Sci.* (1958) **68,** 727.
581. Roberts, J. J., Warwick, G. P., *Biochem. Pharmacol.* (1961) **6,** 217.
582. Roberts, J. J., Warwick, G. P., *Nature* (1959) **183,** 1509.
583. Jones, A. R., Campbell, I. S. C., *Biochem. Pharmacol.* (1972) **21,** 2811.
584. Edwards, K., Jones, A. R., *Biochem. Pharmacol.* (1971) **20,** 1781.
585. Addison, I., Berenbaum, M. C., *Br. J. Cancer* (1971) **25,** 172.
586. Hendry, J. A., Homer, R. F., Rose, F. L., Walpole, A. L., *Br. J. Pharmacol.*
     (1951) **6,** 235.
587. *Ibid.,* 201.
588. Brookes, P., Lawley, P. D., *Br. Med. Bull.* (1964) **20,** 91.

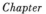

Chapter

Polynuclear Aromatic Carcinogens

Anthony Dipple,[1] Chester Beatty Research Institute of Cancer Research, Royal Cancer Hospital, Fulham Road, London SW3 6JB, England

Nomenclature

IN THE LITERATURE on polynuclear carcinogens a uniform system of nomenclature has not been consistently used, and certain ambiguities, exemplified in the names given to the isomeric benzpyrenes (Figures 1–A and B), have arisen. These ambiguities resulted from the use of different peripheral numbering systems, as illustrated for pyrene (Figure 1–C and D). The system preferred by American scientists (Figure 1–C) gave rise to the 3,4-benzpyrene (Figure 1–A3) and 1,2-benzpyrene (Figure 1–B3) nomenclature for the carcinogenic and noncarcinogenic benzpyrene isomers, respectively, while the system preferred by European workers (Figure 1–D) led to the 1,2-benzpyrene (Figure 1–A2) and 4,5-benzpyrene (Figure 1–B2) nomenclature for these same compounds.

The currently accepted nomenclature, I.U.P.A.C. 1957 Rules, will be used throughout this article, and this gives to pyrene the peripheral numbering illustrated by Figure 1–D. This numbering is dictated by placing the polycyclic system such that:

1. the maximum number of rings lie in a horizontal row;

2. as many rings as possible are above and to the right of the horizontal row;

3. if more than one orientation meets these requirements, the one with the minimum number of rings at the lower left is chosen.

The system is then numbered in a clockwise direction starting with the carbon atom not engaged in ring fusion in the most counterclockwise position of the

[1] Present address: Frederick Cancer Research Center, P.O. Box B, Frederick, MD 21701

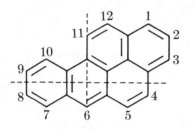

A. 1. Benzo[a]pyrene
   2. 1, 2-Benzpyrene
   3. 3, 4-Benzpyrene
      (carcinogenic)

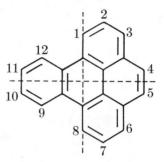

B. 1. Benzo[e]pyrene
   2. 4, 5-Benzpyrene
   3. 1, 2-Benzpyrene
      (noncarcinogenic)

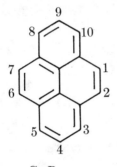

C. Pyrene

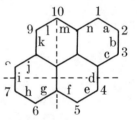

D. Pyrene

Figure 1. Nomenclature for aromatic hydrocarbons

uppermost ring or the uppermost ring which is farthest to the right. Atoms common to two or more rings are not numbered.

This numbering is applied throughout the hydrocarbon field, *e.g.*, the isomeric benzpyrenes (Figure 1–A and B), picene (Figure 2–A), chrysene (Figure 2–B), with the sole exceptions of phenanthrene, anthracene, and cyclopenta[a]phenanthrene, which are numbered as indicated in Figure 3.

The peripheral numbering of the heterocyclic aromatic compounds is dictated by the same principles but with the additional proviso that where a choice of orientation is still available, low numbers are given to the hetero atoms. If a choice still remains, the lowest number is given to oxygen in preference to sulfur and to sulfur in preference to nitrogen. Exceptions to the systematic peripheral numbering system for heterocyclic compounds are the numbering for purine, carbazole (Figure 4–A), and acridine (Figure 4–B).

Thus, apart from a few exceptions, all the polycyclic hydrocarbons and heterocyclic compounds can be systematically numbered according to a few simple rules. The names of structures which have no trivial name are obtained by prefixing the name of a component ring system (the base component,

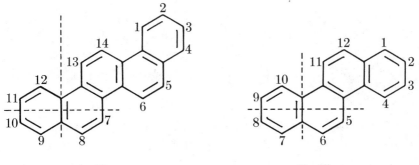

A. Picene   B. Chrysene

*Figure 2. Examples of the peripheral numbering system for
aromatic hydrocarbons*

which should contain as many rings as possible) with designations of the other
component. Isomers are then distinguished by lettering the peripheral sides of
the base component a,b,c, etc. beginning with "a" for the side "1,2," "b" for
the side "2,3," etc. as illustrated earlier for pyrene (Figure 1–D). Thus, the
benzpyrene isomers are distinguished as benzo[*a*]pyrene (Figure 1–A1) and
benzo[*e*]pyrene (Figure 1–B1), and the whole benzpyrene structure is then
numbered according to the rules discussed above.

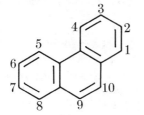

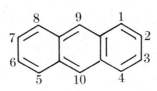

A. Phenanthrene   B. Anthracene

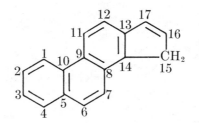

C. 15 *H*-Cyclopenta[*a*]phenanthrene

Figure 3. Exceptions to the systematic numbering for hydrocarbons

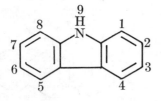
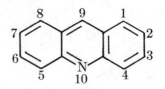

A. Carbazole   B. Acridine

Figure 4. Exceptions to the systematic numbering for heterocyclic compounds

Introduction

The foundations for the scientific study of chemical carcinogenesis in general and hydrocarbon carcinogenesis in particular were laid by Percival Pott in 1775 (1), when he attributed the occurrence of scrotal cancer in chimney sweeps to their occupational exposure to soot. Subsequently, as new industries became established, other industrial carcinogens (coal tar, paraffin, and certain mineral oils) were recognized, again at the expense of much human tragedy. This painful and slow process of developing our knowledge of chemical carcinogenesis was finally curtailed (though unfortunately not concluded) when it was found that coal tar, a proven carcinogen for man, could evoke a carcinogenic response in rabbits (2) and in mice (3). These findings created a first line of defense against the environment and also provided a powerful tool with which the definition of chemical carcinogens could be refined.

In ensuing investigations into the identity of the carcinogenic constituent of coal tar, Bloch and Dreifuss (4) found that carcinogenic activity was concentrated in high boiling fractions which were free from nitrogen, arsenic, and sulfur and which could form a stable picrate. Kennaway (5, 6) subsequently showed that carcinogenic tars could be produced in the laboratory by various procedures which included the pyrolysis of hydrocarbons, such as isoprene and acetylene, in a hydrogen atmosphere. These studies clearly indicated that the carcinogen in these tars was probably some complex aromatic hydrocarbon. Therefore, once Mayneord (7) had shown in 1927 that many carcinogenic mixtures and tars exhibited the same characteristic fluorescence spectrum, the problem was resolved into a search for an aromatic hydrocarbon which manifested these particular spectral characteristics. This search was not immediately successful, but Hieger did find that benz[a]anthracene exhibited a spectrum which was similar to, although not identical with, that of the carcinogenic tars (8). For this reason Kennaway and Hieger (9) tested dibenz[a,h]anthracene for carcinogenic activity in mice shortly after Clar (10) had reported its synthesis. This compound was found to be carcinogenic and thereby, the first carcinogen of defined chemical constitution was recognized.

The fluorescence spectrum of dibenz[a,h]anthracene did not correspond exactly to that of the carcinogenic tars, and Hieger, therefore, undertook a large-scale isolation of the fluorescent carcinogenic constituent starting with two tons of gas works pitch. This work culminated with the identification of this constituent as the hitherto unknown benzo[a]pyrene (Figure 1-A) (*11*).

At this stage the first phase of research into chemical carcinogenesis was complete. An animal test system was available, and it could also be used for screening new compounds. Carcinogenic activity could be ascribed to defined chemical compounds. However, it was soon shown that carcinogenic activity was not confined to just a few types of chemical structures and that many difficult problems still had to be solved. It was not possible, for example, to predict carcinogenic activity from chemical structure since the structural features required for the manifestation of this activity were not defined. It could not be assumed that screening in experimental animals was completely foolproof, and, in any event, this expensive and lengthy process would eventually fail to cope with the vast numbers of new chemicals being produced. Even today, despite the considerable progress which has been made, these basic problems remain. The final solutions for these problems reside, of course, in a complete understanding of the mechanisms of action of the various carcinogens, and most of the research into chemical carcinogenesis has been directed towards this ultimate goal. It seems appropriate, therefore, to attempt to review the literature on polynuclear carcinogens in the context of its relevance to the variety of mechanistic models which have been postulated. The complexity of mechanism through which the application of a chemical to an animal results after many months in the appearance of a tumor requires that mechanistic investigations involve a largely inductive approach. Without the assumptions of this approach little progress could be made. At the same time our outlook must not be narrowed by the unconscious acceptance of these assumptions as proved facts.

It is well established, however, that skin carcinogenesis induced by aromatic hydrocarbons involves at least two stages (*see* Chapter 2). The first stage, initiation, is a fairly rapid process whereby the carcinogen effects a permament change within the cell population. The second stage, promotion, requires a much longer time and can be effected by an agent such as croton oil which is not necessarily a carcinogen. Initiation is then the only stage which absolutely requires the presence of a carcinogen, and in appropriate experiments using the two-stage mouse skin system, the measured carcinogenic potency of a carcinogen accurately reflects its capacity for tumor initiation. However, if a sufficiently large dose of carcinogen is administered to mouse skin, tumors will arise in the absence of any promotion. In this circumstance, or in fact for any measurement of carcinogenic potency other than in the two-stage system above, carcinogenic potency need not necessarily reflect tumor initiating capacity. This follows because the carcinogen itself may be effecting the necessary promotional stimulus, and we cannot assume that all the polynuclear carcinogens are equally effective promoters. However, since most of the approaches to mechanisms involve structure–activity relationships to some extent, it is helpful to think of carcinogenic activity in terms of tumor initiating capacity in the first instance, although the validity of the assumptions implicit in this remains a constant difficulty.

Two general types of mechanisms for chemical carcinogenesis have been conceived. On the one hand, the carcinogen may convert a normal cell into a tumor cell (the instructional theory), and on the other, the carcinogen may modify the environment of preexisting tumor cells so that they are permitted to grow (the selection theory) (12). The instructional theory encompasses several mechanisms through which the carcinogen may effect a heritable change within the cell. For example, the carcinogen may cause a mutational change in the DNA of the cell, may activate a latent oncogenic virus within the cell, or may alter the control systems of the cell in a way that leads to heritable change. Similarly, the selection theory accommodates mechanisms whereby the carcinogen interferes with the immune response and thus permits preexisting cancer cells to grow or where the carcinogen is simply toxic to normal cells and not to the preexisting cancer cells. A full discussion of the evidence relevant to these various views is outside the scope of the present article. However, all these mechanisms require that the carcinogen enter some cell of the host and then interect with some cellular constituent, and that this constitutes the first step in the complex process of chemical carcinogenesis. This first event, tumor initiation, and the various factors which could conceivably modify the ability of a carcinogen to effect it are represented schematically in Figure 5.

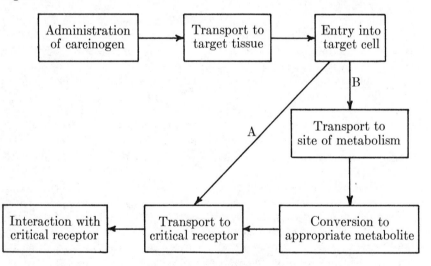

Figure 5. Schematic of factors possibly involved in tumor initiation

Examination of this scheme reveals that a simple relationship between chemical structure and carcinogenic activity need not in fact exist, even though the chemical structure of a carcinogen must ultimately determine its biological activity in a given system. Since it is the only approach available, however, all studies of the mechanism of carcinogenesis by polynuclear carcinogens originate from attempts to correlate the various properties of these carcinogens with their carcinogenic activities.

Chemical Structure and Carcinogenic Activity

In the 1930s a large scale program aimed at defining those structural features of chemical compounds which are necessary for carcinogenic activity was begun. A large number of the compounds synthesized and subsequently screened for carcinogenic activity were polycyclic aromatic hydrocarbons and heterocyclics. All types of chemical carcinogens are covered by Clayson (*13*) and Hueper and Conway (*14*) while Badger (*15, 16*), Arcos and Arcos (*17*), Buu–Hoi (*18*), and Arcos and Argus (*19*) have all contributed excellent reviews of polynuclear carcinogens in general. Lacassagne *et al.* (*20*) dealt specifically with the angular benzacridines. The bibliography, "Survey of compounds which have been tested for carcinogenic activity," (*21, 22, 23, 24*) is of course invaluable, and the current gap in its coverage of the literature (1961–1967) will shortly be filled.

Tables I–VIII present a summary of the status of various polynuclear compounds with respect to carcinogenic activity. Literature references are cited only in cases where these are not readily accessible through the sources above. It should be noted, however, that many compounds are described in the literature by a variety of alternative names.

None of the various proposals for the expression of experimentally determined carcinogenic activities (*14, 15, 25, 26, 27*) has been generally accepted and applied. In Tables II–VIII, therefore, carcinogenic activities are based upon the percentage of treated animals which developed tumors, *i.e.*, up to 33%, slight; 33–66%, moderate; and above 66%, high. The compounds listed in these tables have not necessarily been tested under strictly comparable conditions, and the relative activities given must be regarded as crude approximations. For example, 7-methylbenz[*a*]anthracene and 7,12-dimethylbenz-[*a*]anthracene are both listed under "high activity" (Tables II and III) since either compound can elicit a carcinogenic response in over 90% of the animals exposed to them. Nevertheless, when the activities of the two compounds are compared at relatively low dose levels, the dimethyl derivative is considerably more active than the monomethyl derivative (*23*).

Table I summarizes the carcinogenic activities of unsubstituted aromatic hydrocarbons comprised of six-membered rings, up to and including hexacyclic structures. Most of these compounds were tested in mice either by subcutaneous injections (giving rise to sarcomas) or by topical application to the skin (giving rise to benign papillomas and malignant epitheliomas). The most active carcinogens have been the subject of numerous studies, but in several cases the status of inactive compounds depends upon surprisingly limited experimentation. The initiating activities of some compounds in this category were recently studied by Scribner (*31*) who found that considerable activity was associated with benz[*a*]anthracene, chrysene, benzo[*e*]pyrene, and dibenz[*a,c*]anthracene while phenanthrene, picene, and benzo[*b*]chrysene also showed some activity.

In addition to the compounds listed in Table I, a number of larger structures have been examined. No carcinogenic activity was demonstrated for pyranthrene (*28*), benzo[*a*]coronene, dibenzo[*a,l*]pentacene, phenanthro-

Table I.   Carcinogenic Activities of

Inactive

Benzene[a]

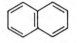
Naphthalene[b]

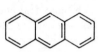
Anthracene[b]

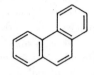
Phenanthrene[a]

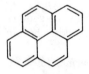
Pyrene[a]

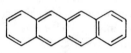
Naphthacene[c]

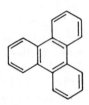
Triphenylene[c]

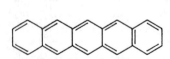
Pentacene[c]

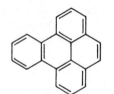
Benzo[e]pyrene[a,c]

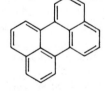
Perylene

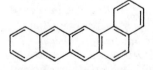
Benzo[a]naphthacene
(2',3'-Naphtho-2,3-
phenanthrene)[c]

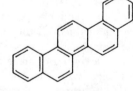
Picene

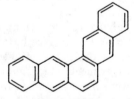
Pentaphene
(2',3'-Naphtho-1,-
2-anthracene)[c]

Unsubstituted Polycyclic Aromatic Hydrocarbons

| *Disputed* | *Moderate* | *High Activity* |

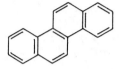

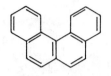

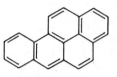

Chrysene[e]

Benzo[c]phenanthrene
(3, 4-Benzphenanthrene)

Benzo[a]pyrene

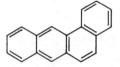

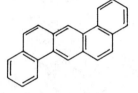

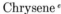

Benz[a]anthracene
(1,2-Benzanthracene)

Dibenz[a, h]anthracene
(1,2:5,6-Dibenzanthracene)[g]

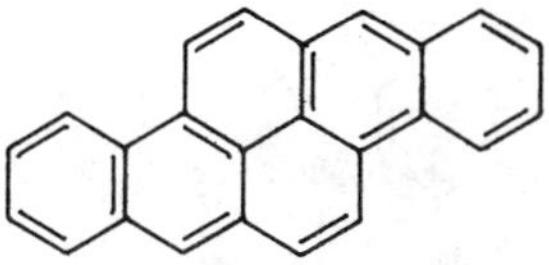

Dibenzo[b, def]chrysene
(Dibenzo[a, h]pyrene)

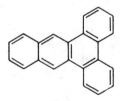

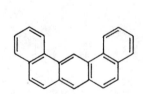

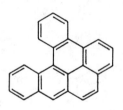

Dibenz[a, c]an-
thracene (1,2:3,4-
Dibenzanthracene)[f]

Dibenz[a,j]anthracene
(1,2:7,8-Dibenzanthracene)[c, g]

Dibenzo[def,p]chrysene
(Dibenzo[a,l]pyrene)

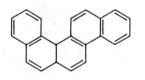

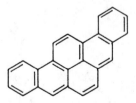

Benzo[c]chrysene (1,2:5,6-
Dibenzphenanthrene)[c, h]

Benzo[rst]pentaphene
(Dibenzo[a,i]pyrene)

Table I.

Inactive

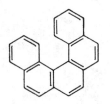

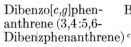

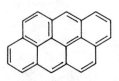

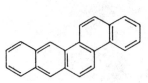

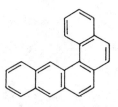

Dibenzo[c,g]phen-
anthrene (3,4:5,6-
Dibenzphenanthrene) [c]

Benzo[b]chrysene(2′,3′-Naph-
tho-1,2-phenanthrene) [c]

Dibenzo[b,g]phenan-
threne (1,2-(1′,2′-Na-
phth)anthracene) [c]

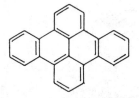

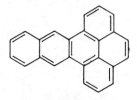

Dibenzo[def,mno]-
chrysene
(Anthanthrene) [a]

Dibenzo[fg,op]naphthacene
(Dibenzo[e,l]pyrene) [c]

Dibenzo[de,qr]naph-
thacene(Naphtho-
[2,3-e]pyrene) [c, d]

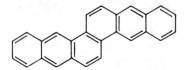

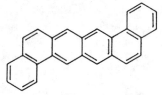

Dibenzo[b,k]chrysene

Dibenzo[a,j]naphthacene [c, i]

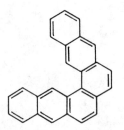

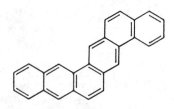

Anthra[1,2-a]anthracene

Benzo[c]pentaphene [e]

Continued

Disputed   *Moderate*   *High Activity*

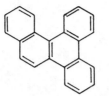

Benzo[g]chrysene(1,2:3,4–
Dibenzphenanthrene)[h]

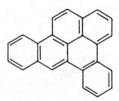

Naphtho[1,2,3,4–
def]chrysene (Di-
benzo[a,e]pyrene)

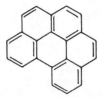

Benzo[ghi]perylene

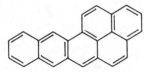

Naphtho[8,1,2-cde]naphthacene
(Naphtho[2,3-a]pyrene)[c]

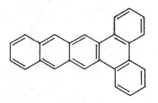

Dibenzo[a,c]naphthacene[j]

Table I. Continued

Inactive

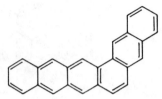

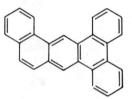

Benzo[b]pentaphene[c,i]   Naphtho[1,2-b]triphenylene

[a] Occasional skin papillomas have been reported.
[b] Tumors have been reported after very high doses.
[c] This compound has been subjected to limited testing only.
[d] Dibenzo[de,qr]naphthacene is referred to as naphtho-[2,3:1,2]pyrene by Arcos and Argus (19) and is said to be inactive although Hoffmann and Wynder (33) have demonstrated weak initiating activity.
[e] The activity exhibited by chrysene in early experiments (34, 35) was subsequently attributed to impurities (36). Recently, however, Van Duuren et al. (37) found chrysene to be an effective initiator in the mouse skin system.
[f] Dibenz[a,c]anthracene, long regarded as inactive, recently exhibited some activity after topical application to mouse skin (38,39) although it remains inactive if administered by subcutaneous injection to mice (40).
[g] Dibenz[a,j]anthracene is less active than dibenz[a,h]anthracene (38).
[h] Benzo[g]chrysene is slightly more active than benzo[c]chrysene (14).
[i] See Lacassagne et al. (30).
[j] Produces leukemia and ovarian tumors but not sarcoma (18).

[9,10-b]triphenylene, benzo[b]naphtho[1,2-k]chrysene, dinaphtho[1,2-b:-1,2-k]chrysene, or dinaphtho[1,2-b:2,1-n]perylene. Coronene was inactive after subcutaneous injections in mice (28) but has produced skin papillomas after topical applications (29). Benzo[a]naphtho[2,1,8-hij]naphthacene (30), benzo[a]naphtho[8,1,2-cde]naphthacene, and dibenzo[cd,lm]perylene exhibit slight carcinogenic activity while tribenzo[a,c,j]naphthacene is inactive at the injection site in mice but elicits leukemia and ovarian tumors (18). Dibenzo[h,rst]pentaphene, though not particularly potent, is perhaps the most active carcinogen among these large molecules (32).

Tables II and III list the carcinogenic activities of the various substituted benz[a]anthracenes that have been examined, Tables IV and V cover derivatives of other aromatic hydrocarbons, and Table VI lists the activities of some hydrocarbons that contain a five-membered ring. These tables do not represent a comprehensive survey of the literature. Major ommissions are the partially hydrogenated derivatives of the compounds in the tables (19, 38), amino substituted compounds (see Chapter 8), and several compounds containing five-membered rings such as fluoranthene derivatives (19), fluorene derivatives, acephenanthrene derivatives, and aceanthrene derivatives.

Table VII presents the structures of some heterocyclic carcinogens. Although a number of derivatives of compounds in this table have been tested, the only compounds for which information on a substantial number of derivatives is available are the inactive benz[a]acridine and benz[c]acridine (Table VIII). The isochromeno derivatives in Table VII contain a lactone ring and should be regarded, perhaps, as carcinogenic alkylating agents rather than heterocyclic compounds.

It is clear that no general structure–activity relationship which would account for all the experimental data can be formulated. This is not surprising in view of the variety and complexity of the numerous compounds examined, for it is conceivable that the limiting factor for the expression of carcinogenic activity (Figure 5) may be different for different groups of compounds. Therefore, relationships which extend over only a limited series of compounds are still worthy of consideration and do represent valuable information, although the current lack of understanding of carcinogenesis precludes the direct interpretation and application of this information.

Derivatives of benz[a]anthracene constitute the most extensive series of polynuclear compounds for which structure–activity relationships have been examined (Tables II, III). The carcinogenic activity of the parent hydrocarbon can be enhanced by substitution with either electron-donating or electron-withdrawing groups, and the magnitude of the effect depends upon the position of substitution (Table II). In most cases, a methyl substituent effects a more pronounced increase in carcinogenic activity (relative to that of benz[a]-anthracene) than do higher alkyl substituents. While methyl substitution at positions 6, 7, 8, and 12 is particularly effective, substitution at positions 1, 2, 3, and 4 on the angular benzene ring results in compounds which are inactive in most of the test systems. This is also reflected, to some extent, in the carcinogenic activities of the dimethylbenz[a]anthracenes (Table III). All such compounds with a methyl group on the angular ring are inactive except 4,5-dimethylbenz[a]anthracene. This holds for the 1,7-, 1,12-, 4,7-, and 4,12-dimethyl compounds even though the 7- and 12-monomethylbenz[a]anthracenes are both potent carcinogens. Similarly, the high carcinogenic activity of 7-12-dimethylbenz[a]anthracene can be destroyed or reduced by a variety of further substitutions (Table III).

Examinations of structure–activity relationships have generated a number of more general observations. It has been suggested that carcinogenic activity depends upon the molecular size of polynuclear compounds (*17, 19*), or upon their molecular thickness (*41, 47*). The relationship between steroid and polynuclear carcinogen structures has excited interest over a number of years, largely because the steroids might be converted into polycyclic hydrocarbons *in vivo*, thereby accounting for the incidence of "spontaneous" tumors (*18, 59, 69*).

More recent studies tend to emphasize the alternative possibility—*i.e.*, that polynuclear carcinogens interfere with normal steroid hormone action. For example, Williams and Rabin (*70*) have shown that several carcinogens interfere with membrane–ribosome association. These authors suggested that the carcinogens produced this effect by occupying or destroying sites on the membrane which are normally available to steroid hormones. Similarly, Lit-

Table II.   Carcinogenic Activities of

Substituent Giving Rise to Compounds of Carcinogenic Activity:

Site of Sub- stitution	*Inactive*
1	$-CH_3{}^{a,b,d}$
2	$-CH_3{}^{a,c,d}$
3	$-CH_3{}^{a,d}$
4	$-CH_3{}^{a,d}$; $-CH_2COOC_2H_5{}^c$; $-OH^{a,b,c}$; $-OCOCH_3{}^b$; $-SO_2Cl^c$; $-SO_3K^c$; $-SO_3C_2H_5{}^c$; $-OCH_3{}^{a,b,c}$
5	$-CH_3{}^d$; $-CH(CH_3)_2{}^a$; $-OCH_2COOH^b$; $-OCOC_6H_5{}^b$; $-OCO(CH_2)_{16}CH_3{}^b$; $-NCO^b$; $-F^{a,b,c,i}$
6	
7	$-CH_2CHCH_2{}^b$; $-(CH_2)_2CH_3{}^b$; $-CH(CH_3)_2{}^{a,b}$; $-(CH_2)_3CH_3{}^b$; $-(CH_2)_4CH_3{}^b$; $-CH_2C_6H_5{}^a$; $-CH_2COOH^{b,c}$; $-CH_2COONa^e$; $-CH_2CH(OCOC_6H_5)CH_2OCOC_6H_5{}^b$; $-CH(OH)CH_3{}^b$; $-CHO^d$; $-CH_2Cl^b$; $-CH_2OCH_3{}^b$; $-CH_2OC_2H_5{}^b$; $-COCH_3{}^{a,b}$; $-COONa$; $-CH_2SH^b$; $-CH_2SCH_2CH(NH_2)COOH^b$; $-CH_2SCN^b$; $-CH_2NCS^b$; $-CH_2N(CH_3)_2{}^b$; $-CH_2N(C_2H_5)_2{}^b$; $-SCN^b$; $-SCH_2CH(NH_2)COOH^b$; $-NCO^b$; $-NO_2{}^b$; $-OH^b$; $-Cl^c$; $-Pb(C_6H_5)_3{}^b$
8	$-(CH_2)_3CH_3{}^c$; $-(CH_2)_4CH_3{}^b$; $-(CH_2)_5CH_3{}^b$; $-(CH_2)_6CH_3{}^b$; $-CH_2COONa^b$; $-COONa^{a,b,f}$
9	$-CH_3{}^d$; $-C_6H_5{}^a$
10	$-CH_3{}^{a,d}$; $-CH(CH_3)_2{}^a$
11	$-CH_3{}^{b,c,d}$; $-C_2H_5{}^b$; $-CH(CH_3)_2{}^b$; $-OH^b$
12	

[a] Painting on mouse skin.
[b] Subcutaneous injections in mice.
[c] Subcutaneous injections in rats.
[d] Intramuscular injections in rats (*41*).
[e] Intravenous injections in mice.

Table III.   Carcinogenic Activities of

Inactive	*Slight*

Carcinogenic Activities of Dimethylbenz[a]anthracenes

Inactive	*Slight*
$1,7^b$; $1,12^d$; $2,9^{a,b}$; $2,10^a$; $3,9^{a,d}$; $3,10^a$; $4,7^{d,m}$; $4,12^{d,m}$; $5,12^{b,d,m}$; $8,11^b$	$9,10^{a,d}$; $9,11^a$

Monosubstituted Benz[*a*]anthracenes

Substituent Giving Rise to Compounds of Carcinogenic Activity:

Slight	*Moderate*	*High*
$-CH_3{}^c$		
$-CH_3{}^c$		
$-CH_3{}^c$; $-F^{b,i}$		$-F^{c,i}$
$-CH_3{}^{a,c}$; $-OH^b$; $-OCH_3{}^b$	$-CH_3{}^b$	
$-CH_3{}^a$		$-CH_3{}^{b,c,d}$
$-C_2H_5{}^d$; $-CH_2CH_2OH^{a,b}$; $-CH_2Br^g$; $-CH_2CN^b$; $-CH_2OC_2H_5{}^a$; $-CH_2COONa^c$; $-CN^{a,b}$; $OCH_3{}^d$; $-SH^b$; $-Br^c$	$-CH_3{}^a$; $-CH_2OH^a$; $-CHO^b$; $-CH_2Br^h$; $-CH_2OCOCH_3{}^{a,b}$; $-CH_2COOH_3{}^b$; $COCl_3{}^{b,c}$; $-OCH_3{}^b$	$-CH_3{}^{b,c,d}$; $-C_2H_5{}^b$; $-CH_2OH$
$-C_2H_5{}^a$; $-(CH_2)_2CH_3{}^a$; $-CH(CH_3)_2{}^{a,b}$; $-(CH_2)_3CH_3{}^a$; $-(CH_2)_4CH_3{}^a$; $-(CH_2)_5CH_3{}^a$; $-(CH_2)_6CH_3{}^a$; $-C_6H_5{}^a$	$-CH_3{}^a$; $-OCH_3{}^b$	$-CH_3{}^{b,c,d}$
$-CH_3{}^{a,c}$	$-CH(CH_3)_2{}^a$	
$-CH_3{}^{b,c}$		
$-CH_3{}^a$		
$-CH_3{}^a$; $-C_2H_5{}^d$	$-CH_3{}^{c,d}$	$-CH_3{}^b$

[f] Intraperitoneal injections in mice.
[g] Tested for initiating activity in mouse skin (*42*).
[h] Subcutaneous injections in newborn mice (*43*).
[i] Miller and Miller (*44*).

Substituted Benz[*a*]anthracenes

Moderate	*High*
Carcinogenic Activities of Dimethylbenz[a]anthracenes	
$6,7^b$; $6,12^b$; $7,8^b$; $7,11^b$	$4,5^c$; $6,7^d$; $6,8^d$; $6,12^d$; $7,8^d$; $7,11^{d,m}$; $7,12^{a,b,c,d,h}$; $8,9^a$; $8,12^{b,d}$

Table III.

Inactive   *Slight*

Carcinogenic Activities of 7-Methylbenz[a]anthracene Derivatives

1-CH$_3$[b]; 3-CH(CH$_3$)$_2$[b]; 4-CH$_3$[d, m]; 4-F[b, c, i];   3-F[a, g, k]; 4-F[g]; 5-F[g];
5-F[a, b, c]; 5-NCO[b]; 5-OH[b]; 9-COOCH$_3$[b];   9-F[b, c, k]; 10-Cl[b];
9-Cl[b]; 9-CN[b]; 9-COOH[b]; 10-COOCH$_3$[b];   12-OCOCH$_3$[b];
10-COOH[b]; 12-CH$_2$OH[h, u]; 12-SCN[b];   5, 12-di-CH$_3$[d, m]
2,3-di-CH$_3$[d, m]; 2,12-di-CH$_3$[d, m];   6, 12-di-CH$_3$[a, b];
3, 12-di-CH$_3$[d, m]; 4-OH, 12-CH$_3$[c, p];   9, 10, 12-tri-CH$_3$[b]
4-OCH$_3$, 12-CH$_3$[a, b, c, p]; 5-OCH$_3$,-
12-CH$_3$[c, p]; 8-C$_2$H$_5$,12-CH$_3$[a, b]

Carcinogenic Activities of 7, 12-Disubstituted Benz[a]anthracenes

7,12-di-C$_2$H$_5$[d, n]; 7,12-di-CN[d, m];   7, 12-di-C$_2$H$_5$[a];
7,12-di-OCH$_3$[b]; 7,12-di-CH$_2$OH[h];   7, 12-di-CH$_2$OH[b];
7,12-di-(CH$_2$)$_2$CH$_3$[b]; 7,12-di-C$_6$H$_5$[a];   7, 12-di-CH$_2$OCOCH$_3$[a, b];
7,12-di-OCOCH$_3$[b]; 7-SCN,12-CH$_3$[b];   7-CH$_2$OH, 12-CH$_3$[d, l]
7-(CH$_2$)$_2$OH,12-CH$_3$[d, l]; 7-(CH$_2$)$_3$OH,-   7-CH(OH)CH$_3$,
12-CH$_3$[d, l]; 7-(CH$_2$)$_3$CH$_3$,12-CH$_3$[d, n];   12-CH$_3$[d, l];
7-CH$_2$OCH$_3$,12-CH$_3$[d, n];   7-CH$_2$OCH$_3$, 12-CH$_3$[c, p]
7-CH$_3$,12-SCN[b]; 7-CH$_3$,12-CH$_2$OH[h, u]   7-CH$_2$CHO, 12-CH$_3$[c, t]

Carcinogenic Activities of 7,12-Dimethylbenz[a]anthracene Derivatives

2-CH$_3$[d, m]; 3-CH$_3$[d, m]; 4-OH[c, p];   5-CH$_3$[d, m]; 6-CH$_3$[a, b];
4-OCH$_3$[a, b, c, p]; 5-OCH$_3$[c, p];   9,10-di-CH$_3$[b]; 5-F[v]
8-C$_2$H$_5$[a, b]

Carcinogenic Activities of Other Substituted Benz[a]anthracenes

5,7-di-OCH$_3$[b]; 7,8-di-C$_2$H$_5$[d, o];   1-CH$_3$,7-CH$_2$Br[g, r];
7,9-di-C$_2$H$_5$[d, o]; 4-Cl,7-CH$_2$Br[b, g, r, s];   4-Br,7-CH$_2$Br[g, r];
5-OCH$_3$,7-(CH$_2$)$_2$CH$_3$[b, e];   5-OCH$_3$,7-C$_2$H$_5$[b];
7-CH$_2$OH,5,12-di-CH$_3$[d, m];   7-CH$_2$OH,4,-
5-F,9-CH$_3$[v]   12-di-CH$_3$[d, m]

[a] Painting on mouse skin.
[b] Subcutaneous injection in mice.
[c] Subcutaneous injections in rats.
[d] Intramuscular injections in rats.
[e] Intravenous injections in mice.
[f] Intraperitoneal injections in mice.
[g] Tested for initiating activity in mouse skin.
[h] Intragastric administration in rats giving mammary tumors.
[i] Intravenous injection in rats giving mammary tumors.
[j] Adequate testing was precluded by high toxicity.
[k] Miller and Miller (44)

Continued

| *Moderate* | *High* |

Carcinogenic Activities of 7-Methylbenz[a]anthracene Derivatives

3-F[b,c,k]; 5-OCH$_3$[b]; 6-F[b,k]; 6-CH$_3$[b];   6-F[a,c,k]; 6-CH$_3$[d]; 8-Cl[b]; 8-CN[b];
8-CH$_3$[b]; 8-OCH$_3$[b]; 8-CONH$_2$[b];   8-CH$_3$[d]; 11-CH$_3$[d,m];
9-F[a,g,k]; 10-F[a,b,c,g,k]; 10-CN[b];   12-CH$_3$[a,b,c,d,h]; 4,12-di-
11-CH$_3$[b]; 12-C$_2$H$_5$[d,n]; 12-CH$_2$OH[b,t];   CH$_3$[d,m]; 6,8-di-CH$_3$[d];
8-CN, 12-CH$_3$[b]; 8-(CH$_2$)$_2$CH$_3$,   6,12-di-CH$_3$[d]; 8,12-di-
12-CH$_3$[a,b]; 9,12-di-CH$_3$[a,b]; 8,9,12-   CH$_3$[a,b,d,i]; 9,12,di-CH$_3$[d,m];
tri-CH$_3$[a,b]; 9,10,12-tri-CH$_3$[a]   10,12-di-CH$_3$[d,m];
     8-Br,12-CH$_3$[b]

Carcinogenic Activities of 7, 12-Disubstituted Benz[a]anthracenes

7, 12-di-Cl[a]; 7,12-di-OCH$_3$[d,n];   7,12-di-CH$_3$[a,b,c,d,h]; 7-OC$_2$H$_5$,-
7-CN,12-CH$_3$[a,b]; 7-CH$_2$OC$_2$H$_5$,   12-CH$_3$[d]; 7-OCH$_3$,12-CH$_3$[d];
12-CH$_3$[b]; 7-C$_2$H$_5$,12-CH$_3$[b];   7-CHO,12-CH$_3$[c,d,p];
7-(CH$_2$)$_2$CH$_3$,12-CH$_3$[d,n]; 7-CH$_2$I,   7-C$_2$H$_5$,12-CH$_3$[d,l];
12-CH$_3$[c,p]; 7-CH$_2$OH,12-CH$_3$[b,h,t,u];   7-CH$_2$OH,12-CH$_3$[c,p];
7-CH$_2$OCOCH$_3$,12-CH$_3$[b,t];   7-CH$_2$Br,12-CH$_3$[c,g,q,r];
7-CH$_3$,12-C$_2$H$_5$[d,n]; 7-CH$_3$,   7-CH$_2$OCOCH$_3$, 12-CH$_3$[c,p];
12-CH$_2$OH[b,t]   7-CH$_2$Cl, 12-CH$_3$[c,p];
     7-CH$_2$OCOC$_6$H$_5$, 12-CH$_3$[c,p]

Carcinogenic Activities of 7,12-Dimethylbenz[a]anthracene Derivatives

8-CN[b]; 8-(CH$_2$)$_2$CH$_3$; 9-CH$_3$[a,b];   4-CH$_3$[d,m]; 6-CH$_3$[d];
8,9-di-CH$_3$[a,b]; 9,10-di-CH$_3$[a]   8-CH$_3$[a,b,d,i]; 8-Br[b];
     9-CH$_3$[d,m]; 10-CH$_3$[d,m]

Carcinogenic Activities of Other Substituted Benz[a]anthracenes

8,12-di-C$_2$H$_5$[d,o]; 6-F, 7-CH$_2$Br[g,r]   6,8-di-C$_2$H$_5$[d,o];
     4,5,10-tri-CH$_3$[c];
     6,8,12-tri-CH$_3$[d];
     5-F,12-CH$_3$ [v]

[l] Pataki and Huggins (*45*).
[m] Pataki *et al.* (*46*).
[n] Huggins *et al.* (*41*).
[o] Pataki and Balick (*47*).
[p] Flesher and Sydnor (*48*).
[q] Dipple and Slade (*49*).
[r] Dipple and Slade (*42*).
[s] Roe *et al.* (*43*).
[t] Boyland and Sims (*50*).
[u] Boyland *et al.* (*51*).
[v] Bergmann *et al.* (*52*).

Table IV.   Carcinogenic Activities of Tri- and

Inactive

Anthracene Derivatives

1-C_6H_5[a]; 2-CH_3[a]; 2-C_6H_5[a]; 9-CH_3[a,b]; 9-C_2H_5[a]; 9-C_6H_5[a]; 9-(9'-anthryl)[a];
1,2-di-CH_3[a,b]; 1,3-di-CH_3[a,b]; 1,4-di-CH_3[a,b]; 2,3-di-CH_3[a,b]; 9,10-di-
CH_3[b]; 1,5-di-$C(CH_2)CH_3$[a]; 9,10-di-C_6H_5[a]; 9, 10-di-$CH_2C_6H_5$[a]; 9,10-di-
(1'-naphthyl)[a]; 9-C_6H_5,10-$COOCH_3$[a]; 9-C_6H_5,10-COOH[a]; 9-C_6H_5,10-
(1'-naphthyl)[a]; 2,9,10-tri-CH_3[b]; 3-CH_3,1,8,9-tri-OH[a]; 2,3,6,7-
tetra-CH_3[a,b]

Phenanthrene Derivatives

1-CH_3,3-$CH(CH_3)_2$[b]; 1-CH_3,7-$CH(CH_3)_2$[a]; 1,9-di-CH_3[a,b]; 3,4-di-COOH[a];
3,4-di-COONa[b]; 3,4-di-$COOCH_3$[b]; 1,2,3,4-tetra-CH_3[b]

Chrysene Derivatives

1-CH_3[a,b]; 1-OCH_3[b]; 1-OH[b]; 1-$OCOCH_3$[b]; 2-OCH_3[b]; 2-$CH(CH_3)_2$[a,b];
3-OCH_3[b]; 4-OCH_3[b]; 4-OH[b]; 6-OCH_3[b]; 6-OH[b]; 2,3-di-CH_3[b]; 5,6-di-
OCH_3[b]; 5,6-di-$OCOCH_3$[b]; 5,6-di-C_6H_5[a]

Benzo[c]phenanthrene Derivatives

3-CH_3[b]; 4-CH_3[b]; 5-CHO[a]; 5-$(CH_2)_2CH_3$[b]; 5-$CH(CH_3)_2$[b]; 6-CH_3[b];
6-$CH(CH_3)_2$[a,b]; 2,3-di-CH_3[b]; 2-CH_3,6-COONa[b]; 5,8-di-CH_3[b];
5,8-di-C_2H_5[b]

Inactive Derivatives of Pyrene

2-CH_3[a]; 3-$O(CH_2)_2COOH$[a]; 4-SO_3Na[a]; 3-OH,1,6,8-tri-SO_3Na[a]

[a] Painting on mouse skin.
[b] Subcutaneous injection in mice.

Table V.   Carcinogenic Activities of Penta- and

Inactive

Substituted Benzo[a]pyrene Derivatives

6-OH[a,b]; 6-NO_2; 6-$CHC(CN)C_6H_4Br$[b]; 7-OH[a,b]; 7-OCH_3[a,b]; 7-$OCOCH_3$[b];
7-$OCOC_6H_4NH_2$[b]; 8-CH_3[a]; 11-OH[b]; 7,8-di-COOK[b]; 7,8-di-COONa[b,c];
1,3,6-tri-Cl[a,b]

Tetracyclic Aromatic Hydrocarbon Derivatives

Slight   *Moderate*

Anthracene Derivatives

9,10-di-CH$_3$^{a}; 1,8,9-tri-OH^a

Phenanthrene Derivatives

1-CH$_3$,3-CH(CH$_3$)$_2$^{a}; 1,2,4-tri-CH$_3$^{a};
1,2,3,4-tetra-CH$_3$^{a}

Chrysene Derivatives

3-OH^b; 4-CH$_3$^{b}; 6-CH$_3$^{b}; 4,5-di-CH$_3$^{b};   5-CH$_3$^{b}
5,6-di-CH$_3$^{a,b}

Benzo[c]phenanthrene Derivatives

2-CH$_3$^{a,b}; 3-CH$_3$^{a}; 4-CH$_3$^{a}; 5-CHO^b;   5-CH$_3$^{a,b}; 5-CH(CH$_3$)$_2$^{a};
5-C$_2$H$_5$^{a}; 5-COCH$_3$^{a,b} 5-(CH$_2$)$_2$CH$_3$^{a}; 6-CH$_3$^{a}

Inactive Derivatives of

Triphenylene   *Naphthacene*

1-CH$_3$^{b}; 1,4-di-CH$_3$^{b} 2-CH(CH$_3$)$_2$^{a}; 5,6,11,12-
                                                   tetra-C$_6$H$_5$^{a}

Hexacyclic Aromatic Hydrocarbon Derivatives

Slight   *Moderate*   *High*

Substituted Benzo[a]pyrene Derivatives

1-COCH$_3$^{a}; 1-C(CH$_2$)CH$_3$;   5-CH$_3$^{b}; 7-CH$_3$^{b};   2-CH$_3$^{b,e}; 3-CH$_3$^{b,e};
3-OH^{a,b}; 4-OCH$_3$^{b};   1, 3, 6-tri-CH$_3$^{b} 3-OCH$_3$^{a,b}; 4-CH$_3$^{b};
5-OH^b; 5-Cl^{a,b};   6-CH$_3$^{b}; 6-CHO^b;
6-OH^{b,k}; 1, 6-di-OCH$_3$^{b};   6-CHCHC$_6$H$_5$^{b};
3, 6-di-OCH$_3$^{b} 11-CH$_3$^{b}; 12-CH$_3$^{b};
                                                                   1, 2-di-CH$_3$^{b};
                                                                   1, 3-di-CH$_3$^{b};
                                                                   1, 4-di-CH$_3$^{b};
                                                                   1, 6-di-CH$_3$^{b};
                                                                   2, 3-di-CH$_3$^{b};
                                                                   3, 6-di-CH$_3$^{b};
                                                                   3, 12-di-CH$_3$^{b};
                                                                   4, 5-di-CH$_3$^{b}

Table V.

Inactive

Substituted Dibenz[a,h]anthracene Derivatives

7-OH[a]; 7-OCOCH$_3$[a]; 7-NO$_2$[a]; 3,10-di-OH[b]; 3,11-di-OH[b]; 4,11-di-OH[m];
5,12-di-OCH$_3$[a,b,l]; 5,12-di-OCOCH$_3$[a,b,l]; 7,14-di-OCH$_3$[b]

Derivatives of Other Compounds

Benzo[g]chrysene	9-CH$_3$[b]; 10-CH$_3$[b]
Picene	2,9-di-CH$_3$[b]
Benzo[b]chrysene	7,12-di-CH$_3$[b]
Perylene	3-CH$_3$[a,b]
Pentaphene	2,11-di-CH$_3$[a]
Dibenz[a,c]anthracene	9,14-di-CH$_3$[a,b]
Dibenz[a,j]anthracene	
Dibenzo[b,def]chrysene	7,14-di-CH$_3$[b,i]; 7,14-di-OSO$_2$Na[a,b]
Dibenzo[def,p]chrysene	10-C$_6$H$_5$
Benzo[rst]pentaphene	5,8-di-CH$_3$[b,i]
Benzo[pqr]picene	7-CH$_3$[b,h]
Naphtho[1,2,3,4-def]chrysene	
Anthanthrene	

[a] Painting on mouse skin.
[b] Subcutaneous injections in mice.
[c] Intraperitoneal injections in mice.
[d] Tested for initiating activity in mouse skin.
[e] Cook and Schoental (*53*).
[f] Lacassagne *et al.* (*54*).
[g] Bergmann *et al.* (*52*).

Table VI.   Carcinogenic Activities of Some Hydrocarbon

Inactive

Cholanthrene and Its Derivatives

1-oxo[b]; 11,12-dihydro[b]; 6-12b-dihydro[a]; 3-CH$_3$,8-OCH$_3$[b]; 3-CH$_3$,8-OH[b];
3-CH$_3$,9-Cl[b]; 3-CH$_3$,9-OH[a,b]; 3-CH$_3$,9-OCH$_3$[a,b]; 3-CH$_3$,11-Cl[b];
3-CH$_3$,11-CN[b]

Continued

Slight	*Moderate*	*High*

Substituted Dibenz[a,h]anthracene Derivatives

2-CH$_3$[a]; 3-CH$_3$[a];	6-CH$_3$[a];	6-F[g]; 7-NCO[b];
5-OCH$_3$[a,b,l]; 7-OCH$_3$[a];	7-OCH$_3$[a,l];	7-OCH$_3$[b,l];
5, 6-di-OCH$_3$[a,b,l];	7, 14-di-CH$_3$[a,b,l]	7-CH$_3$[b]
7, 14-di-(CH$_2$)$_3$CH$_3$[a]		

Derivatives of Other Compounds

10-CH$_3$[b]		
	7,14-di-CH$_3$[a,b]	
7-CHO, 14-CH$_3$[b,f]	7-CH$_3$[b,i];	
	7-CHO[b,f]	
10-CHO[b,i]		10-CH$_3$[b,i]
8-NO$_2$[b]; 5-CHO,8-CH$_3$[b,f]	5-CH$_3$[a,b,i]	5-CHO[b,f]
	7-CH$_3$[d]	
	6-CH$_3$[b,i]	5-CH$_3$[b,i]
6-CH$_3$[b,d,i]; 6-CHO[b,f];		
6-CHO,12-CH$_3$[b,f];		
6,12-di-CH$_3$[b,i]		

[h] Lacassagne *et al.* (*55*).
[i] Lacassagne *et al.* (*56*).
[j] Lacassagne *et al.* (*32*).
[k] Nagata *et al.* (*57*).
[l] Heidelberger *et al.* (*58*).
[m] Badger (*15*).

Derivatives Containing Five-Membered Rings

Slight	*Moderate*	*High*

Cholanthrene and Its Derivatives

3-C(CH$_3$)[b];	cholanthrene[a,c];	cholanthrene[b];
1-oxo,3-CH$_3$[a,b]	3-CH(CH$_3$)$_2$[b];	3-CH$_3$[a,b,c,d,e,f,g,h];
	1,3-di-CH$_3$[b];	4-CH$_3$[b]; 5-CH$_3$[b];
	1-OH,3-CH$_3$[b]	3-C$_2$H$_5$[b]; 2,3-di-CH$_3$[b];
		6,12b-dihydro[b];
		6,12b-dihydro, 3-CH$_3$[b]

Table VI.

Inactive

16,17-Dihydro-15H-cyclopenta[a]phenanthrene and Its Derivatives

16,17-dihydro-15H-cyclopenta[a]phenanthrene[a,b,c]; 1-CH$_3$[a]; 2-CH$_3$[a];
4-CH$_3$[a]; 6-CH$_3$[a,b]; 11-CH$_3$[b]; 12-CH$_3$[a,b]; 15-oxo[a,i]; 17-oxo[a,b,i];
17-CH$_3$[a,b]; 2,12-di-CH$_3$[a,b]; 6,7-di-CH$_3$[a]; 4,12-di-CH$_3$[a];
3-OCH$_3$, 17-CH$_3$[a,i]; 4,17-di-CH$_3$[a]; 6,17-di-CH$_3$[a,b]; 11-OCH$_3$,-
17-CH$_3$[a,i]; 12,17-di-CH$_3$[a,i]; 2-CH$_3$,17-oxo[a,i]; 3-CH$_3$, 17-oxo[a,i];
3-OCH$_3$,17-oxo[a,i]; 4-CH$_3$,17-oxo[a,i]; 6-CH$_3$,17-oxo[a,i]; 12-CH$_3$,-
17-oxo[a,i]; 11,12-dihydro,11-CH$_3$,17-oxo[a,i]; 6,17,17-tri-CH$_3$[a,b]

Cyclopenta[a]phenanthrene and Its Derivatives

17H-cyclopenta[a]phenanthrene[a,i]; 17H,17-C(CH$_3$)$_2$[a,i];
15H,3-OCH$_3$,17-CH$_3$[a,i]

[a] Painting on mouse skin.
[b] Subcutaneous injections in mice.
[c] Subcutaneous injections in rats.
[d] Intramuscular injections in rats.
[e] Intravenous injections in mice.

Table VII.   The Activities of Some

Slight

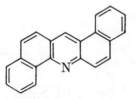

Dibenz[a,h]acridine 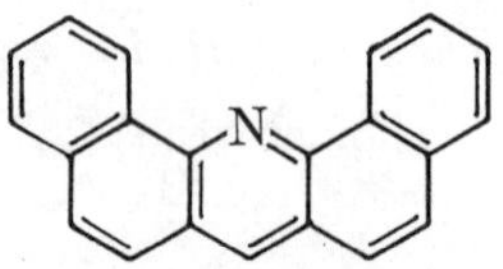   Dibenz[c,h]acridine   Dibenz[a,j]acridine

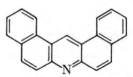

Continued

| *Slight* | *Moderate* | *High* |

16,17-Dihydro-15H-cyclopenta[a]phenanthrene and Its Derivatives

7-CH$_3$^{a}; 11-CH$_3$^{a};
  17-CH$_2$^{a,i}; 11,12-di-CH$_3$^{a};
  11,17-di-CH$_3$^{a,i};
  11,12,17-tri-CH$_3$^{a,i};
  7-CH$_3$,17-oxo^{a,i};
  11-C$_2$H$_5$,17-oxo^{a,i};
  11-(CH$_2$)$_3$CH$_3$,17-oxo^{a,i};
  11-OCOCH$_3$,17-oxo^{a,i};
  11-CH$_3$,16-OH,
  17-oxo^{a,i};
  11-CH$_3$,15-oxo^{a,i}

11-CH$_3$,17-OH^{a,i};
  11-CH$_3$,-
  17-oxo^{a,b,i};
  11-OCH$_3$,-
  17-oxo^{a,i};
  6-OCH$_3$,-
  11-CH$_3$,
  17-oxo^{a,i}; 7-CH$_3$,-
  11-OCH$_3$,-
  17-oxo^{a,i};
  11, 12-di-CH$_3$,-
  17-oxo^{a,b,i}

Cyclopenta[a]phenanthrene and Its Derivatives

15H,17-CH$_3$$^{a, i}$;
  15H,12,17-di-CH$_3$^{a,i};
  15H,11-OCH$_3$,17-CH$_3$^{a,i}

15H,11,17-di-CH$_3$^{a,i};
  15H,11,12,17-tri-
  CH$_3$^{a,i}

^{f} Intraperitoneal injections in mice.
^{g} Intragastric administration in rats giving mammary tumors.
^{h} Oral administration to rats and mice.
^{i} Coombs and Croft (*59*).
^{j} Coombs *et al.* (*60*).

Carcinogenic Heterocyclic Compounds

| *Moderate* | *High* |

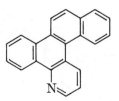

Benzo[*h*]naphtho-
[1,2-*f*]quinoline^c

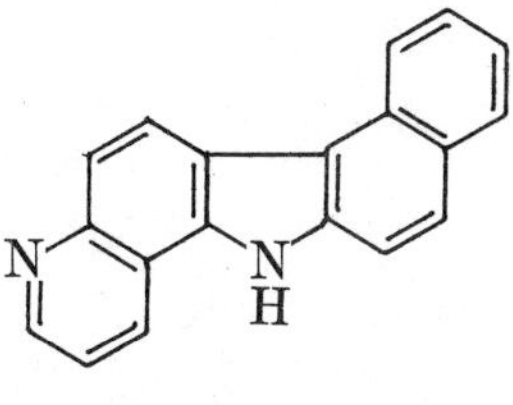

7H-Benzo[*g*]pyrido-
[3,2-*a*]carbazole^a

Table VII.

Slight

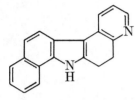

7*H*-Benzo[*a*]pyrido-
[3,2-*g*]carbazole[a]

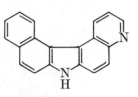

7*H*-Benzo[*c*]pyrido-
[3,2-*g*]carbazole[a]

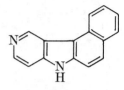

7*H*-Benzo[*g*]-
γ-carboline[d]

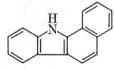

11*H*-Benzo-
[*a*]carbazole

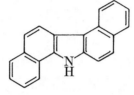

7*H*-Dibenzo-
[*a*,*g*]carbazole

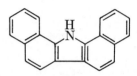

13*H*-Dibenzo-
[*a*,*i*]carbazole

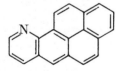

10-Azabenzo-
[*a*]pyrene[c]

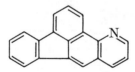

Fluoreno[9,9a,1-*gh*]
quinoline[c]

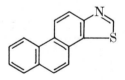

Phenanthro-
[2,1-*d*]thiazole

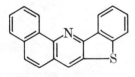

Benzo[*h*]benzo[2,3]-
thieno[3,2-*b*]quinoline

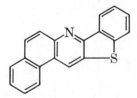

Benzo[*f*]benzo[2,3]-
thieno[3,2-*b*]quinoline

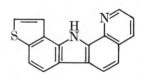

Pyrido[2,3-*a*]thieno-
[2,3-*i*]carbazole[d]

Continued

Moderate	*High*

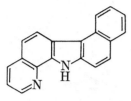

7*H*-Benzo[*g*]pyrido-
[2,3-*a*]carbazole[a]

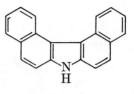

7*H*-Dibenzo-
[*c,g*]carbazole[f]

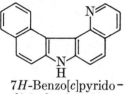

7*H*-Benzo[*c*]pyrido-
[2,3-*g*]carbazole[b]

4,11-Diazadibenzo-
[*b,def*]chrysene[a]

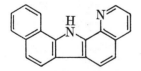

13*H*-Benzo[*a*]pyrido-
[3,2-*i*]carbazole[b]

5-Oxo-5H-benzo[*e*]-
isochromeno[4,3-*b*]indole[g]

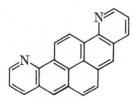

1,12-Diazabenzo-
[*rst*]pentaphene[e]

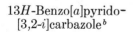

Table VII.

Slight

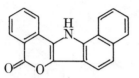   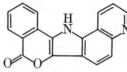

5-Oxo-5*H*-benzo[*g*]–   8-Oxo-8*H*-isochromeno–
isochromeno[4,3-*b*]indole[h]   [3′,4′:4,5]pyrrolo[2,3-*f*]quinoline[g]

[a] Lacassagne *et al.* (*61*).
[b] Lacassagne *et al.* (*62*).
[c] Lacassagne *et al.* (*63*).
[d] Lacassagne *et al.* (*64*).

Table VIII.   Carcinogenic Activities

Inactive

Benz[a]acridines

9-CH₃[b]; 10-CH₃[a]; 10-C₆H₅[b]; 12-CH₃[a,b]; 12-CHO[b]; 8,9-di-CH₃[a,b]; 8-C₆H₅,-
12-CH₃[b]; 9-Cl,12-C₂H₅[a]; 9-CF₃,12-CH₃[b]; 10-CH₃,12-CH(CH₃)₂[b];
10-F,12-C₂H₅[b]; 10-F,12-(CH₂)₂CH₃[b]; 10-F,12-(CH₂)₄CH₃[b]; 10-F,-
12-C₆H₅[b]; 2,9,12-tri-CH₃[b]; 8,9,12-tri-CH₃[a,b]; 8,11,12-tri-CH₃[a,b];
9,11,12-tri-CH₃[a,b]; 2,9-di-CH₃,12-C₂H₅[b]; 2,12-di-CH₃,10-F[b]; 8,9-di-
CH₃,12-CH(CH₃)₂[b]; 8,12-di-CH₃,9-Cl[b]; 9,12-di-CH₃,10-F[b]; 10,11-di-
CH₃,12-CH(CH₃)₂[b]; 8-CH₃,9-Cl,12-C₂H₅[b]; 8-CH₃,9-Cl,12-
CH(CH₃)₂[a,b]; 2,8,10,12-tetra-CH₃[b]; 3,8,10,12-tetra-CH₃[b]; 2,8,12-
tri-CH₃,9-Cl[b]; 2,8,12-tri-CH₃,11-C₂H₅[b]; 2,3,8,10, 11-penta-CH₃[b];
2,3,9,10,12-penta-CH₃[b]; 2,3,8,10,11,12-hexa-CH₃[b]

Benz[c]acridines

7-CHO[b]; 7-(CH₂)₂CH₃[a]; 8-CH₃[b]; 9-CH₃[a]; 9-C₆H₅[b]; 10-CH₃[b]; 5,7-di-CH₃[a,b]
10,11-di-CH₃[a,b]; 7-CH₃,9-C₂H₅[b]; 7-CON(C₂H₅)₂,9-CH₃[b]; 7-C₂H₅,-
9-F[a,b]; 7-(CH₂)₂CH₃,9-F[b]; 7-(CH₂)₄CH₃,9-F[a,b]; 7-CH₂C₆H₅,9-F[b];
7-CH₃,10-CF₃[b]; 7-C₂H₅,11-CH₃[a]; 5,7,11-tri-CH₃[b]; 7,8,11-tri-CH₃[b];
7,9,10-tri-CH₃[b]; 7,11-di-CH₃,10-Cl[b]; 7-C₂H₅,10-Cl,11-CH₃[a]

[a] Painting on mouse skin.
[b] Subcutaneous injections in mice.

Continued

Moderate   *High*

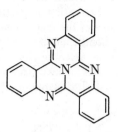

Tricycloquinazoline

[e] Zajdela *et al.* (*65*).
[f] Sellakumar and Shubik (*66*).
[g] Lacassagne *et al.* (*67*).
[h] Lacassagne *et al.* (*68*).

of Substituted Benzacridines

Slight	*Moderate*	*High*
	Benz[a]acridines	
8,12-di-CH$_3$[b];	8,10,12-tri-CH$_3$[a];	
9,12-di-CH$_3$[a];	9,10,12-tri-CH$_3$[b]	
10-F,12-CH$_3$[a,b];		
3,8,12-tri-CH$_3$[b];		
8,12-di-CH$_3$,9-Cl[a];		
10-F,9,12-di-CH$_3$[a]		

Benz[c]acridines		
7-CN[b]; 7,11-di-CH$_3$[a,b];	7,9-di-CH$_3$[a,b];	7-CH$_3$[a]; 7-CHO,9-CH$_3$[b];
7-C$_2$H$_5$,9-CH$_3$[a];	7,10-di-CH$_3$[a,b];	7,8,9,11-tetra-CH$_3$[a]
7-CH$_3$,9-C$_6$H$_5$[a];	7-CH$_3$,9-C$_2$H$_5$[a];	
7-CH$_3$,11-F[b];	7-CH$_3$,9-F[a,b];	
5,7,11-tri-CH$_3$[a];	7-CHO,11-CH$_3$[b];	
7,8,11-tri-CH$_3$[a];	7,9,10-tri-CH$_3$[a];	
7-C$_2$H$_5$,10-Cl,11-CH$_3$[b];	7,9,11-tri-CH$_3$[a,b]	
7,8,9,11-tetra-CH$_3$[b]		

wack *et al.* (*71*) have found that a corticosteroid binding protein of rat liver (ligandin) also binds the polynuclear carcinogen, 3-methylcholanthrene.

The most generally applicable structure–activity relationship for polynuclear carcinogens is that most of the carcinogenic hydrocarbons can be regarded as phenanthrene derivatives (*72*). This observation is particularly important because it is consistent with the conclusions of the theoretical chemists who have indicated that a bond of high double bond character [analogous to the 9,10-bond in phenanthrene (Figure 3)] is essential for carcinogenic activity. The notable exceptions to this generalization not included in Tables I–VIII are 6,12-dimethylbenzo[*b*]thionaphtheno[3,2-*f*]-

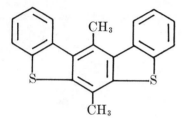

6,12-Dimethylbenzo–
[*b*]thionaphtheno-
[3, 2-*f*]thionaphthen

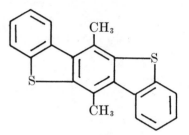

6, 12-Dimethylbenzo-
[*b*]thionaphtheno-
[2, 3-*f*]thionaphthen

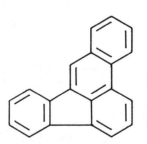

Benzo[*b*]fluoranthene

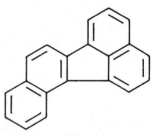

Benzo[*j*]fluoranthene

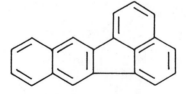

Benzo[*k*]fluoranthene

Figure 6. Polynuclear aromatic carcinogens which are not phenanthrene derivatives

thionaphthen and 6,12-dimethylbenzo[b]thionaphtheno[2,3-f]thionaphthen which are both potent sarcomagens in mice (73), together with the carcinogens, benzo[b]fluoranthene, benzo[j]fluoranthene, and benzo[k]fluoranthene (74, 75) (Figure 6).

Although contributions to and modifications of our knowledge of the carcinogenic activities of polynuclear carcinogens are still being made today, much of the work over the last 25 years has been directed primarily at the mechanism of action of these compounds. This work can be somewhat arbitrarily classified into two main approaches. A great deal of work has been done on chemical carcinogens apart from any biological system. This largely involves the implicit assumption that the critical step in the carcinogenic process is the interaction of the unmodified carcinogen with some cellular receptor (e.g., scheme A, Figure 5). The other approach involves the properties of carcinogens within a biological system together with the attendant response of the biological system to the carcinogen. This relates more closely, but not exclusively, to scheme B of Figure 5.

There has been a considerable interaction between these two approaches over the years, and each has undoubtedly stimulated further development of the other. Nevertheless, it is convenient to deal with most of this work in separate sections under the arbitrary headings of either chemistry or biochemistry of polynuclear carcinogens.

Chemistry of Polynuclear Carcinogens

A comprehensive survey of the chemistry of polycyclic hydrocarbons can be found in the two volumes by Clar (76). However, a few points which are particularly relevant to the carcinogenic action of these compounds are outlined below.

Aromatic compounds cannot be accurately described by the conventional structural formulae given in Tables I and VII. These formulae represent only one of the possible Kekulé structures and erroneously suggest that aromatic compounds contain a framework of carbon atoms linked together by alternating single and double bonds. This would be totally inconsistent with the chemical properties of these compounds and, in fact, all the carbon–carbon bond lengths lie at various values between those of an isolated single bond and an isolated double bond. Furthermore, aromatic compounds exhibit a greater stability (i.e., a lower energy) than that which would be expected for the structure represented by the most stable canonical form. The difference between the energy of the actual compound and that of the most stable hypothetical Kekulé structure is defined as resonance energy. This latter may be computed from experimental values for heats of combustion, heats of hydrogenation, etc., or calculated by the application of quantum mechanics. Resonance energy has no absolute meaning, however, since it merely reflects an increase in the stability of an actual compound over that which would be expected for a hypothetical structure. This stability is not related to chemical reactivity; this is determined by the difference in free energy between the reactants and the transition states for specific chemical reactions. Thus, resonance energy increases along the series: benzene (36 kcal/mole), naphthalene (61 kcal/mole), and anthracene (84 kcal/mole). Chemical reactivity also increases along this series.

The inconsistencies between the properties of aromatic compounds and those expected for the structural representations of these compounds arise because, contrary to the tacit assumption made in drawing conventional structural representations, the pi electrons of aromatic compounds are not localized in discrete bonds but are delocalized over the whole aromatic molecule. The pi electron density distribution varies from compound to compound and is determined for any given aromatic hydrocarbon by the geometry of the carbon atom framework. It is this distribution which primarily determines the chemical properties of aromatic hydrocarbons, and many methods of visualizing this distribution have been devised. The most useful of these is resonance theory which describes the real structures of aromatic compounds as weighted averages of the possible conventional structures with the greatest weights being given to the most stable conventional structures. More detailed descriptions can be obtained by the application of the valence bond and molecular orbital methods of quantum mechanics (77), and the localization theory of chemical reactions is of particular value for predicting chemical reactivity (78).

The chemical stability of benzene arises from the even distribution of the six pi electrons over the ring. This results in hexagonal symmetry so that, in the ground state, the length of each bond is 1.39 A. For a Kekulé structure, alternating single bonds (1.54 A) and double bonds (1.33 A) would be expected. Benzene is not particularly reactive and appears to undergo substitution reactions (which preserve its aromatic character) more readily than addition reactions. The polycyclic aromatic hydrocarbons which most closely resemble benzene with respect to their chemical stability are triphenylene, dibenzo[fg,op]naphthacene (Table I), and phenanthro[9,10-b]triphenylene. All of these can be formulated as condensed polyphenyls, and their chemical properties clearly indicate that this reasonably approximates their actual structures. These compounds are inactive in carcinogenesis experiments.

In general, the most reactive class of polycyclic aromatic hydrocarbons is the acenes [naphthalene, anthracene, naphthacene, pentacene (Table I)]. Reactivity increases with increasing molecular weight, and heptacene is so unstable that it has been impossible to prepare this compound in a pure state. The most notable feature of the chemical reactions of the acenes is the relative ease with which additions across para positions can occur. Maleic anhydride adds across the 1,4-positions of naphthalene to only a very small extent, but an extensive 9,10-addition occurs with anthracene, and the reaction across the 5,12-positions of naphthacene and the 6,13-positions of pentacene occurs very readily. These chemical reactions of the acenes indicate that a pair of pi electrons can be localized across para positions relatively easily. Again, no compound of this group has been shown to be carcinogenic.

In the phene series, i.e., phenanthrene, benz[a]anthracene, pentaphene, and benzo[b]pentaphene (all in Table I), general reactivity is usually lower than in the isomeric acene. In contrast to the acenes, addition reactions across a double bond occur fairly easily, e.g., across the 9,10-bond of phenanthrene

(Figure 3). This double bond in the central ring of phenanthrene exhibits properties which are similar to those of an isolated ethylenic double bond, and it is clear that, to a large extent, a pair of pi electrons is localized in this double bond. However, in addition to a reactive double bond, the higher phenes also contain reactive para positions (*e.g.*, the 7 and 12 positions of benz[*a*]anthracene) which will add reagents such as maleic anhydride. With the exception of benz[*a*]anthracene none of the phenes above have been reported to be carcinogenic (Table I), but many potent carcinogens can be found among substituted benz[*a*]anthracenes (Tables II, III), and many carcinogenic hydrocarbons can be considered to be phenanthrene derivatives (as noted earlier).

Many of the more complex hydrocarbon carcinogens (Table I) also contain a reactive double bond, such as the 4,5-bond in benzo[*a*]pyrene. None of the highly carcinogenic pyrene derivatives undergo facile para addition reactions, however, although substitutions occur very readily in some cases (*e.g.*, at the 6-position of benzo[*a*]pyrene).

It was from this background that attention was directed towards a possible relationship between the chemical reactivity of a specific bond in a polycyclic hydrocarbon (*i.e.*, a bond with high double bond character like the 9,10-bond in phenanthrene) and carcinogenic activity. The early work on the application of theoretical chemistry to predicting chemical reactivity for polynuclear carcinogens has been reviewed by Coulson (*79*). Pullman (*80, 81*) introduced the term, K-region, to describe that bond in a polynuclear compound which has the greatest double bond character, *e.g.*, the 9,10-bond in phenanthrene and the 5,6-bond in benz[*a*]anthracene (Figure 7). She later used the term, L-region, to describe that region of a hydrocarbon which exhibits properties similar to the 9 and 10 positions of anthracene (*82*), *e.g.*, carbons 7 and 12 in benz[*a*]anthracene (Figure 7). Although it is chronologically incorrect, the use of this terminology simplifies the following discussion.

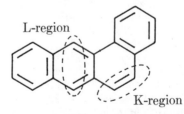

L-region

K-region

Figure 7.   Regions of high chemical reactivity in polycyclic aromatic hydrocarbons

Schmidt (*83, 84, 85*) originated the attempts to relate the carcinogenic activities of polycyclic hydrocarbons to their pi electron density distributions. His methods were crude and qualitative, but regions of high pi electron density (particularly at L-regions) were indicated, and he related the presence of such regions to biological activity. Svartholm (*86*) developed this approach further by applying the ideas of resonance, but the major contributions undoubtedly came later on with the work of the Daudels and the Pullmans and their colleagues (detailed documentation of individual contributions may be found in Coulson's review). These workers applied the more sophisticated quantum mechanical approaches of the valence-bond method (and later the molecular-orbital method) to studies of polynuclear compounds and calculated many molecular parameters so that correlations between carcinogenic activity and electronic structure could be more precisely evaluated.

Pullman (80, 81) showed that an index describing the electrical properties of the K-region (i.e., the "total charge on the K-region" which was defined as the sum of twice the mobile bond order plus the two free valence numbers) seemed to vary with carcinogenic potency for several methylbenz[a]anthracenes, methylbenzo[c]phenanthrenes, methylbenz[a]acridines, and methylbenz[c]arcidines. For example, Table IX lists some benzacridines in roughly increasing order of carcinogenic potency (see Table VII) along with experimentally determined pK_a values and some calculated indices for the pi electron distribution at the K-region. The relationship between the K-region indices and carcinogenic activity is really quite convincing.

For many compounds, carcinogenic activity seemed to relate to a fairly high pi electron density at the K-region, and this indicated that the interaction between the hydrocarbon and the cell which was responsible for initiating the carcinogenic process took the form of an addition reaction at the K-region.

Table IX.   Properties of Some Benzacridines

Compound	K-Region		Excess Charge[b]	pK_a[c]
	Total Charge[a]			
	A	B		
Benz[a]acridine	1.260	1.973	−0.039	3.95
10-Methylbenz[a]acridine			−0.039	4.22
Benz[c]acridine	1.270	1.984	−0.003	3.24
12-Methylbenz[a]acridine	1.273	1.989	−0.036	4.60
10-Methylbenz[c]acridine		1.998		3.68
8-Methylbenz[c]acridine		2.00		3.67
10,11-Dimethylbenz[c]acridine		2.008		3.74
8,9,12-Trimethylbenz[a]acridine		2.018		4.59
9,12-Dimethylbenz[a]acridine	1.284	2.002	−0.023	5.13
8,12-Dimethylbenz[a]acridine	1.286		−0.033	
7,11-Dimethylbenz[c]acridine	1.302	2.022	0.035	
8,10,12-Trimethylbenz[a]acridine	1.298		0.038	
7,10-Dimethylbenz[c]acridine	1.304	2.025	0.049	3.99
7,9-Dimethylbenz[c]acridine	1.304	2.024	0.039	4.26
7,9,11-Trimethylbenz[c]acridine	1.312		0.039	
7,8,9,11-Tetramethylbenz[c]acridine				3.98

[a] Values given under A are from Pullman (81) where total charge is defined as the sum of twice the mobile bond order plus the two free valence numbers. Values given under B are from Lacassagne et al. (20) and arise from the modified definition of total charge from Buu-Hoi et al. (87). Both sets of figures were obtained from the valence bond method.

[b] Values are taken from Greenwood (88) and represent the sum of the charges (which arise upon the introduction of a nitrogen atom or a methyl group into benz[a]anthracene) of the two atoms at the K-region. These values were obtained from the molecular orbital method.

[c] Values taken from Pagès-Flon et al. (89).

There were, however, numerous exceptions to the original relationship, and most of these were unsubstituted polycyclic compounds (Tables I and X). It had been shown that the rate of osmium tetroxide addition to the K-region of these unsubstituted hydrocarbons followed the theoretical predictions reasonably well (*16*) and that the exceptions did not arise from any inadequacies in the theoretical prediction of chemical reactivity. Similarly, experimentally determined reaction rates of unsubstituted hydrocarbons with trichloromethyl radicals were correlated with the highest free valence numbers for these compounds (*98*). Kooyman and Heringa (*99*) then suggested that carcinogenic potency might depend on both the highest free valence number and the highest bond order for a given molecule.

Pullman (*82*) arrived at a similar conclusion, but she suggested that the presence in a polynuclear compound of an L-region (*see* Figure 7), which always contains the two carbon atoms of highest free valence, could inactivate that compound, even though the properties of its K-region were consistent with carcinogenic activity. This proposition (the K- and L-region theory), which was based on calculations related to the ground states of these polynuclear compounds, was then restated more explicitly in terms of the localization theory of chemical reactions (*78, 100*). Thus, for a polynuclear compound to exhibit carcinogenic properties, it had to have a reactive K-region (the sum of the bond localization energy and the minimum carbon localization energy had to be less than a certain value) and an unreactive L-region (the sum of the para localization energy and the minimum carbon localization energy at the para positions had to be greater than another fixed value). This accommodated the known carcinogenic activities of unsubstituted aromatic hydrocarbon tolerably well, and it was concluded that the critical reaction (or the rate determining step in the reaction) between the carcinogen and the cell involved an addition at the K-region. However, in cases where a reactive L-region was present, an addition at this latter region would occur rendering the compound ineffective as a carcinogen (*78*). A number of theoreticians, some using different indices to describe chemical reactivity, have reexamined this structure–activity relationship, but all seem to confirm the general concept that a reactive K-region and an unreactive L-region are associated with carcinogenic activity (*101–106*). Several unsubstituted aromatic hydrocarbons, which for many years were regarded as inactive, are now known to be carcinogenic, e.g., naphtho[8,1,2-*cde*]naphthacene and dibenz[*a,c*]anthracene (Table I). These now make this relationship seem somewhat less convincing (Table X).

The Pullman complex indices for unsubstituted hydrocarbons are given in Table X where the compounds are listed in increasing order of carcinogenic activity. Also given are the bond orders and the coefficients of the highest filled or lowest empty molecular orbitals. The latter describe the electron donor and electron acceptor properties of these molecules (*93*). The compounds with the lowest coefficients should be the most effective electron donors or electron acceptors. These properties are of interest because several workers have suggested that the critical molecular event in carcinogenesis might be the formation of a charge–transfer complex between the carcinogen and a cellular

Table X.   Properties of Some

		K-Region		L-Region
			C.L.E._{min}	C.L.E._{min}
		Bond	+	+
Compound[a]	Bond[b]	Order[c]	B.L.E.[b]	P.L.E.[b]
Benzene	1,2	1.667	4.07	6.54
Naphthalene	1,2	1.725	3.56	5.98
Anthracene	1,2	1.738	3.53	5.38
Phenanthrene	9,10	1.775	3.36	—
Pyrene	4,5	1.777	3.33	—
Naphthacene	1,2	1.741	3.33	5.25
Triphenylene	1,2	1.690	3.81	—
Pentacene	1,2	1.742	3.27	5.03
Picene	5,6	1.758	3.37	—
Pentaphene	6,7	1.790	3.23	5.56
Dibenzo[c,g]phenanthrene	5,6		3.38	—
Benzo[b]chrysene	5,6		3.27	5.47
Dibenzo[b,g]phenanthrene	7,8		3.30	5.48
Dibenzo[def,mno]chrysene	4,5		3.20	—
Dibenzo[b,k]chrysene	6,7		3.24	5.44
Dibenzo[a,j]naphthacene	5,6		3.24	5.42
Chrysene	5,6	1.754	3.38	—
Benz[a]anthracene	5,6	1.783	3.29	5.53
Dibenz[a,c]anthracene	10,11	1.727	3.51	5.67
Dibenz[a,j]anthracene	5,6	1.780	3.31	5.66
Benzo[c]phenanthrene	5,6	1.762	3.41	—
Dibenz[a,h]anthracene	5,6	1.778	3.30	5.69
Benzo[c]chrysene	7,8	1.764	3.41	—
Naphtho[8,1,2-cde]naphthacene	4,5		3.14	5.30
Benzo[a]pyrene	4,5	1.787	3.23	—
Dibenzo[b,def]chrysene	5,6		3.17	—
Benzo[rst]pentaphene	6,7		3.16	—

[a] See Table I for structures and carcinogenic activities.
[b] Pullman and Pullman (78). C.L.E., B.L.E., and P.L.E. are carbon localization energy, bond localization energy, and para localization energy, respectively. The Pullmans' requirements for carcinogenic activity were: C.L.E._{min} + B.L.E. should be equal to or smaller than 3.31 β and, if an L-region is present, C.L.E._{min} + P.L.E. should be equal to or greater than 5.66β.

receptor (107, 108, 109, 110). Pullman and Pullman (93) pointed out that there is no correlation between electron donor or acceptor properties of aromatic hydrocarbons and carcinogenicity when a large series of compounds is studied. This conclusion was also reached from experimental studies on charge–transfer complex formation (111, 112). Table X also lists the experimentally determined affinities of some polycyclic hydrocarbons (in the vapor phase) for thermal electrons (97) and Badger's relative rates of reaction between osmium tetroxide and the K-regions of polycyclic compounds (16). The ionization potentials of these compounds should reflect the ease with which they can be converted to radical cations, but again no correlation with carcinogenic activity is seen (94).

Unsubstituted Aromatic Hydrocarbons

Coefficient of Highest Filled or Lowest Empty M.O.[d]	Ionization Potentials[e]	Absorption Coefficient for Thermal Electrons[f]	Relative Rate of Reaction with OsO_4[g]
1		0.01	
0.618	8.12	0.01	
0.414	7.23	12	
0.605	8.02	0.05	0.1
0.445	7.58	6.0	0.66
0.295	6.64	1.7	
0.684	8.13	0.015	
0.220	6.23		
0.501	7.62		
0.437	7.35		
0.535	—		
0.405	7.29		
0.419	7.11		
0.291	6.84		
0.348	—		
0.358	6.82		
0.520	7.72		slow
0.452	7.35	29	1.0
0.499	7.43		
0.492	7.42		
0.566	7.76	1.3	
0.473	7.42		1.3
0.550	7.71	1.2	slow
0.303	6.70		
0.371	7.15		2.0
0.342	6.75		
0.342	7.06		

[c] By the molecular-orbital method (*90, 91, 92*).
[d] Values taken from Pullman and Pullman (*93*). The lower this coefficient the greater are both the electron donor and electron acceptor properties of the molecule.
[e] Taken from (*94, 95, 96*).
[f] Lovelock *et al.* (*97*).
[g] Badger (*16*).

The carcinogenic activities of the 12 isomeric monomethylbenz[*a*]anthracenes have been studied extensively (Table II), and they can be arranged in order of carcinogenic potency with some confidence (Table XI). The 2- and 3-methyl derivatives are totally inactive, the 6-, 8-, 12-, and 7-methyl derivatives are all highly active carcinogens, and the other isomers have all exhibited some slight activity in one system or another. It can be seen from Table XI that the properties of the K-regions of these molecules do not really distinguish the potent carcinogens from the weakly active or the inactive compounds. However, reasonable relationships with carcinogenic activity exist for the calculated excitation energies for these compounds (*113*), for the conjugating ability of the carbon to which the methyl group is bound [as represented by

Table XI.   Properties of

Position of Methyl Group[a]	Total Charge[b]	K-Region Excess Charge[c]	Rate of OsO_4 Attack[d]	Excitation Energy[e]
2		0.036		0.9116
3		0.011		0.9154
1		0.001		0.9164
4		0.024		0.9134
11	1.292	−0.001		0.9059
10	1.294	0.013		0.9099
9	1.294	0.003	0.64	0.9120
5	1.298	−0.164	0.50	0.9067
6	1.298	−0.164		0.9061
8	1.296	0.009		0.9042
12	1.296	0.003	0.96	0.8984
7	1.306	0.039	0.91	0.8934

[a] For carcinogenic activities *see* Table II.
[b] Defined in footnote a to Table IX and in text. Values from Pullman (81).
[c] Defined in footnote b to Table IX. Values from Greenwood (88).
[d] Experimental values from Badger (117).
[e] Calculated energy change involved in promoting an electron from the highest occupied to the lowest unoccupied molecular orbital, Pullman et al. (113),.

the free valences for benz[a]anthracene (16)], for the bathochromic shift of the 287 nm band of the benz[a]anthracene spectrum as a result of methyl substitution (114), for the nucleophilicites of these compounds for silver ion (115), and for the stabilities of arylmethyl cations derived from these compounds [as represented by decreasing values for the coefficient of the nonbonding molecular orbital at the positive carbon atom (116)] (see Table XI). The best correlation with biological activities appears to lie with the experimentally determined nucleophilicities. All the other properties are undoubtedly interrelated, and it is interesting from this viewpoint that 11-methylbenz[a]-anthracene is an exception in all these cases.

Many polynuclear compounds exhibit the property of photodynamic action, which is the phenomenon whereby a combination of light energy and a chemical sensitizer produces effects which are not induced by either component alone. Studies with limited numbers of polynuclear compounds suggested a possible relationship between the photodynamic action of these compounds and their carcinogenic activities (118, 119). However, when a more extensive range of compounds was studied, no direct link between carcinogenic and photodynamic properties was established (120).

A similar conclusion has been reached from studies of the physical interactions between polycyclic hydrocarbons and cellular constituents. Aromatic hydrocarbons are more soluble in purine solutions (121, 122) or in DNA solutions (123, 124) than in water alone, and many studies have been made on the interactions involved in these phenomena. Most of the data presented

Monomethylbenz[a]anthracenes

Free Valence at Methylation Site[f]	NBMO Coefficient at Methyl Carbon[g]	Equilibrium Constant for Reaction with Ag^+[h]	Bathochromic Shift in nm[i]
0.357	0.693	1.23	
0.352	0.729	1.34	
0.388	0.703		0.5
0.399	0.676		
0.404	0.639	1.34	3.0
0.356	0.693	1.25	1.0
0.355	0.703	1.32	2.0
0.404	0.639	1.25	
0.403	0.639	1.35	1.5
0.406	0.631	1.41	2.0
0.484	0.583	1.64	3.5
0.467	0.561	1.66	4.5

[f] Values from Berthier *et al.* (*91*).
[g] Values from Dipple *et al.* (*116*).
[h] Equilibrium constant for the reaction $Ar + Ag^+ \rightleftharpoons ArAg^+$ (*115*).
[i] The bathochromic shift of the 287 nm band in the spectrum of benz[a]anthracene as a result of methyl substitution (*114*).

appear to support the view that the interaction with DNA involves the insertion of the hydrocarbon molecule between base pairs of the DNA as was proposed for acridine dye–DNA complexes (*125*), although this may not be the only type of interaction involved (*126*). No conclusive proof of this intercalation model for hydrocarbons has been presented yet, but it does seem clear that physical interaction with DNA is related to the size of the hydrocarbons and bears no obvious relationship to their carcinogenic activities (*127*).

Despite these extensive studies of the chemical and physical properties of polynuclear carcinogens, it is reasonably clear that no single property of these compounds can be related quantitatively to their biological activities. This is not surprising in view of the many factors which could potentially modify biological activity (Figure 5), and because of this and the possibility that the process of carcinogenesis may be initiated through various mechanisms, not even the most limited correlation of carcinogenic activity with some chemical or physical property can be totally ignored. Nevertheless, the various relationships reported need to be evaluated, and from this point of view the Pullman relationships between the chemical reactivities of polynuclear compounds and their carcinogenic activities are perhaps the most convincing. However, the fact that many of the more potent carcinogens have low ionization potentials, are good electron donors, readily form charge–transfer complexes, and exhibit quite high photodynamic activities still remain even though many noncarcinogens also exhibit these properties.

Biochemistry of Polynuclear Carcinogens

Metabolism. The earliest and the most extensive studies of polynuclear carcinogens within biological systems were on the metabolic fate of polynuclear compounds. The enzymes primarily responsible for polycyclic hydrocarbon metabolism are the mixed-function oxygenases (*128*). These are membrane bound (found in the microsomal fraction of tissue homogenates) and require NADPH and molecular oxygen to convert the nonpolar hydrocarbons into various hydroxylated derivatives. (Khandwala and Kasper (*129*) recently described enzyme activities for hydrocarbon metabolism in rat liver nuclei.) These derivatives may be conjugated with glucuronic acid to give glucuronides (also a microsomal reaction) or may be converted into sulfates and mercapturic acids (this activity is found in the soluble fraction of the cell). These metabolic reactions occur in various tissues including the skin, but liver is the most active tissue in this respect. Thus, metabolism effects the conversion of nonpolar insoluble foreign compounds into highly polar anionic water-soluble metablolites which can be excreted through the kidneys.

Metabolism studies have involved the assumption that polynuclear compounds themselves do not initiate the carcinogenic process and that the actual initiator is in fact a metabolite of the administered compound (scheme B, Figure 5). In the case of the aromatic amine carcinogens conclusive evidence shows that these assumptions are valid (*130*), but for the polynuclear carcinogens no single class of metabolite has been found to exhibit a higher carcinogenic potency that its parent compound. However, the accumulated indirect evidence for the involvement of metabolism in the carcinogenic action of polynuclear compounds is currently quite impressive.

In the earliest of several reviews of the older literature (*13, 14, 131, 132*) Boyland postulated that, since the dihydro-dihydroxy derivatives resulting from metabolic attack at bonds in naphthalene, anthracene, and phenanthrene were trans diols, the initial metabolic product and the precursor of the diols was probably an epoxide (arene oxide). He also suggested that the reaction of such epoxides with tissue constituents could represent the critical event in the process of carcinogenesis by polycyclic hydrocarbons, and this possibility is currently the subject of intensive study. Boyland's suggestion was supported when that urinary metabolite of naphthalene which was an acid-labile precursor of 1-naphthylmercapturic acid was identified. Boyland and Sims (*133*) showed that this compound was *N*-acetyl-*S*-(1,2-dihydro-2-hydroxy-1-naphthyl)-L-cysteine and noted that the formation of this metabolite and the formation of the 1,2-dihydrodiol could both be accounted for by the proposed 1,2-naphthalene oxide intermediate. In their subsequent extensive studies of aromatic hydrocarbon metabolism these authors showed that most of the metabolic products which they identified could have arisen from intermediate arene oxides (*134*). Newman and Blum (*135*) were the first to synthesize arene oxides, and thereafter, the metabolites obtained from polycyclic hydrocarbons could also be obtained from metabolism of the appropriate arene oxide (*136, 137*). Conclusive proof that arene oxides were transient metabolic intermediates was not provided, however, until Jerina *et al.* (*138*), using a radiotracer trapping technique, demonstrated the metabolic formation of 1,2-naphthalene oxide from naphthalene in a microsomal system.

Holtzman *et al.* (*139*) had previously examined the consequences of subjecting naphthalene to microsomal metabolism in the presence of an atmosphere of isotopic ^{18}O. They found that the 1-naphthol produced contained the heavy isotope and that the *trans*-1,2-dihydrodiol contained one atom of ^{18}O and one atom of ^{16}O which presumably had originated from water. Furthermore, heating the diol in acid gave 95% 1-naphthol and 5% 2-naphthol; only the 1-naphthol contained ^{18}O. Thus, the diol contained ^{18}O exclusively in the 1-hydroxyl group. The mechanistic scheme which these authors postulated to accommodate their data was essentially that in scheme I of Figure 8, where the initially formed cationic species can be regarded as the immediate precursor of 1-naphthol (by loss of a proton from the 1-position) and as the immediate precursor of the dihydrodiol (arising by the attack of water at the 2-position). The intermediacy of the epoxide in the reaction with glutathione (the initial step in mercapturic acid formation) accounted for the fact that glutathione is bound to the 1-position (*142*). It would be expected, therefore, that the glutathione derivative would still retain ^{18}O, now in the 2-hydroxyl group, but this has not yet been investigated.

This scheme accounted perfectly well for the then-known facts, but when Vogel and Klärner (*143*) synthesized 1,2-naphthalene oxide, they found that this compound readily rearranged to 1-naphthol but was not hydrated nonenzymically to a dihydrodiol. Furthermore, Jerina *et al.* (*140*) showed that 1,2-naphthalene oxide in the presence of microsomes and $H_2{}^{18}O$ was enzymically converted to the trans dihydrodiol and that the ^{18}O was located primarily in the 2-hydroxyl group. Thus, their data were consistent with those of Holtzman *et al.* (*139*) but showed that the epoxide was a suitable precursor for the dihydrodiol since the specificity of the attack by water at the 2-position of the epoxide was enzymically directed. In addition, 1,2-naphthalene oxide reacted with glutathione (but not with *N*-acetylcysteine) both enzymically and nonenzymically to yield the same *S*-(1,2-dihydro-2-hydroxy-1-naphthyl)glutathione found as a naphthalene metabolite. These workers (*140*) showed that 1,2-naphthalene oxide could give rise to all the end products of metabolism found for naphthalene in the microsomal system, *i.e.*, 1-naphthol, *trans*-1,2-dihydro-1,2-dihydroxynaphthalene, and *S*-(1,2-dihydro-2-hydroxy-1-naphthyl)-glutathione (this latter is only formed of course when a liver supernatant fraction and glutathione are added to the microsomal system). Moreover, the presence of styrene oxide (a competitive substrate for epoxide hydrase) during the microsomal metabolism of naphthalene decreased the dihydrodiol yield and concomitantly increased the naphthol yield. Increased concentrations of glutathione increased the yield of glutathione derivative at the expense of both dihydrodiol and phenol during the metabolism of naphthalene in the microsomes plus liver supernatant system. This strongly supported the view that all the metabolites arose from a common intermediate, namely 1,2-naphthalene oxide (*see* Figure 8, scheme II).

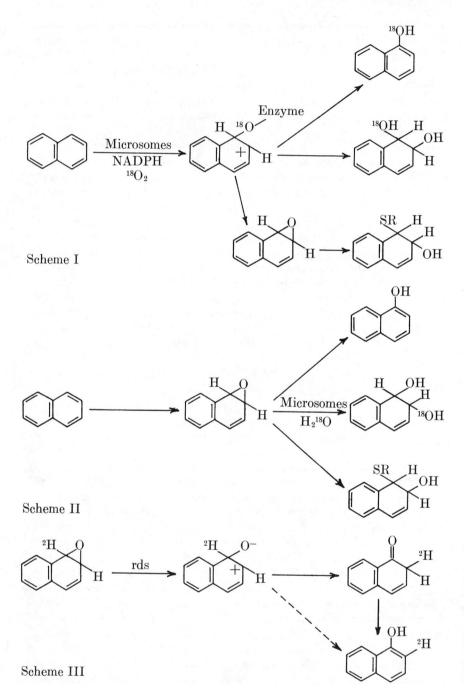

Figure 8. Mechanisms involved in the microsomal metabolism of naphthalene (138, 139, 140, 141). R—SH = glutathione.

One consequence of the discovery of the hydroxylation-induced migration of aromatic substituents [the NIH shift of Guroff *et al.* (*144*)] was a further refinement of the mechanistic description of these metabolic reactions. Jerina *et al.* (*145*) had shown that the isomerization of [4-^{2}H]3,4-toluene oxide to [3-^{2}H]4-hydroxytoluene exhibited a deuterium retention as great as that observed in the enzymic conversion of [4-^{2}H]toluene to [3-^{2}H]4-hydroxytoluene. They suggested, therefore, that arene oxides were likely metabolic intermediates in the enzymic formation of phenols. Similar findings were obtained from a study of the microsomal conversion of naphthalene to 1-naphthol (*146*), where both [1-^{2}H]naphthalene or [2-^{2}H]naphthalene were converted to [2-^{2}H]1-naphthol with approximately 64% of the original deuterium being retained in either case. Under the same conditions both [1-^{2}H]- and [2-^{2}H]1,2-naphthalene oxide rearranged to [2-^{2}H]1-naphthol with approximately 72–75% deuterium retention. These results suggested the formation of a common intermediate during the metabolism of either deuterated naphthalene and the isomerization of either deuterated 1,2-naphthalene oxide. It was proposed that the common intermediate is the keto form of 1-naphthol which arises by the migration of either hydrogen or deuterium from the 1- to the 2-position. Deuterium is retained depending on an isotope effect in the subsequent enolization.

Further investigation of the mechanism of isomerization of arene oxides to phenols (*141*) indicated that for 1,2-naphthalene oxide a stepwise rather than a concerted mechanism is involved. The current view of this mechanism is described in scheme III, Figure 8. The deuterium retentions of 1,2-naphthalene oxide under physiological conditions require that all the phenol should arise from its keto form. However, for other arene oxides (or for 1,2-naphthalene oxide in acid solution) some phenol arises from direct loss of a proton at the cation stage.

Since the route to the phenol does involve a cation intermediate, the distinction between schemes I and II for naphthalene metabolism becomes less clear, *i.e.*, is the epoxide a necessary intermediate *en route* from naphthalene to 1-naphthol? These detailed mechanistic studies have not been carried out for the more complex carcinogenic hydrocarbons although they should serve as a sound basis to interpret the findings on metabolism of these compounds.

The metabolism of aromatic hydrocarbons has been studied in systems ranging from the microsomal preparations discussed above to liver homogenates, liver slices, cultured cells, and whole animals. The metabolites found vary with the system used since all the *in vitro* systems are metabolically deficient with respect to the whole animal. It is necessary, therefore, to discuss the results of metabolic studies in the context of the system used.

The metabolism in animals of a number of aromatic hydrocarbons has been studied, and, in general, the findings with either rats or rabbits are comparable. The situation is far more complex than in microsomal systems because conjugations with sulfuric and glucuronic acids occur, and the conjugates can then give rise to other metabolites. However, most of the metabolites reported for naphthalene in animals can be seen to have arisen through one or other of the primary routes indicated in Figure 8 for the microsomal metabolism. Sims (*147*) pointed out that the naphthalene metabolites in rabbits appear to arise from three routes. The first involves the direct generation of 1-naphthol which is found in urine as either sulfuric acid or glucuronic acid conjugates and not as the phenol. The second route involves the primary production of the *trans*-1,2-dihydrodiol. This is then conjugated with either sulfuric acid or glucuronic acid, and these conjugates break down, as originally proposed by Corner and Young (*148*), to yield 1-naphthyl sulfate, 1-naphthyl glucosiduronate, and the 2-naphthol which is found unconjugated in the urine (Figure 9). The dehydrogenation of the dihydrodiol or its conjugates leads to another group of urinary metabolites, *i.e.*, sulfuric acid conjugates and glucuronic acid conjugates of 1,2-dihydroxynaphthalene. The third primary metabolic route involves the formation of the glutathione derivative, *S*-(1,2-dihydro-2-hydroxy-1-naphthyl)glutathione, which appears to be the starting point for the formation of the urinary mercapturic acid (*N*-acetyl-*S*-(1,2-dihydro-2-hydroxy-1-naphthyl)L-cysteine). In rat biles a series of amino acid conjugates of naphthalene were found, and from these the precursor–product relationship of the glutathione derivative and the mercapturic acid was established by Boyland *et al.* (*149*).

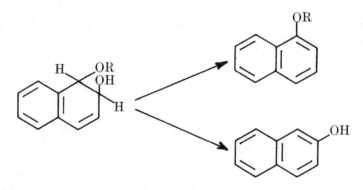

Figure 9.   Metabolic breakdown of sulfates or glucosiduronates of trans-*1,2-dihydro-1,2-dihydroxynaphthalene* (148). $R = SO_3H$ *or* $C_6H_9O_6$.

All the naphthalene metabolites arise from metabolic attack at the 1,2-bond, but when more complex molecules are examined several sites of metabolic attack are detected. However, in view of the potential importance of the K-regions in polycyclic aromatic hydrocarbon carcinogeneisis, the metabolic reactions which occur at this region for various compounds should be compared. The compounds which have been studied in whole animals will be dealt with in order of increasing reactivity of their K-regions as indicated by bond orders and complex indices listed in Table X (p. 278–279).

The results of studies of the products of metabolic attack at the K-region (1,2-bond) of anthracene in rats differ dramatically from those found for naphthalene in that neither 1- nor 2-hydroxyanthracene nor conjugates thereof are detected (*150*). On the other hand, *trans*-1,2-dihydro-1,2-dihydroxyanthracene and 1,2-dihydroxanthracene are produced and excreted mainly as sulfuric acid and glucuronic acid conjugates. A mercapturic acid, *N*-acetyl-*S*-(1,2-dihydro-2-hydroxy-1-anthryl)cysteine, is also excreted in the urine.

A similar situation obtains for the K-region of phenanthrene (9,10-bond). No 9-hydroxyphenanthrene or conjugate thereof is present in the untreated urine of either rats or rabbits (*151*). The major metabolite is *trans*-9,10-dihydro-9,10-dihydroxyphenanthrene which is also excreted as sulfuric acid and glucuronic acid conjugates (*134*). A sulfuric acid conjugate of 9,10-dihydroxyphenanthrene is found in the urine, as is *N*-acetyl-*S*-(9,10-dihydro-9-hydroxy-10-phenanthryl)cysteine (*152*).

For the K-region of pyrene (4,5-bond), no evidence of phenol formation is found, the 4,5-dihydrodiol is detected in relatively small amounts, and no 4,5-dihydroxypyrene derivatives are found. The major metabolite appears to be the mercapturic acid, *N*-acetyl-*S*-(4,5-dihydro-4-hydroxy-5--pyrenyl)L-cysteine (*153*).

In the case of benz[*a*]anthracene (*154*) the major metabolite at the K-region (5,6-bond) is again a mercapturic acid, *N*-acetyl-*S*-(5,6-dihydro-6-hydroxy-5-benz[*a*]anthracenyl)cysteine, and whereas the dihydrodiol at the K-region of phenanthrene was the major metabolic product, the 5,6-dihydrodiol of benz[*a*]anthracene is only a minor metabolite. Phenols are not formed at the K-region of benz[*a*]anthracene.

For both phenanthrene and benz[*a*]anthracene Boyland and Sims (*134, 154*) estimate that the extent of metabolic attack at any given bond increases with increasing bond order, *i.e.*, the most extensive metabolic attack occurs at the K-region. It can be seen from the summary above that the final products of metabolic attack at K-regions vary with the bond order of this region. Thus, for naphthalene all the three primary metabolic routes (Figure 8, scheme II) are followed, and phenol, dihydrodiol, and mercapturic acid are formed. However, as the double bond character of the K-region increases on going to anthracene, the phenol route becomes inoperative. Similarly, as double bond character increases further on going to pyrene and then benz[*a*]anthracene, it appears that the dihydrodiol route is less favored also, and the main metabolic route becomes mercapturic acid formation.

It is interesting to consider these observations with respect to the mechanistic schemes of Figure 8. It appears that phenols are formed only at bonds where the energy required to localize a pair of electrons at that bond (bond localization energy) is fairly high. This is to be expected since the higher the bond localization energy, the greater the gain in energy on reverting from the arene oxide or cation intermediates in Figure 8 to the fully aromatic system. However, the rate-determining step in the formation of 1-naphthol from 1,2-naphthalene oxide (scheme III, Figure 8) does not involve regeneration of the fully aromatic system (*141*); this only occurs during the enolization step. In fact, ketones are usually much more stable than their enolic forms, and 2-tetralone was isolated (*155*) from an acid hydrolysis of a mercapturic acid metabolite of 1,2,3,4-tetrahydro-1,2-naphthalene oxide. This is a somewhat extreme example because the bond localization energy for the isolated double bond in a dihydronaphthalene would be very low, but it does illustrate the point that phenol formation could be interrupted at the enolization step of scheme III, Figure 8, for compounds with relatively low bond localization energies. Raha (156) isolated a compound presumed to be the keto-form of a K-region phenol of benzo[a]pyrene, and Pullman and Pullman (157) calculated that for the K-region double bond of this compound the keto-form of a phenol would be the most stable form while at any other bond in the molecule, the enol form would be favored.

These isolated reports are noteworthy because of the subsequent description of the arene oxide–phenol rearrangement mechanism. However, Kasperek and Bruice (158) have shown that 9,10-phenanthrene oxide is stable in the absence of acid, although benzene oxide and 1,2-naphthalene oxide will rearrange to phenols under these conditions. In contrast, Boyland and Sims (136) report that 9,10-phenanthrene oxide is partially converted to 9-hydroxyphenanthrene and the trans diol by a heat-inactivated liver homogenate, and subsequently, many other K-region epoxides have been shown to rearrange to phenols in biological systems. Since the keto form of these phenols were not found, this may suggest that arene oxide–phenol rearrangements at K-regions involve primarily the direct loss pathway of scheme III, Figure 8 and that no NIH shift would be involved.

The preponderance of K-region dihydrodiols as metabolic products in animals also appears to decrease with decreasing bond localization energies at the K-region. Pandov and Sims (159) have shown that this is consistent with the behavior of the epoxide intermediates, since 9,10-phenanthrene oxide is converted to a dihydrodiol by the enzyme epoxide hydrase in rat liver homogenates or microsomes much more rapidly than is 5,6-dibenz[a,h]anthracene oxide.

The more active carcinogens are found among the compounds with low bond localization energies at the K-region. The metabolism studies discussed so far, therefore, suggest that carcinogenic activity is associated with the absence of K-region phenols and dihydrodiols as metabolites and with the presence of glutathione derivatives and mercapturic acids as metabolites. This could suggest that these latter metabolites are instrumental in initiating the carcinogenic process, or alternatively, that the epoxide fulfills this role since for the more carcinogenic compounds less epoxide is being bled off into phenols and diols (160).

The first possibility was suggested by Kuroki and Heidelberger (161) who pointed out that the h-protein in mouse skin [a soluble protein for which the extent of binding of polycyclic hydrocarbons correlates with carcinogenic potency (162) and to which dibenz[a,h]anthracene-5,6-oxide is extensively bound (161)] may be an enzyme involved in glutathione conjugation of arene oxides. Their argument was based on similarities in structure between h-protein and the azo-dye binding protein in rat liver (163), together with the observation of Ketterer et al. (164), that the purified azo-dye–protein complex could be dissociated under appropriate conditions to yield a component with the amino acid analysis of a glutathione conjugate. The difference in chemistry between the mercapturic acid formed from naphthalene and from benz[a]anthracene is also of interest. In the studies cited earlier, Boyland and Sims found that the mercapturic acid from naphthalene was converted by acid into 1-naphthylmercapturic acid plus traces of 1-naphthol, 2-naphthol, and naphthalene. The mercapturic acid from benz[a]anthracene gave primarily benz[a]anthracene and N,N'-diacetylcystine along with a trace of the arylmercapturic acid.

Changes in the spectrum of metabolites produced with changes in the chemistry of the bond attacked can also be seen in the metabolic reactions at bonds other than the K-region, as in benz[a]anthracene, for example. Thus, 3,4-dihydro-3,4-dihydroxybenz[a]anthracene, 8,9-dihydro-8,9-dihydroxybenz[a]anthracene, and 3-, 4-, 8- and 9-hydroxybenz[a]anthracene were detected as metabolites in animals. Metabolic reactions at these bonds are, therefore, similar to those found at the 1,2-bond of naphthalene. Although 10,11-dihydro-10,11-dihydroxybenz[a]anthracene was also detected, no 10- or 11-hydroxybenz[a]anthracene was found; the metabolic reactions at this bond appear to relate more closely to those at the 1,2-bond of anthracene than to those at the 1,2-bond of naphthalene. Another pattern of products results from metabolic attack at the 1,2-bond of pyrene. In this case the only metabolite detected is 1-hydroxypyrene.

Some metabolic products resulting from attack at the L-region of benz[a]anthracene have been found and identified as 7-hydroxybenz[a]anthracene and possibly 7,12-dihydro-7,12-dihydroxybenz[a]anthracene. According to Boyland and Sims (154), these could have arisen from an initial epoxidation across the 7- and 12-positions. Metabolism also occurs at the methyl groups of methylated hydrocarbons yielding hydroxymethyl derivatives and carboxylic acids (165, 166). The mechanism of the first step in these reactions involves the direct displacement of a proton by a positive oxygen species rather than the generation of an intermediate aralkyl carbonium ion. This follows because studies with ^{18}O have shown that in the microsomal conversion of ethylbenzene to methylphenyl carbinol, the oxygen atom in the carbinol originates from atmospheric oxygen rather than from water (167).

Most of the more recent studies of the metabolism of polycyclic hydrocarbons (which include studies of the more carcinogenic hydrocarbons, 7,12-dimethylbenz[a]anthracene, benzo[a]pyrene, dibenz[a,h]anthracene, and 3-methylcholanthrene) have used only the *in vitro* systems of rat liver slices, rat liver homogenates, cultured cells, and liver microsomal preparations. The results of these experiments are consistent with the generalizations made on the basis of the animal studies, but a number of possible contradictions are also raised. In general, the *in vitro* systems yield the same, but not all, the metabolites found in animal studies. In line with the previous generalizations, it is found that K-region phenols are not produced and that the more carcinogenic compounds are not converted to any large extent into K-region dihydrodiols (168). Although it might be expected that the more carcinogenic compounds would be converted fairly extensively to K-region glutathione conjugates, no evidence has been presented so far to justify this expectation.

Glutathione conjugates are not formed in the simple microsomal system because the necessary enzyme activity and glutathione are not present. However, liver homogenates are competent in this respect, and glutathione conjugates at the K-regions of benz[a]anthracene, dibenz[a,h]anthracene (136), and 3-methylcholanthrene (137) are detected in this system, but analogous conjugates at the K-region of the potent carcinogen 7,12-dimethylbenz-[a]anthracene are not detected (165). At present there is no quantitative data on the amounts of glutathione conjugates produced, and this metabolism route, like phenol and dihydrodiol formation, may become increasingly inoperative with increasing carcinogenic activity of the hydrocarbon concerned. This would leave most of the reactive metabolic intermediate (arene oxide?) free to react with various cellular constituents and to initiate the carcinogenic process. The alternative explanation for the apparent absence of K-region metabolites for 7,12-dimethylbenz[a]anthracene is that metabolic attack at the K-region does not occur. This does not seem likely because Keysell et al. (170) have recently identified 7,12-dimethyl-5,6-benz[a]anthracene oxide as a microsomal metabolite of 7,12-dimethylbenz[a]anthracene. Similarly, it has been shown that in microsomal systems, K-region oxides of dibenz-[a,h]anthracene, phenanthrene, benz[a]anthracene, pyrene, and benzo[a]-pyrene are produced (171, 172, 173).

The intermediacy of arene oxides in the metabolism of polycyclic hydrocarbons is established beyond question, but the detailed mechanisms of the metabolic reactions must eventually account for the observations that the metabolism of K-region oxides always leads to the isolation of some K-region phenols, whereas K-region phenols are never found as metabolic products of the parent hydrocarbon except in the case of naphthalene (136, 137, 174). Very recently the syntheses of several arene oxides at bonds other than K-region bonds have been described. The relationship between the metabolism of these compounds and the metabolic reactions occurring at the appropriate bond in the parent compound is similar to that for the K-region oxides (175, 176, 177, 178).

In summary, the primary metabolic fates which befall the polycyclic aromatic hydrocarbons can be classified according to the chemistry of the sites which are modified (Table XII).

1. Metabolic reactions occur at L-regions but, since the presence of such regions of low para localization energy is usually associated with an absence of carcinogenic activity, these metabolic reactions are probably not involved in the expression of carcinogenic activity.

2. Metabolic reaction also occurs on saturated carbon atoms in polycyclic aromatic hydrocarbons leading to the sequential formation of hydroxy compounds, ketones and aldehydes (the aldehyde in Table XII has not been found as a metabolite though it is presumably formed as an intermediate), and carboxylic acids. Some of these products, notably the aldehydes and ketones, have exhibited high carcinogenic activities and could, therefore, be

directly involved in the expression of the carcinogenic potential of the parent compounds.

3. Metabolic modification of "aromatic" double bonds is the most predominant and most extensively studied type of metabolic reaction. This yields a spectrum of metabolic products which could be involved in expressing carcinogenic activity. The relative abundance and the chemical properties of the products obtained vary with the bond localization energy of the particular bond concerned as illustrated for the K-regions of several hydrocarbons in Table XII.

Relationship between Metabolism and Carcinogenic Action. Evidence indicating that metabolism is involved in the carcinogenic action of polynuclear carcinogens is circumstantial. It has been known for many years that polynuclear carcinogens become covalently bound to certain tissue constituents of animals treated with these carcinogens. By exploiting the intense fluorescence of benzo[a]pyrene, Miller (181) showed that this carcinogen was covalently bound to epidermal proteins of mouse skin. Such covalent interactions do not occur in the absence of metabolic activity, and these findings required that the carcinogen be metabolized *in vivo* to a chemically reactive form which can react covalently with cellular macromolecules. Wiest and Heidelberger (182) applied radiotracer techniques to studies of hydrocarbon binding to cellular constituents, and Heidelberger and Moldenhauer (183) subsequently showed that there was a positive correlation between carcinogenic activity and the extents to which seven of eight radioactive polycyclic hydrocarbons were bound to soluble mouse skin proteins. The exception was dibenz[a,c]anthracene which was extensively bound and was believed to be noncarcinogenic. Next, binding to a specific electrophoretic fraction of the soluble proteins was compared with carcinogenic activity, and an excellent correlation with carcinogenic activity was found for the 12 compounds studied (162). This established a link between binding and carcinogenic activity and, therefore, a link between metabolism and carcinogenic activity. The binding of polynuclear carcinogens to other cellular macromolecules has also been reported. Heidelberger and Davenport (184) noted that covalent binding of hydrocarbons to nucleic acids occurred in mouse skin, but they experienced difficulty in confirming this observation (185). Brookes and Lawley (186) showed that firm binding of hydrocarbons to DNA, RNA, and proteins of mouse skin did occur and that the extent of binding to DNA was positively correlated with carcinogenic potency.

The respective correlations between carcinogenic potency and protein binding, or carcinogenic potency and DNA binding, have been used to support the protein deletion hypothesis of carcinogenesis (187) and the somatic mutation hypothesis of carcinogenesis (188), respectively. From the present point of view both of these correlations support the concept that a chemically reactive metabolite may be involved in the process of chemical carcinogenesis. More direct evidence for the generation of chemically reactive metabolites comes from the work of Grover and Sims (189) and of Gelboin (190) who independently demonstrated that a covalent interaction between aromatic hydrocarbons and DNA does occur in the presence of liver

Table XII.   Summary of Metabolic Modifications

Metabolism at L-Regions (150)

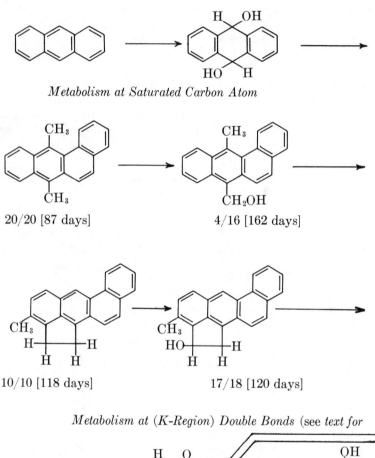

Metabolism at Saturated Carbon Atom

20/20 [87 days]   4/16 [162 days]

10/10 [118 days]   17/18 [120 days]

Metabolism at (K-Region) Double Bonds (see *text for*

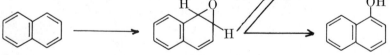

K-Region Metabolites Found in Studies on Whole Animals for:	*Phenol*
Naphthalene	found
Anthracene	absent
Phenanthrene	absent
Pyrene	absent
Benz[a]anthracene	absent

of Polycyclic Aromatic Hydrocarbons

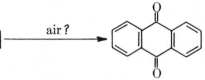

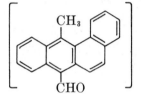

15/15 [102 days]   Sarcoma in rats [mean latent period] (*179*)

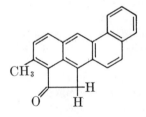

19/19 [132 days]   Sarcoma in mice [mean latent period] (*180*)

references and discussion)

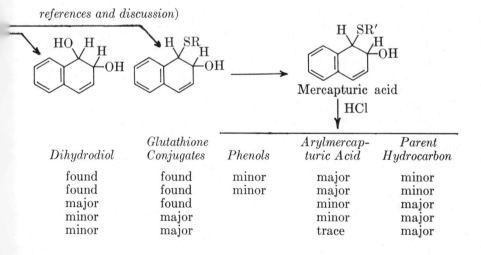

Mercapturic acid

| HCl

Dihydrodiol	*Glutathione Conjugates*	*Phenols*	*Arylmercap-turic Acid*	*Parent Hydrocarbon*
found	found	minor	major	minor
found	found	minor	major	minor
major	found		minor	major
minor	major		minor	major
minor	major		trace	major

microsomal preparations. The subsequent proofs that arene oxides are micro-somal metabolites, together with demonstrations that arene oxides react with nucleic acids and proteins both in chemical reactions (160) and in cells in culture (191, 192) offer one possible explanation of the covalent interactions observed.

Other suggestive evidence for the involvement of metabolism in the carcinogenic action of polynuclear carcinogens arises from various studies of the biological effects of aromatic hydrocarbons. Haddow (193) ob-served that primary tumors are more resistant to the growth-inhibitory prop-erties of aromatic hydrocarbons than are normal cells, and several studies have subsequently confirmed the generality of this observation, which is sub-ject to only a few exceptions [see reviews by Vasiliev and Guelstein (194); Diamond (195)]. Diamond et al. (196) found that cells which are sensitive to the toxic action of 7,12-dimethylbenz[a]anthracene bind considerably more of the carcinogen to their nucleic acids and proteins than do resistant cells. Furthermore, Andrianov et al. (197) demonstrated directly that cells which resist the toxic effects of benzo[a]pyrene exhibit a considerably reduced capacity for metabolizing this carcinogen relative to that of cells which are sensitive. Similarly, Gelboin et al. (198) demonstrated that the levels of arylhydrocarbon hydroxylase activity in various cell types are positively correlated with sensitivity to the toxic effects of benzo[a]pyrene. These workers also provided conclusive proof that the toxic effects of aromatic hydrocarbons require metabolic transformation of the hydrocarbon to a toxic metabolite when they showed that a benzo[a]pyrene metabolite, namely 3-hydroxybenzo[a]pyrene, is cytotoxic to cells irrespective of their capacities for metabolism of the parent hydrocarbon.

A relationship between metabolism and toxicity of aromatic hydro-carbons is, therefore, firmly established but toxicity and carcinogenicity need not necessarily be expressed through similar mechanisms. In fact, from studies analogous to those above, a rather confusing picture of the relationship between metabolism and carcinogenic action emerges.

Many compounds, including the polycyclic hydrocarbons and 5,6-benzoflavone (2-phenylbenzo[f]chromone), will induce the microsomal enzymes involved in hydrocarbon oxidation in a variety of tissues and cell culture systems (199, 200, 201, 202, 203). Many of these compounds also inhibit hydrocarbon carcinogenesis. Thus, the yield of mammary tumors in rats, in response to treatment with 7,12-dimethylbenz[a]anthracene, is decreased by treatment of animals with various polycyclic compounds (204), with 5,6-benzoflavone (205), and with 3-methylcholanthrene (206). The carcinogenic action of benzo[a]pyrene in mouse lung and skin is in hibited by 5,6-benzoflavone (207). In complementary experiments, Wheatley (206) showed that an inhibitor of hydrocarbon metabolism, namely the hydrochloride of β-diethylaminoethyldiphenylpropyl acetate (SKF 525-A), enhances 7,12-dimethylbenz[a]anthracene-induced mammary carcinogenesis in the rat.

A possible conclusion from consideration of these data is that metabo-lism is not involved in the carcinogenic action of polycyclic aromatic hydrocarbons. However, it is known that carcinogenesis by 2-acetylamino-fluorene is inhibited by dietary 3-methylcholanthrene (*208, 209*), yet this aromatic amine does express its carcinogenic potential *via* metabolic activation (*130, 210*). The explanation of this apparent inconsistency was provided by Miller *et al.* (*211*) who showed that dietary 3-methylcholanthrene enhanced the production of some of the noncarcinogenic urinary metabolites of 2-acetylaminofluorene at the expense of the carcinogenic metabolite, *N*-hydroxy-2-acetylaminofluorene.

It is conceivable that similar inductions or inhibitions of specific enzyme activities may be involved in the studies of hydrocarbon carcinogenesis discussed above, and, in a number of recent studies, evidence for the selective inhibition of certain hydrocarbon metabolizing activities has been presented. Diamond and Gelboin (*212*) have found that 7,8-benzoflavone (2-phenylbenzo[*h*] chromone) inhibits hydrocarbon metabolism and hydrocarbon toxicity in hamster embryo cell cultures. Furthermore, this compound inhibits the aryl hydrocarbon hydroxylase activity (this refers to the rate of conversion of benzo[*a*]pyrene into 3-hydroxybenzo[*a*]pyrene) of hamster cell homogenates and rat liver microsomes only when these activities have been induced by prior treatments with benz[*a*]anthracene and 3-methylcholanthrene, respectively. No inhibition of aryl hydrocarbon hydroxylase activities in homogenates and microsomes from noninduced cells and rats is observed.

Several studies exploiting the different properties of the isomeric 5,6- and 7,8-benzoflavones have been reported (*212, 213, 214, 215*). Both compounds can induce the enzyme, aryl hydrocarbon hydroxylase, which converts benzo-[*a*]pyrene to 3-hydroxybenzo[*a*]pyrene, in a variety of tissues. After oral administration of these compounds, the level of this enzyme activity in mouse liver, lung, and small intestine is considerably higher than in control animals, and the induction is greater for 5,6-benzoflavone than for 7,8-benzoflavone. Similarly, the inhibitory effect of dietary 5,6-benzoflavone on the occurrence of 7,12-dimethylbenz[*a*]anthracene-induced lung adenomas in mice is greater than that of 7,8-benzoflavone (*216*).

Somewhat surprising differences between these two flavones were found when their effects on the aryl hydrocarbon hydroxylase activity of mouse skin were examined (*213*). After intraperitoneal injection of either compound in mice, induced levels of aryl hydrocarbon hydroxylase were found in skin homogenates. However, after topical application of these compounds, induced levels of the enzyme were found after treatment with 5,6-benzoflavone but were not found after treatment with 7,8-benzoflavone. In fact treatment with the latter compound reduced the level of this activity considerably with respect to the control values. When either of the benzoflavones is added directly to the mouse skin homogenates used for the enzyme assay, inhibition of the enzyme can be seen, and the inhibitory action of the 7,8-isomer is greater than that of the 5,6-isomer. Subsequent studies with radioactive 7,8-benzoflavone have shown, however, that the previously applied compound is not present in the skin homogenates prepared for the assay of enzyme activity in sufficient amounts for its enzyme-inhibitory activity to account for the apparent lack of enzyme induction (215).

The effects of these benzoflavones on hydrocarbon-initiated skin tumorigenesis are equally fascinating. Thus, Wattenberg and Leong (207) show that topically applied 5,6-benzoflavone induces the level of aryl hydrocarbon hydroxylase present in the skin and inhibits skin carcinogenesis elicited by benzo[a]pyrene. No enzyme induction is observed after topical application of 7,8-benzoflavone, yet this treatment inhibits skin tumorigenesis initiated by a single dose of 7,12-dimethylbenz[a]anthracene by 55–80% (213, 214, 215) and inhibits the covalent binding of this carcinogen to DNA, RNA, and protein in mouse skin by 50–70% (214, 215). 7,8-Benzoflavone does not inhibit skin tumorigenesis initiated by a single dose of benzo[a]pyrene to any appreciable extent (inhibition was seen in one experiment) (214). It does, however, inhibit the covalent binding of benzo[a]pyrene to RNA and protein of skin by about 50% but inhibits the covalent binding of this carcinogen to DNA by only 18% (214).

These findings, together with related studies (217), clearly demonstrate the complexity of the enzyme activities which are involved in hydrocarbon metabolism. In addition, they strongly suggest that metabolic activation is involved in polycyclic hydrocarbon carcinogenesis and that this metabolic activation can be effected by more than one enzyme activity. One important point that these studies have emphasized is the different properties which these benzoflavones exhibit in various tissues and cellular systems.

Confirmation of the indications that metabolism is a necessary step in the mechanism of action of polynuclear carcinogens could be provided by demonstrating that some metabolic products exhibit a greater carcinogenic activity than the compound from which they are derived. However, this has not been demonstrated for the polynuclear carcinogens. A number of hydrocarbon metabolites do exhibit carcinogenic activity, and notable for their high activities are 1- and 2-hydroxy-3-methylcholanthrene and 3-methylcholanthrene-1- and 2-one (180). It is somewhat surprising that this observation has not been examined further since most other hydrocarbon metabolites have been shown to be considerably less carcinogenic than the parent hydrocarbons (various phenols and hydroxymethyl compounds are listed in Tables II–VI).

The arene oxides, which are metabolic intermediates, are less carcinogenic than the parent compounds. The carcinogenic activities of 7-methyl-5,6-benz[a]anthracene oxide and 5,6-benz[a]anthracene oxide, which had been synthesized by Newman and Blum (135), were compared with the activities of the parent hydrocarbons by Miller and Miller (218). 7-Methyl-5,6-benz[a]anthracene oxide was considerably less active than 7-methylbenz[a]anthracene after subcutaneous injections in either rats or mice, after repeated topical applications to mice, and in initiation–promotion experiments in mouse skin. In this last system 5,6-benz[a]anthracene oxide was slightly more active than benz[a]anthracene itself, and this was the only test applied to these compounds. The arene oxides examined by Boyland and Sims (50, 180) were tested only by subcutaneous injection into mice. 3-Methyl-11,12-cholanthrene oxide, 5,6-dibenz[a,h]anthracene oxide, and 5,6-benz[a]anthracene oxide were less active than their parent hydrocarbons while at the dose levels used, 7-methyl-5,6-benz[a]anthracene oxide and 5,6-chrysene oxide evoked tumor incidences comparable to those of the parent hydrocarbons. However, the latent period was longer for the oxides. Van Duuren *et al.* (*219*) showed that the K-region oxides of phenanthrene, 7-methylbenz[a]-anthracene, and dibenz[a,h]anthrene exhibit initiating activity in mouse skin but that this activity is rather feeble compared to that of dibenz[a,h]anthracene.

A number of problems beset the interpretation of carcinogenicity data for chemically reactive compounds like the arene oxides. For example, it is possible that these reactive compounds are destroyed before reaching the appropriate receptor sites, and the low carcinogenic activities of arene oxides do not ncessarily prove that they are not the metabolites responsible for the carcinogenic activity of aromatic hydrocarbons.

Recently, it was shown that many K-region oxides are more effective than their parent hydrocarbons in effecting malignant transformation of cells in culture (*220, 221, 222*) and that some K-region oxides evoke mutations in Chinese hamster cell cultures (*223*), in bacteriophage (*224*), in bacteria (*225*), and in *Drosophila* (*226*). In view of this galaxy of biological activity, it is still possible that arene oxides are intermediates in the metabolic activation of aromatic hydrocarbons to their final carcinogenic forms.

In summary, it appears that a considerable body of evidence indicates that metabolism is involved in the carcinogenic action of polynuclear carcinogens but that there is no incontrovertible proof of this point. Inseparable from this is the fact that the identities of metabolites responsible for the carcinogenic action of polynuclear carcinogens have not been clearly established. In the absence of specific direction from the biological studies, a variety of possible mechanism through which polynuclear carcinogens might conceivably be converted *in vivo* to chemically reactive entities, which can react with cellular receptors and thereby initiate the carcinogenic process, have been considered.

Model Studies for Metabolic Activation of Polynuclear Carcinogens

Numerous studies of covalent interactions occurring *in vitro* have been made in the belief that the *in vivo* covalent binding of polynuclear carcinogens to cellular macromolecules represents an important step in the carcinogenic action of these compounds. This has been necessary because the extent of binding which occurs *in vivo* is too low to permit useful studies of the chemistry of the interaction to be performed on the quantities of products obtainable from the biological sources.

The *in vitro* studies have involved two general approaches. In the first, specific mechanisms of metabolic activation have been postulated, suitable chemically reactive hydrocarbon derivatives have been prepared, and the chemistry and carcinogenic activities of these derivatives have been investigated. The arene oxides fall into this category for, despite the fact that they are now proven metabolic intermediates, their role in the carcinogenic action of their parent hydrocarbons is far from being firmly established. Little can be added to the previous discussion of arene oxides since the chemistry of their interactions with cellular macromolecules has not been extensively studied. Apart from demonstrations that several arene oxides react with DNA, RNA, and histone *in vitro* (*160*) and bind to DNA, RNA, and proteins in cell in culture (*191, 192*), it has been shown that they react more extensively with DNA than with depurinated DNA, more extensively with polyguanylic acid than with polyadenylic acid, and do not react appreciably with polyuridylic acid or polycytidylic acid (*227*).

Miller and Miller (*218*) suggested, by analogy with their findings on the metabolic activation of 2-acetylaminofluorene, that hydroxymethyl metabolites of methyl substituted hydrocarbons might be esterified to reactive benzylic esters and that these could be the carcinogenic metabolites. However, the hydroxymethyl metabolites, like the arene oxides, are now known to be less carcinogenic than the parent hydrocarbons. Dipple *et al.* (*116*), therefore suggested that metabolic precursors of these metabolites might be responsible for the carcinogenic action of polycyclic hydrocarbons. The cationic species of scheme III, Figure 8 were regarded as possible precursors of the K-region oxides, and arylmethyl cations were regarded as possible precursors of the hydroxymethyl derivatives which are found as metabolites of methyl-substituted hydrocarbons. A good correlation between the calculated stabilities of such arylmethyl cations and carcinogenic potency for the 12 isomeric monomethylbenz[a]anthracenes was found (*see* Table XI), and some experimental support for the postulated involvement of cationic species in the carcinogenic process was obtained when it was found that, for the five out of six 7-bromomethylbenz[a]anthracenes, carcinogenic potency increased with an increasing tendency to react through a kinetically first order process (*42*). However, McMahon *et al.* (*167*) have shown that carbocations are not intermediates in the microsomal conversion of ethylbenzene to methylphenyl carbinol, and therefore it would be surprising if the metabolism of methylbenz[a]anthracenes involved arylmethyl cation intermediates.

The carcinogenic activities of several compounds which could be regarded as models for reactive esters of 7-hydroxymethylbenz[a]anthracenes have been studied. Several 7-bromomethylbenz[a]anthracenes are carcinogenic in a variety of animal tests (*42, 43, 49*) as are a number of derivatives of 7-hydroxymethyl-12-methylbenz[a]anthracene (*48*) (data are presented in Table III). Where comparable tests were made, none of these synthetic derivatives was more carcinogenic than the parent hydrocarbon, but Flesher and Sydnor (*228*) have shown that the effective dose of the modified hydrocarbon, in certain cases at least, can be considerably less than that of the parent compound because of differences in transport or diffusion of the two compounds.

The 7-bromomethylbenz[a]anthracenes are useful tools for investigating various aspects of chemical carcinogenesis (*229, 230, 231*), and the chemistry of reaction of both 7-bromomethylbenz[a]anthracene and 7-bromomethyl-12-methylbenz[a]anthracene with nucleic acids has been studied (*232, 233*). The reaction of 7-bromomethylbenz[a]anthracene with nucleosides in dimethylacetamide results in the aralkylation of ring nitrogens of purine and pyrimidine nucleosides, as is found in studies with most alkylating agents (*234*). However, when reactions with nucleosides or nucleic acids in aqueous solutions are examined, a completely different and novel set of aralkylation products, resulting from substitutions on the amino groups of guanine, adenine, and cytosine residues, are found (I, II, and III, Figure 10). These products are also found in the DNA of mouse skin which has been exposed to these bromo compounds (*231*), and to date, they represent the only polycyclic hydrocarbon–nucleic acid products that have been characterized.

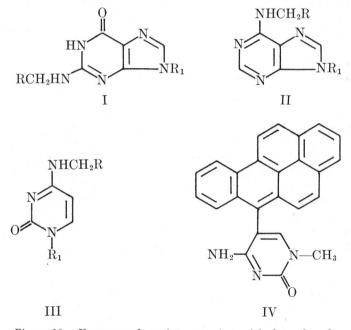

Figure 10. Known products from reactions of hydrocarbon derivatives with nucleic acid constituents (232, 233, 249). RCH_2 = benz[a]anthracenyl-7-methyl or 12-methylbenz[a]anthracenyl-7-methyl, R_1 = DNA.

If DNA is the critical target with which carcinogenic metabolites must react to initiate the carcinogenic process, it seems that for 7-methylbenz[a]anthracene, neither an ester of 7-hydroxymethylbenz[a]anthracene nor 7-methyl-5,6-benz[a]anthracene oxide can be the final carcinogenic metabolite. This follows from the studies of Baird *et al.* (*235*) who showed that after enzymic conversion to deoxyribonucleosides, the reaction products of both 7-bromomethylbenz[a]anthracene and 7-methyl-5,6-benz[a]anthracene oxide with DNA are chromatographically separable from analogous products obtained from the DNA of cell cultures which had been exposed to [³H] 7-methyl-benz[a]anthracene.

Another possible mechanism for metabolic activation of polycyclic hydrocarbon carcinogens involves their conversion into free radicals. Nagata et al. (236) have observed that after stirring benzo[a]pyrene with mouse skin homogenates for several days, a free radical may be detected by electron spin resonance spectroscopy. Furthermore, a radical is similarly produced from another carcinogen, 3-methylcholanthrene, but not from pyrene, phenanthrene, and dibenz[a,c]anthracene. The benzo[a]pyrene radical is also obtained after stirring with albumin solution, and the electron spin resonance spectrum of this radical is identical to that of the 6-phenoxy radical obtained by the oxidation of 6-hydroxybenzo[a]pyrene (237). Photoirradiation of benzo[a]pyrene in organic solvents can also yield the 6-phenoxy radical (238). It is found that this radical is also present in benzene solutions of 6-hydroxybenzo[a]pyrene and that this benzo[a]pyrene metabolite will react covalently with DNA at room temperature (239). The chemistry of this interaction has not been elucidated so far, and it is known that 6-hydroxybenzo[a]pyrene exhibits no notable carcinogenic activity (Table V).

The second general approach to these model studies has involved studies of various mechanisms through which the parent hydrocarbons themselves may become covalently linked to cellular macromolecules in vitro. Benzo[a]pyrene is covalently bound to DNA or to DNA constituents after irradiation of mixtures or physical complexes of these components with light at or near the wavelength of the absorption bands of the hydrocarbon (240, 241). Covalent interactions similarly occur when hydrocarbon–DNA physical complexes are irradiated with x-rays (242), treated with hydrogen peroxide (243, 244), treated with iodine (244, 245), or exposed to the ascorbic acid model hydroxylating system of Udenfriend et al. (246) as described by Lesko et al. (245). More detailed studies of the iodine-induced reactions revealed that carcinogenic hydrocarbons are more extensively bound to DNA than are noncarcinogenic hydrocarbons and that iodine-induced binding of benzo[a]pyrene occurs more readily with polyguanylic acid than with other homopolyribonucleotides (247). Comparisons of the hydrocarbon–DNA products obtained in these in vitro systems and the hydrocarbon–DNA products formed in vivo have not been reported.

Although the chemistry of these various covalent interactions is not yet fully understood, the number of studies of these reactions suggests that this situation will not obtain for very long. Rice (241) and Antonello et al. (248) thought that the photochemical reaction between benzo[a]pyrene and pyrimidines involved the formation of a cyclobutane ring in which the 5,6-double bond of the pyrimidine is fused with a double bond of the hydrocarbon. However, by applying elemental analysis, infra red, ultraviolet, and nuclear magnetic resonance spectroscopy, Cavalieri and Calvin (249) have shown that the photoproduct from benzo[a]pyrene and 1-methylcytosine is, in fact, 6-(1-methylcytos-5-yl)benzo[a]pyrene (IV, Figure 10). An analogous structure has been assigned to the major photoproduct from thymine and benzo[a]-

pyrene, although this was thought to be contaminated with an isomeric product in which the thymine is linked to either the 1- or 12-position of the hydrocarbon (*250*). Hoffman and Müller (*251*) reported that one of the products formed by irradiation of benzo[a]pyrene and DNA involves the formation of a covalent bond between the 6-position of benzo[a]pyrene and the 8-position of guanine nucleotides.

The 6-position of benzo[a]pyrene is also involved in the iodine-induced reactions discussed above. Benzo[a]pyrene forms a charge transfer complex with iodine which exhibits a strong electron spin resonance signal (*109, 111*). Furthermore, exposure of benzo[a]pyrene to iodine vapor generates the 6,12-, 3,6-, and 1,6-benzo[a]pyrene quinones together with benzo[a]pyrene dimers linked together through the 6-positions (*252*). It was suggested that radical cation intermediates are involved in these reactions, and it was subsequently shown that, in the presence of iodine, benzo[a]pyrene reacts covalently with pyridine to yield benzo[a]pyren-6-ylpyridinium salts (*253*). Evidence for similar covalent interactions with purines and pyrimidines has also been presented (*254*).

Since the metabolism of polycyclic hydrocarbons is an oxidative process, chemically reactive intermediates or potentially carcinogenic metabolites have been sought in *in vitro* oxidations of polycyclic hydrocarbons. The study by Jeftic and Adams (*255*) of the electrochemical oxidation of benzo[a]pyrene is particularly interesting with respect to the observations on the *in vitro* covalent interactions of this carcinogen. The initial step in this oxidation involves a one-electron process which yields the benzo[a]pyrene radical cation. This latter is consumed either by dimerization to 6,6'-bibenzo[a]-pyrenyl followed by further oxidation or by reaction with water to form a neutral radical which is oxidized further to 6-hydroxybenzo[a]pyrene. The hydroxy compound is then oxidized to a neutral phenoxy radical which is ultimately transformed into a mixture of benzo[a]pyrene quinones. Thus, if cellular oxidations occur through analogous mechanisms, a number of reactive radical intermediates (both neutral and cationic) would be generated, and any one of these might be the carcinogenic metabolite.

The one-electron transfer oxidation of 7-12-dimethylbenz[a]anthracene effected by manganese dioxide, ferricyanide, or Ce^{IV} has also been described by Fried and Schumm (*256*). All the identified reaction products could be accounted for by the generation of the radical cation followed by attack of solvent at positions 7 and 12 and at the methyl groups. This observation provides an interesting contrast to the iodine-induced reaction of 7,12-di-methylbenz[a]anthracene with pyridine which was reported to yield a 7,12-dimethylbenz[a]anthracen-5-yl-pyridinium salt (*253*). Recently, however, Cavalieri (*258*) reported that the iodine-induced reaction of 7,12-dimethyl-benz[a]anthracene with pyridine yields a 12-methylbenz[a]anthracenyl-7-methylpyridinium salt which is more consistent with expectation based on the report of Fried and Schumm (*256*).

The relevance of chemical oxidations to biological oxidations can now be tested to some extent by looking for equivalent NIH shifts in the two systems [reviewed in Daly *et al.* (*257*)]. This has not been applied so far to the oxidations discussed above, but it is conceivable that NIH shifts might be involved in the metabolic reactions leading to the benzo[*a*]pyrene quinones. Thus, either studies of this nature or comparisons of the reaction products obtained *in vitro* with those obtained *in vivo* will eventually permit the relevance of these model studies to be evaluated.

General Discussion

In order to change normal tissue into tumor tissue, a chemical carcinogen must interact in some way or other with some receptor in the host. This interaction could involve a simple physical interaction, a charge–transfer interaction, or a covalent bond formation (which would presumably be mediated by metabolism of the carcinogen). One primary objective of most of the studies reviewed here has been to define the type of interaction involved in the initiation of chemical carcinogenesis. The fact that the identity of the critical receptor is also unknown has made the achievement of this objective particularly difficult.

In the face of such a formidable task the general approach to the problem of the definition of the initial interaction has necessarily involved the construction of hypotheses and the subsequent testing of these hypotheses by experiment. This appears to be relatively straightforward until the design of the critical tests for various hypotheses is attempted. It can then be seen that there are, in fact, only two general types of test which can be applied and that these are neither totally independent nor critical.

If an interaction requiring no metabolic activation is postulated as the initiating event, this can be tested only by structure–activity relationships; *i.e.*, the more potent carcinogens should interact more strongly or more extensively than the weaker carcinogens. Even if this criterion is met, the test is not critical since the identity of the receptor is not known. Alternatively, if metabolic activation to a reactive intermediate is postulated, this can be tested by showing that the metabolic intermediate is more carcinogenic than the parent compound. However, a negative result in such a test is not conclusive, particularly if the intermediate is chemically unstable.

For these reasons, an evaluation of the current status of knowledge about the mechanism of action of polynuclear carcinogens can only be made on a tentative basis. No incontrovertible evidence has showed that metabolic activation of aromatic hydrocarbons plays any role in their carcinogenic action. The arguments consistent with the idea that metabolic activation is involved are that:

1. Correlations are found between binding to cellular macromolecules and carcinogenic potency;

2. The existence of chemically reactive metabolites (arene oxides) has been demonstrated;

3. Arene oxides exhibit high biological activities;

4. Carcinogenesis can be inhibited by the inhibition of metabolism;

5. Metabolism is involved in the toxic action of aromatic hydrocarbons. These could perhaps be considered to outweigh the arguments against this idea which are that:

1. No class of metabolite (including arene oxides) exhibits higher carcinogenic activity than the parent hydrocarbons;

2. Non-covalent interactions between carcinogens and cellular macromolecules do occur;

3. Inhibition of carcinogenesis can be effected by inducing metabolizing enzymes;

4. Carcinogenic activity may be enhanced by the inhibition of metabolizing enzymes.

If it is assumed that the metabolic activation of polycyclic hydrocarbons is obligatory for carcinogenic action, it must be admitted that the identity of the active metabolite involved remains unknown. The current favorites are the arene oxides but again, evidence for and against requires a careful evaluation. On the positive side, arene oxides are known metabolic intermediates, react *in vitro* or in cell cultures with cellular macromolecules, and exhibit a wide range of biological activities *in vitro*. This must be weighed against the contraindications which are that arene oxides are not generally more effective carcinogens than the parent hydrocarbons and that, for the one arene oxide studied (7-methyl-5,6-benz[a]anthracene oxide), the products of reaction with DNA *in vitro* are different from the products of binding of the parent hydrocarbon to DNA in cells.

Another possibility is that reactive esters of hydroxymethyl metabolites might be the active agents for methyl-substituted hydrocarbons. There is little evidence in favor of this postulate since such esters are not known metabolites, model compounds for such esters are not more effective carcinogens than the parent compounds, and although these models do react with cellular macromolecules, the products of these reactions are not the same as those formed when the parent compound is bound in cells.

Many other possible structures have been suggested for active metabolites. These include carbocations, free radicals, and radical cations, but there is not enough experimental data available to evaluate these. In their studies of the one-electron transfer oxidation of 7,12-dimethylbenz[a]anthracene, Fried and Schumm (256) directed attention towards 7-formyl-12-methylbenz[a]anthracene and 12-formyl-7-methylbenz[a]anthracene as possible active metabolites of this polycyclic hydrocarbon. The former compound is certainly a potent carcinogen (Table III).

Experimental studies of the carcinogenic activities of hydrocarbon metabolites indicate that the 3-methylcholanthrene-1- and 2-ones are probably the most active metabolites identified to date. The carcinogenic activities of these metabolites has not stimulated further research. The reason for this is that similar metabolites could not be envisaged for most of the polycyclic hydrocarbon carcinogens since they do not contain the five-membered ring of cholanthrene. However, it is now known that certain arene oxides can rearrange to phenols through a ketone intermediate, that K-region arene oxides are formed metabolically from many potent hydrocarbon carcinogens, and that a K-region ketone should not rearrange to a phenol very easily. Another class of potentially active metabolites of the polycyclic hydrocarbons is, therefore, the K-region ketones.

Before leaving this particular aspect of hydrocarbon carcinogenesis, the studies of 2-acetylaminofluorene should be mentioned once more. Metabolic activation is involved in the carcinogenic action of this carcinogen [see Miller and miller (130)]. This is perhaps the most compelling evidence in favor of the idea that metabolic activation is involved in the carcinogenic action of other carcinogens, such as the polynuclear compounds.

The most outstanding contemporary achievement in the polynuclear carcinogen field is the recent clarification of the detailed mechanisms involved in the microsomal metabolism of polynuclear carcinogens. Further developments in this area, particularly in the extension of the detailed kinetic and mechanistic analyses to the more complex (but also more carcinogenic) tetra- and pentacyclic compounds will be of interest. Knowledge of the products of metabolism of polycyclic hydrocarbons in animals and in various *in vitro* systems has also grown considerably over the years and has provided the necessary foundation and mechanistic outline for these recent developments. However, with regard to the identification or quantitation of hydrocarbon metabolites, the conflicting evidence on the extent of metabolic attack at the K-regions of the highly carcinogenic compounds, such as 7,12-dimethylbenz-[a]anthracene, seems to require further clarification.

Another general worry concerns the limited experimental evidence upon which the "noncarcinogenic" status of many polynuclear compounds depends. Recent reexaminations of "inactive" compounds have revealed that several such compounds exhibit initiating activity, even if they have not been found to be complete carcinogens.

In conclusion, perhaps the current central issue in the mechanism of action of polynuclear carcinogens should be restated. Does a metabolite mediate in the carcinogenic action of polynuclear carcinogens? If this is so, the metabolite has not yet been identified. However, the lack of definitive proof of the involvement of a metabolite cannot be construed as proof that a metabolite is not involved.

Addendum

The published work on polynuclear aromatic carcinogens since the completion of the original chapter (March 1973) is too extensive for comprehensive review. However, papers which have resolved some of the questions raised or which have led to major changes in or additions to the knowledge presented at that time are summarized below.

Recent studies on the chemistry of polynuclear aromatic carcinogens have been concerned largely with the synthesis and properties of arene oxides. The original route to K-region oxides (135) was the closure of the appropriate dialdehyde with tris[dimethylamino]phosphine, and non-K-region oxides were obtained by dehydration of the trans diols with the dimethylacetal of dimethylformamide (*260, 261*) or by converting the more readily obtainable cis diols *via* 2-alkoxy-1,3-dioxolanes into halohydrin esters. These yield the oxides after treatment with base (*262*). Halohydrin esters in a saturated ring of a polycyclic hydrocarbon are now used to synthesize non-K-region oxides also (*263, 264*).

The suggestion that K-region ketones might mediate the carcinogenic action of polycyclic hydrocarbons (p. 303) was put forward independently by Newman and Olson (*265*). They isolated tautomeric mixtures of phenols and ketones in attempts to prepare the K-region phenols of 7,12-dimethylbenz[a]anthracene. Harvey *et al.* (*261*) also isolated the 5-oxo-5,6-dihydro derivative after reductive cleavage of 5-acetoxy-7,12-dimethylbenz[a]anthracene. Dipple *et al.* (*266*) prepared both the 5- and 6-oxo-5,6-dihydro derivatives *via* acid-catalyzed dehydration of the cis diol but these ketones did not exhibit any carcinogenic activity in mice. Since these authors could not confirm the earlier report (*156*) of the K-region ketones of benzo[a]pyrene, the predominance of K-region ketones over phenols at ambient temperature may be confined to the methylbenz[a]anthracenes. Although the keto form of 9-phenanthrol has not been isolated, its existence at low temperature (77°K) is evident from infrared spectra of uv-irradiated suspensions of the 9,10-oxide in Nujol (*267*).

Studies of the reaction of 1,2-naphthalene oxide with various nucleophiles indicate that substitution usually occurs on the 2-position (*268, 269*). This has cast doubt on the earlier structural assignment for the glutathione conjugate formed metabolically from this oxide (*see* Figure 8 and Table XII). The glutathione residue was assigned to the 1-position because a 1-substituted naphthalene was obtained after dehydration (*133, 140, 149*). However, Jeffrey and Jerina (*269*) have shown that dehydration of *trans* 1-hydroxy-2-thioethyl-1,2-dihydronaphthalene yields 1-thioethylnaphthalene. This results from migration of the thioethyl group *via* a cyclic sulfonium intermediate. A similar migration was also implicated in the dehydration of the analogous glutathione derivative. The glutathione residues in Figure 8 and Table XII might be more correctly assigned, therefore, to the 2-position. This simplifies scheme II of Figure 8 in that the 1,2-naphthalene oxide is now combined with both water or glutathione by reaction through the 2-position. It is no longer necessary to attribute to the epoxide hydrase and the glutathione transferase enzymes specificities for directing nucleophilic attack at the 1-position and 2-position of the oxide, respectively, (*see* p. 283). A variety of studies testify to the involvement of arene oxides in the metabolism of aromatic substrates by hepatic tissues. In the formation of meta-hydroxylated metabolites from nitrobenzene, methyl phenyl sulfide, and methyl phenyl sulfone, however, it appears that arene oxides are not necessarily involved (*270*).

A direct hydroxylation mechanism for the formation of hydroxymethyl metabolites from methyl-substituted hydrocarbons was inferred earlier (p. 289) from extrapolations of the studies with ethyl benzene (*167*). This has been confirmed by Grandjean and Cavalieri (*271*) who examined the microsomal metabolites produced from 7-methylbenz[a]anthracene and 7,12-dimethylbenz[a]anthracene in the presence of $H_2{}^{18}O$ or ${}^{18}O_2$.

It has now been established, in contrast to some earlier reports (*168*), that the potent carcinogens, 7,12-dimethylbenz[*a*]anthracene and benzo[*a*]-pyrene, are subject to metabolic attack at their K-regions (*169, 272*). Moreover, the earlier expectation that the glutathione conjugate should be the major metabolite (p. 291) at the K-region for these compounds seems to be justified for metabolism in rat liver preparations (*169*). The general theme which arose in the original discussion of the metabolic products formed at double bonds in aromatic hydrocarbons (p. 286–291, Table XII) was that the distribution of metabolic products depended upon the bond localization energy of the particular bond concerned. This holds true for 7,12-dimethyl-benz[*a*]anthracene where a glutathione conjugate is the major metabolic product at the K-region and a dihyrodiol is the major metabolic product at the 8,9-double bond (*169*). A similar situation obtains for benz[*a*]anthracene. Booth and Sims (*273*) have shown that the presence of glutathione and soluble enzymes have little effect on the rate of microsomal conversion of the hydrocarbon to the 8,9-dihydrodiol, but the rate of production of the 5,6-dihydrodiol is markedly inhibited. Furthermore, in a system containing both epoxide hydrase and glutathione transferase activities, benz[*a*]anthracene 5,6-oxide, was converted to a glutathione conjugate more rapidly than was the 8,9-oxide while the 8,9-oxide was converted to a diol more rapidly than the 5,6-oxide (*273*).

The predominance of dihydrodiols as metabolites at some of the non-K-region double bonds may well be an important factor in the activation of the polycyclic hydrocarbons to carcinogenic metabolites. Recent developments in this area have arisen through further studies of the interaction of these carcinogens with DNA (p. 299). Brown *et al.* (*247*) found that the microsome-catalyzed binding of 7,8-dihydro-7,8-dihydroxybenzo[*a*]pyrene to DNA was 10-fold greater than that of the hydrocarbon itself. This suggested that this non-K-region diol might be an intermediate in the binding of benzo[*a*]-pyrene to DNA. Subsequently, Sims and his co-workers (*275*) showed that the analogous 8,9-dihydrodiol of benz[*a*]anthracene was metabolically converted to 8,9-dihydro-8,9-dihydroxybenz[*a*]anthracene 10,11-oxide. This compound reacted with DNA to yield products which were chromatographically inseparable from those formed when benz[*a*]anthracene was bound to DNA cells or when the diol was bound to DNA in microsomal systems (*275*). In studies with the more potent carcinogen, benzo[*a*]pyrene, similar observations implicating 7,8-dihydro-7,8-dihydroxybenzo[*a*]pyrene 9,10-oxide in the binding reaction with DNA were made (*276*).

If DNA is the cellular receptor which is modified in the initiation stage of carcinogenesis, it appears that a possibly general mechanism of metabolic activation of polycyclic hydrocarbons has now been defined. This involves the initial formation of a non-K-region diol which is subsequently converted to a diol-epoxide. Hulbert (*277*) has pointed out that two geometrical isomers of such diol-epoxides are possible and has deduced that, in the preferred conformation of one of these isomers, internal hydrogen bonding could lead to the generation of a stabilized internal ion pair. Although the suggestion that carbonium ions may be the ultimate carcinogens for polycyclic hydrocarbons is not new (*116*), the generation of such species through diol-epoxides is a very attractive concept. The diol-epoxide isolated by Booth and Sims (*275*) was relatively stable, and these authors may not have been studying the highly reactive geometrical isomer.

The recent switch of interest away from the K-regions of the polycyclic hydrocarbons was prompted by the low carcinogenic potencies of the K-region oxides and the different products obtained when the reaction of a K-region oxide with DNA was compared to the binding of the parent hydrocarbon to DNA in cellular systems (*235*). This difference in products has subsequently been confirmed for two other hydrocarbons (*259, 276*). Exogenously supplied K-region oxides will react with DNA of cells in culture (*235*), but a similar reaction of endogenously produced K-region oxide does not take place. The reason for the latter must presumably be that the oxide produced by metabolism is completely consumed by further metabolic reactions yielding glutathione conjugates and dihydrodiols. Similarly, the non-K-region oxides, 8,9-benz[*a*]anthracene oxide and 7,8-benzo[*a*]pyrene oxide, appear to be consumed by further metabolism to yield the corresponding dihydrodiols. These, however, undergo further metabolism to diol-epoxides and, for reasons not yet apparent, these escape further metabolism and are able to react with the cellular DNA.

Further confirmation of the role played by diol-epoxides in the carcinogenic action of the hydrocarbons requires a study of the carcinogenic potencies of these metabolites. These studies are in progress in some laboratories at this time, and the results will no doubt be availble before publication of this discussion.

Acknowledgments

The author wishes to express his gratitude to Helen Anton for her expert assistance in the preparation of this manuscript, to his colleagues, P. Sims, W. M. Baird, and P. D. Lawley for valued discussions, and to M. M. Coombs for a preview of one of his papers. The Chester Beatty Research Institute receives grants from the Medical Research Council and the Cancer Research Campaign.

Literature Cited

1. Pott, P., "Chirurgical Observations" (1775), Reprinted in *Natl. Cancer Inst. Monogr.* (1963) **10**, 7.
2. Yamagiwa, K., Ichikawa, K., *Mitt. Med. Fak. Tokio* (1915) **15**, 295.
3. Tsutsui, H., *Gann* (1918) **12**, 17.
4. Bloch, B., Dreifuss, W., *Schweiz. Med. Wochenschr.* (1921) **51**, 1033.
5. Kennaway, E. L., *J. Pathol. Bacteriol.* (1924) **27**, 233.
6. Kennaway, E. L., *Br. Med. J.* (1925) **2**, 1.
7. *Ibid.* (1955) **2**, 749.
8. Hieger, I., *Biochem. J.* (1930) **24**, 505.
9. Kennaway, E. L., Hieger, I., *Br. Med. J.* (1930) **1**, 1044.
10. Clar, E., *Ber. Dtsch. Chem. Ges.* (1929) **62**, 350.
11. Cook, J. W., Hewett, C. L., Hieger, I., *J. Chem. Soc.* (1933) 395.
12. Prehn, R. T., *J. Natl. Cancer Inst.* (1964) **32**, 1.

13. Clayson, D. B., "Chemical Carcinogenesis," J. and A. Churchill, London, 1962.
14. Hueper, W. C., Conway, W. D., "Chemical Carcinogenesis and Cancers," C. C. Thomas, Springfield, 1964.
15. Badger, G. M., *Br. J. Cancer* (1948) **2**, 309.
16. Badger, G. M., *Adv. Cancer Res.* (1954) **2**, 73.
17. Arcos, J. C., Arcos, M., *Prog. Drug Res.* (1962) **4**, 407.
18. Buu-Hoï, N. P., *Cancer Res.* (1964) **24**, 1511.
19. Arcos, J. C., Argus, M. F., *Adv. Cancer Res.* (1968) **11**, 305.
20. Lacassagne, A., Buu-Hoï, N. P., Daudel, R., Zajdela, F., *Adv. Cancer Res.* (1956) **4**, 315.
21. Hartwell, J. L., "Survey of Compounds Which Have Been Tested for Carcinogenic Activity," U.S. Public Health Service Publication No. **149**, Washington, D.C., 1951.
22. Shubik, P., Hartwell, J. L., "Survey of Compounds Which Have Been Tested for Carcinogenic Activity," Supplement 1, U.S. Public Health Service, Publication No. **149**, Washington, D.C., 1957.
23. *Ibid.*, Supplement 2, U.S. Public Health Service, Publication No. **149**, Washington, D.C., 1969.
24. Thompson, J. I. and Company, "Survey of Compounds Which Have Been Tested for Carcinogenic Activity," 1968–1969 Volume, U.S. Public Health Service Publication No. **149**, Washington, D.C., 1968–1969.
25. Iball, J., *Am. J. Cancer* (1939) **35**, 188.
26. Fieser, L. F., *Am. J. Cancer* (1938) **34**, 37.
27. Berenblum, I., *Cancer Res.* (1945) **5**, 561.
28. Lacassagne, A., Buu-Hoï, N. P., Zajdela, F., Lavit-Lamy, D., *C.R. Acad. Sci. Paris* (1961) **252**, 826.
29. Van Duuren, B. L., Sivak, A., Langseth, L., Goldschmidt, B. M., Segal, A., *Natl. Cancer Inst. Monogr.* (1968) **28**, 173.
30. Lacassagne, A., Buu-Hoï, N. P., Zajdela, F., *C.R. Acad. Sci. Paris* (1960) **250**, 3547.
31. Scribner, J. D., *J. Natl. Cancer Inst.* (1973) **50**, 1717.
32. Lacassagne, A., Buu-Hoï, N. P., Zajdela, F., Lavit-Lamy, D., *C.R. Acad. Sci. Paris* (1964) **259**, 3899.
33. Hoffmann, D., Wynder, E. L., *Z. Krebsforsch.* (1966) **68**, 137.
34. Barry, G., Cook, J. W., Haslewood, G. A. D., Hewett, C. L., Hieger, I., Kennaway, E. L., *Proc. Roy. Soc. B* (1935) **117**, 318.
35. Bottomley, A. C., Twort, C. C., *Am. J. Cancer* (1934) **20**, 781.
36. Bachmann, W. E., Cook, J. W., Dansi, A., De Worms, C. G. M., Haslewood, G. A. D., Hewett, C. L., Robinson, A. M., *Proc. Roy. Soc. B* (1937) **123**, 343.
37. Van Duuren, B. L., Sivak, A., Segal, A., Orris, L., Langseth, L., *J. Natl. Cancer Inst.* (1966) **37**, 519.
38. Lijinsky, W., Garcia, H., Saffiotti, U., *J. Natl. Cancer Inst.* (1970) **44**, 641.
39. Van Duuren, B. L., Sivak, A., Goldschmidt, B. M., Katz, C., Melchionne, S., *J. Natl. Cancer Inst.* (1970) **44**, 1167.
40. Lacassagne, A., Buu-Hoï, N. P., Zajdela, F., *Eur. J. Cancer* (1968) **4**, 123.
41. Huggins, C. B., Pataki, J., Harvey, R. G., *Proc. Natl. Acad. Sci. U.S.A.* (1967) **58**, 2253.
42. Dipple, A., Slade, T. A., *Eur. J. Cancer* (1971) **7**, 473.
43. Roe, F. J. C., Dipple, A., Mitchley, B. C. V., *Br. J. Cancer* (1972) **26**, 461.
44. Miller, J. A., Miller, E. C., *Cancer Res* (1963) **23**, 229.
45. Pataki, J., Huggins, C. B., *Biochem. Pharmacol.* (1967) **16**, 607.
46. Pataki, J., Duguid, C., Rabideau, P. W., Huisman, H., Harvey, R. G., *J. Med. Chem.* (1971) **14**, 940.
47. Pataki, J., Balick, R., *J. Med. Chem.* (1972) **15**, 905.
48. Flesher, J. W., Sydnor, K. L., *Cancer Res.* (1971) **31**, 1951.

49. Dipple, A., Slade, T. A., *Eur. J. Cancer* (1970) **6**, 417.
50. Boyland, E., Sims, P., *Int. J. Cancer* (1967) **2**, 500.
51. Boyland, E., Sims, P., Huggins, C., *Nature (London)* (1965) **207**, 816.
52. Bergmann, E. D., Blum, J., Haddow, A., *Nature (London)* (1963) **200**, 480.
53. Cook, J. W., Schoental, R., *Br. J. Cancer* (1952) **6**, 400.
54. Lacassagne, A., Buu-Hoï, N. P., Zajdela, F., Lavit-Lamy, D., *C.R. Acad. Sci. Paris* (1961) **252**, 1711.
55. Lacassagne, A., Buu-Hoï, N. P., Zajdela, F., Saint-Ruf, G., *C.R. Acad. Sci. Paris* (1968) **266**, 301.
56. Lacassagne, A., Buu-Hoï, N. P., Zajdela, F., *C.R. Acad. Sci. Paris* (1958) **246**, 95.
57. Nagata, C., Tagashira, Y., Inomata, M., Kodama, M., *Gann* (1971) **62**, 419.
58. Heidelberger, C., Baumann, M. E., Griesbach, L., Ghobar, A., Vaughan, T. M., *Cancer Res.* (1962) **22**, 78.
59. Coombs, M. M., Croft, C. J., *Prog. Exp. Tumor Res.* (1969) **11**, 69.
60. Coombs, M. M., Bhatt, T. S., Croft, C. J., *Cancer Res.* (1973) **33**, 832.
61. Lacassagne, A., Buu-Hoï, N. P., Zajdela, F., Périn, F., Jacquignon, P., *Nature (London)* (1961) **191**, 1005.
62. Lacassagne, A., Buu-Hoï, N. P., Zajdela, F., Jacquignon, P., Périn, F., *C.R. Acad. Sci. Paris* (1963) **257**, 818.
63. Lacassagne, A., Buu-Hoï, N. P., Zajdela, F., Mabille, P., *C.R. Acad. Sci. Paris* (1964) **258**, 3387.
64. Lacassagne, A., Buu-Hoï, N. P., Zajdela, F., Perrin-Roussel, O., Jacquignon, P., Périn, F., Hoeffinger, J-P., *C.R. Acad. Sci. Paris* (1970) **271**, 1474.
65. Zajdela, F., Buu-Hoï, N. P., Jacquignon, P., Dufour, M., *Br. J. Cancer* (1972) **26**, 262.
66. Sellakumar, A., Shubik, P., *J. Natl. Cancer Inst.* (1972) **48**, 1641.
67. Lacassagne, A., Buu-Hoï, N. P., Zajdela, F., Jacquignon, P., Mangane, M., *Science* (1967) **158**, 387.
68. Lacassagne, A., Buu-Hoï, N. P., Zajdela, F., Stora, C., Mangane, M., Jacquignon, P., *C.R. Acad. Sci. Paris* (1971) **272**, 3102.
69. Haddow, A., Kon, G. A. R., *Br. Med. Bull.* (1947) **4**, 314.
70. Williams, D. J., Rabin, B. R., *Nature (London)* (1971) **232**, 102.
71. Litwack, G., Ketterer, B., Arias, I. M., *Nature (London)* (1971) **234**, 466.
72. Hewett, C. L., *J. Chem. Soc.* (1940) 293.
73. Waravdekar, S. S., Ranadive, K. J., *J. Natl. Cancer Inst.* (1957) **18**, 555.
74. Wynder, E. L., *Br. Med. J.* (1959) **1**, 317.
75. Wynder, E. L., Hoffmann, D., *Cancer* (1959) **12**, 1194.
76. Clar, E., "Polycyclic Hydrocarbons," Vols. 1 and 2, Academic, London, 1964.
77. Coulson, C. A., "Valence," University Press, Oxford, 1952.
78. Pullman, A., Pullman, B., *Adv. Cancer Res.* (1955) **3**, 117.
79. Coulson, C. A., *Adv. Cancer Res.* (1953) **1**, 1.
80. Pullman, A., *C.R. Acad. Sci. Paris* (1945) **221**, 140; *Compt. rend. soc. biol.* (1945) **139**, 1056.
81. Pullman, A., *Ann. Chim. (Paris)* (1947) **2**, 5.
82. Pullman, A., *C.R. Acad. Sci. Paris* (1953) **236**, 2318.
83. Schmidt, O., *Z. Phys. Chem.* (1938) **39**, 59.
84. *Ibid.* (1939) **42**, 83; **43**, 185; **44**, 193.
85. Schmidt, O., *Naturwissenschaften* (1941) **29**, 146.
86. Svartholm, N. V., *Arkiv. Kemi. Minerol. Geol.* (1941) **A15**, No. 13.
87. Buu-Hoï, N. P., Daudel, P., Daudel, R., Lacassagne, A., Lecocq, J., Martin, M., Rudali, G., *C.R. Acad. Sci. Paris* (1947) **225**, 238.
88. Greenwood, H. H., *Br. J. Cancer* (1951) **5**, 441.
89. Pagès-Flon, M., Buu-Hoï, N. P., Daudel, R., *C.R. Acad. Sci. Paris* (1953) **236**, 2182.
90. Coulson, C. A., Longuet-Higgins, H. C., *Rev. Sci.* (1947) **85**, 929.

91. Berthier, G., Coulson, C. A., Greenwood, H. H., Pullman, A., *C.R. Acad. Sci. Paris* (1948) **226,** 1906.
92. Baldock, G., Berthier, G., Pullman, A., *C.R. Acad. Sci. Paris* (1949) **228,** 931.
93. Pullman, B., Pullman, A., *Nature (London)* (1963) **199,** 467.
94. Pullman, B., Pullman, A., Umans, R., Maigret, B., *Jerusalem Symp. Quantum Chem. and Biochem.* (1969) **1,** 325.
95. Matsen, F. A., *J. Chem. Phys.* (1956) **24,** 602.
96. Hedges, R. M., Matsen, F. A., *J. Chem. Phys.* (1958) **28,** 950.
97. Lovelock, J. E., Zlatkis, A., Becker, R.S., *Nature (London)* (1962) **193,** 540.
98. Kooyman, E. C., Farenhorst, E., *Nature (London)* (1952) **169,** 153.
99. Kooyman, E. C., Heringa, J. W., *Nature (London)* (1952) **170,** 661.
100. Pullman, A., *Bull. Soc. Chim. (France)* (1954) **21,** 595.
101. Koutecky, J., Zahradnik, R., *Cancer Res.* (1961) **21,** 457.
102. Flurry, R. L., *J. Med. Chem.* (1964) **7,** 668.
103. Mainster, M. A., Memory, J. D., *Biochim. Biophys. Acta* (1967) **148,** 605.
104. Scribner, J. D., *Cancer Res.* (1969) **29,** 2120.
105. Sung, S.S., *C.R. Acad. Sci. Paris* (1971) **273,** 1247.
106. *Ibid.* (1972) **274,** 1597.
107. Mason, R., *Br. J. Cancer* (1958) **12,** 469; *Nature (London)* (1958) **181,** 820.
108. Chalvet, O., Mason, R., *Nature (London)* (1961) **192,** 1070.
109. Szent–Györgyi, A., Isenberg, I., Baird, S. L., *Proc. Natl. Acad. Sci. U.S.A.* (1960) **46,** 1445.
110. Allison, A. C., Nash, T., *Nature (London)* (1963) **197,** 758.
111. Epstein, S. S., Bulon, I., Koplan, J., Small, M., Mantel, N., *Nature (London)* (1964) **204,** 750.
112. Laskowski, D. E., *Cancer Res.* (1967) **27,** 903.
113. Pullman, A., Berthier, G., Pullman, B., *Acta Unio Contra Cancrum* (1951) **7,** 140.
114. Jones, R. N., *J. Am. Chem. Soc.* (1940) **62,** 148.
115. Kofahl, R. E., Lucas, H. J., *J. Am. Chem. Soc.* (1954) **76,** 3931.
116. Dipple, A., Lawley, P. D., Brookes, P., *Eur. J. Cancer* (1968) **4,** 493.
117. Badger, G. M., *J. Chem. Soc.* (1950) 1809.
118. Mottram, J. C., Doniach, I., *Lancet* (1938) **234,** 1156.
119. Santamaria, L., *Acta Unio Contra Cancrum* (1963) **19,** 591.
120. Epstein, S. S., Small, M., Falk, H. L., Mantel, N., *Cancer Res.* (1964) **24,** 855.
121. Brock, N., Druckrey, H., Hamperl, H., *Arch. Exp. Pathol. Pharmakol.* (1938) **189,** 709.
122. Weil-Malherbe, H., *Biochem. J.* (1946) **40,** 351.
123. Liquori, A. M., deLerma, B., Ascoli, F., Botré, A., Trasciatti, M., *J. Mol. Biol.* (1962) **5,** 521.
124. Boyland, E., Green, B., *Br. J. Cancer* (1962) **16,** 507.
125. Lerman, L., *J. Mol. Biol.* (1961) **3,** 18.
126. Nagata, C., Kodama, M., Tagashira, Y., Imamura, A., *Biopolymers* (1966) **4,** 409.
127. Craig, M., Isenberg, I., *Biopolymers* (1970) **9,** 689.
128. Mason, H. S., *Adv. Enzymol.* (1957) **19,** 79.
129. Khandwala, A. S., Kasper, C. B., *Biochem. Biophys. Res. Comm.* (1973) **54,** 1241.
130. Miller, J. A., Miller, E. C., *J. Natl. Cancer Inst.* (1971) **47,** V.
131. Boyland, E., *Biochemical Soc. Symp.* (1950) **5,** 40.
132. Williams, R. T., "Detoxication Mechanisms," Wiley, New York, 1959.
133. Boyland, E., Sims, P., *Biochem. J.* (1958) **68,** 440.
134. *Ibid.* (1962) **84,** 571.
135. Newman, M. S., Blum, S., *J. Am. Chem. Soc.* (1964) **86,** 5598.

136. Boyland, E., Sims, P., *Biochem. J.* (1965) **97,** 7.
137. Sims, P., *Biochem. J.* (1966) **98,** 215.
138. Jerina, D. M., Daly, J. W., Witkop, B., Zaltzman-Nirenberg, P., Udenfriend, S., *J. Am. Chem. Soc.* (1968) **90,** 6525.
139. Holtzman, J., Gillette, J. R., Milne, G. W. A., *J. Am. Chem. Soc.* (1967) **89,** 6341.
140. Jerina, D. M., Daly, J. W., Witkop, B., Zaltzman-Nirenberg, P., Udenfriend, S., *Biochemistry* (1970) **9,** 147.
141. Kasperek, G. J., Bruice, T. C., Yagi, H., Jerina, D. M., *J.C.S. Chem. Comm.* (1972) 784.
142. Booth, J., Boyland, E., Sims, P., *Biochem. J.* (1960) **74,** 117.
143. Vogel, E., Klärner, F. G., *Angew. Chem. Int. Ed. Eng.* (1968) **7,** 374.
144. Guroff, G., Daly, J. W., Jerina, D. M., Renson, J., Witkop, B., Udenfriend, S., *Science* (1967) **158,** 1524.
145. Jerina, D. M., Daly, J. W., Witkop, B., *J. Am. Chem. Soc.* (1968) **90,** 6523.
146. Boyd, D. R., Daly, J. W., Jerina, D. M., *Biochemistry* (1972) **11,** 1961.
147. Sims, P., *Biochem. J.* (1959) **73,** 389.
148. Corner, E. D. S., Young, L., *Biochem. J.* (1955) **61,** 132.
149. Boyland, E., Ramsay, G. S., Sims, P., *Biochem. J.* (1961) **78,** 376.
150. Sims, P., *Biochem. J.* (1964) **92,** 621.
151. *Ibid.* (1962) **84,** 558.
152. Boyland, E., Sims, P., *Biochem. J.* (1962) **84,** 564.
153. *Ibid.* (1964) **90,** 391.
154. *Ibid.,* **91,** 493.
155. *Ibid.* (1960) **77,** 175.
156. Raha, C. R., *Bull. Soc. Chim. Biol.* (1970) **52,** 105.
157. Pullman, A., Pullman, B., *Jerusalem Symp. Quantum Chem. Biochem.* (1969) **1,** 9.
158. Kasperek, G. J., Bruice, T. C., *J. Am. Chem. Soc.* (1970) **94,** 198.
159. Pandov, H., Sims, P., *Biochem. Pharmacol.* (1970) **19,** 299.
160. Grover, P. L., Sims, P., *Biochem. Pharmacol.* (1970) **19,** 2251.
161. Kuroki, T., Heidelberger, C., *Biochemistry* (1972) **11,** 2116.
162. Abell, C. W., Heidelberger, C., *Cancer Res.* (1962) **22,** 921.
163. Ketterer, B., Ross-Mansell, P., Whitehead, J. K., *Biochem. J.* (1967) **103,** 316.
164. Ketterer, B., Beale, D., Litwack, G., Hackney, J. F., *Chem. Biol. Interactions* (1971) **3,** 285.
165. Boyland, E., Sims, P., *Biochem. J.* (1965) **95,** 780.
166. *Ibid.* (1967) **104,** 394.
167. McMahon, R. E., Sullivan, H. R., Craig, J. C., Pereira, W. E., *Arch. Biochem. Biophys.* (1969) **132,** 575.
168. Sims, P., *Biochem. Pharmacol.* (1970) **19,** 795.
169. Booth, J., Keysell, G. R., Sims, P., *Biochem. Pharmacol.* (1973) **22,** 1781.
170. Keysell, G. R., Booth, J., Sims, P., Grover, P. L., Hewer, A., *Biochem. J.* (1972) **129,** 41p.
171. Selkirk, J. K., Huberman, E., Heidelberger, C., *Biochem. Biophys. Res. Comm.* (1971) **43,** 1010.
172. Grover, P. L., Hewer, A., Sims, P., *Febs. Letters* (1971) **18,** 76.
173. Grover, P. L., Hewer, A., Sims, P., *Biochem. Pharmacol.* (1972) **21,** 2713.
174. Boyland, E., Sims, P., *Biochem. J.* (1965) **95,** 788.
175. Sims, P., *Biochem. J.* (1971) **125,** 159.
176. *Ibid.* (1972) **130,** 27.
177. Sims, P., *Xenobiotica* (1972) **2,** 469.
178. Waterfall, J. F., Sims, P., *Biochem. J.* (1972) **128,** 265.
179. Pataki, J., Huggins, C. B., *Cancer Res.* (1969) **29,** 505.
180. Sims, P., *Int. J. Cancer* (1967) **2,** 505.
181. Miller, E. C., *Cancer Res.* (1951) **11,** 100.

182. Wiest, W. G., Heidelberger, C., *Cancer Res.* (1953) **13**, 250.
183. Heidelberger, C., Moldenhauer, M. G., *Cancer Res.* (1956) **16**, 442.
184. Heidelberger, C., Davenport, C. R., *Acta Unio Contra Cancrum* (1961) **17**, 55.
185. Heidelberger, C., *J. Cell Comp. Physiol.* (1964) **64**, 129.
186. Brookes, P., Lawley, P. D., *Nature (London)* (1964) **202**, 781.
187. Miller, J. A., Miller, E. C., *Adv. Cancer Res.* (1953) **1**, 339.
188. Boveri, T. H., *Zur Frage der Entstehung maligner Tumoren*, Gustav Fischer, Jena, 1914.
189. Grover, P. L., Sims, P., *Biochem. J.* (1968) **110**, 159.
190. Gelboin, H. V., *Cancer Res.* (1969) **29**, 1272.
191. Grover, P. L., Forrester, J. A., Sims, P., *Biochem. Pharmacol.* (1971) **20**, 1297.
192. Kuroki, T., Huberman, E., Marquardt, H., Selkirk, J. K., Heidelberger, C., Grover, P. L., Sims, P., *Chem. Biol. Interactions* (1971/72) **4**, 389.
193. Haddow, A., *J. Pathol. Bacteriol.* (1938) **47**, 581.
194. Vasiliev, J. M., Guelstein, V. I., *J. Natl. Cancer Inst.* (1963) **31**, 1123.
195. Diamond, L., *Trans. N.Y. Acad. Sci.* (1970) **32**, 234.
196. Diamond, L., Defendi, V., Brookes, P., *Cancer Res.* (1967) **27**, 890.
197. Andrianov, L. N., Belitsky, G. A., Ivanova, O. J., Khesina, A. Y., Khitrovo, S. S., Shabad, L. M., Vasiliev, J. M., *Br. J. Cancer* (1967) **21**, 566.
198. Gelboin, H. V., Huberman, E., Sachs, L., *Proc. Natl. Acad. Sci. U.S.A.* (1969) **64**, 1188.
199. Conney, A. H., Miller, E. C., Miller, J. A., *J. Biol. Chem.* (1957) **228**, 753.
200. Wattenberg, L. W., Leong, J. L., *J. Histochem. Cytochem.* (1962) **10**, 412.
201. Gelboin, H. V., Blackburn, N. R., *Cancer Res.* (1964) **24**, 356.
202. Wattenberg, L. W., Page, M. A., Leong, J. L., *Cancer Res.* (1968) **28**, 934.
203. Nebert, D. W., Gelboin, H. V., *J. Biol. Chem.* (1968) **243**, 6250.
204. Huggins, C., Grand, L., Fukunishi, R., *Proc. Natl. Acad. Sci. U.S.A.* (1964) **51**, 737.
205. Wattenberg, L. W., Leong, J. L., *Proc. Soc. Exp. Biol. Med.* (1968) **128**, 940.
206. Wheatley, D. N., *Br. J. Cancer* (1968) **22**, 787.
207. Wattenberg, L. W., Leong, J. L., *Cancer Res.* (1970) **30**, 1922.
208. Miyaji, T., Moskowski, L. I., Senoo, T,. Ogata, M., Odo, T., Kawai, K., Sayama, Y., Ishida, H., Matsuo, H., *Gann* (1953) **44**, 281.
209. Miller, E. C., Miller, J. A., Brown, R. R., MacDonald, J. C., *Cancer Res.* (1958) **18**, 469.
210. Miller, E. C., Miller, J. A., Hartmann, H. A., *Cancer Res.* (1961) **21**, 815.
211. Miller, J. A., Cramer, J. W., Miller, E. C., *Cancer Res.* (1960) **20**, 950.
212. Diamond, L., Gelboin, H. V., *Science* (1969) **166**, 1023.
213. Gelboin, H. V., Wiebel, F., Diamond, L., *Science* (1970) **170**, 169.
214. Kinoshita, N., Gelboin, H. V., *Proc. Natl. Acad. Sci. U.S.A.* (1972) **69**, 824.
215. Kinoshita, N., Gelboin, H. V., *Cancer Res.* (1972) **32**, 1329.
216. Diamond, L., McFall, R., Miller, J., Gelboin, H. V., *Cancer Res.* (1972) **32**, 731.
217. Wiebel, F. J., Leutz, J. C., Diamond, L., Gelboin, H. V., *Arch. Biochem. Biophys.* (1971) **144**, 78.
218. Miller, E. C., Miller, J. A., *Proc. Soc. Exp. Biol. Med.* (1967) **124**, 915.
219. Van Duuren, B. L., Langseth, L., Orris, L., Baden, M., Kuschner, M., *J. Natl. Cancer Inst.* (1967) **39**, 1217.
220. Grover, P. L., Sims, P., Huberman, E., Marquardt, H., Kuroki, T., Heidelberger, C., *Proc. Natl. Acad. Sci. U.S.A.* (1971) **68**, 1098.
221. Marquardt, H., Kuroki, T., Huberman, E., Selkirk, J. K., Heidelberger, C., Grover, P. L., Sims, P., *Cancer Res.* (1972) **32**, 716.
222. Huberman, E., Kuroki, T., Marquardt, H., Selkirk, J. T., Heidelberger, C., Grover, P. L., Sims, P., *Cancer Res.* (1972) **32**, 1391.

223. Huberman, E., Aspiras, L., Heidelberger, C., Grover, P. L., Sims, P., *Proc. Natl. Acad. Sci. U.S.A.* (1971) **68,** 3195.
224. Cookson, M. J., Sims, P., Grover, P. L., *Nature New Biol.* (1971) **234,** 186.
225. Ames, B. N., Sims, P., Grover, P. L., *Science* (1972) **176,** 47.
226. Fahmy, O. G., Fahmy, M. J., *Cancer Res.* (1973) **33,** 2354.
227. Grover, P. L., Sims, P., *Biochem. J.* (1972) **129,** 41p.
228. Flesher, J. W., Sydnor, K. L., *Int. J. Cancer* (1970) **5,** 253.
229. Lieberman, M. W., Dipple, A., *Cancer Res.* (1972) **32,** 1855.
230. Venitt, S., Tarmy, E. M., *Biochim. Biophys. Acta* (1972) **287,** 30.
231. Rayman, M. P., Dipple, A., *Biochemistry* (1973) **12,** 1538.
232. Dipple, A., Brookes, P., Mackintosh, D. S., Rayman, M. P., *Biochemistry* (1971) **10,** 4323.
233. Rayman, M. P., Dipple, A., *Biochemistry* (1973) **12,** 1202.
234. Lawley, P. D., *Prog. Nucleic Acid Res. Mol. Biol.* (1966) **5,** 89.
235. Baird, W. M., Dipple, A., Grover, P. L., Sims, P., Brookes, P., *Cancer Res.* (1973) **33,** 2386.
236. Nagata, C., Kodama, M., Tagashira, Y., *Gann* (1967) **58,** 493.
237. Nagata, C., Inomata, M., Kodama, M., Tagashira, Y., *Gann* (1968) **59,** 289.
238. Inomata, M., Nagata, C., *Gann* (1972) **63,** 119.
239. Lorentzen, R., Caspary, W., Ts'o, P. O. P., "Abstracts of Papers," 162nd National Meeting, ACS, 1971, Biol. **26.**
240. Ts'o, P. O. P., Lu, P., *Proc. Natl. Acad. Sci. U.S.A.* (1964) **51,** 272.
241. Rice, J. M., *J. Am. Chem. Soc.* (1964) **86,** 1444.
242. Rapaport, S. A., Ts'o, P. O. P., *Proc. Natl. Acad. Sci. U.S.A.* (1966) **55,** 381.
243. Morreal, E. C., Dao, T. L., Eskins, K., King, C. L., Dienstag, J., *Biochim. Biophys. Acta* (1968) **169,** 224.
244. Umans, R. S., Lesko, S. A., Ts'o, P. O. P., *Nature (London)* (1969) **221,** 763.
245. Lesko, S. A., Ts'o, P. O. P., Umans, R. S., *Biochemistry* (1969) **8,** 2291.
246. Udenfriend, S., Clark, C. T., Axelrod, J., Brodie, B. B., *J. Biol. Chem.* (1954) **208,** 731.
247. Hoffmann, H. D., Lesko, S. A., Ts'o, P. O. P., *Biochemistry* (1970) **9,** 2594.
248. Antonello, C., Carlassare, F., Musajo, L., *Gazz. Chim. Ital.* (1968) **98,** 30.
249. Cavalieri, E., Calvin M., *Photochem. Photobiol.* (1971) **14,** 641.
250. Blackburn, G. M., Fenwick, R. G., Thompson, M. H., *Tetrahedron Lett.* (1972) **7,** 589.
251. Hoffmann, H. D., Müller, W., *Jerusalem Symp. Quantum Chem. Biochem.* (1969) **1,** 183.
252. Wilk, M., Bez, W., Rochlitz, J., *Tetrahedron* (1966) **22,** 2599.
253. Rochlitz, J., *Tetrahedron* (1967) **23,** 3043.
254. Wilk, M., Girke, W., *Jerusalem Symp. Quantum Chem. Biochem.* (1969) **1,** 91.
255. Jeftic, L., Adams, R. N., *J. Am. Chem. Soc.* (1970) **92,** 1332.
256. Fried, J., Schumm, D. E., *J. Am. Chem. Soc.* (1967) **89,** 5508.
257. Daly, J. W., Jerina, D. M., Witkop, B., *Experientia* (1972) **28,** 1129.
258. Cavalieri, E., "Abstracts of Papers," 166th Natl. Meeting, ACS, 1973, Biol. 193.
259. Swaisland, A. J., Hewer, A., Pal, K., Keysell, G. R., Booth, J., Grover, P. L., Sims, P., *Febs. Letters* (1974) **47,** 34.
260. Goh, S. H., Harvey, R. G., *J. Am. Chem. Soc.* (1973) **95,** 242.
261. Harvey, R. G., Goh, S. H., Cortez, C., *J. Am. Chem. Soc.* (1975) **97,** 3468.
262. Dansette, P., Jerina, D. M., *J. Am. Chem. Soc.* (1974) **96,** 1224.
263. Yagi, H., Jerina, D. M., *J. Am. Chem. Soc.* (1973) **95,** 243.
264. *Ibid.* (1975) **97,** 3185.
265. Newman, M. S., Olson, D. R., *J. Am. Chem. Soc.* (1974) **96,** 6207.
266. Dipple, A., Levy, L. S., Iype, P. T., *Cancer Res.* (1975) **35,** 652.

267. Jerina, D. M., Witkop, B., McIntosh, C. L., Chapman, O. L., *J. Am. Chem. Soc.* (1974) **96,** 5578.
268. Jeffrey, A. M., Yeh, H. J. C., Jerina, D. M., DeMarinis, R. M., Foster, C. H., Piccolo, D. E., Berchtold, G. A., *J. Am. Chem. Soc.* (1974) **96,** 6929.
269. Jeffrey, A. M., Jerina, D. M., *J. Am. Chem. Soc.* (1975) **97,** 4427.
270. Tomaszewski, J. E., Jerina, D. M., Daly, J. W., *Biochemistry* (1975) **14,** 2024.
271. Grandjean, C., Cavalieri, E., *Biochem. Biophys. Res. Commun.* (1974) **61,** 912.
272. Kinoshita, N., Shears, B., Gelboin, H. V., *Cancer Res.* (1973) **33,** 1937.
273. Booth, J., Sims, P., *Biochem. Pharmacol.* (1974) **23,** 2547.
274. Borgen, A., Darvey, H., Castagnoli, N., Crocker, T. T., Rasmussen, R. E., Wang, I. Y., *J. Med. Chem.* (1973) **16,** 502.
275. Booth, J., Sims, P., *Febs Letters* (1974) **47,** 30.
276. Sims, P., Grover, P. L., Swaisland, A., Pal, K., Hewer, A., *Nature (London)* (1974) **252,** 326.
277. Hulbert, P. B., *Nature (London)* (1974) **256,** 146.

Chapter

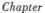

6

Soots, Tars, and Oils as Causes of Occupational Cancer

M. D. Kipling, Department of Employment, Employment Medical Advisory Service, Auchinleck House, Broad Street, Birmingham, B15 1DL, England

THE OBSERVATION THAT the incidence of skin cancer increased in workers exposed to soot, tar, and oil and that it was possible to induce similar cancers in animals resulted in world wide research to isolate the active carcinogenic constituents. Population studies have been particularly fruitful in Britain where notification of occupational skin cancers to the Factory Inspectorate has been obligatory for over 50 years.

Cancer of the skin occurring in chimney sweeps and caused by soot was first described in 1775 by Pott (1). Since then tar (2), pitch (3), and mineral oil (4) have been shown to be carcinogenic to the skin. There is also evidence that internal organs may be affected (5, 6, 7).

Domestic soots are the products of imperfect combustion of carbonaceous materials, such as wood, coal, and oil. They consist of finely divided carbon particles, hydrocarbons, and tars. The presence of carcinogens was first shown experimentally in mice (8). Later benzo(a)pyrene (formerly 3,4-benzpyrene) was identified as a carcinogenic constituent (9). Wood soot in a smoked-sausage factory was also shown to be carcinogenic (10). Industrial soots (carbon blacks for industry) are produced by the incomplete combustion of natural gas or oil residues and were also shown to contain benzo(a)pyrene (11).

Coal tar and pitch are the residual products of coal distillation. Contact with them has led to an increased incidence of skin cancer (12) and, in gas workers, of lung cancer (13, 14). Tar was first shown to be a carcinogen experimentally in 1915 by Yamagiwa and Ichikara (15) who painted it on a rabbit's ears for 11 years. Later, similar results were produced in mice (16, 17). Coal tar pitch (18), anthracene oil (19), and creosote derivatives of coal tar (20) were also shown to be carcinogenic, and skin cancers were pro-

315

duced from blast furnace tar (21). Carcinogenic tars were manufactured synthetically from various sources such as isoprene, acetylene, skin, yeasts, and cholesterol. It was shown that carcinogenicity increased coincidentally with the temperature involved in the distillation of tars (19) and that the carcinogenic potency of tars prepared at temperatures of 500°, 600°, and 750°C materially increased with the preparation temperature (22).

The observation that carcinogenic tars fluoresced with a spectrum similar to that of benz(a)anthracene led, in 1932, to the identification of benzo(a)-pyrene as a carcinogenic agent (23). Later dibenzo(a,h)pyrene, dibenzo(a,i)-pyrene, benzo(b)fluoranthene, and dibenz(a,h)anthracene (24) were shown also to be carcinogenic constituents (see Figure 1). This important class of carcinogens is reviewed separately in Chapter 5, and carcinogenic hazards associated with smoking and air pollution are covered in Chapter 7.

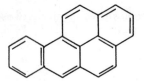

Benzo[a]pyrene

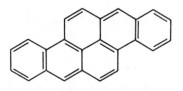

Dibenzo[a,h]pyrene

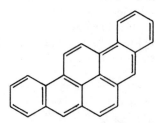

Dibenzo[a,i]pyrene

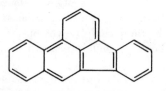

Benzo[b]fluoranthene

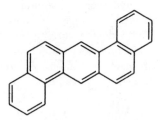

Dibenzo[a,h]anthracene

Nature, London
Figure 1.   Hydrocarbons isolated from coal-tar pitch (23, 24)

Shale Oil

Shale oil is derived from shale formed at the bottom of shallow lakes out of inorganic material and the debris of plants and aquatic organisms. Its final composition varies in different parts of the world. Oil has been distilled from shale, and it may be an important industry in the future.

The first case of carcinoma attributed to shale oil was described in 1876 (*4*). Its carcinogenicity was shown experimentally (*25*), and the presence of benzo(*a*)pyrene and other polycyclic hydrocarbons was later demonstrated (*26*). These substances could not be demonstrated in the parent rock shale, suggesting that the heat used in production was important in the formation of carcinogens. Shale oil distilled below 250°C contained carcinogenic compounds other than benzo(*a*)pyrene (*27*).

Petroleum Oils

Petroleum oils are formed by the decomposition of animal and vegetable matter affected by heat and pressure in the earth's crust. They vary in final composition in different parts of the world and consist of hydrocarbons (paraffinic and naphthenic) with compounds of sulfur, oxygen, and nitrogen. Sulfur is in the highest concentration (up to 6%) and nitrogen the lowest (about 0.1%). Benzo(*a*)pyrene was isolated in a specimen of cracked oil (*28*), and its presence was demonstrated in crude oil (*29*).

In 1968 the Medical Research Council in the United Kingdom published their report (*30*) on the "Carcinogenic Action of Mineral Oils," based on work done in several British universities. In an attempt to isolate specific carcinogens, crude oils from fields in Kuwait, Oklahoma, and Lagunillas were steam distilled under reduced pressure. The most biologically active fractions (boiling range 300°–400°C) were distilled further. Aliquots of the fractions (350°–390°C) obtained on a Stedman still were treated with maleic anhydride, picric acid, and chromatographed on alumina (*31*). Other fractions (390°–410°C) were extracted in a small vacuum column. The carcinogenic activity appeared to lie in materials boiling above 350°C (presence in lower boiling fractions was possibly the result of azeotropism), and it was still present in fractions boiling at 420°C. It was extracted with acetone–water and appeared with the polycyclic aromatic fraction during absorption chromatography. Over 40 chemical compounds were isolated from mineral oil fractions, many for the first time, by repeated chromatography, complexing with picric acid and trinitrobenzene, and fractional crystallization. Further studies of the nature of the active compounds did not identify any single highly potent carcinogen. Several of the compounds separated were structurally similar to very potent carcinogens, and the total activity of the oil could be caused by the combined effect of several individually weak carcinogens.

Compounds isolated included a wide range of aromatic hydrocarbons, *e.g.*, di-, tri-, and tetramethylnaphthalenes and phenanthrenes, chrysene and methyl derivatives, perylene, triphenylene, and tetramethylfluorene. Heterocyclic compounds included di- and tetramethyldibenzothiophenes, thiabenzofluorene, and tetra- and pentamethylcarbazoles. A few representative compounds are shown in Figure 2.

Three-ring compounds are generally not carcinogenic, and the dimethylanthracenes isolated were all inactive except for 9,10-dimethylanthracene. Benz(a)anthracene, although only weakly active, is the parent compound of several known carcinogens. For example, 10-methylbenz(a)anthracene, also isolated and positively identified, is weakly active on rabbit skin but apparently not on mouse skin. Another member of this "family," 9,10-dimethylbenz(a)-anthracene, was isolated but not positively identified and is a weak carcinogen. The isomeric 7,12-dimethylbenz(a)anthracene (formerly 9,10-dimethylbenz-1,2-anthracene, the standard strong carcinogen, but never identified in the oil fractions) was used in this work. The activity of chrysene, which was also identified, is variously reported in the literature; it may be slightly active. Several of the dimethyl derivatives of chrysene, but not any identified in the oil, are active. Of the heterocyclic compounds separated from the oil, only 1,3,6,7-tetramethyldibenzothiophene is weakly active.

In 1971 the problem of carcinogens in oil was reviewed (29). Since it appeared that solvent or other comparable refining processes reduced the amounts of polycyclic aromatic hydrocarbons in oil, it was concluded that they would reduce or eliminate the risk of skin cancer. The reliability of tests for the total polycyclic aromatic content of oil or of those compounds that might cause skin cancer was investigated. The results of new laborious techniques that isolate benzo(a)pyrene from crude oil were compared with the simpler measurement of ultraviolet absorbance (derived from FDA 121, 2589(c) of the United States Code of Federal Regulations, Title 21), measurement of total aromatic carbon by infrared spectroscopy (32), or mass spectrometry (33). The measurement of ultraviolet absorbance was the most satisfactory and the infrared determination of aromatic carbon content the least. No method was accurate enough to be of value.

Soots

Today, exposure to domestic chimney soot is not significant, and chimney sweeps' cancer is rare, because chimney sweeps no longer climb inside chimneys. However, exposure to carbon black occurs among its manufacturers and users, notably rubber and paint makers. No increased incidence of cancer has been attributed to exposure to carbon black in this work probably because polycyclic hydrocarbons are adsorbed onto the carbon black particles (11). It is not established that the polycyclics in rubber from carbon black and oil used as an extender are released by the action of heat and solvents in molding to produce a carcinogenic risk.

Pitch and Tar

Exposure to pitch and tar occurs mainly in the coal, gas, and coke industries, in steel-making plants, and in the manufacture of patent fuels. The development of pitch and tar warts is not uncommon in these industries.

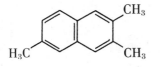

2,3,6-Trimethylnaphthalene

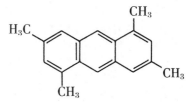

1,3,5,7-Tetramethylanthracene

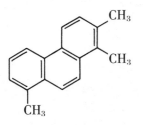

1,2,8-Trimethylphenanthrene

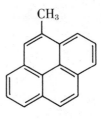

4-Methylpyrene

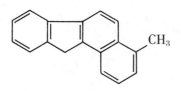

4-Methylbenzo[a]fluorene

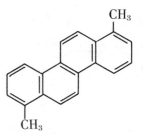

1,7-Dimethylchrysene

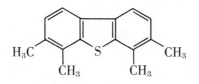

1,2,7,8-Tetramethyldibenzothiophene

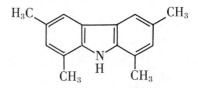

1,3,6,8-Tetramethylcarbazole

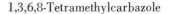

Medical Research Council (Great Britain) Specialist Report Series
Figure 2. Representative compounds isolated from mineral oil fractions (30)

Sporadic cases of skin cancer occur among workers engaged in embedding optical lenses, jointing drain pipes, creosoting railroad sleepers, and manu-facturing accumulator cases, carbon electrodes, brushes, pitch fiber pipes, and roofing material. Pipe benders and dippers, manufacturers of felt, crucibles, and clay pigeons from clay and pitch have also been affected. Recently attention has been drawn to the occurrence of growths on the lips of fishermen who hold the twine for net making in their teeth (34). Gas workers exposed to products of coal carbonization showed increased incidence of lung (and probably also bladder) cancer. Mortalities were 3.06 per 1000 for retort workers compared with 1.81 for lung cancer in the comparable age and sex groups of the general population and 0.31 per 1000 as compared with 0.14 for bladder cancer. Work as topman on the retorts was a particular hazard (35). Among steelworkers in the United States the mortality from respiratory cancer increased two-fold in coke oven workers (13).

Lubricating and Cutting Oils

The first description of cancer of the scrotum in a Scottish shale oil worker was in 1876 (4). Later, a user of shale oil in cotton mule spinning died from the disease (36). During 22 years 19 cases of skin cancer, of which three were scrotal, occurred in paraffin process workers, and 46 cases, of which 28 were scrotal, occurred among the other workers such as retortmen and stillmen (36).

The cotton mule spinning industry in Great Britain originally used shale oil to lubricate the spindles. Mules are machines on which a carriage moves back and forth requiring the operator to lean over so that his groin is con-taminated by the spray from the spindles and from direct contact with oil on the carriage. From 1920 to 1943 there were 1303 recorded cases of skin cancer in the British textile industry, of which 824 were scrotal. There were 615 fatal cases of scrotal cancer recorded between 1911 and 1938 (37).

Cancer from oil in the metal-working industry, particularly among work-ers in automatic machine shops, was first found to be an appreciable risk in a survey carried out in Birmingham, England (38, 39). Between 1950 and 1967, 187 cases of scrotal cancer occurred in this region, the majority of which could be attributed to oil (40). In 1966, for example, 16 of 19 recorded cases of scrotal cancer in Birmingham were caused by oil (41).

Toolsetters or setter operators in an automatic shop using neat (i.e., not emulsified) cutting oil run the greatest risk of skin cancer because their work requires them to constantly lean over the machine with subsequent contamina-tion of the groin. In Birmingham, England, bar automatic machine workers showed a high incidence of cancer from oil. Other metal-working occupational sources of scrotal cancer include metal rolling, tube drawing, metal hardening, and general machine operating. The major risk is from exposure to neat oils, but occasionally soluble emulsions have been incriminated. The industries with automatic shops and the nut-and-bolt manufactuers are affected most. Cases have also arisen from exposure by changing transformer oil in electrical substations, painting or spraying of mold oil for brick and tile making or concrete molding, drop forging, rubber mixing, wire drawing, rope making, in the jute industry, and from grease in metal working (*42*). No cases occurred from handling oil in garages or from diesel oil (*43*).

In the United States, studies showed that 9 out of 14 (*44*), 13 out of 27 (*45*), and 22 out of 28 (of whom 12 cotton workers and 10 machinists) (*46*) victims of scrotal cancer had been exposed to oil. Other cases occurred in a works pressing process (*47*).

In the valley of the river Arve in the Savoy Alps of France, at least 60 cases of scrotal cancer and many cases of skin cancer among the bar automatic machine workers (*décolleteurs*) have occurred since 1955. The high incidence in the relatively small population of the valley occurred mainly among the self-employed or workers in small premises (*48*). Contact with neat cutting oils probably caused the epidemic, but other undetected factors might be involved since similar contact in many other centers did not cause a comparable high incidence (*49*).

In females, an increased incidence of cancer of the vulva was found in cotton operatives in the United Kingdom and in silver polishers using cloths impregnated with mineral oil (*50*). An excess incidence of cancers other than on the skin (*e.g.*, larynx, lung, and stomach) was attributed to oil mist in mule spinning (*51*). Recent evidence indicates that victims of scrotal cancer show a significant increase in cancers of the respiratory tract or upper digestive tract (*52*).

Preventive measures have reduced the incidence and severity of skin cancers in industry (*53*). In Britain the Mule Spinning Regulations of 1952 have ensured that since 1953 only oil drastically refined with sulfuric acid is used in cotton spinning and that mule spinners are examined medically every six months. These measures and the marked decline of mule spinning have resulted in a sustained decline in the incidence of scrotal cancer in Great Britain (*54*). Voluntary medical examinations were provided in the shale oil and gas industries and, along with shower baths, are required by law in patent-fuel plants. In the metal-working industry routine medical examinations were arranged in a few plants where experience has shown that there is a special risk. Warning leaflets (SHW 259A) with colored illustrations of the early stages of lesions caused by oil on the hands and scrotum are distributed to all people exposed to oil. This information has enhanced early detection and treatment in many cases of scrotal cancer. The use of solvent-refined oils is also strongly recommended. The recent award of damages to the widow of a man who had scrotal cancer has led to widespread publicity that has aided in educating workers and management. A high standard of cleanliness and the use of guards on the machinery are advised, but a survey of the hygienic conditions in machine shops showed the condition is not necessarily connected with poor hygienics among the workers (*42*).

The great disparity of the number of reported cases caused by pitch, tar, and oil in the United Kingdom and other countries is not easily explained. Only in the French Alps has the incidence of scrotal cancer been comparable with that in England (*49*). The high incidence of skin cancer in British workers has been attributed to lack of hygiene, but a factor of real importance may be that legal notification since 1923, compensation by the State since 1910, and registration of tumors at the Regional Cancer Registries since 1936 have provided a greater knowledge of its occurrence than elsewhere. This theory is supported by the apparent great excess of bladder tumors in rubber workers and cancers from asbestos exposure in Great Britain as compared with other countries—an excess that cannot readily be attributed to other causes.

Literature Cited

1. Pott, P., "Chirurgical Works," Vol. 5, p. 63, London, 1775.
2. Volkmann, R., *Beitr. Chirurg., Leipzig* (1875) **370.**
3. Manouviriez, A., *Ann. Hyg. Publique* (1876) **45,** 459.
4. Bell, J., *Edinburgh Med. J.* (1876) **22,** 135.
5. Butlin, H. T., *Br. Med. J.* (1892) **1,** 1341.
6. Southam, A., *Rep. Int. Conf. Cancer* (1928), 280.
7. Kennaway, E. L., Kennaway, N. M., *Brit. J. Cancer* **1,** 260.
8. Passey, R. D., *Br. Med. J.* (1922) **2,** 112.
9. Goulden, F., Tipler, M. M., *Brit. J. Cancer* (1949) **3,** 157.
10. Sulman, E., Sulman, F., *Cancer Res.* (1946) **6,** 366.
11. Falk, H. L., Steiner, P. E., *Cancer Res.* (1952) **12,** 30.
12. Heller, J., *J. Ind. Hyg.* (1930) **12,** 169.
13. Lloyd, J. W., *J. Occup. Med.* (1971) **13,** 53.
14. Doll, R., *Br. J. Ind. Med.* (1952) **9,** 180.
15. Yamagiwa, K., Ichikawa, K., *J. Jap. Path. Ges.* (1915) **5,** 142.
16. Tsutsui, H., *Gann* (1918) **12,** 17.
17. Murray, J. A., *Br. Med. J.* (1921) **2,** 795.
18. Passey, R. D., Woodhouse, J. L., *J. Pathol. Bacteriol.* (1925) **28,** 145.
19. Kennaway, E. L., *Br. Med. J.* (1925) **2,** 1.
20. Lenson, N., *New Engl. J. Med.* (1956) **254,** 520.
21. Bonser, G. M., *Lancet* (1932) **I,** 775.
22. Twort, C. C., Fulton, J. D., *J. Pathol. Bacteriol.* (1930) **33,** 119.
23. Cook, J. W., Hewett, C., Hieger, I., *Nature, Lond.* (1932) **130,** 926.
24. Badger, G. M., "The Chemical Basis of Carcinogenic Activity," p. 9, Thomas, Springfield, Ill., 1962.
25. Leitch, A., *Brit. Med. J.* (1922) **2,** 1104.
26. Berenblum, I., Schoental, R., *Br. J. Exp. Pathol.* (1943) **24,** 232.
27. Bogovski, P., *Vop. Onkol.* (1959) **5,** 486.
28. Tye, R., Graf, M. J., Horton, A. W., *Anal. Chem.* (1955) **27,** 248.
29. Catchpole, W. M., MacMillan, E., Powell, H., *Ann. Occup. Hyg.* (1971) **14,** 171.
30. *Med. Res. Counc. (G. Brit.) Spec. Rep. Ser.* (1968) **306,** 10.
31. King, P. J., *Ind. Lubric. Tribology* (Aug., 1969) 231.
32. Brandes, G., *Brennst. Chem.* (1956) **37,** 263.
33. Gallegus, E. T., *Anal. Chem.* (1967) **39,** 1833.
34. Haddow, A. J., *Ann. Rept., Regional Cancer Committee, Univ. Glasgow, 8th,* (1968) 33.
35. Doll, R., Fisher, R. E. W., Gammon, E. J., Gunn, W., Hughes, G. O., Tyrer, F. H. Wilson, W., *Br. J. Ind. Med.* (1965) **22,** 1.
36. Henry, S. A., "Cancer of the Scrotum in Relation of Occupation," p. 16, Oxford Univ. Press, Oxford (1946).
37. *Ibid.,* p. 43.
38. Cruickshank, C. N. D., Squire, J. R., *Br. J. Int. Med.* (1950) **7,** 1.
39. Cruickshank, C. N. D., Gourevitch, A., *Br. J. Ind. Med.* (1952) **9,** 74.

40. Waterhouse, J. A. H., *Ann. Occup. Hyg.* (1971) **14,** 161.
41. Kipling, M. D., *Trans. Soc. Occup. Med.* (1969) **19,** 39.
42. Kipling, M. D., *Ann. Roy. Coll. Surgeons* (1974) **55,** 74.
43. Kipling, M. D., *Ann. Rep., H.M. Chief Inspector Factories, (1967),* (1968) 113.
44. Graves, R., Flo, S., *J. Urol.* (1940) **43,** 309.
45. Dean, A. L., *J. Urol.* (1948) **61,** 511.
46. Kickham, C. J., Dufresne, M., *J. Urol.* (1967) **98,** 108.
47. Hendricks, N. V., *Arch. Ind. Health* (1959) **19,** 524.
48. Thony, C., Thony, J., "Le Cancer du Décolleteur," Centre de Médecine du Travail de Cluses, 1970.
49. Kipling, M. D., *Trans. Soc. Occup. Med.* (1971) **21,** 73.
50. Cooke, M. A., Kipling, M. D., *Arch. Mal. Prof.* (1973) **34,** 244.
51. Henry, S. A., *Br. Med. Bull.* (1947) **4,** 392.
52. Holmes, J. G., Kipling, M. D., Waterhouse, J. A. H., *Lancet* (1970) **II,** 214, 967.
53. Kipling, M. D., *Ann. Roy. Coll. Surgeons* (1974) **55,** 79.
54. Waterhouse, J. A. H., *Ann. Occup. Hyg.* (1971) **14,** 164.

Chapter

7

Environmental Respiratory Carcinogenesis

Dietrich Hoffmann and Ernst L. Wynder, Divisions of Environmental Carcinogenesis and Epidemiology, Naylor Dana Institute for Disease Prevention, American Health Foundation, Valhalla, N.Y., 10595

In 1912, ADLER PUBLISHED a monograph on lung cancer (*1*). The rarity of the disease at that time prompted the author to ask: "Is it worthwhile to write a monograph on primary malignant tumors of the lung?" Today, cancer of the respiratory tract is one of the commonest causes of death in developed countries (*2*). In the United States, England, and Wales, for instance, it is now the most common cause of cancer death among males.

A detailed study of the epidemiological history of lung cancer illustrates that environmental factors play a crucial role in the incidence of this disease. Thirty years ago, more women than men died of cancer; today the reverse is true (Figure 1). This remarkable change is mainly due to a sharp increase in the incidence of lung cancer in men. With the exception of cancer of the pancreas, the death rates of other types of human cancer have decreased or remained relatively stable (Figure 2) (*2*).

Prospective and retrospective studies have implicated three factors in the overall increase of lung cancer—tobacco (especially cigarette smoking), urban pollution, and (to a minor extent) the emergence of new industrial environments. The epidemiological studies which demonstrated the dramatic increase in lung cancer provided the main impetus for the bioassays and chemical–analytical studies in tobacco and air pollution carcinogenesis and occupational cancer of the respiratory tract. In addition to these research activities, increased emphasis has been placed on the reduction and removal of carcinogens from the human respiratory environment.

Industrial Carcinogens

Carcinogenic stimuli in occupational respiratory environments appear to have relatively little effect on the overall incidence of human cancers (Table I). Whatever influence does exist must be separated from the tumor-

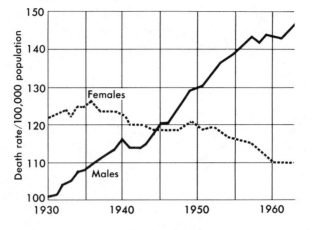

Cancer Mortality for Selected Sites

Figure 1.   Age adjusted cancer death rate by sex;
U.S., 1930–1963 (2)

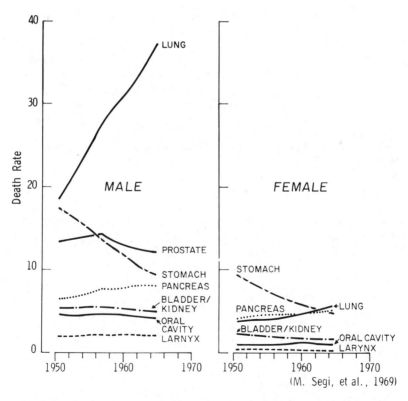

Cancer Mortality for Selected Sites

Figure 2.   Time trends for cancers reportedly related to tobacco smoke and
other air pollutants; U.S. white (2)

Table I.   Relative Contribution of Suggested Carcinogenic
Inhalants to Cancer Death Rates[a]

Cancer Site	Tobacco Smoke	Polluted Air	Occupational Environment
Respiratory tract			
oral cavity	++++	−	−
larynx	++++	−	?
lung	++++	+?	+
Gastrointestinal tract			
esophagus	+++	−	−
stomach	−	?	−
pancreas	++	−	−
liver	−	−	+
Genitourinary tract			
kidney	+++	−	+
bladder	+++	−	+
prostrate	−	?	?

[a] Excess death as percentage of total cancer deaths at specific site: ++++ = >50%, +++ = 10–50%, ++ = 1–10%, + = 0.1–1%, − = 0.0%.

igenic stimulus of tobacco smoke. Nevertheless, for specific industrial groups, certain exposures to inhaled pollutants are of obvious importance, especially since such exposure is usually preventable (Table II). Furthermore, the study of occupational cancer results often in leads to the actual chemical nature of human carcinogens and their elimination, or at least reduction, from the environment.

Radioactive Aerosols. The oldest known occupational respiratory cancer hazard has been associated for centuries with the mining of radio-active ores. However, it was only in 1879 that Härting and Hesse recognized that the primarly ailment of Schneeberg miners was lung cancer (3). A follow-up of the miners from the Schneeberg and Joachimsthal regions in Germany showed that lung cancer represented between 41.5 and 83.0% of all deaths from all causes. It has been estimated that during a miner's life-time, the total radiation exposure of the nuclei of the basal cells of the respiratory epithelium amounts to 14,000–257,000 rads (4). These miners might have inhaled also as much as 6 g of dust, silica, arsenic, and cobalt during every 7-hr working day.

Another group of miners of radioactive ores, those working in Saint Lawrence, Newfoundland, were the subjects of a retrospective study covering 1933–1961 (5). Of the 630 miners studied, 69 died—36.2% of them from lung cancer. For these miners, it was estimated that the average radiation dose to the bronchial epithelium ranged between 1,000 and 18,000 rads, although the maximum exposure could have been much higher.

Uranium workers provide a recent example of occupational lung cancer in the U.S. (6). Among 3314 white miners, 10 deaths from lung cancer were expected based on the incidence of lung cancer in the general population.

However 62 deaths were observed. It is of more than academic interest that all but two of the lung cancer patients were smokers. Of the remaining 60 cases, 56 smoked 20–50 cigarettes a day, and 4 smoked as few as 10 cigarettes daily.

In the case of the uranium miners from the United States, and most likely also of those from Newfoundland, we are probably not dealing with an irradiation insult alone. Synergistic effect appears to exist between radiation and cigarette smoke and/or mining dust. However, the population at risk was exposed concurrently to several carcinogenic factors in these instances as well as in other cases of environmental carcinogenesis. Cancer of the bronchi in asbestos workers (7), and perhaps in some selective urban populations, represents another example of concurrent exposure to several carcinogens. This subject is discussed in another chapter of this monograph (8).

Arsenicals. Inorganic arsenicals have been long suspected to act as carcinogens in the respiratory tract following their introduction into occupational environments and their use as drugs, in food, and in drinking water (9, 10). In most cases where arsenicals are the suspected lung carcinogen, the workers had also been exposed to radioactive materials or dust from

Table II.   Epidemiological and Experimental Evidences for Carcinogenicity of Industrial Inhalants

Carcinogens	Site[a]	Evidences[b] Epidemiological	Evidences[b] Experimental
Aromatic amines	bladder (1895)	++	++
Arsenic	skin (1820)	++	?
	bronchi (1951)	++	—
Asbestos	bronchi (1935)	++	++
	mesothelium (1955)	++	++
Beryllium	lung (1954)	?	+
Chloromethyl ethers	bronchi (1968)	++	++
Chromate	bronchi (1936)	++	++
	nose (1953)	?	?
Coke oven fumes	bronchi (1971)	++	++
	kidney (1972)	+	?
Isopropyl oil	nasal cavity (1946)	+	?
Mustard gas	bronchi (1925)	++	+
Nickel	bronchi (1933)	++	++
	nasal cavity (1933)	++	—
Radioactive aerosols	lung (1879)	++	++
Vinyl chloride	angiosarcoma of the liver (1974)	++	++
Wood dust	nasal cavity (1951)	++	?

[a] Number in parenthesis is the year the agent was first suspected to be a human carcinogen.

[b] ++ = established, + = suggestive, — = negative, ? = questionable or not tested.

gold, nickel, or cobalt. The fact that several of the arsenic-containing materials alone are carcinogens in certain occupational settings motivated Doll and Shubik to place arsenicals in the group of suspected carcinogens (11, 12). This classification is supported by inconclusive data from bioassays for carcinogenicity of arsenicals (13).

We have, however, listed arsenic as an established skin and lung carcinogen (Table II). Several considerations suggested the more cautious conclusion. First, the studies by Doll, Shubik, and others were not intended to disqualify arsenicals as possible carcinogens in man at this time, but rather to point to the many still unresolved problems related to the carcinogenic effect of materials containing arsenic. Secondly, Roth has reported excess deaths from lung cancer in German vineyard workers who used arsenic as pesticides (14). He studied 27 deaths among workers in the Moselle region who developed chronic arsenic poisoning after being exposed to arsenic insecticides over 12–14 years. Death occurred 8–14 years after these pesticides had been banned in the vineyards and involved 12 cases of lung cancer, one of which was bilateral.

This and other observations caused arsenicals to be prohibited as insecticides in many developed countries. This ban included their use on tobacco plants. In 1950–51, Satterlee reported an average of 46 μg of arsenic in popular American types of cigarettes (15), whereas the last available data for 1967 showed average values of 7.7 $\pm$ 0.5 μg of arsenic (16). Hopefully, this downward trend will continue, and increased attention will be given to reducing occupational exposure to arsenicals and their intake in food and water.

Chromium. A now classical example of occupational cancer is cancer of the lung in chromate workers. For the past 60 years, a steady increase occurred in the production and use of chromite ore, chromium metal, chromium alloys, and chromium compounds. After the first reports from Germany in 1936–38 (17), several retrospective studies confirmed a steady increase of lung cancer among chromium workers in Europe and the U.S. (10). About 80% of the reported lung cancers were squamous cell carcinomas and the rest adenocarcinomas. In 1948, Machele and Gregorius reported that the incidence of cancer of the respiratory tract in workers in the chromate-producing industry in the U.S. was about 16 times higher than in the general population (18). This finding suggests that monochromate is a causative factor for the high death rate from lung cancer. The chromate plant study by Mancuso and Hueper reported similar findings based on six cases of lung cancer among 33 individuals who died (19). The average latent period of exposure was 10.6 years.

Most of the epidemiological studies on cancer of the respiratory tract in chromate workers did not record the smoking history. This led researchers to question the specific role of chromium compounds in the production of cancer (20). Fisher and Riekert studied this aspect and found that among a group of 38 chromate workers with lung cancer, two were nonsmokers, three smoked only pipe and/or cigar, three smoked less than one pack of cigarettes per day, and only five smoked two packs per day (21). The rarity of lung cancer among nonsmokers (22), the low percentage of heavy smokers among this group of lung cancer patients, and the absence of data supporting a different smoking pattern for chromate workers compared with the general population lead us to conclude that in special occupational settings, chromate is a respiratory carcinogen to man (23). It is clear that where respiratory cancer is causally linked to factors in the occupational environment, the smoking history of the patients needs to be recorded. At the same time, we should continue our efforts to inhibit the induction of occupational lung cancer by strict preventive measures.

In the experimental setting, various chromium compounds have been carcinogenic. Compounds yielding the most significant results include chromium oxides and certain chromates, particularly calcium chromate introduced intrapleurally or intramuscularly (24). The most convincing experimental data in support of the human findings are the studies in which pellets containing several forms of chromates and chromic oxides were implanted into bronchi of rats (25). The chromium oxides tested were inactive; however, calcium chromate induced six squamous cell carcinomas and two adenocarcinomas in a group of 100 rats. The observed tumors were histologically comparable with tumors found in the lungs of chromate workers.

Nickel. At the beginning of this century, one of the largest nickel refineries was constructed in Clydach, Wales. This factory used the Mond process as a major step in the purification of nickel. The process is based on the reaction of unrefined nickel powder with carbon monoxide at about 50°C and the decomposition of the separated vapors of nickel tetracarbonyl at 180°C resulting in highly purified nickel.

About 30 years after the opening of the Clydach facility, the Chief Inspector of Factories in England reported 10 cases of nasal cancer among workers on the Mond process (26). The 1948 report listed a total of 82 cases of lung cancer and 47 cases of nasal cancer among the refinery workers in Clydach (27).

In 1968, Sunderman reviewed the occurrence of respiratory cancer in the nickel industry and found that to date, 254 cases of lung cancer and 79 cases of nasal cancer have been reported among nickel workers (process: Mond, smelting, and electrolysis) in Wales, Norway, Germany, Canada, Russia, and Japan (28). Doll examined the death certificates of nickel workers in England for 1938–1947 and 1948–1956 (29, 30) and found that the death rate among nickel workers from lung cancer was 4.9 times that of the general population while the death rate from nasal cancer was 196 times higher. Workers employed at factories using the Mond process had as much as 7.1 and 297 times the risk for lung and nose cancer, respectively, compared with that of the general population. No data on tobacco consumption were available. Doll confirmed that the increased incidence in the rate of cancer among nickel workers is limited to the respiratory tract. The older age distribution observed by Doll for the second period he studied (1948–1956) indicates that the greatest risk occurred some time in the past. Among workers who died in the latter period, there were no excess deaths from the two types of cancer in men under the age of 50.

Morgan, in a report on a particular refinery in South Wales, concluded that no excess deaths from either lung or nose cancer occurred in workers hired after 1924 (*31*). In that year, the manufacturing process was changed in this particular plant. In subsequent years, improvements were made in plant equipment and methods, resulting in less dusty working conditions. At the same time, more careful preventive medical controls were instituted. This supports the concept that an industrial process can be modified to reduce or completely eliminate suspected carcinogenic hazards.

The carcinogenic properties of nickel compounds have been established by numerous experiments (*28*). Nickel metal in pellets or powder form, nickel oxide, nickel sulfide, nickelocene, and nickel carbonyl have been tested and induced tumors in the experimental animal. A large group of additional nickel compounds, as yet untested, are also expected to be carcinogenic. Sunderman's study supports the human findings by reporting the induction of squamous cell carcinoma and adenocarcinomas in the lungs of rats exposed to vapors of nickel carbonyl (*28, 32*). The biochemical alterations which develop in rats after nickel carbonyl exposure were also explored, and from this study, it was suggested that this compound inhibits DNA-dependent RNA synthesis and therefore alters the expression of genetic information (*28*).

Coke Oven Effluents. Coal tar was indicated to be a skin carcinogen as early as 1875 (*33*). Since that time, skin tumors have been reported in various countries among workers handling coal tar and several of its products (*34*). In 1916, Yamagiwa and Ichikawa first found coal tar to be carcinogenic to the animal skin by inducing papillomas and carcinomas in rabbit ears (*35*). In 1933, Cook *et al.* isolated and identified benzo[*a*]-pyrene, a potent carcinogen, from coal tar and, in fact, with it the first carcinogen from an environmental agent (*36*). Since then, about a dozen other carcinogenic polynuclear aromatic hydrocarbons (PAH) have been isolated from coal tar (Table III) (*37*).

In 1936, Kawahata and Kuroda reported the occurrence of 61 cases of lung cancer among workers of one steel company in Japan (*38, 39*). Since then, lung cancer has also been reported in coke oven and gas retort workers in England, the U.S., Canada, and Norway (*10*). However, it was

Table III.

Carcinogens in coal tar[a]

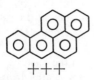

+++

Benzo[*a*]pyrene

+

Benzo[*e*]pyrene

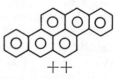

++

Dibenzo[*a,h*]pyrene

Table III.   (Continued)

Carcinogens in coal tar[a] (*continued*)

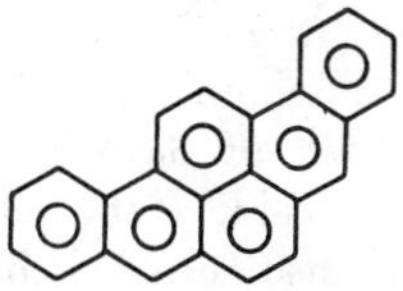

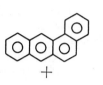

$++$

Dibenzo[*a,i*]pyrene

Benz[*a*]anthracene

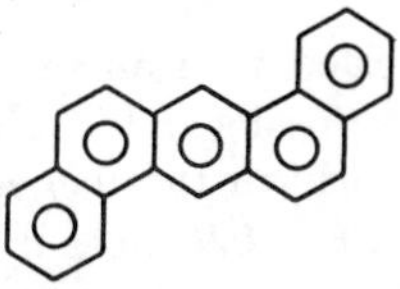

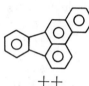

$++$

Dibenz[*a,h*]anthracene

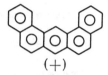

$(+)$

Dibenz[*a,i*]anthracene

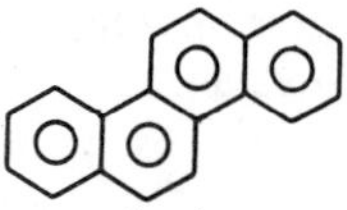

$(+)$

Chrysene

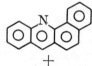

$++$

Benzo[*b*]fluoranthene

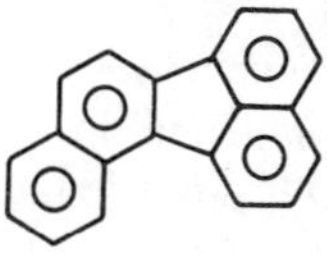

$++$

Benzo[*i*]fluoranthene

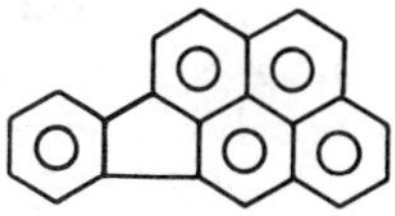

$+$

Indeno[1,2,3-*cd*]pyrene

$+$

Benz[*c*]acridine

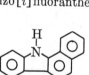

$(+)$

11 H-Benzo[a]carbazole

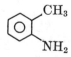

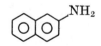

o-Toluidine

β-Naphthylamine

Quinoline

[a] $+++$ = high, $++$ = moderate, $+$ = weak, $(+)$ = possibly weak. Relative carcinogenic activity on mouse skin. Chrysene is present in the coal tar of the Ruhr district (Germany) with an average concentration of 1.5%.

not until 1971–1972 that detailed background information became available for coke oven workers who developed lung cancer (40, 41). At this time, Lloyd and his group presented specific mortality data for 4661 workers from 12 steel plants in the U.S. and Canada. The workers were employed during 1951–1955 at various coke oven sites. A total of 69 lung cancer cases were reported with an overall risk of developing lung cancer of about 2.5 times that predicted for the general population. The relative risk of developing lung cancer for men employed five or more years at the full top side of the coke oven was 6.9 times that predicted. Unexpectedly, the study also revealed that coke oven workers have a 7.5 times greater risk of dying from kidney cancer. The relatively small number of cases involved and the lack of histological verification require further explanation of this interesting epidemiological lead. Despite the absence of smoking data, coke oven workers face unquestionably higher risks of death from lung and kidney cancer.

A study of the high concentration of PAH in the coke oven effluents during the loading period strongly supports the concept that carcinogenic hydrocarbons at least contribute to the high incidence of lung cancer (42).

Chloromethyl Ethers. Clues on the occurrence and nature of environmental carcinogens have been derived almost entirely from human observations. Percival Pott first associated scrotal cancer with soot in chimney sweeps in 1775 (43), radioactive aerosols were first identified as respiratory carcinogens in uranium miners in 1879 (3), and the first conclusive studies implicating cigarette smoke as a lung carcinogen were completed in 1950 (44, 45). Since then, great progress has been made in our knowledge of chemical carcinogenesis and in our ability to predict potential carcinogens. We have also made great strides in developing methods to reduce or even eliminate specific carcinogens from industrial or general environments. An apt example is the identification of chloromethyl ethers as respiratory carcinogens in man and their drastic curtailment in industrial use.

For the last decade, Van Duuren and his associates at the New York University have studied the relationship between the structure of alkylating agents and their carcinogenicity. These investigations have led them to postulate that halo ethers act as potential carcinogens. Of these agents, chloromethyl ether (CMME) was a weak carcinogen, and bis(chloromethyl) ether (BCME) was a powerful carcinogen (46, 47). Furthermore, Laskin et al. subsequently reported the production of bronchiogenic carcinomas and esthesioneuroepitheliomas in relatively high incidence levels by exposure of rats to concentrations of as little as 0.1 ppm of BCME (48). Subsequent investigations at a single factory in which CMME and BCME are widely used as intermediates in organic synthesis and in the preparation of certain ion exchange resins revealed a high incidence rate of lung cancer in CMME workers (49). Commercial CMME contains 1–7% BCME. Of the reported 14 cases of lung cancer, 13 were examined histologically; of these, 12 had oat cell carcinoma, a relatively rare form of lung cancer, and one had a squamous cell carcinoma. With one exception, the time of exposure to the chloromethyl ethers was between 3 and 14 years. The age of first diagnosis varied between 33–55 years with an average age of 45 years. This age is far below the average age of 60 years for male lung cancer patients in general (*50*).

Today the industrial use of chloromethyl ethers has been widely curtailed or stopped altogether (*51*). Bis(chloromethyl) ether is now among the group of 10 carcinogens for which zero tolerance has been proposed (*52*) (Table IV). It is advisable that the laboratory chemist exercise greatest caution in the future use of chloromethyl ethers for experimental purposes.

Table IV.   Ten Carcinogens with Suggested Zero Tolerance for Occupational Environments

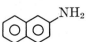

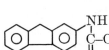

N-Nitrosodi-methylamine   Bis(chloro-methyl) ether   β-Propiolactone

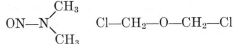

2-Naphthylamine   2-Fluorenylacetamide   4-Dimethylaminoazobenzene

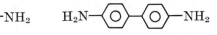

4-Nitrobiphenyl   4-Aminobiphenyl   Benzidine

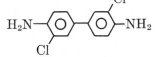

3,3′-Dichlorobenzidine

Vinyl Chloride. At the 10th International Cancer Congress in 1970, Viola reported the induction of skin (Zymbal's) epidermoid carcinomas, lung adenocarcinomas, and some osteochondromas of the limbs in rats exposed to high concentrations of vinyl chloride (VC) (*53, 54*). The animals were exposed to 30,000 ppm of VC for 10 months for 20 hr each week. This and subsequent studies including those by industry have demonstrated the carcinogenicity of VC to mice, rats, and hamsters (*55, 56*). Maltoni and Lefemine induced Zymbal's gland carcinomas, nephroblastomas, and angiosarcomas of the liver and of other locations in rats following 52 weeks of exposure for 20 hr each week. The concentrations of VC were 10,000 ppm (69 rats), 6000 ppm (72 rats), 2500 (74 rats), 500 ppm (67 rats), and 50 ppm (64 rats), with angiosarcomas in 7, 13, 14, 7, 4, and 1 rats, respectively (air controls were negative) (55). The authors also found some liver angiosarcomas in mice exposed to the same concentrations of VC; this has also been reported by Keplinger et al. (56). They exposed three groups of 100 mice each to 2500 ppm, 200 ppm, and 50 ppm VC, respectively, for 7 hr each day for eight months. At that time, the authors found 28, 11, and 2 animals in each group, respectively, with angiosarcomas of the liver.

These experimental data as well as the observation that long-term exposure to VC has induced liver damage and scleroderma-like skin changes ("vinyl chloride disease") (58) in workers have attracted the attention of industrial and governmental hygienists. At the beginning of 1974, seven cases of angiosarcomas in VC workers were reported in the U.S., two cases each in the Federal Republic of Germany and Sweden, and one each in England and Rumania. For the U.S., the incidence rate for angiosarcoma of the liver is 0.0014/100,000 per year (20–30 cases). Based on this rate, one would expect 0.027 cases per 20,000 VC workers. However, the actual number of cases was 13, or about 400 times higher than the rate for the general population (59). Since this figure is calculated on the basis of only 13 cases (May 1974), it is possible that future reporting of cases will significantly increase the risk factor for VC workers.

The case of the carcinogenic activity of vinyl chloride clearly demonstrates that the dissemination of data on carcinogenicity from the laboratory to the public and to industrial and health authorities must be improved. Our health officials must evaluate data immediately and if caution is indicated, actions must be taken to protect workers. The general public and the international community should be informed of such actions as expediently as possible. In the case of VC, the urgency of such data dissemination to all concerned is obvious, since in 1971 alone 7.0×10^9 kg of the monomer vinyl chloride were produced in 73 factories in 26 countries, involving thousands of workers (60).

In the case of angiosarcoma of the liver induced by vinyl chloride, the impact has been relatively easy to detect since we are dealing with a very rare type of cancer and a well defined population. In cases where a newly detected or produced agent is inducing a more common form of cancer, such as carcinoma of the lung, it would be more difficult to detect the increased risk of such a carcinogen for an occupational group. Studies on animals should, however, help to increase our awareness. Tobacco smoke contains up to 16 ng of VC per cigarette and 27 ng per cigar, but it was not detected in ambient laboratory air (149).

The need for quick dissemination of data on carcinogenicity becomes even more urgent in the case the agent is not limited to occupational environments. For example, the Environmental Protection Agency recently estimated that until 1974 U.S. plants were discharging 9×10^7 kg of VC monomer annually into the atmosphere and that 1–2 ppm of VC were detected in the air near these plants (61).

Nitrosamines. Today more than 80 nitrosamines are known to be carcinogenic in experimental animals (62). Another chapter of this monograph (Chapter 11) notes that, at present, there is no direct evidence that the nitrosamines cause cancer in man. In view of the fact, however, that nitrosamines are carcinogenic to the usual laboratory animals, as well as monkeys, birds, amphibia, and fish, and because of the existence of similarities in the metabolism of *N*-nitrosodimethylamine (dimethylnitrosamine) in human and animal tissues *in vitro*, there is a strong possibility that some nitrosamines are carcinogenic to man.

These considerations alone dictate that the greatest cautions be exercised in the industrial use of nitrosamines and that these agents be excluded from household goods and from food. In order to meet these goals, a selective nitrosamine detector was developed by Fines *et al.* which permits detection of nitrosamines at nanogram levels (*63*). Furthermore, we need also new analytical instrumentation to detect trace amounts of those secondary and tertiary amines, and quarternary ammonium salts which in the body can be nitrosated, or dealkylated and nitrosated, to carcinogenic nitrosamines. In the past few years, several studies have demonstrated that certain amines can serve as precursors for nitrosamines and can induce tumors in the experimental animal when fed together with alkali nitrites (*62, 64*). Recently, one study even reported the induction of squamous cell carcinomas in the lungs of rats which were fed high concentrations of heptamethyleneimine hydrochloride and sodium nitrite (*65*).

Although these studies do not prove the carcinogenicity of nitrosamines in man, they should activate our attention to the possibility that in specific cases, ingested nitrosamines or their precursors can induce lung cancer. Certainly, as will be discussed later under "Tobacco Smoke," inhalation remains the most likely route of entry into our respiratory tract for environmental carcinogens and procarcinogens. Nevertheless, lung carcinogens and their precursors may also enter the body *via* the skin or the digestive tract.

Other Industrial Respiratory Carcinogens. It certainly is beyond the scope of this review to discuss all the known or suspected industrial lung carcinogens. We have omitted those carcinogens or suspected carcinogens which occur primarily in only isolated instances in occupational environments. This group of compounds includes such materials as beryllium, isopropyl oil, mustard gas, and wood dust (Table II). One of the more important industrial carcinogens which is receiving wide-spread attention, asbestos, is discussed in another chapter of this monograph (*8*). For information on other industrial respiratory carcinogens, we refer the reader to the subject literature (*10, 34, 66, 67*).

Air Pollution

The effect of atmospheric pollution on the induction of respiratory cancer is difficult to evaluate because of the overriding effect of cigarette smoke (*68, 69*). Lung cancer, however, does occur more commonly in cities, and in fact, a recent committee of the National Academy of Sciences estimated that urban dwellers may have twice as high an incidence rate of lung cancer as those in rural areas (*70*).

Epidemiological Considerations. A number of retrospective and prospective studies have been concerned with the relative influence and nature of the "urban factor" in the etiology of lung cancer. It appears that the urban factor is not only a consequence of atmospheric pollution but also of several other variables (Table V).

The urban excess in lung cancer may in part arise from occupational factors. As discussed above, several occupations face an increased risk of cancer of the respiratory tract; the number of men employed in these, however, is small. Doll stated, "the number of men employed in occupations which are known to carry specific risks of the disease is small and unless new risks are discovered among men employed in common occupations, this factor cannot be of major importance" (71).

Furthermore, rural residents, when chronically or critically ill, will seek help in the more advanced urban medical centers (68, 71, 72). This circumstance appears to account for only a small portion of the urban factor and should, in the future, become negligible with the provision of comprehensive medical care in rural areas. Immigrants to the U.S. settle predominantly in cities and have shown striking alterations in their likelihood of developing cancer (73). The changes were always in the direction of the U.S. incidence rates. For instance, immigrants from England and Wales exhibit a decrease of lung cancer incidence more nearly approximating the lower U.S. level. However, the diagnoses reported on death certificates may be more accurate in urban than in rural areas.

Several studies have shown differences between the smoking habits of rural and urban populations with the cigarette consumption higher for city dwellers (69, 74). These differences were at least partially responsible for the increased urban mortality from lung cancer. In a prospective study the American Cancer Society noted a 50% narrowing of the urban/rural difference in lung cancer mortality after corrections were made for smoking habits (74). A similar investigation in England also demonstrated the decrease but not the disappearance of the urban factor after adjustment for smoking habits (75).

Investigations of these various contributors to the "urban factor" in respiratory carcinogenesis may not eliminate the role of polluted air. Within each urban/rural grouping, lung cancer death rates increase strongly with cigarette smoking and show always somewhat higher rates for the city smokers (Figure 3) (74). Atmospheric pollution appears to offer a reasonable explanation for the persistence in the urban–rural ratio of lung cancer even though the precise degree of this effect remains to be determined.

Table V. Contributors to the "Urban Factor" in Respiratory Carcinogenesis

More accurate reporting and recording of death certificates
Higher degree of atmospheric pollution
More industrial exposure
More cancer diagnosed and treated
Different immigration/migration patterns
Differences in socioeconomic factors
More cigarettes smoked

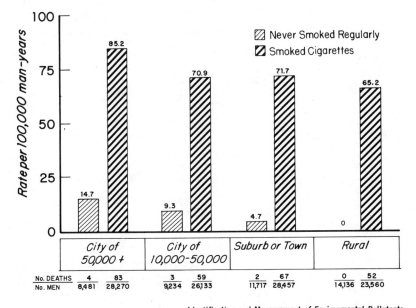

Identification and Measurement of Environmental Pollutants

Figure 3.   Age-standardized rates for well established cases of bronchio-genic carcinoma, by rural–urban classification. Rates for cigarette smokers are compared with those for men who never smoked regularly (105).

Laboratory Studies. The findings from bioassays and physiochemical studies are equally significant to the epidemiological data in relating atmospheric pollution to the pathogenesis of respiratory cancer. The elucidation of the mechanisms leading to lung cancer induction remains primarily the domain of the physical and biological sciences. In environmental carcinogenesis, demonstrable parallelism between epidemiological data and laboratory findings add to both. In air pollution, carcinogenesis bioassay data from mammalian species lend support to the concept that air pollution represents one factor in the increased risk of urban dwellers to develop lung cancer. Above all, laboratory studies offer the possibility of reducing the emission of potentially harmful carcinogens into our environment.

BIOASSAY FOR CARCINOGENICITY. The respiratory system admits the bulk of air pollutants to the human body. Studies of particulate matter and toxic volatile agents from atmospheric pollutants have dealt with their passage, deposition, and retention in the respiratory tract. Depending on the air pollution situation, the particles may range from 0.1–10^4 μm in diameter. Figure 4 shows the size range for various pollutants and depicts particles ranging from 0.25–10 μm as "lung damaging." Particles less than 0.25 μm are seldom retained in the lung, and if so, they remain located in the alveolar regions. Particles with diameters greater than 10 μm are lodged in the upper respiratory tract and thus do not reach the bronchi (76, 77). Before the carcinogenic agent can be eluted from the particles trapped in the lung and can come in contact with the bronchial epithelium,

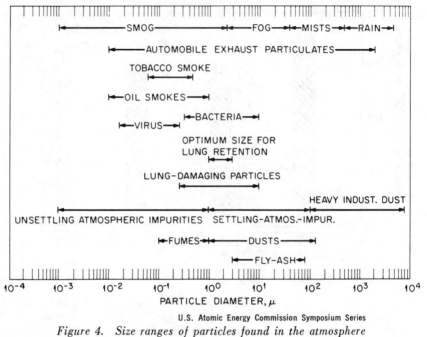

U.S. Atomic Energy Commission Symposium Series

Figure 4.   Size ranges of particles found in the atmosphere
(77)

the physiochemical defense mechanism of the tracheobronchial tree has to be impaired. This defense mechanism consists of a mucus layer which is propelled upwards by ciliated cells. In the non-diseased lung and in the lung in which mucus flow is not already altered, it appears unlikely that the residence time is long enough to elute the carcinogenic agents from the pollutants after which they may enter the underlying cells of the bronchus. However, it has been amply demonstrated that several environmental irritants can inhibit the mucus flow (Table VI) and thus facilitate the uptake of carcinogens by the bronchial epithelium. Questions then arise about the nature and amount of carcinogens in the respiratory pollutants and the chemical nature of such carcinogens. Leiter *et al.* and Leiter and Shear were among the first to induce subcutaneous sarcomas following injection of the organic matter of atmospheric dusts and soot originating from different cities in the U.S. (*78, 79*). Skin cancers and sarcomas in mice have also been produced with organic pollutants by several groups in the U.S. and England (*70, 80*). In one study, organic pollutants even induced lesions in the uterine cervix of mice which were histologically undistinguishable from those induced by carcinogenic hydrocarbons (*81*). In recent years, tumors in the liver and adenomas in the lung were also induced by applying organic particulates from various U.S. cities to newborn mice (*82, 83*). Several potential contributors to urban pollution, such as extracts from chimney soot, road dust, and gasoline and diesel exhaust tars were carcinogenic in the experimental animal (*70, 80*).

IDENTIFICATION OF CARCINOGENS. Several attempts have been made to correlate the tumorigenicity of urban pollutants with the activities of known animal carcinogens. Hueper and co-workers fractionated organic particulates from eight U.S. cities and bioassayed them for tumorigenicity by subcutaneous injection into mice (*84*). They applied the total organic matters as well as the aliphatic aromatic and oxygenated neutral subfractions from each of the eight samples. The total organic matter of six of the eight samples induced a significant number of sarcomas as did two aromatic and two oxygenated neutral subfractions; the eight aliphatic fractions were all inactive. In our own studies, we fractionated organic air pollutants from Detroit and New York City into insoluble, acidic, and basic portion and into aliphatic, aromatic, and oxygenated neutral subfractions (Figure 5). Of the materials, the total organic matter and the aromatic, neutral subfractions induced papillomas and carcinomas in the skin of 50–95% of the mice. The insoluble and acidic portions and the aliphatic and oxygenated neutral subfractions were inactive as complete carcinogens. The basic portions were not tested since they amounted to only 0.55–3.4% of the total organic matter.

Recently, Epstein *et al.* tested fractions of organic pollutants from New York City in newborn mice and found significant tumorigenic activities for the aromatic neutral subfraction as well as for the basic portion (*83*). A detailed chemical analysis of the aromatic neutral subfraction revealed

Table VI. Some Identified Cilia Toxic and Mucus Coagulating Agents in Air Pollutants

Chemical Classification	Urban Pollution	Tobacco Smoke
Paraffins	2-methylpentane	
Olefins	2-methylbut-2-ene	
	2-methylpent-2-ene	
Aromatic hydrocarbons	benzene	benzene
	toluene	toluene
	xylenes	xylenes
Aldehydes	formaldehyde	formaldehyde
	acetaldehyde	acetaldehyde
	propionaldehyde	propionaldehyde
		isobutyraldehyde
	acrolein	acrolein
		furfural
Carboxylic acids	formic acid	formic acid
	acetic acid	acetic acid
Phenols	phenol	phenol
	cresols	cresols
Peroxides	acetyl peroxide	
	peracetic acid	
Epoxides	propylene oxide	
	cyclohexene oxide	
Inorganic chemicals	sulfur dioxide	hydrogen cyanide
		nitrous acid

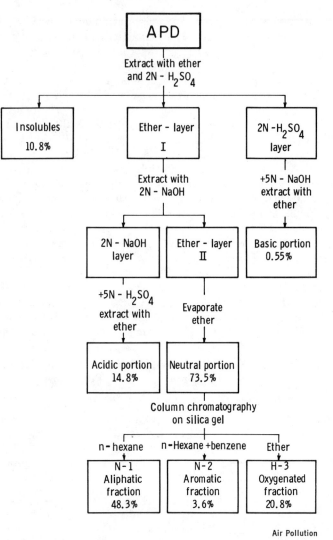

Air Pollution

*Figure 5. Separation scheme of organic particulate matter
(Detroit) (80)*

the enrichment of practically all of the PAH from the total particulates in
this subfraction and also revealed the presence of at least six known carcinogenic PAH in the organic pollutants. In the bioassayed organic particulates
from four different locations in Detroit and New York, the concentrations
of the strong carcinogen, benzo[a]pyrene (BaP), varied between 0.011,
and 0.035% and of the weak carcinogen, benz[a]anthracene (BaA), varied
between 0.017 and 0.06%. Using chemically purified BaP as positive controls, we estimated that 45–55% of the carcinogenicity of the total organic
particulates and of the aromatic neutral subfractions could be explained by

Table VII. Polynuclear Aromatic Hydrocarbons in Urban Atmospheres

PAH	Carcino- genicity[a]	µg/1000 m³	Location
Benzo[a]pyrene	+++	0.05–74	U.S. cities (1958)
		6	average of 100 U.S. cities (1958)
		≤54	London (1968)
		18–37	Belfast (1961–62)
		5–18	Dublin (1961–62)
		5–11	Oslo (1962–63)
		2–5	Helsinki (1962–63)
		2.5–6.5	Sydney (1962)
Benzo[b]fluoranthene	++	2.3–7.4	U.S. cities (1958)
		0.5–1.5	Sydney (1962)
Benzo[j]fluoranthene	++	0.8–4.4	Detroit (1962–63)
Dibenzo[a,h]pyrene	++		presence questionable
Tribenzo[a,e,i]pyrene	++		presence questionable
Dibenz[a,h]anthracene	++	3.2–32	German cities (not detected in U.S. cities) (1966)
Benz[a]anthracene	+	0.1–21.6	U.S. cities (1958)
		4	average of 100 U.S. cities (1958)
Chrysene	(+)	1.5–13.3	Cincinnati (1965)
		1.3–11.6	Detroit (1962–63)
Benzo[e]pyrene	+	1–25	12 U.S. cities (1958)
		5	average of U.S. cities (1958)
		≤37	London (1967–68)
		5–8	Oslo (1962–63)
Indeno[1,2,3-cd]pyrene	+	1.5–8.2	Detroit (1962–63)
Benzo[g,h,i]perylene	−	2–35	12 U.S. cities (1958)
		18–26	Belfast (1961–62)
		12–46	London (1962)
Anthanthrene	−	0.26	average of U.S. cities (1958)
		2–6	London (1962)
Coronene	−	2	average of U.S. cities (1958)
		4–20	London (1962)
Perylene	−	0.7	average U.S. cities (1958)
Pyrene	−	trace–35	12 U.S. cities (1958)
		1.3–19.3	Detroit (1962–63)
Fluoranthene	−	4	U.S. average (1958)
		0.9–15.0	Detroit (1962–63)

[a] Relative carcinogenic activity on mouse skin: +++ = high, ++ = moderate, + = weak, (+) = possibly weak, − = inactive.

BaP alone (*80*). In Table VII, we have listed the PAH identified in urban air and their reported concentrations (*70, 80, 85, 86*).

The presence of tumorigenic agents in the oxygenated neutral subfractions, as observed by Hueper *et al.* in their bioassay in the connective tissue of mice (*84*), is considerably important since it demonstrates that PAH-free fractions contain tumorigenic agents. It appears likely that the tumors induced by these fractions were at least partially caused by still-unidentified epoxides and peroxides of similar structure as proposed by Kotin and Falk (*87*). These oxygenated neutral compounds are probably formed from unsaturated hydrocarbons after emission and from ozone and/or other oxidizing agents in the atmosphere under the influence of sunlight. The observation that tumors can be induced by applying the basic portion of organic pollutants (*84*) to newborn mice suggests the presence of aza-heterocyclic hydrocarbons. Sawicki *et al.* identified this type of compound in polluted air (*87, 88*) (Table VIII). Dibenz[*a,j*]acridine and dibenz[*a,h*]-acridine are known animal carcinogens.

One of the shortcomings of animal bioassay techniques in determining the carcinogenic potential of atmospheric pollutants is their disregard for the nature of the insoluble portions of the particulates. Only 8–24% of the urban particulates are organic matter (*89*), and so far, only these matters have been bioassayed (*80*). The major portion of the remaining particulates, however, are made up of silicates, metal oxides, and carbon. As expected, the particulate matter contains a large spectrum of metallic oxides (*90, 91*). Depending on the collection site, iron oxides may account for up to 15% of total urban particulates. In recent years, certain iron oxides facilitated the carcinogenicity of active PAH as carriers for the induction of bronchogenic carcinomas in hamsters (*92*). It is hoped that future bioassays with air pollutants will use this or similar techniques for estimating the importance in respiratory carcinogenesis of the inert materials in pollutants.

From the bioassays of the organic particulates, one can conclude that polluted air contains trace amounts of carcinogens. The most important types of these carcinogens are the active species of the PAH group. BaP is

Table VIII.   Concentrations of Aza-heterocyclic Compounds in the Average American Urban Atmosphere (*88*)

Compound	Benzene-soluble Fraction (µg/g)	Airborne Particulates	µg/1000 m³ Air
Benzo[*f*]quinoline	20	2	0.2
Benzo[*h*]quinoline	30	3	0.3
Benz[*a*]acridine	20	2	0.2
Benz[*c*]acridine	50	4	0.6
11 *H*-Indeno[1,2-*b*]quinoline	10	1	0.1
Dibenz[*a,h*]acridine	7	0.6	0.08
Dibenz[*a,j*]acridine	4	0.3	0.04

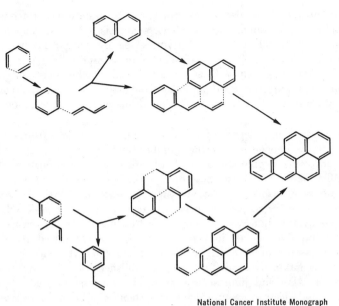

National Cancer Institute Monograph

Figure 6.   Pathways for the pyrosynthesis of benzo[a]pyrene
(94)

the most active compound of this group. Minor carcinogens are aza-hetero-cyclic hydrocarbons and certain types of epoxides and peroxides. However, the total amount of carcinogens in urban pollutants is very small. The highest amount reported for the U.S. is 74 μg BaP in 1000 m^3 polluted air [320 mg total particulates; (85)]. Taking this value, if one stayed outdoors for 24 hr, there would be approximately 0.9–1.5 μg BaP in the air one breathes (11–20 m^3). The U.S. city average would amount to 0.07–0.12 μg. These very low values certainly do not conflict with the human data showing only slightly elevated lung cancer risk for the urban nonsmoker and a somewhat more elevated lung cancer risk for the urban cigarette smoker compared with rural cigarette smokers (70, 74, 93). Whatever the demonstrated increase in the relative risk factor for lung cancer caused by present day urban pollution, the established presence of potentially harmful carcinogens in the atmosphere should increase our efforts to remove the agents to whatever degree possible.

Sources for Atmospheric Carcinogens. Carcinogenic PAH are formed primarily during the incomplete combustion of organic matter by a few distinct mechanisms. The prevailing pyrolytic route for PAH is the initial formation of C,H-radicals in zones with highly elevated temperatures ($> 600°$) and the subsequent combining of C,H-radicals to the thermodynamically preferred aromatic hydrocarbons including those of carcinogenic hydrocarbons with four to six condensed aromatic rings (**Figure 6**) (94). This route is enhanced during the burning of precursors with an aromatic ring system. Alkylated PAH are formed primarily during incom-

plete combustion from specific precursors, such as steroids, or from unsaturated organic compounds *via* the diene synthesis (95). Carcinogenic aza-
heterocyclic hydrocarbons are pyrosynthesized by similar mechanism from
certain nitrogen-containing organic compounds, especially from precursors
with a pyridine ring. These facts suggest that all combustions can contribute
to urban pollution with PAH and the combustion of certain nitrogen containing precursors, as well as to the pollution with aza-heterocyclic hydrocarbons.

The sources and degree of PAH pollution vary widely from community
to community depending on the number and types of heat and power
generation plants, degree and methods of refuse burning, industrial activities,
and traffic patterns. It is, therefore, unrealistic to generalize for urban
communities in respect to the emission sources of PAH. An exception,
however, is seen for national efforts to reduce the emission of PAH. In this
case, some overall figures are needed. Most estimates for the release of PAH
are based on BaP as an indicator. BaP is prosynthesized by the same
mechanism as the other carcinogenic hydrocarbons. It is a strong carcinogen, its isolation methods are well established, and it induces strong
responses in UV- and fluorescence-spectrophotometers, as well as in flame
ionization and electron capture detector systems of gas chromatographs.

In Table IX, BaP emission data are presented for the U.S. as compiled
by the National Academy of Sciences (70). These data are only estimates
and may no longer apply in their entirety. They, nevertheless, permit an
overall impression of the PAH pollution in the U.S. In summary, the
following relative contributions are suggested for the major source categories
of total PAH emissions (expressed in terms of annual estimated benzo[a].
pyrene emission): heat and power generation, 500 tons/year; refuse burning,
600 tons/year; coke production, 200 tons/year; and motor vehicles, 20
tons/year (70).

The nation-wide estimates cannot be applied to individual areas. For
example, the major emission sources for the coal mining and steel producing
states are coal-fired furnaces, coal refuse burning, and coke production. In
our major cities, motor vehicles contribute significantly to the PAH atmospheric burden. This applies specifically to downtown areas of New York
City and Los Angeles (96, 97). The only motor vehicle data available for
Detroit show a surprisingly small contribution of 5% of the BaP in the
downtown area, 18% of which was located in the freeway area and 42% in
the suburban atmosphere (98).

Indoor Pollution. Since most people now spend a major portion of
the day in homes and offices, some background information on indoor
pollution is indicated. Based on the limited literature available, we assume
that the major sources for pollution within residential structures are
improperly vented furnaces, incinerators, leakage from outdoors, and
tobacco smoke.

The data published by Stocks *et al.* suggest that offices have 25–70%
lower PAH concentrations than found in the immediate outdoor atmosphere
(99, 100). The degree to which tobacco smoke can pollute indoor air is

Table IX. Estimated Benzo[*a*]pyrene Emission in the United States (*61*)

Heat and Power Generation Sources

Type of Unit	Gross Heat (Btu/hr)	BaP (μg/10⁶ Btu)	BaP (tons/yr)
Coal			
residential furnaces	0.1×10^6	$1.7\text{--}3.3 \times 10^6$	420
intermediate units	$60\text{--}250 \times 10^6$	15–40	10
coal-fired steam			
power plant	$1000\text{--}2000 \times 10^6$	20–400	1
Oil			
low-pressure air-			
atomized	0.7×10^6	900 ⎱	
other	$0.02\text{--}21 \times 10^6$	100 ⎰	2
Gas			
premix-burners	$0.01\text{--}9 \times 10^6$	20–200	2
Wood		50,000	40

Estimated subtotal: approximately **500**

Refuse Burning

Enclosed incinerators	
municipal	<1
commercial and industrial	23
institutional	2
apartment	8
Open burning	
municipal	4
commercial and industrial	10
domestic	10
forest and agricultural	140
vehicle disposal	50
coal refuse fires	340

Estimated subtotal: approximately **600**

Coke Production 200

Transportation

Vehicle Type	Fuel Consumed (gal/yr)	BaP (μg/gal)	BaP (tons/yr)
Gasoline-powered			
automobiles	56.4×10^9	170	10
trucks	24.2×10^9	≈500	≈12
Diesel fuel-powered			
trucks and buses	5.8×10^9	62	0.4

Estimated subtotal: approximately **22**

Chemical Week

Table X.   Chemical Analytical Data: Situations

Geographic Location	Ethnic Group	Tribe and Hut No.	Sample Size[a]
Mountain	Bantu	Nyeri 2	A
Mountain	Bantu	Nyeri 3	A
Coast	Bantu	Wadigo 1	A
Coast	Bantu[b]	Wadigo 1[b]	B
Mountain	Nilohamitic	Nandi 1	B
Mountain	Nilohamitic	Nandi 2	B
Central plateau	Nilohamitic	Samburu	A

[a] Total sample size: $A = 3,300$ ft^3 $= 93,446$ m^3; $B = 3,710$ ft^3 $= 105,050$ m^3.
[b] Sample was obtained in a bedroom adjacent to the kitchen.

indicated in a report from a beer hall in Prague where the BaP concentration was 28–144 μg per 1000 m^3. This figure more than doubles the highest reported outdoor pollution (101). Recently, public health authorities and the scientific community have been concerned with pollution by tobacco sidestream smoke in buses, trains, and public buildings (102, 103). Some research interest in this area is now apparent (104).

Another more rare example of indoor pollution relates to a high incidence of nasopharyngeal cancer among natives of certain tribes in the mountains of Kenya. The incidence rate of this type of cancer was relatively low for natives of Kikuyu related tribes inhabiting the coastal regions of Kenya (105, 106). One major difference between the living conditions of the mountain and coast line tribes is the construction and ventilation of their huts. The mountain tribes live in a cold, rainy climate and spend large portions of the day in very poorly ventilated dwellings, with only one small door and no windows. The huts are constantly heated by an open wood and cow dung fire, resulting in high levels of pollution (Table X). As a result, the concentrations of phenols, BaA, and BaP greatly exceed the values reported for most urban areas. These data suggest that pollution problems do not always go hand-in-hand with industrial development.

Reduction of Atmospheric Carcinogens. In recent years, some progress has been made in reducing urban pollution. London represents one example of such progress after her citizens suffered through air pollution episodes in 1952 and in 1962 (107). Since then, the British Government and the city have enforced strict regulations for industry and a change from coal to oil heating for private and public housing. The United Kingdom has, furthermore, made emission control devices mandatory. The maximal emission values for motor vehicles per km are 4.2 g of hydrocarbons and 48 g of carbon monoxide; the U.S. standards are 2.1 g and 24 g, respectively (108). These regulations led to a significant reduction of gaseous air pollutants, especially of the cilia-toxic sulfur dioxide as well as to a reduction of particulate matter, including that of carcinogenic hydrocarbons (109).

Analyzed During Cooking in Huts (105)

TPM Collected (mg)[c]	TOM Extracted (mg)[d]	TOM (mg/m³)	BaP (µg/1000 m³)	BaA (µg/1000 m³)
731.2	632.0	6.763	166	515
252.4	240.6	2.575	85	79
140.2	75.5	0.808	24	29
33.0	31.9	0.304	no BaP found	16
431.0	289.3	2.754	291	268
592.0	409.5	3.898	140	225
246.2	93.9	1.005	37	33

[c] TPM = total particulate matter collected.
[d] TOM = total organic matter extracted.

National Research Council, Canada

In the U.S., many communities and counties have enacted new ordinances which set limits for the sulfur content of coal and heating oil. Industries have shown initiative in controlling the emission of pollutants (110). Nevertheless, new control measures are still needed. As discussed under "Sources for Atmospheric Carcinogens," coal refuse burning represents still a major source of atmospheric pollution in the coal-mining states. Coal refuse is a major by-product of the coal mining industry resulting in large dumps or heaps of rocks intermixed with small pieces of coal. Unfortunately, once or twice a year, these dumps can self-ignite and release very dense smoke for weeks. Hopefully, the mining industry will increase the use of coal refuse for filling abandoned mine shafts or find new applications for this by-product and thereby reduce a major source of atmospheric pollution.

In the last decade, some cars have been equipped with emission control devices. These devices have been estimated to reduce the emission of PAH by 85% (Table XI) (70). The central reason for the lower PAH yields from current emission controlled vehicles is the shifting from rich carburation (2.85% carbon monoxide) to lean carburation (0.9–1.4% carbon monoxide). However, aging of an internal combustion engine can increase PAH emissions. Hangebrauck et al. reported five times the BaP emission for a car after 50,000 mi compared to the emission after 5000 mi of operation

Table XI.   Automotive Benzo[a]pyrene Emission Factors (70)

Source	Benzo[a]pyrene Emission Factors (µg/gal of Fuel Consumed)
Uncontrolled car (1956–1964)	170
1966 Uncontrolled car	45–70
1968 Emission-controlled vehicle	20–30
Advanced systems	<10

National Academy of Sciences

Table XII.   Emission Rates of Polynuclear Aromatic Hydrocarbons from a Gasoline Engine (80)

	"Tar" Emission		"Tar" Analysis (ppm)			
	(g/hr)	(g/gal fuel)	BaP[c]	BaA[c]	Py	Flu
Standard run[a]	4.4	2.2	100	180	2400	1330
Run with high oil consumption[b]	10.2	4.8	566	925	4100	2200

[a] 1 qt/1600 mi.
[b] 1 qt/200 mi.
[c] Quantitative values (±5%) determined by isotype dilution technique using BaP-6-C^{14} and BaA-9-C^{14}, respectively.

Air Pollution

(111). A significantly higher emission of PAH also correlated with an increased oil consumption (Table XII) (112). Hopefully, future developments will make annual emission rate inspections mandatory in all states for cars, trucks, buses, and motorcycles. The measure should significantly reduce atmospheric pollution in urban communities.

In recent years, the public has been increasingly concerned with the emission of lead from gasoline engines, which has led to the introduction of low lead fuels. In order to keep the anti-knock number high, the aromatic portion (benzene, toluene, and xylenes) in some of these fuels has been significantly increased. Experimental engines operated only on aromatic fuels have demonstrated that this will increase PAH emission. (Table XIII). The recent practice of synthesizing isooctane (anti-knock number 100) from cracking gases and adding it to gasoline will eventually reduce the aromatic portion in fuels.

Summary. Atmospheric pollution most likely represents one factor for the increased risk of the urban population, especially of cigarette smokers, to develop lung cancer. This concept is supported by laboratory studies which demonstrated that polluted air contains agents which can inhibit the physiological defense mechanism of the tracheobronchial tree, that air pollutants can induce carcinomas and sarcomas in the experimental animal,

Table XIII.   Benzo[a]pyrene, Benz[a]anthracene, and Phenol Emission Rates with Gasoline and Hydrocarbon Fuels (1-Min. Run) (105)

Fuel	B[a]P (μg)	B[a]A (μg)	Phenol (mg)
Gasoline	9.6	17.3	1.4
2,2,4-Trimethylpentane	2.6	0.8	0.013
2,2,4-Trimethyl-1-pentene	0.7	0.4	0.059
50% o-Xylene + 50% benzene	25.8	56.3	5.56
25% 2,2,4-Trimethylpentane +25% 2-Methylbutane +50% o-Xylene	9.0	32.3	0.46

National Research Council, Canada

and that pollutants contain trace amounts of carcinogenic agents. The major carcinogens identified belong to the PAH group; minor carcinogens are found with some aza-heterocyclic compounds and suspected with some epoxides and peroxides.

The major sources for PAH pollution in the U.S. expressed as BaP are—heat and power generation, 500 tons/year; refuse burning, 600 tons/ year; coke production, 200 tons/year; and motor vehicles, 20 tons/year. Whereas these are national estimates, there exist great differences in the sources of atmospheric pollution in individual communities. In large cities, vehicular exhaust becomes a major polluter. Measures should be increased to reduce the emission of pollutants from transportation and stationary sources.

Tobacco Smoke

Table I lists the degree of evidence for each agent suspected to induce respiratory cancer. Cigarette smoke is by far the most important single factor contributing to an increased risk of developing cancer of the respiratory tract, especially of the lung. The Royal College of Physicians concluded, "Cigarette smoking is an important cause of lung cancer." In 1971, they added: ". . . the quantitative association between cigarette smoking and development of cancer is most simply explained on a causal basis and no other explanations account for the fact" (*113, 141*). The Advisory Committee of the U.S. Surgeon General stated in 1964 that, "Cigarette smoking is causally related to lung cancer in men," and that, ". . . the magnitude of the effect of cigarette smoking far outweighs all other factors related to the disease" (*115*). These conclusions are based on more than 100 prospective and retrospective studies from more than 15 countries and are supported by extensive experimental investigations (*115, 116, 117*).

Some Epidemiological Observations. The relative risk of developing lung cancer increases with the number of cigarettes consumed (Figure 3). Prospective and retrospective studies support the concept that the earlier an individual starts smoking, the higher the risk of developing cancer of the respiratory tract. Lung cancer death risks in women are presently much lower than in men. Important factors contributing to this difference are the overall lower cigarette consumption by women in the age group at which lung cancer is most likely to occur, that women smoke more filter-tip and "low tar and nicotine" cigarettes than men, and also that women began to smoke later than men. The extent of the influence of endocrine factors in the variation in the incidence of lung tumors is still unknown (*113, 114, 115, 116*).

Pipe and cigar smokers experience only a slightly higher risk of developing lung cancer than nonsmokers. Apparently, the lungs of these smokers are exposed to less tobacco smoke than those of cigarette smokers, because they tend to smoke in general less heavily and because most of them consider themselves to be non-inhalers. Those who do inhale, do so infrequently and only slightly. Consequently, the harmful effects of cigar and pipe smoking appear to be limited to those sites which are directly exposed to the smoke. Mortality rates from cancer of the oral cavity, extrinsic larynx, pharynx, and esophagus are significantly higher than the rates for nonsmokers and are approximately equal for cigar, pipe, and cigarette smokers (*113, 114, 115, 116*).

Several studies indicate a more common occurrence of cancer of the kidney and the urinary bladder in cigarette smokers than in nonsmokers (*113, 114, 115, 116*). In a more recent publication, it was shown that male and female cigarette smokers face about twice the relative risk of developing bladder cancer and that the increased risk is correlated with both the number of cigarettes smoked per day and the various degrees of inhalation (*118*). Several mechanisms have been suggested for this correlation; however, these findings are still inconclusive (*133*).

The mortality rate of carcinoma of the pancreas in the U.S. has risen from 2.9 to 8.2 per 100,000 per year from 1920 to 1965 (*116*). Epidemiological evidence suggests an association between cigarette smoking and cancer of the pancreas (*116, 119*). At present, not a single biochemical study has concerned itself with the underlying mechanism of this association (*119*).

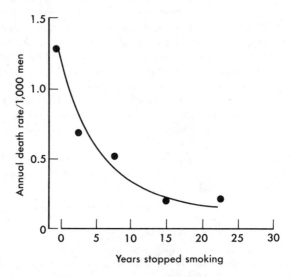

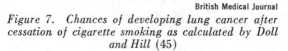

British Medical Journal

Figure 7.   Chances of developing lung cancer after cessation of cigarette smoking as calculated by Doll and Hill (45)

One of the strongest supports for the causal association between cigarette smoking and lung cancer is found in the decreased risk of ex-smokers' developing lung cancer (Figure 7) (*120*). It is estimated that the ex-smoker faces about the same very low risk as the nonsmoker after 12–15 years of smoke cessation (*113, 114, 115, 116*). As shown in Figure 3, the smoker faces an increased risk of developing cancer of the lung with increasing daily cigarette consumption. Epidemiological as well as experimental data suggest that it is primarily the particulate matter ("tar") of inhaled tobacco smoke which is correlated with this dose–response curve. Since we know from extensive analytical studies throughout the world that, in general, filter cigarettes deliver 10–50% less "tar" than plain cigarettes, it is of great practical importance to know the relative lung cancer risk of filter cigarette smokers.

To date, two studies have explored this question. Both support the concept that a smoker who changes from plain to filter cigarettes and who does not increase his daily cigarette consumption has after about 10 years of smoking filter cigarettes a reduced lung cancer risk compared with the smoker who continues to consume plain cigarettes (50, 121).

Characteristics of Tobacco Smoke. When tobacco is smoked, as is true in most organic combustion, the organic matter is incompletely burned. The result is the formation of a dense aerosol with a total smoke weight (average of 10 puffs) per cigarette of 400–500 mg, containing 5×10^9 particles per ml with a size distribution between 0.1 and 1.0 μm and a medium size of 0.4 μm. The major components by weight of the total smoke are: nitrogen (50–66%), oxygen (10–15%), carbon dioxide (8–14%), carbon monoxide (3–6%), and wet particulate matter (4–9%). Hydrogen, argon, methane, volatile hydrocarbons, aldehydes, ketones, hydrogen cyanide, and water vapor are minor constituents (117, 122).

Given the particle size distribution noted above, the particulate portion of tobacco smoke is almost entirely within the range of lung damaging particles (Figure 4). These particles are also slightly charged and dipolar. The separation of gas phase constituents from particulate matter is arbitrarly achieved by smoking through a specific glass fiber filter. Those compounds which are retained by more than 50% on the filter are considered as particulate constituents, the rest as gas phase compounds. It is estimated that the gas phase contains less than 150 compounds whereas in the particulate phase, so far more than 2000 compounds have been identified (123).

The pH of the smoke of U.S. cigarettes varies between 5.6 and 6.2 depending on the puff measured and on the type of tobacco blend used. Cigarettes made exclusively from Burley tobacco as well as cigars deliver a smoke which ranges between 6.2 and 8.0 with the higher values for the final puffs of a tobacco product (124). The temperature reached in the burning cone during puffing of cigarettes varied between 850°–900°C, with peak temperatures on the periphery bypass zone of up to 1200°C (117, 125).

In the literature, a distinction is made between mainstream smoke and sidestream smoke. Mainstream smoke or smoke (terms which are used interchangeably) is formed during puffing. Sidestream smoke is formed in between puffs.

Most laboratory studies are based on tobacco smoke which is produced by machine smoking. The standard smoking conditions for cigarettes adapted in the U.S. and most foreign countries derived their average parameters from human observations. These are one puff a minute, with a puff volume of 35 ml, a puff duration of 2 sec, and a butt length of 23 mm for plain cigarettes.

Experimental Tobacco Carcinogenesis. Today, the evidence that an environmental agent increases the risk for cancer in man can be derived only from epidemiological studies. Experimental investigations can not only support or weaken the correlations observed in man, but they can also contribute to an understanding of the mechanism(s) leading to the induction of a specific type of cancer by an environmental agent. Above all, laboratory tests have the unique function of determining the chemical nature of tumorigenic agent(s) and developing methods to reduce the active factor(s). Experimental tobacco carcinogenesis is a good example for this concept.

BIOASSAY FOR CARCINOGENICITY. The first experiments which established tobacco smoke as carcinogenic to laboratory animals were completed in 1953 and 1957 with tar applications to epithelial tissues of mice and rabbits (Figure 8) (*126, 127*). Since that time, a large number of studies have been published which demonstrated the carcinogenicity of tobacco smoke (*116, 117*).

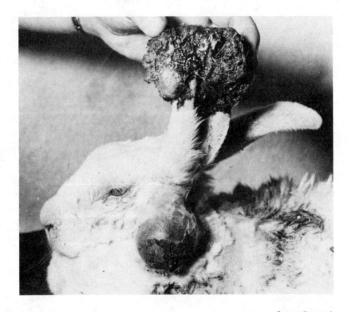

Cancer Research

*Figure 8.   Carcinoma of rabbit ear with metastasis to cervical
gland induced with cigarette smoke condensate* (127)

Ideally, a suspected carcinogen should be tested at the site corresponding to its site of action in man and by the same mode of exposure as in man. In tobacco carcinogenesis the route of choice would be voluntary inhalation of smoke by laboratory animals. Studies using Rhesus monkeys have shown that some monkeys may voluntarily smoke cigarettes, but they were not willing to inhale as man (*128*). The forced exposure of dogs to cigarette smoke by means of tracheotomy have led to hyperplastic and metaplastic changes in the bronchi. However, the observed carcinomas *in situ* need reconfirmation and are presently pursued by refined techniques (*129*).

In passive inhalation experiments, small mammals can be exposed to freshly generated tobacco smoke. Using this method, one can induce adenomas and, in isolated cases, also adenocarcinomas in mouse lungs. These types of tumors, however, cannot be compared with those tumors which occur in the bronchial epithelium of smokers. Recently, new inhalation chambers attached to smoking machines were developed, especially designed to accommodate Syrian hamsters (*77*). Dontenwill and his associates in the Tobacco Research Institute in Hamburg, Germany, have used these machines on large scale tests. The hamsters were exposed to diluted smoke (1:7) for about 10 min twice daily for at least 18 months. Of the animals which survived total exposure time, about 30% developed precancerous lesions, 10% carcinomas of the larynx, and 5% tumors of the esophagus (*131*). None of the animals developed carcinomas of the trachea or bronchus. This later finding was expected since only less than 1% of the smoke particles bypassed the larynx and reached the lung. In the animals which were exposed to the gas phase of cigarette smoke alone, no pathological change was observed in the upper or lower respiratory tract. This observation supports earlier findings that the gas phase alone does not contain enough carcinogens to induce neoplastic changes (*77, 131*).

The particulate phases of cigarette, cigar, and pipe smoke are carcinogenic to the skin of mice, the bronchial epithelium of dogs and rats, and the connective tissue of rats as demonstrated by more than 100 studies from more than 10 countries (*116, 117*). The dose–response effects observed when tar is applied to epithelial tissue are quite comparable with those of pure carcinogenic compounds (*132*).

IDENTIFICATION OF CARCINOGENS. *Gas Phase.* As discussed earlier, tobacco smoke is arbitrarily separated into a gas phase and a particulate phase by a glass fiber filter. The gas phase alone does not induce tumors in the experimental animal. It is likely, however, that some of the carcinogenic gas phase constituents are trapped on the filter together with the particulate or perhaps that they are present below the threshold level of a carcinogen.

Two approaches immediately appear promising for the identification of volatile carcinogens. One is the systematic bioassay of the gas phase fraction. Model studies, however, have shown that fractionation of the gas phase can lead to a number of artifacts (*133*). The second and more promising approach is the search for volatile carcinogens which theoretically could be present in tobacco smoke. Table XIV lists the identified and suspected volatile carcinogens in tobacco smoke.

Particulate Phase. The first fractionation experiments with the particulate matter of cigarette smoke were published in 1957 and have been repeated by at least five groups (*117, 133, 136, 137, 138*). These studies have shown that the neutral portion and those neutral subfractions which contain the PAH are the only carcinogenic fractions. The carcinogenic PAH and aza-heterocyclic hydrocarbons so far identified, however, can account

Table XIV. Identified and Some Theoretically Possible Carcinogens in the Gas Phase of Tobacco

Carcinogens	Chemical Formula	Identification	Reference to Carcinogenicity
Arsine	H_3As	−	124
Bis(chloromethyl)ether	$ClCH_2O—CH_2Cl$	−	46, 47, 48
Hydrazines	$H_2N—NH_2$	+	13
	$H_3C—NH—NH_2$	+	13
Nickel carbonyl	$Ni(CO)_4$	−	32
Nitro olefins	$R—C{=}CH—R'$ $\quad$		
	$\quad\quad|$	−	125
	$\quad\quad NO_2$		
Volatile nitrosamines	$R—CH_2{\searrow}$	+	13, 150
	$\quad\quad\quad N—NO$		
Vinyl chloride	$R'—CH_2{\nearrow}$	+	149

for only a small portion of the observed activity (Figure 9). The acidic portion, on the other hand, is inactive by itself. However, it promotes the activity of the neutral fraction and its PAH-containing subfractions significantly.

These data have led to the working concept that the particulate matter of tobacco smoke contains trace amounts of carcinogenic hydrocarbons and aza-heterocyclic hydrocarbons which serve as tumor initiators. The activity of these tumor initiators is increased by several of the tumor promoters and co-carcinogens which are found primarily in the acidic portion.

During the burning of tobacco, a major portion of the tumor-initiating hydrocarbons are pyrosynthesized from unspecific precursors (117, 133). The tumor promoting agents, on the other hand, are formed from specific precursors. Comparative bioassays with the smoke condensates from tobacco leaves and tobacco stems have shown that these specific precursors reside primarily in the wax layer of the tobacco leaf (139). Not only do these wax layer constituents contribute to the flavor of tobacco smoke, they are at least partially responsible for the tumor-promoting activity of the smoke. Fractionation studies have shown, in fact, that in the absence of tumor-promoting agents tobacco smoke would hardly induce tumors in the experimental animal.

In Table XV, we have listed the tumorigenic agents so far identified in the particulate matter of cigarette smoke. Other active constituents, especially tumor promoters and co-carcinogens, remain to be identified.

Reduction of Tumorigenicity. During the last 15 years an increasing number of studies have been concerned with the reduction of the tumorigenic activity of tobacco smoke. Since in man and in the experimental animal dose–response effects have been observed, the simplest way to reduce the carcinogenic potential of tobacco smoke is to reduce the number of cigarettes and/or to smoke cigarettes with active filters. At present, the tips of commercial filter cigarettes do not remove or reduce selectively carcinogenic agents from the smoke. However, several opportunities are open for the selective reduction of the tumorigenicity of tobacco tar as measured on the experimental animal (*140, 141, 142*).

In the U.S. and in many European countries, commercial cigarettes use blends of Bright, Burley, Turkish, and Maryland tobaccos as fillers. In general, cigarettes made up exclusively from Burley and Maryland varieties form not only less tar (20–50%) than Bright and Turkish varieties but also less carcinogenic hydrocarbons (B*a*P reduced by 40–60%). In addition, the tars from Burley and Maryland cigarettes have significantly lower

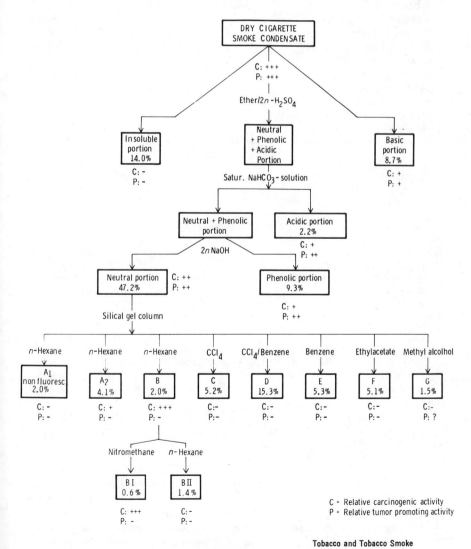

Tobacco and Tobacco Smoke

Figure 9.   Fractionation scheme of cigarette smoke condensate (117)

Table XV.   Tumorigenic Agents Identified in the Particulate Phase of Tobacco Smoke[a]

Component	Relative Activity	$\mu g/100$ Cigarettes
Tumor Initiators		
PAH		
benzo[a]pyrene	+++	3.0–4.0[b]
5-methylchrysene	+++	0.06
dibenz[a,h]anthracene	++	0.4
dibenzo[a,i]pyrene	++	traces
dibenzo[a,l]pyrene	++	traces
benzo[b]fluoranthene	++	0.3
benzo[j]fluoranthene	++	0.6
indeno[1,2,3-cd]pyrene	+	0.4
benz[a]anthracene	+	6.0–8.0[b]
benzo[c]phenanthrene	+	traces
2-methylfluoranthene	+	0.2
3-methylfluoranthene	+	0.2
chrysene	+	4.0[b]
1-, 2-, 3-, and 6-methylchrysenes	+	2.0
Aza-heterocyclics		
dibenz[a,h]acridine	+	traces
dibenz[a,j]acridine	+	1.0[b]
dibenzo[c,g]carbazole	+	traces
Tumor Promoters		
Phenols		
phenol	+	10,000[b]
o-, m-, and p-cresols	+	7,200[b]
2,4- and 2,5-dimethylphenols	+	2,000[b]
catechol	co-carcinogen	30,000
Fatty acids		
stearic acid	+	7,500[b]
oleic acid	+	5,800[b]
Other Identified Tumorigenic Agents		
Polonium-210	carcinogen	traces
Nitrosonornicotine	carcinogen	14–550[b]
Arsenic	carcinogen	?
2-Naphthylamine	bladder carcinogen	22[b]

[a] The values were determined in the mainstream smoke of a popular U.S. cigarette without filter tip (85 mm).
[b] Quantitative values; the other values are isolated amounts.

tumorigenic activities (40–60%) as measured on mouse skin (*117*). England, Wales, and Finland, which use Bright tobacco in their cigarettes, have significantly higher mortality rates from lung cancer (1966–67; 61.0–78.1/ 100,000 per year) than those countries which use predominantly Burley tobaccos (France; 27.7/100,000; (*2*)). One reason for this difference lies in the higher ammonia and pH values (>6.2) for the smoke of Burley cigarettes, and with it, the presence of unprotonated nicotine, the most toxic form of this alkaloid (*124*). These smoke factors seem to be important for the low degree of inhalation by smokers of Burley tobacco compared with smokers of other cigarettes.

One major difference between Burley tobaccos and Bright tobaccos is the relatively high nitrate content of the Burley varieties (1.2–3.5%) and the actual absence of nitrate in Bright tobaccos (<0.1%). Experimental studies with the smoke of Burley cigarettes rich in nitrate or artificially enriched with alkali nitrates, have demonstrated significantly lower values for tar, volatile phenols, carcinogenic PAH, highly reduced tumorigenicity, and elevated values for ammonia (with nitrate as a major precursor) and pH (>6.2) compared with the smoke of the appropriate controls (*124, 140, 142*).

The nitrate content of Burley leaves decreases with their elevated position on the stalk. The higher the stalk position, however, the higher the leaf content of nicotine and waxes (primarily paraffins, terpenes, certain esters, and alkaloids), and therefore, the upper leaves are better precursors for tar, alkaloid, phenols, and carcinogenic hydrocarbons (*143*). This fact suggests that the upper leaves should not be used after curing as such, but rather in the preparation of reconstituted tobacco sheets or for freeze-dried tobacco.

The preparation of reconstituted tobacco sheets which include the use of tobacco stems leads to a tobacco product which delivers smoke reduced in tar and selectively reduced in volatile phenols, carcinogenic hydrocarbons, and tumorigenicity to the experimental animal compared with genuine tobacco (*117, 140, 141, 142, 114, 145*). The development of the tobacco freeze-drying process enables the tobacco manufacturer to about double the filling power of tobacco by opening the leaf structure (*146*). The top leaves with high wax layers are especially suited for this process. It appears that the freeze-drying process significantly increases the filling power of tobacco and thus reduces unselectively the yield of particulate compounds. Table XVI summarizes the various approaches used to reduce the tar yields of tobacco products which in many cases also lead to the selective reduction of carcinogenic agents and tumorigenicity of the tar as measured on the experimental animal. Today, many of these processes are used to manufacture tobacco blends for cigarettes and have, in fact, already led to a significant reduction in the tar and nicotine yields of U.S. cigarettes (*147*) and even to a selective reduction of the tumorigenicity of the particulate matter (*148*).

Conclusions. Cigarette smoking is causally associated with the increased risk of developing lung cancer. Cigar and pipe smokers have only a slightly higher lung cancer risk than nonsmokers; however, they face approximately the same risk of developing cancer of the oral cavity, extrinsic larynx, pharynx, and esophagus as do cigarette smokers. Cigarette smokers appear to have a somewhat increased risk of developing cancer of the kidney, urinary bladder, and pancreas. The risk of ex-smokers developing lung cancer decreases as the years they have refrained from smoking accumulate.

Table XVI.   Some Experimental Approaches for the

Experimental Cigarette	Control	Reduction (% "Tar")
Tobacco selection		
I tobacco type—Burley	bright	20–50
II stalk position—low	high	40–60
III nitrate content—high	low	10–40
IV tobacco part—stem	lamina	30–70
Cigarette paper		
I perforated	unperforated	20–60
II ammonium sulfamate treated	untreated	10–30
Filter tips		
I cellulose acetate	nonfilter	20–60
II charcoal and cellulose acetate	nonfilter	15–50
III charcoal	nonfilter	10–40
Modified tobacco products		
I reconstituted tobacco sheet	standard	0–70
II expanded tobacco	standard	40–60
Tobacco substitutes		
I new smoking product	standard	50–80

[a] Reduction in tumorigenicity as measured on mouse skin: ++ reduction $\geq 50\%$, + significant, but $<50\%$, (+) some reduction, n.d.—not determined, − no selective reduction.

After 12–15 years of nonsmoking, they have about the same risk of lung cancer as do nonsmokers. Preliminary epidemiological data indicate that long-term smokers of filter cigarettes face a lower lung cancer risk than smokers of plain cigarettes.

Inhalation studies have not yet clearly demonstrated that the exposure of animals to tobacco smoke leads to carcinoma of the lung. This is true because animals are able to avoid particulates entering the lower respiratory tract if exposed to smoke in chambers. However, inhalation experiments have led to tumor induction in the larynx and esophagus. The tar of tobacco smoke is carcinogenic to the experimental animal at various sites such as the trachea, bronchi, skin, and connective tissue.

The particulate matter of tobacco smoke contains traces of carcinogens which act as tumor initiators and tumor promoters. The carcinogens of major importance thus far identified belong to the group of polynuclear aromatic hydrocarbons while the importance of aza-heterocyclic hydrocarbons and nitrosamines, as well as polonium-210 and arsenic, remains to be determined. Some volatile phenols and some fatty acids have been identified as tumor promoters. However, the major promoters have not been designated yet. The gas phase contains traces of carcinogenic volatile nitrosamines, hydrazines, and possibly arsine, chloromethyl ethers, nitro olefins, and nickel carbonyl.

Reduction of the Tumorigenicity of Cigarette Smoke

Maximal Reported Reduction

(%) Nicotine	(%) Phenol	(%) BaP	Tumorigenicity[a]
—	50	60	++[b]
85	75	50	n.d.
40	50	50	n.d.
90	40	50	++[b]
50	55	50	—
10–30	20	20	(+)
55	90	60	—
50	75	50	n.d.
40	40	40	—
70	80	80	++[b]
60	60	60	n.d.[c]
100	80	60	+

[b] Highly selective reduction of tumorigenicity.
[c] Filling power of tobacco highly increased; no selective reduction.

Significant progress has been made on the selective reduction of tumorigenic agents in tobacco smoke. The methods of achieving such a reduction include the selection of tobacco varieties and leaves, the incorporation of tobacco stems and ribs, of reconstituted tobacco sheets, and of freeze-dried tobaccos into the blend. Some of these tobacco modifiers are today already part of the blended U.S. cigarette. Basic research on tobacco and tobacco smoke and on the modification of tobacco smoke should lead towards a less harmful cigarette.

Outlook

Detailed epidemiological and experimental evidence exists that the environment significantly influences the incidence of human cancer, that the effect is especially notable in the production of squamous cell cancer, and that environmental carcinogens play a significant role in cancer of the respiratory tract. Long before we understand the precise mechanisms of carcinogenesis, alterations of certain environmental factors will reduce cancer incidence.

We have already witnessed a reduction of industrial cancers. The future will bring further reductions if we continue to place emphasis on reducing contacts of the workers with suspended carcinogens. This is of special importance for industrial lung cancer. As recently seen with bis(chloromethyl) ether, trace amounts of volatile carcinogens can lead to the induction of lung cancer after only short term exposure. If a synthetic product is indicated to be correlated with human cancer, its production should be curtailed immediately. Hopefully, in the future the production or isolation of new materials made possible by technological advances will not be initiated before animal bioassay tests assure that the intermediates and final substances are not carcinogenic.

Air pollution, another factor which is incriminated as a respiratory carcinogen, should be controlled at its sources. The incidental burning of refuse coal is an example in which a major source of pollution can be prevented. This can be done by filling the exploited mining shafts with the refuse coal. The burning of refuse, a major source of atmospheric pollution, should be reduced with large scale installation of new and efficient incinerators and, whenever needed, by enforcement of city ordinances.

In the future, however, this type of air pollution control may not suffice. For example, new types and increasing amounts of inexpensive plastics and polymers will add to urban refuse and may generate new pollutants when incinerated. The use of polyvinyl chloride and other chlorinated polymers which produce hydrochloric acid upon combustion is increasing. Since it is possible that hydrochloric acid together with formaldehyde forms the very powerful lung carcinogen, bis(chloromethyl) ether, we must control the future use of chlorinated polymers and plastics, especially as long as these materials are not biodegradable. Similar considerations are also indicated for nitrile-group containing polymers, since they are known to form hydrocyanic acid upon incomplete combustion. It is expected that in the future the urban pollution resulting from the operation of gasoline and diesel engines will decrease with the wide scale use of emission control devices and with the decrease of aromatic portions of the fuels.

The major factor for the steady increase of lung cancer during the last three to four decades is, however, the increased consumption of tobacco products, especially cigarettes. The obvious way to reverse this trend is the large scale and voluntary cessation of smoking. Extensive educational campaigns by public and voluntary health organizations have shown, however, that a large proportion of today's smokers is not willing to, or cannot, give up this habit. The awareness of this fact and the steady emergence of new smokers should encourage us to develop and market less harmful tobacco products. The application of efficient filter material, selection of tobacco types and leaves, the use of stems, ribs, reconstituted tobacco sheets, and freeze-dried tobacco have already yielded encouraging results. New processes, such as the production of tobacco substitutes and other modifications should be explored to reduce further the carcinogenicity of tobacco products.

We conclude our review with the hope that we have shown that the environment is a major factor for the steep increase in lung cancer and that respiratory carcinogenesis offers the scientist and, especially the chemist, a unique opportunity to apply his knowledge and imagination towards the time when preventable illness is no longer an acceptable way of life.

Acknowledgment

The major part of our studies were supported by National Cancer Institute Grant NIH-NCI-70-2087; Cancer Society Grant BC 56P; U.S. Dept. of Agriculture Contracts 12-14-100-10283(34) and 12-14-100-10295(34); and Environmental Protection Agency Grant R-800985.

Literature Cited

1. Adler, I., "Primary Malignant Growths of the Lungs and Bronchi," Longmans, Green & Co., New York, 1912.
2. Segi, M., Kurihara, M., "Cancer Mortality for Selected Sites," No. 6 (1966–1967), Japan Cancer Society, Tokyo, Japan, 1972.
3. Härting, F. H., Hesse, W., *Vjochr. Med. Ger. K.* (1879) **30**, 296; **31**, 102; **31**, 313.
4. Lorena, E., *J. Natl. Cancer Inst.* (1944) **5**, 1.
5. de Villiers, A. J., Windish, J. P., *Br. J. Ind. Med.* (1964) **21**, 94.
6. Gundin, P. E., Jr., Lloyd, J. W., Smith, E. U., Archer, V. E., Holaday, D. A., *Health Phys.* (1970) **16**, 105.
7. Selikoff, I. J., Hammond, E. C., Chung, J., *J. Am. Med. Assoc.* (1968) **204**, 106.
8. Wagner, J. C., "Chemical Carcinogens," *ACS Monogr.* (1976) **173**, Chapter 15.
9. Buchanan, W. D., "Toxicity of Arsenic Compounds," Elsevier, Amsterdam, 1962.
10. Hueper, W. C., "Occupational and Environmental Cancers of the Respiratory System," Springer-Verlag, Berlin, 1966.
11. Doll, R., *Br. J. Ind. Med.* (1959) **16**, 181.
12. Shubik, P., "Environment and Cancer," p. 142, Williams & Williams, Baltimore, 1972.
13. "Survey of Compounds Which Have Been Tested for Carcinogenic Activity," No. **149**, Suppl. 1, Suppl. 2, DHEW (NIH) 72-35, DHEW (NIH) 73-35, Sect. I and Sect. II. U.S. Public Health Service (1951, 1957, 1969, 1972, 1973).
14. Roth, F., *Dtsch. Med. Wochenschr.* (1957) **82**, 211.
15. Satterlee, H. S., *New Engl. J. Med.* (1956) **254**, 1149.
16. Lee, B. K., Murphy, G., *Cancer* (1969) **23**, 1315.
17. Alwens, W., *Rrch. Gewerbepath. Gewerbehyg.* (1937) **7**, 69.
18. Machele, W., Gregorius, F., *Public Health Rep. U.S.* (1948) **63**, 1114.
19. Mancuso, T. F., Hueper, W. C., *Ind. Med. Surg.* (1951) **20**, 358.
20. Oettel, H., *Proc. 5th Conf. Occup. Cancer* (1960) German Res. Council, 25.
21. Fisher, R. S., Riekert, P. W., *Am. J. Pathol.* (1959) **35**, 699.
22. Wynder, E. L., Berg, J. W., *Cancer* (1967) **20**, 1161.
23. Bidstrap, P. L., Case, R. A. M., *Br. J. Ind. Med.* (1956) **13**, 260.
24. Payne, W. W., *A.M.A. Arch. Ind. Health* (1966) **21**, 530.
25. Kuschner, M., *Am. Rev. Respir. Dis.* (1968) **98**, 573.
26. Bridge, J. C., "Annual Report of the Chief Inspector of Factories for the Year 1932," H. M. Stationery Office, London, 1933.
27. Barrett, G. P., "Annual Report of the Chief Inspector of Factories for the Year 1948," H. M. Stationery Office, London, 1949.
28. Sunderman, F. W., Jr., *Dis. Chest* (1968) **54**, 41.
29. Doll, R., *Br. J. Ind. Med.* (1958) **15**, 217.
30. Doll, R., "Industrial Pulmonary Diseases," E. J. King, C. M. Fletcher, Eds., p. 208, Little, Brown and Co., Boston, 1957.
31. Morgan, J. G., *Br. J. Ind. Med.* (1958) **15**, 224.
32. Sunderman, F. W., Donnelly, A. J., West, B., Kinkaid, J. F., *A.M.A. Arch. Ind. Health* (1959) **20**, 36.

33. Volkmann, R., *Beitr. Chir.* (1875) 370.
34. Eckhardt, R. E., "Industrial Carcinogens," Grune & Stratton, New York, 1959.
35. Yamagiwa, K., Ichikawa, K., *Mitt. Med. Fak. Tokyo* (1916) **15,** 295.
36. Cook, J. W., Hewett, C. L., Hieger, I., *J. Chem. Soc.* (1933) **1,** 395.
37. Lang, K. F., Eigen, I., *Fortschr. Chem. Forsch.* (1967) **8,** 91.
38. Kawahata, K., *Gann* (1936) **30,** 341.
39. Kuroda, S., Kawahata, K., *Z. Krebsforsch.* (1936) **45,** 36.
40. Lloyd, J. W., *J. Occup. Med.* (1971) **13,** 53.
41. Redmond, C. K., Ciocco, A., Lloyd, J. W., Rush, H. W., *J. Occupat. Med.* (1972) **14,** 621.
42. Searl, T. D., Cassidy, F. J., King, W. H., Brown, R. A., *Anal. Chem.* (1970) **42,** 954.
43. Pott, P., "Chirurgical Observations Relative to the Cataract, the Polyps of the Nose, the Cancer of the Scrotum, the Different Kinds of Ruptures and the Mortification of the Toes and Feet," Hawes, Clarke and Collins, London, 1775.
44. Wynder, E. L., Graham, E. A., *J. Am. Med. Assoc.* (1950) **143,** 329.
45. Doll, R., Hill, A. B., *Br. Med. J.* (1950) **2,** 739.
46. Van Duuren, B. L., Goldschmidt, B. M., Katz, B. S., Langseth, L., Mercado, M. S., Sivak, A., *Arch. Environ. Health* (1968) **16,** 472.
47. Van Duuren, B. L., Katz, B. S., Goldschmidt, B. M., Frenkel, K., Sivak, A., *J. Natl. Cancer Inst.* (1972) **48,** 1431.
48. Laskin, S., Kuschner, M., Drew, R. T., Cappiello, Nelson, N., *Arch. Environ. Health* (1971) **23,** 135.
49. Figueroa, W. G., Raszkowski, R., Weiss, W., *New Engl. J. Med.* (1973) **288,** 1056.
50. Wynder, E. L., Mabuchi, K., Beattie, D. J., *J. Am. Med. Assoc.* (1970) **213,** 2221.
51. Nelson, N., *New Engl. J. Med.* (1973) **388,** 1123.
52. Health Research Group and Oil, Chemical, and Atomic Workers, International Union, "Petition Requesting a Zero Tolerance for Ten Carcinogens Through an Emergency Temporary Standard Issued Under the Authority of the Occupational Safety and Health Act," Washington, D.C., 1973.
53. Viola, P. L., *Int. Cancer Congr. Abstr. 10* (1970) 20.
54. Viola, P. L., Bigotti, A., Caputo, A., *Cancer Res.* (1971) **31,** 516.
55. Maltoni, C., Lefemine, G., *Ann. N.Y. Acad. Sci.* (1975) **246,** 195.
56. Keplinger, M. L., Goode, J. W., Gordon, D. E., Calandra, J. C., *Ann. N.Y. Acad Sci.* (1975) **246,** 219.
57. Marsteller, H. J., Lelbach, W. K., Müller, R., Jühe, S., Lange, C. E., Rohner, H. G., Veltman, G., *Dtsch. Med. Wochenschr.* (1973) **48,** 2311.
58. Lange, C. E., Jühe, S., Stein, G., Veltman, G., *Int. Arch. Arbeitsmed* (1974) **32,** 1.
59. Heath, C. W., Jr., Falk, H., Creech, J. L., Jr., N.Y. Acad. Sci. (1975) **246,** 231.
60. Keane, D. P., Stehaugh, R. B., Townsend, P. L., *Hydrocarbon Process.* (1973) 99.
61. *Chem. Week* (1974) 19.
62. Magee, P. N., Montesano, R., Preussmann, R., "Chemical Carcinogens," *ACS Monogr.* (1976) **173,** Chapter 11.
63. Fine, D. H., Rufeh, F., Lieb, D., Rounbehler, D. P., *Anal. Chem.* (1975) **47,** 1188–1190.
64. Sander, J., "Environment and Cancer," Williams & Wilkins Co., Baltimore, 1972.
65. Lijinsky, W., Taylor, H. W., Snyder, C., Nettesheim, P., *Nature* (1973) **244,** 176.
66. Clayson, D. B., "Chemical Carcinogenesis," Little, Brown, & Co., Boston, 1962.

67. Schmähl, D., "Entstehung, Wachstum und Chemotherapie Maligner Tumoren," Cantor, K. G., Aulendorf, Germany, 1970.
68. Royal College of Physicians, "Air Pollution and Health," Pitman Med. Sci. Publishing Co., Ltd., London, 1970.
69. U.S. Public Health Service, "The Health Consequences of Smoking," *DHEW Publ. No. (HSM)* (1971) **71-7513.**
70. National Academy of Sciences "Particulate Polycyclic Organic Matter: Biological Effects of Atmospheric Pollutants," National Resource Council, Washington, D.C., 1972.
71. Doll, R., "Carcinoma of the Lung," J. R. Bignall, Ed., Vol. **1**, p. 81, Livingstone, Edinburgh, 1958.
72. Clemmensen, J., Nielsen, A., Jensen, E., *Br. J. Cancer* (1953) **7,** 1.
73. Haenzel, W., *J. Natl. Cancer Inst.* (1961) **26,** 37.
74. Hammond, E. C., Horn, D., *J. Am. Med. Assoc.* (1958) **166,** 1159, 1294.
75. Stocks, P., Campbell, J. M., *Br. J. Med.* (1955) **2,** 923.
76. Hatch, T. F., Gross, P., "Pulmonary Deposition and Retention of Inhaled Aerosols," Academic, New York, 1964.
77. Hoffmann, D., Wynder, E. L., *U.S. A. E. C. Symp. Ser.* (1970) **18,** 173.
78. Leiter, J., Shimkin, M. B., Shear, M. J., *J. Nat. Cancer Inst.* (1942) **3,** 155.
79. Leiter, J., Shear, M. J., *J. Natl. Cancer Inst.* (1942) **3,** 167.
80. Hoffmann, D., Wynder, E. L., "Air Pollution," Vol. **2,** p. 187, A. C. Stern, Ed., Academic, New York, 1968.
81. Bogacz, J., Koprowska, I., *Acta Cytol.* (1961) **5,** 311.
82. Epstein, S. S., Joshi, S., Andrea, J., Mantel, N., Sawicki, E., Stanley, T., *Nature* (1966) **212,** 1305.
83. Ashina, S., Andrea, J., Carmel, A., Arnold, E., Bishop, Y., Yoshi, S., Coffin, D., Epstein, S. S., *Cancer Res.* (1972) **32,** 2263.
84. Hueper, W. C., Kotin, P., Tabor, E. C., Payne, W. W., Falk, H., Sawicki, E., *Arch. Pathol.* (1962) **74,** 89.
85. Sawicki, E., *Arch. Environ. Health* (1967) **14,** 46.
86. International Agency for Research on Cancer "Evaluation of Carcinogenic Risk," Vol. **3,** Lyon, France, 1973.
87. Kotin, P., Falk, H. L., *Radiat. Res. Suppl.* (1963) **3,** 193.
88. Sawicki, E., McPherson, S. P., Stanley, T. M., Meeker, J., Elbert, W. C., *Int. J. Air Water Pollut.* (1965) **9,** 515.
89. Lindsey, A, J., *Natl. Cancer Inst. Monogr.* (1962) **9,** 235.
90. Corn, M., "Air Pollution," Vol. **1,** p. 47, A. C. Stern, Ed., Academic, New York, 1968.
91. Mueller, P. K., Kothny, E. L., *Anal. Chem.* (1973) **45,** 112.
92. Saffiotti, U., *U.S.A.E.C. Symp. Ser.* (1970) **18,** 27.
93. Hitosugi, M., *Bull. Inst. Public Health Tokyo* (1968) **17,** 237.
94. Badger, G. M., *Natl. Cancer Inst. Monogr.* (1962) **9,** 1.
95. Hoffmann, D., Wynder, E. L., *J. Natl. Cancer Inst.* (1972) **48,** 1855.
96. Collucci, J. M., Begeman, C. R., *Environ. Sci. Tech.* (1971) **5,** 145.
97. Collucci, J. M., Begeman, C. R., *Proc. Int. Clear Air Congr., 2nd* (1971) 28.
98. Collucci, J. M., Begeman, C. R., *J. Air Pollut. Control Assoc.* (1965) **15,** 113.
99. Stocks, P., *Int. J. Air Pollut.* (1958) **1,** 1.
100. Stocks, P., Commins, B. T., Aubrey, K. V., *Int. J. Air Water Pollut.* (1961) **4,** 141.
101. Galuškinová, V., *Neoplasma* (1961) **11,** 465.
102. U.S. Public Health Service, "The Health Consequences of Smoking," *DHEW Publ. No. (HSM)* (1972) **72-7516.**
103. Abelson, P. H., *Science* (1967) **158,** 1527.
104. Schmeltz, I., Hoffmann, D., Wynder, E. L., *Prev. Med.* (1975) **4,** 66.
105. Hoffmann, D., Wynder, E. L., "Identification and Measurement of Environmental Pollutants," Int. Symp. Nat. Res. Council, Canada (1971) 9.

106. Clifford, P., *Proc. Roy. Soc. Med.* (1972) **65,** 1.
107. Scott, J. A., *Med. Officer* (1963) **109,** 1963.
108. American Automobiles Manufacturers Assoc., "International Standards for Emission Control," p. 3, 1974.
109. Ashby, E., "Report Royal Comm. Environ. Pollution," HM Stationery Office, London, 1971.
110. Stern, A. C., "Air Pollution," Vol. **III,** Sources of Air Pollution and Their Control, Academic, New York, 1968.
111. Hangebrauck, R. P., von Lehmden, D. J., Meeker, J. E., *Public Health Serv. Publ.* (1966) **999-AP-33.**
112. Hoffmann, D., Theisz, E., Wynder, E. L., *J. Air Pollut. Control Assoc.* (1965) **15,** 155.
113. Royal College of Physicians, "Smoking and Health," Pitman Medical, London, 1962.
114. Royal College of Physicians, "Smoking and Health Now," Pitman Medical and Scientific, London, 1971.
115. U.S. Public Health Service, "Smoking and Health," *Public Health Serv. Publ.* (1964) **1103.**
116. U.S. Public Health Service, "The Health Consequences of Smoking," *Public Health Serv. Publ.* (1967, 1968, 1969, 1971, 1972, 1973, 1974) **1696, 1696,** Suppl. 1968, **1696-2,** (HSM) **71-7513,** (HSM) **72-7516,** (HSM) **73-8704,** (CDC) **74-8704.**
117. Wynder, E. L., Hoffmann, D., "Tobacco and Tobacco Smoke: Studies in Experimental Carcinogenesis," Academic, New York, 1967.
118. Cole, P., Monson, R. R., Haning, H., Friedell, G. H., *New Engl. J. Med.* (1971) **284,** 129.
119. Wynder, E. L., Mabuchi, K., Maruchi, N., Fortner, J. G., *J. Natl. Cancer Inst.* (1973) **50,** 645.
120. Doll, R., Hill, A. B., *Br. Med. J.* (1964) **1,** 1399.
121. Bross, I. D. J., *Natl. Cancer Inst. Monogr.* (1968) **28,** 35.
122. Keith, C. H., Derrick, J. C., *J. Colloid Sci.* (1960) **15,** 340.
123. Schmeltz, I., Hoffmann, D., *Chem. Rev.* (1977) **77,** 295–311.
124. Brunnemann, K. D., Hoffmann, D., *Food Cosmet. Toxicol.* (1974) **12,** 70.
125. Wakeham, H., "The Chemistry of Tobacco and Tobacco Smoke," I. Schmeltz, Ed., p. 1, Plenum, New York, 1972.
126. Wynder, E. L., Graham, E. A., Croninger, A. B., *Cancer Res.* (1953) **13,** 855.
127. Graham, E. A., Croninger, A. B., Wynder, E. L., *Cancer Res.* (1957) **17,** 1058.
128. Jarvik, M. E., *Ann. N.Y. Acad. Sci.* (1967) **142,** 280.
129. Auerbach, O., Hammond, E. C., Kirman, D., Garfinkel, L., *Arch. Environ. Health* (1970) **21,** 754.
130. Dontenwill, W., *U.S.A.E.C. Symp. Ser.* (1970) **18,** 389.
131. Dontenwill, W., Chevalier, H. J., Harke, H. P., Lafrenz, U., Reckzeh, G., Schneider, B., *J. Natl. Cancer Inst.* (1973) **51,** 1781.
132. Bock, F. G., *Natl. Cancer Inst. Monogr.* (1968) **28,** 57.
133. Hoffmann, D., Wynder, E. L., "The Chemistry of Tobacco and Tobacco Smoke," I. Schmeltz, Ed., p. 123, Plenum, New York, 1972.
134. Holland, R. H., Acevedo, A. R., *Cancer* (1966) **19,** 1248.
135. Deichmann, W. B., MacDonald, W. E., Lampe, W. E., Dressler, I., Anderson, W. A. D., *Ind. Med. Surg.* (1965) **34,** 800.
136. Wynder, E. L., Wright, G. F., *Cancer* (1957) **10,** 255.
137. Dontenwill, W., Elmenhost, H., Harke, H. R., Reckzeh, G., Weber, K. H., Misfeld, J., Timm, J., *Z. Krebsforsch.* (1970) **73,** 265.
138. Bock, F. G., *J. Natl. Cancer Inst.* (1972) **48,** 1849.
139. Wynder, E. L., Hoffmann, D., *Cancer* (1969) **24,** 289.
140. Hoffmann, D., Wynder, E. L., *Natl. Cancer Inst. Monogr.* (1968) **28,** 151.

141. Hoffmann, D., Wynder, E. L., *J. Natl. Cancer Inst.* (1972) **48,** 1855.
142. Dontenwill, W., Chevalier, H. J., Harke, H. P., Klimisch, H. J., Lafrenz, U., Reckzeh, G., Fleischmann, G., Keller, W., *Z. Krebsforsch.* (1972) **78,** 236.
143. Rathkamp, G., Tso, T. C., Hoffmann, D., *Beitr. Tabakforsch.* (1973) **7,** 179.
144. Moshy, R. J., Halter, H. M., *Natl. Cancer Inst. Monogr.* (1968) **28,** 133.
145. Halter, H. M., Ito, T. I., *J. Natl. Cancer Inst.* (1972) **48,** 1869.
146. Johnson, W. H., *Proc. Int. Tobacco Sci. Congr., 5th* (1971) 142.
147. Wynder, E. L., Hoffmann, D., *J. Natl. Cancer Inst.* (1972) **48,** 1749.
148. Wynder, E. L., Hoffmann, D., *Science* (1968) **162,** 862.
149. Hoffman, D., Patrianakos, C. P., Brunnemann, K. D., Gori, G. B., *Anal. Chem.* (1976) **48,** 47–50.
150. Brunneman, K. D., Yu, L., Hoffman, D., *Cancer Res.* (1977) **37,** 3218–3222.

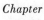

Carcinogenic Aromatic Amines and Related Compounds

D. B. Clayson[1] and R. C. Garner,[2] Department of Experimental Pathology and Cancer Research, School of Medicine, Leeds LS2 9NL, Yorkshire, England

A CORRELATION BETWEEN aromatic amine exposure and human cancer was reported first by Rehn (*1*) in 1895. He observed that three men, who were employed in making magenta (fuchsin) (**1**) from commercial aniline at the same factory in Basel, had bladder cancer. A fourth bladder cancer patient was engaged in the same process at another factory. Bladder cancer is sufficiently rare to make a cluster of a few cases noteworthy. Rehn called this condition "aniline cancer," but we now know that this name is inappropriate. This occupational disease was reported subsequently in all countries with an established chemical industry. Experienced medical officers concluded that aniline (**2**), benzidine (**3**), 2-naphthylamine (**4**), and 1-naphthylamine (**5**) were the probable causative agents (*2*).

An epidemiological survey of bladder cancer in parts of the British chemical industry has greatly clarified this position. Case and his colleagues (*3*) listed all men who had worked in the industry making or using the suspect chemicals between 1921 and 1950. Those who had been employed for less than six months were excluded. The working histories of the more than 4000 remaining names were assembled, and the men were divided into groups that had worked with aniline, benzidine, 2-naphthylamine, 1-naphthylamine, or a mixture of two or more of these chemicals. The incidence of the disease in each group was determined from death certificates, hospital records, reports of coroners' inquests, and by inquiry from the patient or his relatives. Death

---

[1] Present address: Eppley Institute for Cancer Research, University of Nebraska Medical Center, Omaha, Neb. 68105

[2] Present address: Cancer Research Unit, University of York, Heslington, York, Y01 5DD, England

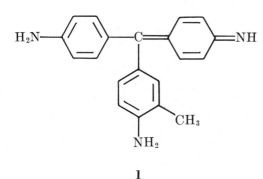

1

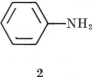

2

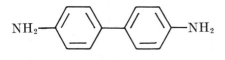

3

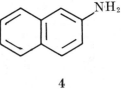

4

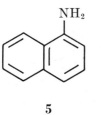

5

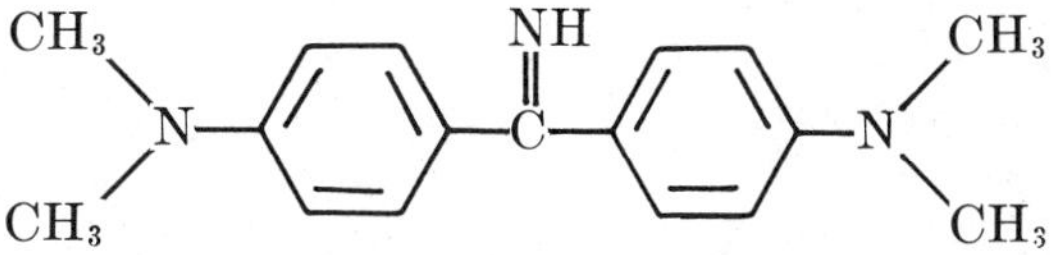

6

certificates are an unreliable way to determine the incidence of bladder cancer because many cases have a long prognosis and patients may die of intercurrent disease while their tumor is in remission. In such cases bladder cancer is not shown on the death certificate. As a control for this working population, Case and his colleagues used the entire male working population of England and Wales. The reason for this is referred to below; it meant that statistical comparisons could be made only between the number of death certificates for each group. Fortunately the position was sufficiently clearcut for this not to confuse the situation. It was first shown that aniline induced excess bladder tumors only when used to manufacture auramine (**6**) and magenta (**4**).

Subsequent work showed that a bladder cancer hazard was demonstrable in the manufacture of these two chemicals but not with aniline in other circumstances. Therefore, it was possible to enlarge the groups of men who had worked with the other suspect chemicals by adding those who had worked with aniline and only one other suspect chemical to the group exposed to the suspect chemical alone. 2-Naphthylamine was the most hazardous material, followed by benzidine and 1-naphthylamine. Even six-months exposure to 2-naphthylamine demonstrably increased the risk of bladder cancer while five years or more appeared necessary for 1-naphthylamine. The average latent period from first entry into the industry to diagnosis of the disease was 17–18 years for 2-naphthylamine and benzidine and 22 years for 1-naphthylamine (3). Commercial 1-naphthylamine, in the time covered by the survey, normally contained 4–10% 2-naphthylamine; thus, it is not possible to be sure that the apparent effect of the 1-naphthylamine was not the result of the contaminating 2-isomer it contained. Animal experiments have clarified this position (see page 408).

Case's first intention was to use the incidence of bladder cancer in men in an English county borough as a control population for the men in the chemical industry. A section of this control population had an unexpectedly high incidence of the disease, and this was traced to men who had worked in a large rubber factory (5). The causative agent was identified as a rubber compounding ingredient containing 1- and 2-naphthylamines (Nonox S). Further research indicated the manufacture of electric cables which were coated with rubber containing the same noxious compounding ingredient and which also led to bladder cancer (6). Suspicion of human bladder cancer induced by aromatic amines was reported for rat catchers working with α-naphthylthiourea (7); for medical personnel, chiefly nurses, who may have used benzidine in the test for occult blood (8); laboratory workers; and tire remolders, who may be exposed to aromatic amine fumes when the tires are heated. Furthermore, some patients receiving 2-naphthylamine mustard (8) for the blood condition *polycythaemia vera* succumbed to bladder cancer 2½–11 years later (9). Confirmation of the industrial hazard in the manufacture of the naphthylamines and benzidine came from other countries (*e.g.*, Japan, France, U.S.A., Russia, and Germany).

One further chemical, 4-biphenylamine (9), has been shown to be a bladder carcinogen in man (10). It was used in the United States between 1935

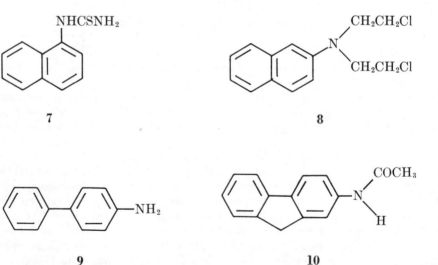

NHCSNH₂

7

CH₂CH₂Cl
N
CH₂CH₂Cl

8

NH₂

9

COCH₃
N
H

10

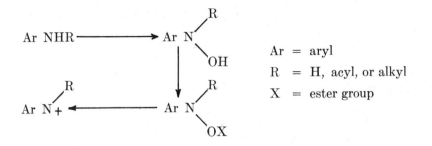

$$Ar\ NHR \longrightarrow Ar\ N \begin{smallmatrix} R \\ \\ OH \end{smallmatrix}$$

Ar = aryl

R = H, acyl, or alkyl

X = ester group

$$Ar\ N+ \overset{R}{\longleftarrow} Ar\ N \begin{smallmatrix} R \\ \\ OX \end{smallmatrix}$$

Figure 1.   Scheme for metabolic activation of aromatic amines

and 1954 when Melick and his colleagues reported that of the 171 men they knew had been exposed to the chemical, 19 developed bladder tumors. Since 1960, this series has been followed by exfoliative cytology (the examination of cells in freshly collected urine to see if their appearance, after staining, indicates that they may have come from a tumor). Of a population of 315 known to have been exposed, 53 have bladder tumors (*11, 12*).

The investigation of tumor induction in animals by the aromatic amines helped to confirm the epidemiological conclusions and provide experimental models for further study. Hueper *et al.* (*13*) provided the first successful model for human bladder cancer by injecting and then feeding large quantities of commercial 2-naphthylamine to dogs. After two years, bladder tumors were identified either at autopsy or cystoscopy in a substantial proportion of the animals. Partially purified and rigorously purified 2-naphthylamine were as effective bladder carcinogens as the commercial chemical (*14, 15*), thus indicating that the pure amine is likely to be the carcinogen rather than an impurity in it.

Further animal experiments proved the existence of many more carcinogenic aromatic amines since Hueper's classic experiment, and these are the basis of this chapter. Unlike the polycyclic hydrocarbons, aromatic amines do not induce tumors at the site of their administration but usually at a distant site such as the liver, intestine, or urinary bladder. Similarly the response to aromatic amines is species specific. 2-Naphthylamine, for example, is a potent bladder carcinogen in men and dogs but is virtually noncarcinogenic in rats and rabbits. These differences lead to the concept that the aromatic amines need metabolic activation to induce tumors. This concept has been demonstrated in detail by James and Elizabeth Miller and their group at the University of Wisconsin (*16*).

On present evidence *N*-hydroxylation is a prerequisite for carcinogenicity for this group of compounds; this may be followed by esterification of the hydroxyl group in some but probably not all cases. The final intermediate is unstable and breaks down to an electrophile which interacts with the tissues (Figure 1).

It might be expected that with this knowledge we could predict the stability and carcinogenicity of the activated metabolites of aromatic amines in animals, but this has yet to be achieved. Because metabolic activation explains the interrelationships among the chemicals discussed here, the mechanism of their activation is considered first. The details of the carcinogenicity of the various molecular species and the effects of different modifying factors follow.

Mechanisms of Activation of Aromatic Amines

In this section the reasons why some aromatic amines are not potently carcinogenic to all laboratory animals are discussed in the light of their metabolism. Certain structural features of aromatic amines important for carcinogenicity are shown, and some of the known activation steps for some laboratory animal carcinogens are described. Much of the discussion centers on the metabolism of N,2-fluorenylacetamide (2-FAA) (10), which is the most intensively investigated of all animal carcinogens. Activation of other amine carcinogens is also reviewed since the investigations on 2-FAA have been described extensively in recent years (17, 18, 19).

Real progress in understanding the structural diversity of chemical carcinogens was made only in the last decade. Prior to this period many hypotheses were advanced to explain why carcinogens were active at sites distant to their application. Metabolism of the compounds was considered to be important for carcinogenic activity, but all the metabolites isolated were less active than the parent compound when tested by well tried methods.

In 1960 a new urinary metabolite of 2-FAA was identified in rats. This metabolite had a faster mobility on paper chromatography than any previously identified hydroxy derivative (20). Compounds excreted in the urine are often conjugated with a polar group such as sulfate or glucuronic acid, and this new metabolite was no exception. After enzymic hydrolysis with glucuronidase it was identified as N-hydroxy-2-FAA (11).

The oxidation of aromatic amines to hydroxylamines is chemically well known. Biological N-hydroxylation was demonstrated (21) during studies on the mechanism of methemoglobin formation by aromatic amines, although as early as 1915, it was suggested that N-hydroxylation of aromatic amines might take place biologically (22). At that time it was thought that o- and p-aminophenols were the methemoglobin inducing agents which oxidized hemoglobin to the ferric state, but Heubner questioned this because p-chloroaniline (12) induced methemoglobinemia but could not be para-hydroxylated. In 1948, Brodie and Axelrod (23) suggested that phenylhydroxylamine might be formed during the metabolism of acetanilide (13) and assigned the methemoglobin production by acetanilide to this metabolite.

After these early observations of N-hydroxylation, Uehleke studied the metabolism of a series of para-substituted aniline derivatives and found that all such derivatives were N-hydroxylated faster than aniline and that the resulting N-hydroxy derivatives induced methemoglobinemia proportional to the amount of N-oxidation (24). Many other examples of N-hydroxylation have since been reported during the metabolism of aromatic amines, and these are discussed next.

Formation of N-Hydroxy Derivatives. Oxidation of primary and secondary aromatic amines is a long-recognized and well documented reaction which takes place easily because of electron availability (*25*). Electron withdrawing substituents such as nitro groups inhibit the ease of oxidation. Biological oxidation of foreign compounds is also a long-recognized reaction; as early as 1867 conversion of benzene to phenol was found in both man and dog (*26*). However, biological N-oxidation of aromatic amines has been recognized for only just over 20 years.

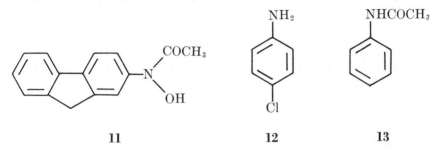

11   **12**   **13**

N-Hydroxylation is one important step in converting an aromatic amine to its ultimate carcinogenic form, that is to a metabolite, which is directly responsible for tumor formation. It appears now that all carcinogenic aromatic amines must be converted to N-hydroxy compounds although all N-hydroxy compounds are not necessarily carcinogenic. There are two major routes to N-hydroxy derivatives—oxidation of a primary or secondary amino group or reduction of a nitro, nitroso, or N-oxide group.

OXIDATION. Oxidation of either a primary or secondary aromatic amine is the major route to N-hydroxy compounds in animals. The oxidation can take place within a number of organs in the body, but it occurs primarily in the liver. The enzymes responsible for oxidation in the liver are in a network of intracellular membranes known as the endoplasmic reticulum. These membranes have a number of functions but are important chiefly as sites of protein synthesis. They can be obtained by ultracentrifuging a liver homogenate at 10,000 g for 10 min, to remove nuclei and mitochondria, and at 100,000 g for 60 min, which precipitates them as a pellet at the bottom of the centrifuge tube. The pellet consists of endoplasmic reticulum membrane fragments known as microsomes. Microsomes, which are spheroids of endoplasmic reticulum, are artefacts of the preparation procedure and do not exist as such within the cell. However, the microsomal fraction can carry out several enzymic conversions if supplemented with the necessary cofactors. The endoplasmic reticulum membranes contain an electron transport system, known as the mixed function oxidases, which can metabolize a variety of drugs, carcinogens, steroids, etc. Using the microsomal fraction, these conversions are carried out *in vitro* with a number of aromatic amines as shown by Kiese and Uehleke (*21*). The microsomal fraction has to be supplemented with $NADPH_2$ as this is essential for all mixed function oxidations, and atmospheric oxygen is required. In a series of these conversions, p-aminopropiophenone (**14**), p-phenetidine (**15**), p-chloroaniline (**12**), and p-toluidine (**16**) the production of the nitroso

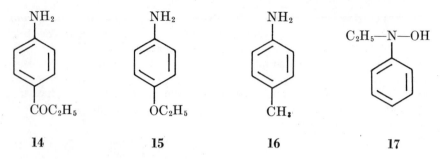

14   **15**   **16**   **17**

derivative from the aromatic amine paralleled methemoglobin production by these compounds in the cat. With a number of carcinogenic aromatic amines the formation of nitroso derivatives by rat liver microsomes decreased in the order—4-biphenylamine, 2-fluorenylamine, aniline and 2-naphthylamine equivalently, and 4-stilbenamine (27).

N-Hydroxy derivatives of primary aromatic amines are somewhat unstable and are often further oxidized to nitroso derivatives. On the other hand, N-hydroxy derivatives of acylated aromatic amines are stable; hence, they are more amenable to isolation. This made it possible for the Millers to demonstrate N-hydroxy-N-2-FAA formation *in vivo*, and Irving to demonstrate N-hydroxy-N-2-FAA production by rabbit liver microsomes *in vitro* (28). The rabbit is particularly suited to such studies because of its high activity in converting 2-FAA to the N-hydroxy form; as much as 22–30% of a dose of FAA is excreted in the urine as the glucuronide conjugate of N-hydroxy-N-2-FAA (29).

It was originally thought that N-hydroxylation *in vivo* or *in vitro* of 2-FAA was proportional to the amount of cytochrome P-450, the terminal cytochrome of the mixed function oxidase electron transport chain. However, although higher activities of this enzyme increase the ring hydroxylation of 2-FAA (30), there is often no proportionate increase in N-hydroxylation. A number of compounds, such as the polycyclic hydrocarbons can increase ring hydroxylation activity when administered previously to the living animal. As will be discussed later, such agents profoundly alter the susceptibility of animals to aromatic amine carcinogenesis, because they alter the overall balance of the metabolic pathways.

Repeated exposure to an aromatic amine carcinogen can sometimes increase the metabolism rate. If rats are exposed repeatedly to 2-FAA, there is a gradual increase in the rate of N-hydroxy-N-2-FAA excretion in the urine until by 18 weeks the quantity has increased nine fold (31). This is an important consideration when investigating the metabolism of any compound in animals. Repeated exposure, as opposed to a single administration, may alter the amount of toxic or carcinogenic metabolites formed.

Although N-hydroxylation is a prerequisite for tumor induction by carcinogenic aromatic amines, not all N-hydroxy derivatives are carcinogenic. Thus, N-phenylhydroxylamine, N-ethyl-N-phenylhydroxylamine (**17**) (32), and N-hydroxy-N-1-fluorenylacetamide (**18**) (33) were all noncarcinogenic when tested.

Like most enzyme reactions, there appears to be some substrate specificity in the N-hydroxylation of aromatic amines. Some amines cannot be N-hydroxylated enzymically and are therefore noncarcinogenic. However, if the N-hydroxy derivative is prepared chemically, carcinogenic activity may be found, e.g., N-hydroxy-7-OH-N-2-FAA (**19**) (*33*). N-Hydroxylation also can be increased by suitable ring substitution. 7-OH-2-FAA is one of the main ring hydroxylated metabolites of 2-FAA and is noncarcinogenic. If the 7 position is fluorinated, hydroxylation is blocked at that position, and N-hydroxylation and carcinogenic activity are increased (*32*).

Other aromatic amines similar in structure to 2-FAA are N-hydroxylated by the rat, and all the N-hydroxy derivatives have greater carcinogenic activity than the parent compound. These include 4-biphenylacetamide (**20**) (*34*), 4-stilbenylacetamide (**21**) (*35*), and 2-phenanthrenylacetamide (**22**) (*32*).

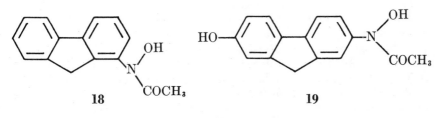

18   19

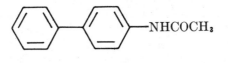

20

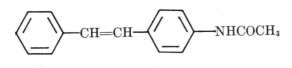

21

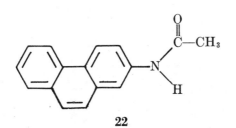

22

Further evidence for the importance of *N*-hydroxylation is provided by the failure of 3-methylcholanthrene to inhibit *N*-hydroxy-2-FAA carcinogenesis whereas 2-FAA carcinogenicity is considerably reduced (*36*). Enzyme induction by the hydrocarbon reduces the overall production of the *N*-hydroxy compound.

2-Naphthylamine is a proven bladder carcinogen in man. At one time it was thought to be active through the formation of ortho hydroxy derivatives as metabolites (*37*). The validity of these experiments has been questioned, and current thought is that *N*-oxidation products are the active metabolites. There is a good correlation between appearance of *N*-oxidation products in the urine and carcinogenicity in animals (*38*). The dog, monkey, and hamster exhibit bladder tumors after 2-naphthylamine administration (*39*). The mouse develops liver tumors, but no tumors are induced in rats and rabbits. Administration of *N*-2-naphthylhydroxylamine (**23**) to dogs results in a greater tumor incidence than with the parent compound (*40*). 2-Nitrosonaphthalene (**24**) also has been identified as a metabolite of 2-naphthylamine in the dog. It too is carcinogenic (*41*).

Chemical synthesis of 1-naphthylhydroxylamine (**25**) showed that this compound is tumorigenic in the rat and more potent than 2-naphthylhydroxylamine. Neither compound induces bladder tumors in the rat, but both cause liver tumors. 1-Naphthylamine is noncarcinogenic, or only weakly carcinogenic, in animals. However, its *N*-hydroxy derivative is considerably more potent than 2-naphthylamine (*40*).

N-Hydroxylation is probably important for carcinogenicity of the aminoazo dyes. *N*-Hydroxy-*N*-4-monomethylaminoazobenzene (**26**) (*N*-hydroxy-MAB) could not be synthesized although its benzyloxy ester (**27**) is an extremely potent carcinogen (*see* page 425). *N*-Hydroxy-4-aminoazobenzene (**28**) was noncarcinogenic (*44*) as was its *N*-acetyl derivative (**29**), indicating the importance of an *N*-methyl group. Ring substitutents can affect the carcinogenicity of the azo dye series of compounds. For example, substitution of

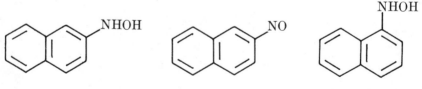

23   24   25

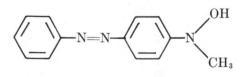

26

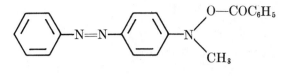

27

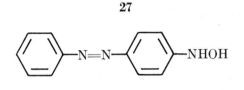

28

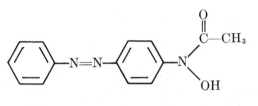

29

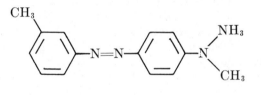

30

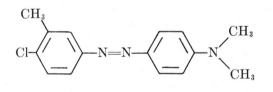

31

methyl in the 3′ position profoundly increases the carcinogenicity of DAB (**30**). In a series of DAB derivatives, 3′-methyl-4′-chloro DAB (**31**) was the most potent tumor-inducing agent when fed for 50 days, but 3′-methyl-4′-ethyl-DAB (**32**) was the most potent when fed continuously for 12 months (*43, 44*).

REDUCTION. N-Hydroxy derivatives can be formed by reduction. Within the tissues there are many reductases, some of which reduce nitro, nitroso, or N-oxide groups to N-hydroxy derivatives. The best characterized of these are those that act on 2-FAA congeners. 2-Nitrosofluorene (**33**), an oxidation

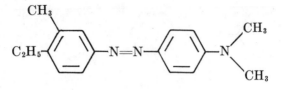

32

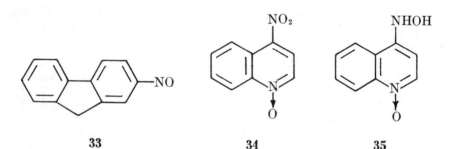

33   **34**   **35**

product of N-hydroxy-2-FA, can be converted back to the parent compound enzymatically. Hamster and rabbit liver soluble enzymes had considerably more activity in carrying out this reduction than those from the rat (45).

Interest was recently revived in nitrosofluorene because it is a powerful frame-shift mutagen in *Salmonella typhimurium* (46). There is now thought to be a correlation between compounds that are mutagenic for bacteria and those which are directly carcinogenic for animals. However, 2-nitrosofluorene is only weakly carcinogenic (47). Its mutagenicity could be caused by the ability of the bacteria to reduce the compound to N-hydroxy FA, reductase activity having been shown in this group of bacteria (48). The increased mutagenic activity of the nitroso compound over the N-hydroxy derivative may be caused by an increased lipid solubility.

4-Nitroquinoline-1-oxide (NQO) (**34**) is a potent carcinogen in the rat and mouse. Repeated subcutaneous injection of 4-hydroxyaminoquinoline-1-oxide (HAQO) (**35**) results in more sarcomas than after injection of the parent compound (50). Also a single injection of HAQO induced tumors while the nitro derivative did not (51). NQO is a potent mutagen for *Salmonella typhimurium* but is unable to mutate phage (52). On the other hand, HAQO is mutagenic for both. A reductase was identified in *Salmonella* which will reduce NQO to its N-hydroxy derivative. A similar enzyme was identified in rat liver soluble fraction. It appears to be a diaphorase and not the nitroreductase responsible for p-nitrobenzoic acid reduction (53).

Japanese workers did many structure–activity studies on NQO and its derivatives. Apparently the nitro group must be in the 4 position for carcinogenicity (*see* Tables XI and XII for structures and carcinogenicity).

Reduction of a nitro group also appears to be important for the carcinogenicity of some nitrofuran compounds. Urinary bladder tumors were found after feeding N-(4-[5-nitro-2-furyl]2-thiazolyl)formamide (**36**) to rats and mice (*54*). The same compound induced both bladder and renal pelvic tumors in the dog (*55*). Many other 5-nitrofuran compounds were tested for carcinogenicity (Table XIV); certain structural features are important for activity. It is essential that the nitro group be in the 5 position of the furan ring. Several enzymes reduced nitrofurans to their corresponding *N*-hydroxy derivatives. One of these occurs in the liver-soluble fraction and requires NADPH (*56*). Two other enzymes which are able to reduce nitrofurazone (**37**) and furazolidone (**38**) were found in the liver microsomal fraction. One of these appeared to be xanthine oxidase, since it was inhibited by allopurinol, and the other was NADPH-cytochrome c reductase (*57*).

Importance of *N*-Hydroxylation for Tumor Induction. After isolation of *N*-hydroxy-2-FAA as a metabolite of 2-FAA, this compound was tested for carcinogenicity (*58*). It was a more potent carcinogen in the rat than the parent compound. In the guinea pig, it induced tumors at the injection site while 2-FAA did not (*59*). Originally it was proposed that the resistance of the guinea pig to 2-FAA was the result of an inability to carry out the *N*-hydroxylation step. However, many other aromatic *N*-hydroxy derivatives were noncarcinogenic. *N*-Hydroxylation is a prerequisite for tumor initiation, but it is not the sole requirement. It appears that at least two aromatic rings, either fused as in 2-naphthylamine or joined as in 4-biphenylamine, are required for potent carcinogenicity. The more complicated structural requirement is probably necessary to stabilize a positive charge on the amine nitrogen (Figure 2).

If *N*-hydroxy derivatives are the "ultimate" form of the carcinogen, they should react *in vitro* with cellular macromolecules to give derivatives similar

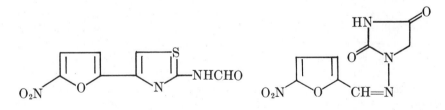

36   37

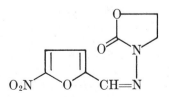

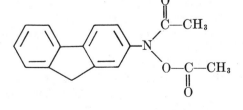

38   39

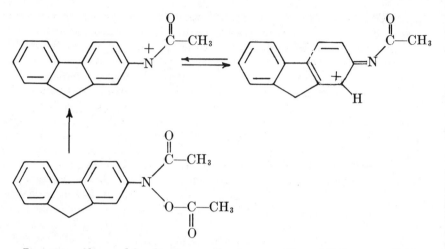

Figure 2.   Charge delocalization on the decomposition of N-2-acetoxy FAA

to those found *in vivo* after administration of the parent compound. This is
not the case since there are only a few reports in the literature of *N*-hydroxy
derivatives binding to macromolecules *in vitro* (*60, 61*). These reports do not
exclude the possibility of esterification of the *N*-hydroxy derivative by the
buffer in the assay medium as described below.

Except for the latter binding studies, it appears that *N*-hydroxy derivatives are not the ultimate carcinogenic form but a proximate form which must
be further metabolized.

Esterification. A clue to these further metabolites was provided when
the Millers and their co-workers (*62*) were attempting to synthesize the
N-hydroxy derivative of MAB. They found this synthesis impossible and
therefore synthesized the benzoyloxy ester. The idea was that the ester would
break down in the tissues to yield *N*-hydroxy MAB. When the ester was tested
for carcinogenicity, it was found to be extremely potent, particularly as a
subcutaneous carcinogen. Incubation of the benzoyloxy ester with macromolecules *in vitro* gave covalently bound derivatives which were similar to those
found after MAB administration *in vivo* (*47*). This was the first indication
that esters might be the ultimate form of carcinogenic aromatic amines.

FORMATION OF *N*-ACETATES. After it was realized that esters of *N*-hydroxy
compounds might be the ultimate forms of these carcinogens, the *N*-acetoxy
ester of 2-FAA (**39**) was synthesized. This compound was an extremely
potent carcinogen subcutaneously, giving tumors at the injection site. It was
equipotent with the polycyclic hydrocarbons, the most potent compounds
known at that time. Also *N*-2-acetoxy FAA reacted *in vitro* with cellular
macromolecules to give covalently bound derivatives identical to those found
after administration of 2-FAA to animals. For example, *N*-2-acetoxy FAA
reacts with methionine to yield 3-methylmercapto-2-FAA *in vitro* (*40*) (*63*).
3-Methylmercapto-2-FAA is also found on alkaline hydrolysis of liver protein
after 2-FAA administration *in vivo*. *N*-2-Acetoxy FAA also reacts with guano-

sine monophosphate to give 8-guanyl-2-FAA *in vitro*. A similar conjugate was isolated from a hydrolysate of DNA after 2-FAA administration (*47*).

In a study of the mechanism of nucleophilic attack in a series of acethydroxamic acids, 2-fluorenyl- and 4-stilbenyl-*N*-acetoxy-acetamides dissociated unimolecularly to form acetate ions and carbonium ions whereas the corresponding biphenyl and phenanthrene compounds underwent bimolecular dissociation (*63*).

Esterification by acetate is a common conjugation mechanism in the metabolism of amines, sulfonamides, and some aromatic amino acids. It can take place nonenzymically as in the reaction of *N*-hydroxy-2-FAA with acetyl CoA (*64*). However, the pH optimum for this reaction is about 10.0 so that at physiological pH only a minute amount of ester can be formed.

Recently two new mechanisms of enzymic acetylation of *N*-hydroxy compounds were described. *N*-Hydroxy-2-FAA is converted to a free nitroxide radical by a one-electron oxidation process. Both potassium ferricyanide and moist silver oxide catalyze the reaction to produce the radical form (*see* Figure 3). Two nitroxide ions formed dismutate to yield one molecule of 2-nitrosofluorene and one molecule of *N*-acetoxy FAA (*65*). Both molecules have

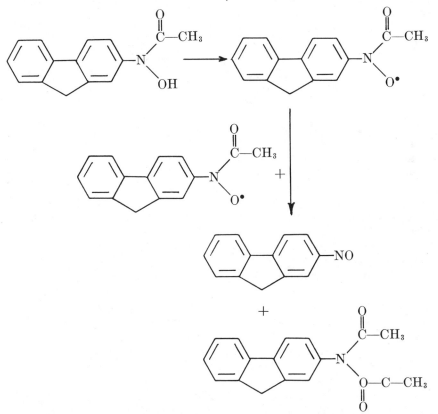

Figure 3.   Formation of N-2-acetoxy FAA by one electron oxidation

carcinogenic activity. Enzymically, the reaction can be catalyzed by various peroxidases: both human myeloperoxidase and lactoperoxidase are active (66). The importance of peroxidase activity for organ specificity of carcinogens is discussed later. Other acethydroxamic acids also undergo one-electron oxidation.

Bartsch *et al.* reported another activation enzyme which is found in liver cell sap and esterifies hydroxamic acids (67). It can transfer an acetyl group from a molecule of N-hydroxy-2-FAA to one molecule of N-hydroxy-2-FA. The acetyl donor need not be N-hydroxy-2-FAA. Other carcinogenic acethydroxamic acids such as 4-N-hydroxybiphenylylacetamide can be used (68).

Acetylation does not always lead to increased carcinogenicity. Diacetylhydroxyaminoquinoline (**41**) is much more reactive with nucleophiles *in vitro*, than NQO, but it was less carcinogenic than NQO (69). Possibly the molecule is so reactive that it is unable to reach the critical target within the cell to initiate tumors; instead, it reacts with noncritical nucleophiles.

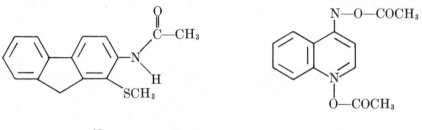

40   41

FORMATION OF N-SULFATES. Although various synthetic esters of N-hydroxy-2-FAA were extremely reactive, they did not appear to be the ones actually generated within the cell. The Millers and their co-workers and King and Phillips (70) independently demonstrated that N-hydroxy-2-FAA could be esterified with 3′-phosphoadenosine-5′-phosphosulfate by an enzyme in the soluble fraction of the liver cell (71). The enzyme activity of this sulfotransferase differed between sexes and between species. Male rats had a higher activity than females, and activity was directly related to sensitivity to the carcinogenic action of 2-FAA in several species (72). The guinea pig, for example, resists the carcinogenic activity of 2-FAA and has low activities of this sulfotransferase. The guinea pig therefore not only poorly N-hydroxylates 2-FAA but also is unable to esterify any N-hydroxy compound formed. These two low enzyme activities probably account for this species' resistance to liver tumor induction by 2-FAA.

The synthetic N-sulfate of 2-FAA is extremely reactive and has a half-life of about 1 min in water. When this compound was tested for carcinogenicity either subcutaneously in rats or on the skin of mice or rats, very few tumors were obtained. This is probably caused by the breakdown of the ester by reaction with extracellular materials before it can reach critical targets within the cell. Confirmatory evidence for the involvement of the N-sulfate in carcinogenesis was the discovery that depletion of the intracellular sulfate level with acetanilide reduces the carcinogenicity of 2-FAA (*73*). Also, the toxicity and reactivity of N-hydroxy-2-FAA are increased by simultaneous administration of sulfate ion (*74*).

FORMATION OF N-CARBAMATE ESTERS. N-Carbamate esters of N-hydroxy compounds are formed nonenzymically by reaction with a suitable donor. Carbamyl phosphate formed carbamate esters with N-hydroxy-2-FAA; the pH optimum of the reaction is 4.5 (*75*). There is only negligible reaction at physiological pH. At pH 7.0, acetylation by acetyl CoA produces more esterification of N-hydroxy-2-FAA than carbamylation by carbamyl phosphate. With N-hydroxy-2-phenanthylacetamide or N-hydroxy-4-stilbenylacetamide one gets more carbamate ester.

FORMATION OF N-PHOSPHATES. Activation of N-hydroxy-2-FAA has been found with ortho phosphate (*76*). Activation of HAQO may occur through phosphate esterification (*77*). Transfer of a phosphate group from ATP to the hydroxamic acid is catalyzed by a soluble enzyme of the liver. The resulting phosphate ester reacts with nucleophiles to form adducts identical to those obtained *in vivo* after administration of the parent compound.

GLUCURONIDE FORMATION. There is considerable debate on the importance of glucuronidation as an activation mechanism for aromatic amines. Glucuronidation of the N-hydroxy group is one of the major routes for excretion of N-hydroxy-2-FAA. The N-glucuronide of N-hydroxy-2-FAA (N-glu-2-FAA) will react *in vitro* with nucleophiles although the reaction rate is much slower than with either N-acetoxy-2-FAA or N-2-FAA-N-sulfate (*78*). This glucuronide also had a much lower carcinogenic potency than N-hydroxy-2-FAA (*79*) and has no mutagenic activity (*80*). The N-glucuronide of 2-FA might be formed by deacetylation of N-glu-2-FAA or by esterification of N-2-hydroxy-FA as discussed next. It is considerably more reactive with nucleophiles than N-glu-2-FAA *in vitro* (*81*). It is also a potent mutagen for bacterial transforming DNA (*82*). However, it is less carcinogenic than N-glu-2-FAA. This can be explained in the same way as the weak carcinogenicity of N-2-FAA-N-sulfate.

Detoxification Mechanisms. All the activation mechanisms described above use enzymes normally involved in the detoxification of foreign compounds. The enzymes carrying out these reactions sometimes generate reactive metabolites but usually produce less toxic derivatives. For example, hydroxylation generally produces a less toxic compound, such as the conversion of aniline to *p*-aminophenol, whereas N-hydroxylation gives a much more toxic compound. These enzymes convert the foreign compound to a more polar molecule and thus facilitate its excretion in the urine and feces. Sulfate esterification of N-hydroxy-2-FAA yields the highly reactive N-sulfate. Sulfate esterification of phenols to give ethereal sulfates leads to a less toxic and a more rapidly excreted product. Since ring hydroxylation is the predominant metabolic route for aromatic amines, there will be a balance between activation and deactivation reactions. This balance can be altered, for example, by pretreatment with 3-methylcholanthrene which increases the rate of ring hydroxylation of 2-FAA without a proportional increase in N-hydroxylation.

Thus the carcinogenicity of 2-FAA in the rat is reduced by prior 3-methyl-cholanthrene administration as mentioned previously.

ORTHO HYDROXYLATION. Ortho hydroxylation of aromatic amines has been recognized for some time. It was once thought that this step was the prime activation mechanism for several aromatic amines (37). This inter-pretation was based on the observation that a number of ortho hydroxy aro-matic amines induced bladder tumors when implanted in a paraffin or choles-terol pellet in the bladder lumen. For example, 2-amino-1-naphthol hydro-chloride (42) induced tumors in this test but 2-naphthylamine did not. The validity of such tests was questioned because the paraffin or cholesterol pellet itself produces profound changes in the bladder epithelium with variable tumor induction (83, 84, 85, 86).

In a series of tests in mice, the cholesterol pellet induced an 8% bladder tumor incidence while 8-methylxanthurenic acid (43), xanthurenic acid (44), 8-hydroxyquinaldic acid (45), 3-hydroxy-L-kynurenine (46), and 3-hydroxy-anthranilic acid (47) (all metabolites of tryptophan) gave a significantly higher incidence. If 8-methylxanthurenic acid, which gave a 30% bladder tumor incidence when implanted in a cholesterol pellet, was injected into animals with a cholesterol bladder implant, a similar bladder tumor incidence was obtained (87).

Among other changes, a pellet induces a hyperplastic and an inflamma-tory response (83), and significantly increases the mitotic rate in the bladder epithelium (84). It appears that the presence of the pellet leads to a carci-nogenic response by the epithelium. This may be because of a co-carcinogenic action of the pellet or because the bladder is sensitized to the action of low levels of extraneous carcinogens present in the urine.

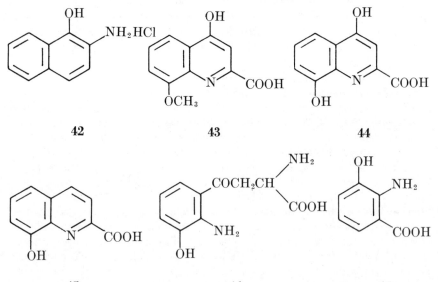

42   43   44

45   46   47

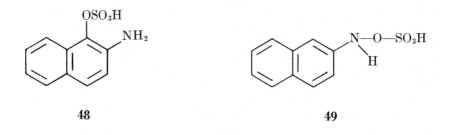

48   49

Nevertheless, Manson (*88*) has noted that 2-amino-1-naphthylhydrogen sulfate (**48**), a principal detoxication product of 2-naphthylamine in dogs, has many properties associated with 2-hydroxylaminonaphthalene sulfate (**49**) *in vitro*. The former metabolite was only a weak carcinogen, even when tested by bladder implantation. This indicates either that it cannot react with the critical targets for carcinogenesis or that its polar nature prevents its entry into cells.

Bladder cancer patients who have not been occupationally exposed to carcinogens may have an abnormal tryptophan metabolism with emphasis on the niacin pathway. It was thought that the tumors might be induced by tryptophan or one of its metabolites since these were active in the bladder implantation test. DL-Tryptophan induced marked hyperplasia of the bladder transitional epithelium (*89*). There are a number of difficulties which weakened the earlier concepts of tryptophan carcinogenesis (*see* page 439).

Hydroxylation ortho to an amino group is commonly found in the metabolism of aromatic amines. The reaction is NADPH-dependent, requires molecular oxygen, and is carried out by the drug metabolizing enzymes in the liver. Ortho hydroxylation also occurs by transfer of the hydroxyl group from the hydroxylamine. Incubation of *N*-hydroxy-2-FAA with rat liver microsomes leads to transfer of the hydroxyl group to the 3 position. A similar reaction is found with the *N*-4-hydroxy derivative of biphenylacetamide (*N*-4-hydroxy BPA) (*90*).

DEACETYLATION AND DEHYDROXYLATION. Administration of ring labeled 2-FAA to animals causes a higher binding of radioactivity to macromolecules than 2-FAA labeled in the acetyl side chain. This difference is the result of deacetylation of 2-FAA to give 2-FA bound residues. Some enzymes identified can deacetylate both 2-FAA and *N*-hydroxy-2-FAA.

One such enzyme in rats is localized in the liver-cell soluble fraction and can be inhibited by fluoride (*91*). Two deacetylating enzymes were found in guinea pig liver microsomes. One of these deacetylates *N*-hydroxy-2-FAA 265 times faster than 2-FAA while the other has a similar activity for both substrates (*92*). A dehydroxylating enzyme was identified in the liver soluble fraction of rats. It was comparatively labile and lost activity after a 60-min incubation at 37°C (*90*). Deacetylation could be considered under certain circumstances to be an activation step, particularly in organs where transacetylation could occur.

ESTERIFICATION. Some esterification enzymes were described in the preceding section on activation. Esterification is normally a deactivating step in the metabolism of a foreign compound. Ring hydroxylation of aromatic amines is the major route of metabolism for these compounds; the phenols formed are often further conjugated with either sulfate, glucuronic acid, or phosphate groups.

Tissue Specificity of Activation Enzymes. The sensitivity of a particular tissue to aromatic amine carcinogenesis depends partly on the ability to convert the proximate carcinogen to its ultimate form. N-Hydroxylation, a liver mixed function oxidase-dependent reaction, is a prerequisite for the further activation of the aromatic amine molecule. Failure to N-hydroxylate will confer resistance against the carcinogenic effect to the animal.

Once the N-hydroxy compound is formed, it is subjected to competing metabolic pathways. It may be sulfated by the soluble sulfotransferase in the liver. Deficiency of this enzyme confers resistance in some cases. However, there are several other activation enzymes besides sulfotransferases which have already been described. Absence of or low sulfotransferase activity does not confer tissue resistance to the carcinogen. Rat ear duct gland and mammary gland have low sulfotransferase activity yet they are sensitive to 2-FAA carcinogenicity (93). These tissues may have some other activating enzyme such as peroxidase or acetyl transferase activity, both of which can produce a reactive ester form.

Esterification is unlikely to be the sole mechanism of activation. N-Acetyl-N-2-naphthylamine did not produce tumors in dogs after two years, but tumors appeared with an equivalent dose of 2-naphthylamine (94). Since the dog is unable to acetylate aromatic amines, N-hydroxy amines may be the ultimate carcinogens for bladder tissue in this species. Similarly, the rabbit is resistant to the hepatocarcinogenic effect of 2-FAA but does develop bladder tumors, possibly through N-hydroxy metabolites without further esterification.

Not only does the level of activating enzymes determine the tissue sensitivity to a particular aromatic amine carcinogen but also the level of detoxification enzymes. It is the balance of the two that is important for sensitivity. Increasing the level of the detoxification enzymes by prior treatment with inducing agents can often decrease the carcinogenicity of the compound under study, but for any particular compound, resistance or sensitivity may often depend on the overall *in vivo* pharmacodynamics or pharmacokinetics of metabolism of the compound. Such studies have not been carried out in detail for any aromatic amine carcinogens.

Structure–Activity Relationships

The carcinogenic potential of the many aromatic amines which have been tested for their ability to induce cancer are discussed in this section. The basic information is recorded in the various volumes published by the United States Public Health Service, "Survey of Compounds Which Have Been Tested for Carcinogenic Activity" (95–100). The information in these valuable volumes is uncritical as everything was recorded in an easily accessible fashion without a specialized assessment of the significance of the experimental data.

We have subdivided the information in the following manner:

A. *Anilines*

B. *Extended anilines*
1. Biphenylamines
2. Benzidine
3. Methylene-bis(aniline)s
4. Stilbenamines

C. *Fused ring amines*
1. Fluorenamines
2. Naphthylamines
3. Anthramines
4. Phenanthramines
5. Others

D. *Aminoazo and other azo compounds*
1. 4-(Phenylazo)aniline
2. N,N-Dimethyl-4-phenylazo-aniline
3. o-Tolylazo-m-toluene
4. Phenylazonaphthol
5. Others

E. *Heterocyclic amines*
1. 4-Nitroquinoline-1-oxides
2. Purine oxides
3. Five-membered heterocyclic amines and nitro compounds
4. Tryptophan and indole
5. Other heterocycles

These different molecular types all have one thing in common; in each case they are probably converted by metabolic activation to aryl hydroxylamines or related compounds. In compiling the data on those compounds which have been shown to be carcinogenic, we have eliminated results in which insufficient numbers of animals were used and those in which the authors, for one reason or another, failed to maintain the animals for enough time to develop tumors. Furthermore, certain techniques and tumors, such as local sarcomas formed in response to the subcutaneous injection of some test substances and bladder tumors after bladder implantation, present difficulties in interpretation. What remains is not claimed to be comprehensive, but demonstrates the major groups of active compounds. Because so much work on aromatic amine carcinogenesis since 1960 has been related to the *in vivo* mechanism of action of these compounds, it is necessary to repeat material already described above.

Anilines. Early experiments, which purported to show that aniline was carcinogenic, were disputed by Bonser (*101*) who drew attention to the inadequacy of the histopathological description of the lesions. Further investigation of this substance was discouraged by the demonstration, using epidemiological methods, that aniline was not a bladder carcinogen in workers exposed during its manufacture, purification, or use (*4*).

The consumption of excessive quantities of analgesics containing phenacetin (**50**), antipyrine (**51**), and caffeine (**52**) in Sweden may be an example of a single ring aromatic amine inducing cancer in man. Analgesic abuse became part of folk medicine in some districts of Sweden after World War I. Abuse is defined as an individual consumption of more than 1 kg of the analgesic over several years. These quantities may result in renal

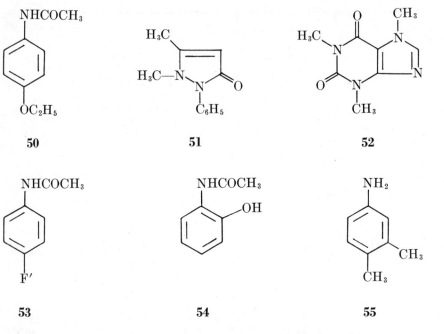

50   **51**   **52**

53   **54**   **55**

papillary necrosis. Bengsston *et al.* (*102*) noted that renal pelvic cancer was also associated with excessive consumption of the drug. In 242 patients with renal papillary necrosis, 142 were abusers. All nine cases of renal pelvic cancer occurred in the latter group, thus establishing a correlation between analgesic abuse and this form of cancer; there were also a few instances of bladder cancer. Bengsston and her colleagues also showed that renal pelvic cancer in abusers occurred at an earlier age than similar tumors in instances where the etiology was unknown. There are two difficulties in assessing this evidence. First, there is still a relative lack of information about similar conditions in countries other than Sweden, although cases of urinary tract carcinoma associated with excessive consumption of analgesics have been reported from Australia (*103*) and the United States (*104*). Secondly, there is no evidence to suggest which components in the analgesic lead to the tumors. Bengsston *et al.* (*102*) indicted phenacetin—a speculation supported by the known predilection of the carcinogenic aromatic amines for the urinary tract in man. However, on present evidence neither antipyrine, a pyrazolone derivative, nor caffeine, a bacterial mutagen, can be excluded.

Morris *et al.* (*105*) claimed that *p*-fluoracetanilide (**53**), *o*-hydroxyacetanilide (**54**), and 3,4-dimethylaniline (**55**) were carcinogenic, because they induced pituitary adenomas in Buffalo rats. No reliance can be placed on this observation because of the variation in the yield of these tumors in the pituitaries of untreated rats used as controls for this and other experiments (*37*).

Yamamoto (*106*) did not find tumors in small numbers of rats fed massive doses of acetanilide and related chemicals as controls for other experiments. Homberger *et al.* (*107, 108*) tested a series of single-ring aromatic amines in rats and mice. Several chemicals induced cancer when the animals were treated at up to the maximum tolerated dose of the amine. *o*-Toluidine hydrochloride (**56**) led to 35 subcutaneous sarcomas in 50 CD rats, and it was shown subsequently to be a bladder carcinogen. It gave tumors of the reticulo-endothelial system in mice. *m*-Toluidine did not induce tumors in these experiments while *p*-toluidine was not a bladder carcinogen. 4-Chloro-*o*-toluidine hydrochloride (**57**) induced 40 hemangiosarcomas in 82 CD mice while 2,4,5-trimethylaniline gave 17 "hepatomas" and 12 lung adenomas in 82 mice. 2,5-Dimethoxy-4-stilbenamine (**58**), used as a positive control, induced 34 ear duct tumors in 50 rats. Similar tumors did not occur in untreated rodents. These results were presented in abstract form from a larger series of tests of single ring aromatic amines. They leave no doubt that single-ring aromatic amines under appropriate dosages may be carcinogenic.

The presumed activated intermediates of these aromatic amines, the phenylhydroxylamines, have received relatively little attention. Phenylhydroxylamine is produced from aniline or nitrobenzene and induces methemoglobinemia. The recent tests of phenylhydroxylamine (*32*) and two analogs (**59, 60**) (*32, 33*) as carcinogens were negative but unsatisfactory in view of the short survival of the animals.

Although aniline is not a bladder carcinogen in man, high doses of other single-ring aromatic amines induce cancers in experimental animals. This must be kept in mind when assessing the safety of compounds of this nature, although the interpretation of the significance of tumors induced by

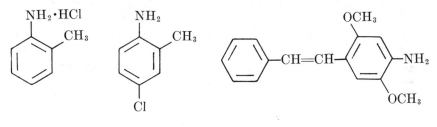

56   57   58

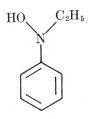

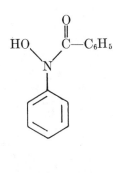

59   60   61

massive doses of chemicals may present considerable difficulties if the results must be judged in terms of safety in man.

There have been reports on the hepatotoxicity of single-ring aromatic amines. For example, paracetamol (**61**), a widely used analgesic, will in large doses induce severe liver necrosis (*109*). Thus, this drug is commonly being used for suicide since it is readily available to the public. Compounds such as cysteamine protect against the liver necrosis, and it was suggested that drug preparations should include this compound as a protecting agent (*110*). Paracetamol toxicity depends on the activity of the liver mixed-function oxidases and on the liver glutathione level (*111*). Although an epoxide may be the necrotizing agent, the possibility that *N*-hydroxylation is important must be considered. Whatever the activation mechanism, there is no doubt that paracetamol does arylate macromolecules (*112*). Liver function tests are normal in people taking therapeutic amounts of the analgesic (*109*).

Extended Anilines. 4-BIPHENYLAMINES. The carcinogenicity of 4-biphenylamine (BPA) (**9**) (4-aminobiphenyl) in man has already been mentioned (*see* page 368). This chemical provides a useful example of a substance which produces varied responses in different experimental species, a property which may indicate that the substance needs metabolic activation. Thus, Walpole and his colleagues (*113*) showed that BPA was a powerful bladder carcinogen in dogs. In rats, BPA induced mainly intestinal and mammary tumors later in life (*114*). The results in dogs were confirmed by Deichmann and his group (*115*) who also demonstrated that as little as 1 mg/kg body weight/day BPA induced bladder carcinomas and papillomas within 33 months in all the six dogs under test (*116*), but that a single dose was ineffective (*117*). 2-Naphthylamine, which is also a powerful bladder carcinogen in dogs, (*see* page 405), was not effective under the former conditions. The same workers also showed that 4-nitrobiphenyl was carcinogenic to the dog bladder (*118*). BPA is only weakly carcinogenic in mice, inducing a low incidence of bladder tumors in each of two strains of mice, and liver tumors in one (*119, 120*). In rabbits, however, it induced bladder tumors in two to five years (*121*).

The derivatives of BPA (Table I) illustrate some of the apparent generalizations that apply to other types of aromatic amines. For example, the position of the amino group relative to the biphenyl appears to be important. Both BPA and 4-biphenylacetamide (BPAA) have moderate carcinogenicity in the rat, but in the same experiment 3- and 2-biphenylacetamide appeared to be only weakly carcinogenic in this, the only treated species (*122*). This result reflects the general observation that aromatic amines with a conjugated para substituent in the same ring tend to be more carcinogenic than amines with this substituent in other positions or absent (*123*).

Substitution of a methyl group ortho to an aromatic amino group often enhances the carcinogenicity of an aromatic amine. This is illustrated by the potency of 3,2'-dimethyl-BPA in the rat intestine; intestinal tumors were formed with a latency of less than 300 days in 75% of male Wistar rats after the chemical was injected subcutaneously to a total dose of 2.8–4.0 g/kg body weight (*114*). Tumors of other tissues, such as the ear duct, were also present. This was the system of choice for the induction of intestinal tumors until 1,2-dimethylhydrazine hydrochloride, cycasin, and methylazoxymethanol acetate (12) were also shown to induce lower intestinal tract tumors. A surgically prepared isolated segment of colon was not susceptible to 3,2′-dimethyl-BPA-induced tumorigenesis. The result indicated that the presence of feces was necessary for tumor formation, but it was not possible to demonstrate whether the fecal metabolite content, the mechanical properties of the feces, or the absence of gut bacteria was responsible (124).

When 3,2′-dimethyl-BPA was given by subcutaneous injection to Wistar rats for limited periods, the intestinal cancer yield was almost abolished, and there were only a small number of bladder papillomas induced. In Slonaker rats more bladder tumors were found (125).

The importance to the carcinogenic action of the methyl group at the position ortho to the amino group is confirmed by the fact that 3-methyl, 3-3′-dimethyl-, 3,2′,5′-trimethyl-, and 3,2′4′,6′-tetramethyl-4-BPA are carcinogenic to intestinal tract and other tissues (114, 126, 127) whereas 2- and 2′-methyl-BPA and their acetylated derivatives failed to induce tumors in similar experiments (114, 122, 126).

The effect of ortho substitution other than methyl in BPA is varied. 3-Methyl-BPA is a bladder carcinogen in rats, but 3-chloro-BPA and 3-hydroxy-BPA apparently have no effect (122, 126).

The bond between a carbon atom in an aromatic ring and fluorine is usually very strong. Fluorine substitution has been used to block positions to metabolic hydroxylation. Since ring C-hydroxylation is believed to be a detoxification mechanism, fluorine substitution in the ring positions in which detoxifying hydroxylation occurs leads to more potent carcinogens. For example, 4′-fluoro-4-BPA (62) with blocked 4′-hydroxylation is a more potent carcinogen than BPA. It produced tumors in most of the rats under test. These tumors included hepatomas, cholangiomas, and renal tumors which developed within six months, as well as injection site sarcomas, intestinal tract adenocarcinomas, and pancreatic and testicular tumors. Some of the latter were possibly unrelated to the chemical because no untreated animals were kept as a control (128, 129).

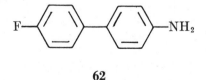

62

As long as feeding tests are relied on, there is no evidence that 3-C- hydroxylation of BPA is other than a detoxification product (122). Nevertheless, if 3-hydroxy-BPA is mixed with paraffin wax to form a pellet and implanted into the lumen of the mouse bladder, carcinomas of the epithelium are formed in a significantly greater yield than in mice implanted with the

Table I.   Carcinogenicity of

Compound	Species	Route[a]	Adequacy[b]
4-Biphenylamine	mouse	O	S
	rat	O	A
	hamster	O	
	rabbit	O	S
	dog	O	A
4-Biphenylhydroxylamine	mouse (new-born)	S.C.	S
N-Acetoxy-4-biphenylacetamide	rat	S.C.	S
4-Biphenylacetamide	rat	O	A
4-Biphenyldimethylamine	rat	O	S
4-Nitrobiphenyl	dog	O	A
4-Biphenylacethydroxamic acid	rat	O	A
2-Fluorophenylaniline	rat	O	S
2-Chloro-4-phenylaniline	rat	S.C.	S
3′-Fluoro-4-phenylaniline	rat	O	S
4′-Fluoro-4-biphenylamine	mouse	O	S
	rat	S.C.	A
2-Methyl-4-phenylaniline	rat	O	S
3-Methyl-4-phenylaniline	rat	O	S
2′-Methyl-4-phenylaniline	rat	O	S
4′-Methyl-4-phenylacetanilide	rat	O	S
3,2′-Dimethyl-4-biphenylamine	rat	S.C./O	A
3,3′-Dimethyl-4-biphenylamine	rat	S.C.	S
3,2′,5′-Trimethyl-4-biphenylamine	rat	S.C.	S
3,2′,4′,6′-Tetramethyl-4-biphenylamine	rat	S.C.	S
3-Methoxy-4-biphenylamine	rat	S.C.	S

[a] O, oral; S.C., subcutaneous injection.
[b] A, tested in more than one institute; S, evidence less convincing.

vehicle alone. 4′-Hydroxy-3-BPA was likewise tumorigenic by this test, but BPA itself was not (*130*). Recently, 3-hydroxy-, 4′-hydroxy-BPA, and BPA induced liver tumors in newborn mice after a limited series of injections (*131*). Whether bladder implantation or injection into newborn mice gives results that can be extrapolated to other situations is not yet established.

N-Hydroxy-BPAA is produced when BPA or BPAA is fed to rats and when the latter compound is fed to dogs. BPA, like other aromatic amines, is not acetylated in dogs. In contrast to findings with 2-FAA, the amount of N-hydroxylated conjugates of BPA (which may be hydrolyzed by taka-diastase to N-hydroxy-BPA) decreased slowly during continuous feeding. Long term animal tests showed that N-hydroxy-BPAA induced more mammary tumors in female weanling rats than did BPAA. This evidence suggests that N-hydroxylation is the first step in the metabolic activation of BPAA (*34*). However, in contrast to 2-FAA (*see* page 446) 3-methylcholanthrene feeding did not greatly influence the yield of tumors induced by either

4-Biphenylamine and Its Derivatives

Tumors Induced in[c]

Local	Bladder	Kidney	Liver	Intestine	Ear Duct	Breast	Other
−	?	−	+	−	−	−	−
−	−	−	?	?	−	+	−
−	−	−	−	−	−	−	−
−	+	−	−	−	−	−	−
−	+	−	−	−	−	−	−
−	−	−	+	−	−	−	−
+	−	−	−	−	−	−	−
−	−	−	−	+	+	+	−
−	−	−	−	+	+	+	−
−	+	−	−	−	−	−	−
+	−	−	−	−	+	+	−
−	−	−	−	−	−	+	−
−	−	−	−	−	−	−	−
−	−	−	−	−	−	+	−
−	−	−	+	−	−	−	−
−	−	+	+	+	−	−	pancreas
−	−	−	−	+	+	−	−
−	−	−	−	−	−	−	−
−	−	−	−	−	−	−	−
−	−	−	−	−	−	−	−
−	+	−	−	+	+	+	salivary gland
−	−	−	−	+	−	−	salivary gland
−	−	−	+	+	−	−	−
−	−	−	+	+	−	−	−
−	+	−	−	−	−	−	−

[c] +, tumors reported; −, tumors not reported.

BPAA or its *N*-hydroxy derivative. *N*-Acetoxy BPAA is a potent locally acting carcinogen. The possibility that the glucuronide of *N*-hydroxy BPAA reacts with nucleic acids and guanosine was discussed by Irving (*132*).

BPA is a potent bladder carcinogen in dogs, but since this species does not acetylate aromatic amines, *N*-hydroxy BPAA probably does not lie on the pathway leading to metabolic activation in this species. Arylhydroxylamines are easily oxidized to nitroso compounds under biological conditions as Radomski and his colleagues showed by chromatographic analysis of both classes of compound (*38*). In dogs the proportion of the dose of BPA, 2-naphthylamine, and 1-naphthylamine converted to hydroxylamines and nitroso compounds together was, in this limited series, proportional to the carcinogenicity of the parent amines to dog bladder (*i.e.*, BPA > 2-naphthylamine ≫ 1-naphthylamine). The active metabolite of BPA in dogs is likely to be the glucuronide of *N*-hydroxy-BPA (*133*), which has been obtained in solution from dog urine but decomposes on concentration. BPA serves as a model for amino derivatives of several important ring systems such as 2-FAA, 3-aminobenzofuran, and 3-aminodibenzothiopene and its oxides.

BENZIDINE (4,4'-DIAMINOBIPHENYL) (3). Benzidine is not only carcinogenic to men who make, purify, or use it in the chemical industry (3, 134), but is also carcinogenic in certain animal species. The pattern, however, differs from that found with 4-BPA. Bladder tumors were found in the dog (136) but only in a proportion of animals after a latent period of seven to nine years and at a time in the life of the dog when spontaneously occurring tumors are common. In rats, subcutaneously injected benzidine induced liver tumors, ear duct carcinomas, and a few adenocarcinomas of the intestine (126), while only hepatomas were induced in mice (136). In rabbits the toxicity of benzidine prevented an equivalent dose to that in other species being given, and it was not possible to obtain comparable results (121).

Several derivatives of benzidine, such as o-tolidine, 3,3'-dichlorobenzidine (63), and o-dianisidine (64), are important as dye intermediates and rubber and plastic compounding ingredients. They are often produced in batches on the benzidine plant and may contribute to the environmental carcinogenic load associated with benzidine in man. Each was investigated experimentally in some depth, especially by Pliss (137, 138, 139, 140, 141), who used rats as his test species (Table II) and induced tumors with each compound.

How benzidine is metabolically activated is not known. Clayson (142) and Meigs et al. (143) investigated its metabolism, but there is no evidence to contradict or support the idea that N-hydroxylation plays the key role

Table II.   Carcinogenicity of

Compound	Species	Route[a]	Adequacy[b]
Benzidine	dog	O	A
	hamster	O	S
	rat	S.C.	A
	mouse	S.C.	S
Diacetylbenzidine	rat	O	S
o,o'-Tolidine	rat	S.C.	A
o,o'-Dianisidine	hamster	O	S
	rat	O	S
3,3'-Dichlorobenzidine	rat	O/S.C.	A
	hamster	O	S
3,3'-Dihydroxybenzidine	rat	O/S.C./ Top	S
3,3'-Benzidinedicarboxylic acid	rat	S.C.	S
	mouse		
2-Methyldiacetylbenzidine	rat	O	S

[a] O, oral; Top, topical; S.C., subcutaneous injection.
[b] A, tested in more than one institute; S, evidence less convincing.

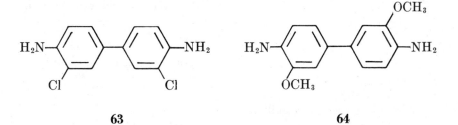

63   64

with these derivatives. The second amino group in the compound makes the synthesis of potential metabolites more difficult.

4,4'-METHYLENEDIANILINE AND ANALOGS. 4,4'-Methylenedianiline (DAPM) (**65**) and 4,4'-methylene-bis(2-chloroaniline) (DACPM, MOCA) (**66**) are used extensively in the plastics industry, especially after conversion to the diisocyanate in the manufacture of polyurethane foams and resins. 4,4'-Methylenebis(2-methylaniline) (DAMPM) (*146*) (**67**) was used experimentally for this purpose but is not manufactured on as large a scale. These chemicals are also used to make dyes such as *p*-rosaniline.

DACPM and DAMPM are carcinogenic when high levels are administered (Table III). DAPM is hepatotoxic and therefore cannot be fed at high levels. The chance contamination of flour which was made into bread led to 84 cases of jaundice and hepatocellular necrosis in the population of an Essex town (*147*). Munn (*148*) reported that DAMPM was far more carcinogenic than

Benzidine and Its Derivatives

			Tumors Induced in[c]				
Local	Blad-der	Kid-ney	Liver	In-testine	Ear Duct	Breast	Other
−	?+	−	−	−	−	−	−
−	−	−	+	−	−	−	−
−	−	−	+	+	+	−	−
−	−	−	+	−	−	−	−
−	−	−	−	−	−	?	
+	−	−	−	−	+	+	lymphoma, skin
−	?	−	−	−	−	−	forestomach
−	−	−	−	−	?	−	−
−	+	−	−	+	+	+	skin, lymphoma
−	+	−	+	−	−	−	bone
−	−	−	−	−	−	−	none significant
−	−	−	?	−	−	?	?
							hemopoietic tissue
−	−	−	−	+	+	+	

[a] +, tumors reported; −, tumors not reported; ?, evidence equivocal.

Table III. Carcinogenicity of

Compound	Species	Route[a]	Adequacy[b]
4,4'-Methylenedianiline	rat	O/S.C.	A
4,4'-Methylenebis(2-methylaniline)	rat	O	A
4,4'-Methylenebis(2-chloroaniline)	rat	O/S.C.	A
	mouse	O	S
4-Aminodiphenylamine	mouse	S.C.	S
Auramine	rat	S.C./O	S
	mouse	O	S

[a] O, oral; S.C., subcutaneous injection.
[b] A, tested in more than one institute; S, evidence less convincing.

DAPM in rats, but since the experiment was uncontrolled, the carcinogenicity of DAPM could not be assessed. Steinhoff and Grundmann (*149*) approximately doubled the incidence of benign and malignant tumors by the subcutaneous administration of DAPM to a total dose of 1.4 g/kg body weight over 1000 days. It is not evident whether DAPM is truly carcinogenic.

Evidence for the carcinogenicity of DACPM and DAMPM comes from experiments by feeding and by subcutaneous injection. DACPM led to

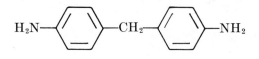

65

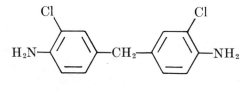

66

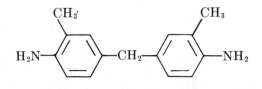

67

Methylenedianiline and Related Compounds

Tumors Induced in[c]

Local	Bladder	Kidney	Liver	Intestine	Ear Duct	Breast	Other
—	—	—	?	—	—	—	—
—	—	—	+	—	—	+	lung, skin
—	—	—	+	—	—	—	lung
—	—	—	+	—	—	—	hemangio-sarcoma
—	—	—	—	—	—	—	—
+	—	—	+	?	—	—	—
—	—	—	+	—	—	—	—

[c] +, tumors reported; —, tumors not reported; ?, evidence equivocal.

vascular and liver tumors in mice and liver and lung tumors in rats. The amount of DACPM used was high: 1000 ppm in one feeding experiment and a total dose of 25–27 g/kg body weight in another (*150, 151*). DAMPM led to tumors of the lung, liver, mammary gland, and skin after administration by gavage to rats at a total dose of 10.2 g/kg body weight. A feeding experiment, carried out by the same authors at 200 ppm in the diet was difficult to assess. An epidemiological evaluation of the effect of DACPM was negative (*152*). However, as the population at risk consisted of only 31 men with defined exposure of 6 months to 16 years and 178 other DACPM workers of unstated exposure duration who were examined cytologically, any conclusions drawn from this study are tentative.

The manufacture of auramine led to bladder cancer in man (*3, 4*). Williams and Bonser (*153*) showed that this substance was hepatocarcinogenic to rats and mice. Attempts to induce tumors in dogs (*154*) or rabbits (*121*) were unsuccessful.

Two other compounds in this series were examined by feeding 1.62 mmoles/kg in the diet to rats (*155*). 3-Benzylacetanilide (**68**) was without activity whereas 4-phenylthioacetanilide (**69**) gave single tumors of the breast and intestine in nine male and nine female rats by 10 months.

STILBENAMINES. The carcinogenic activities of derivatives of 4-stilbenamine (SA) (4-aminostilbene) (**70**) and 4-stilbenylacetamide (SAA) (**71**) are listed in Table IV. Attention was first drawn to this group by Haddow

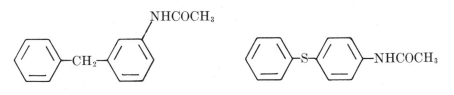

68

69

Table IV.   Carcinogenic Activity of

Compound	Species	Route[a]	Adequacy[b]
4-N-Stilbenamine	rat	SC/O	A
4-N-Stilbenylacetamide	rat	SC/O	A
	mouse	Top	S
N-(4-Styrylphenyl)hydroxylamine	rat	SC	S
N-Hydroxy-4,N-stilbenylacetamide	rat	SC/O/ Top	A
N-Acetoxy-4-N-stilbenylacetamide	rat	SC	S
4-Stilbenyl-N,N-dimethylamine	rat	O	A
4-Stilbenyl-N,N-diethylamine	rat	SC	S
2-Methyl-4-stilbenamine	rat	SC	S*
3-Methyl-4-stilbenamine	rat	SC	S*
N,N,2'-Trimethyl-4-stilbenamine	rat	O	S
N,N,3'-Trimethyl-4-stilbenamine	rat	O	S
N,N,4'-Trimethyl-4-stilbenamine	rat	O	S
4-(2,5-Dimethoxy)stilbenamine	rat	SC	S
2'-Fluoro-4-stilbenyl-N,N-dimethylamine	rat	O	S
4'-Fluoro-4-stilbenamine	rat	SC	S*
4'-Fluoro-4-stilbenyl-N,N-dimethylamine	rat	O	S
2'-Chloro-4-stilbenyl-N,N-dimethylamine	rat	O	S
3'-Chloro-4-stilbenyl-N,N-dimethylamine	rat	O	S
4'-Chloro-4-stilbenyl-N,N-dimethylamine	rat	O	S
4'-Nitro-4-stilbenyl-N,N-dimethylamine	rat	O	S
4,4'-Diaminostilbene	rat	SC	S*
3,3'-Dichloro-4,4'-diaminostilbene	rat	SC	S*
2,2'-Dichloro-4,4'-diaminostilbene	rat	SC	S*
2-Cyano-4-stilbenamine	rat	SC	S
2-(4-N,N-Dimethylaminostyryl)quinoline	rat	O	S
	mouse	IV	S

[a] O, oral; Top, topical; SC, subcutaneous injection; IV, intravenous injection.
[b] A, tested in more than one institute; S, evidence less convincing; S*, preliminary

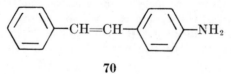

70

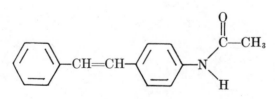

71

Stilbenamines and Related Compounds

Tumors Induced in[c]

Local	Blad-der	Kid-ney	Liver	In-testine	Ear Duct	Breast	Other
?	−	−	−	−	+	+	−
−	−	−	−	−	+	+	−
+	−	−	−	−	−	−	−
+	−	−	−	?	?	−	−
+	−	−	−	?	+	+	−
+	−	−	−	−	+	−	−
−	−	−	−	−	+	−	−
−	−	−	−	−	+	−	−
+	−	−	−	−	−	−	−
+	−	−	−	−	−	−	−
−	−	−	−	−	−	−	−
−	−	−	−	−	+	−	−
−	−	−	−	−	?	−	−
−	−	−	−	−	+	−	−
−	−	−	+	−	+	+	−
−	−	−	+	+	+	−	−
−	−	−	−	−	+	?	−
−	−	−	−	−	+	?	? sarcomas
−	−	−	?	−	+	?	−
−	−	−	−	−	+	−	−
−	−	−	−	−	?	−	−
?	−	−	+	−	−	−	−
+	−	−	−	−	−	−	−
?	−	−	+	?	−	−	−
−	−	−	+	−	−	−	lung
−	−	−	−	−	+	−	? stomach
−	−	−	+	−	−	−	+ leukemia ovary?

communication or abstract.

[c] +, tumors reported; −, tumors not reported; ?, evidence equivocal.

and his colleagues (*156*) who examined them as possible antineoplastic agents. The main feature of this group is its ability to induce acoustic duct carcinomas in rats—a fact which was utilized by Druckrey (*157*) in the study of the dose–response relationship in carcinogenesis. The acoustic duct carcinoma is particularly useful for the purpose since it becomes clinically apparent early in its development. In Druckrey's experiment the smallest dose, 0.5 mg/kg body weight/day 4-stilbenyldimethylamine, led to 39 carcinomas in 50 rats in 560 days.

Comparatively little work has been done on the critical structure for SA carcinogenesis. The ethylenic bond (−CH=CH−) appears to be essential insofar as its replacement by anil (−CH=N−) removes carcinogenicity. 4-Dibenzylylamine is a very weak carcinogen (*63*).

N-Hydroxy-SAA was isolated from the urine of rats fed SAA or SA (*63, 158*). It induces subcutaneous sarcomas on injection in only a few of the treated rats, and it is a more effective mammary gland carcinogen than SAA on feeding to weanling female rates. It should be considered a proximate carcinogen. *N*-Acetoxy–SAA was prepared and gave sarcomas and acoustic duct tumors on subcutaneous injection (*63*). Baldwin and Smith (*158*) identified 4′-hydroxy–SAA as a metabolite. Recent evidence indicates that the epoxidation of the ethylenic bond of stilbene occurs, and this possibly contributes to the carcinogenicity of the stilbenamines (*159*).

Fused Ring Amines. 2-FLUORENYLACETAMIDE. 2-Fluorenylacetamide (2-FAA) (2-acetylamino- or 2-acetamido-fluorene) (**10**) was proposed as an insecticide to replace the highly toxic lead, arsenic, and fluorine sprays which were used before 1940. Tumors of the liver, bladder, renal pelvis, acoustic duct, and (in single instances) of the colon, lung, and pancreas arose in male and female Slonaker rats given 0.03–0.125% 2-FAA in their diet for 95–333 days (*160*). World War II delayed the fuller publication of these results until 1947 (*161, 162, 163, 164*). In the later publications, it was shown also that tumors were induced by 2-FAA in mice. Tumors of liver, bladder, and kidney were produced in C57, C3H, and Bagg albino mice. In rats the importance of the amino group in the action of 2-fluorenamine (2-FA) and 2-FAA was demonstrated; 2-chlorofluorene, fluorene, fluorenone, and xanthone did not induce tumors.

Different species respond to chronic administration of 2-FAA in different ways (Table V). Both guinea pigs and monkeys fail to develop tumors after treatment; in the case of monkeys, it is possible that the correct dosage and length of experiment has not yet been achieved. Guinea pigs may be deficient in the enzyme necessary for the first step of aromatic amine activation. The sites of tumors induced by 2-FAA in other species are variable. For example, bladder and liver tumors have been induced in dogs, mice, and rats; liver tumors (but not bladder tumors) in chickens, fish, cats and hamsters; and bladder tumors but not liver tumors) in rabbits.

There are also variations in the response to 2-FAA in different colonies of inbred animals within a species. Bielschowsky (*165, 166*) found that 2-FAA induced intestinal cancer in his Piebald rats whereas his Wistar strain was less susceptible to this tumor. This contrasts with the bladder tumors described in the Slonaker rat (*160*). In mice, Armstrong and Bonser (*167*) examined the effect of 2-FAA in five inbred strains (Table VI). The variations were reported in comparatively small numbers of mice; nevertheless, the differences between strains in the incidence of hepatomas and bladder papillomas were convincing. Large scale experiments using BALB/c and C57 mice confirmed these results; the incidence of bladder papillomas being both sex and strain dependent (*168, 169*).

Chemical structure and carcinogenic activity relationships in the 2-FAA series, the metabolism of these compounds in rats, and so forth were reviewed by Weisburger and Weisburger in 1958 (*17*). In rats, an equilibrium is set up between the enzymic deacetylation of 2-FAA and the reacetylation of 2-FA. Therefore any fluorene derivative which may be converted enzymically to FA or FAA is carcinogenic as illustrated by N-2-fluorenylmethylamine and 2-nitrofluorene (Table V). N-Fluorenylphthalamic acid led to the induction of smaller yields of transplantable hepatomas which superficially appear to be similar to normal liver. Enzyme measurements, however, have demonstrated important differences between liver and each of these so-called "Morris" hepatomas (*170, 171*). Other substituents on the nitrogen as, for example, with N-fluorenyl-2-benzenesulfonamide or N-fluorenyl-2-p-toluenesulfonamide, failed to induce tumors since they were not hydrolyzed *in vivo*.

The effects of ring substituents on the carcinogenicity of 2-FAA (Table V) were similar to those with 4-BPA. A series of seven carcinogenic fluoro derivatives of 2-FAA indirectly demonstrates that C-hydroxylation of 2-FAA does not lead to tumor formation (*123*).

Studies on the metabolism of FAA established that the most prominent metabolites of 2-FAA were C-hydroxylated derivatives conjugated with glucuronide or sulfate. These metabolites are not concerned with carcinogenesis, but rather are the detoxication products of 2-FAA. The isolation and characterization of these metabolites and the study of their conjugation with sulfate and glucuronic acid were summarized (*20*).

The discovery of the formation of N-hydroxy-2-FAA (2-fluorenylacethydroxamic acid) and the investigation of its carcinogenic properties were discussed in the previous section (*see* page 371). Briefly,

1. N-hydroxy-2-FAA leads to a greater yield of tumors than an equimolecular level of 2-FAA, especially in the mammary gland of weanling rats (*58, 59*);

2. N-hydroxy-2-FAA induces local tumors (*e.g.*, in the forestomach on feeding or in the subcutaneous tissues, especially when injected subcutaneously as the cupric chelate (*172*));

3. N-hydroxy-2-FAA induces tumors in guinea pigs whereas 2-FAA is without effect in this species (*59*);

4. the effect on the tumor yield of feeding a variety of substances with 2-FAA is explicable by the levels of N-hydroxy-2-FAA produced from 2-FAA under these conditions (*see* page 446);

5. the failure of N-hydroxy AAF to react nonenzymically with DNA, RNA, and protein *in vitro* clearly indicates that this compound is a proximate rather than the ultimate carcinogen (*16*);

6. the synthesis and demonstration of the carcinogenicity of the highly reactive N-acetoxyarylacetamides and N-benzoyloxyarylacetamides suggest that the ultimate carcinogen might be an ester of N-hydroxy-2-FAA (*63*);

7. there is evidence that in the liver the sulfate ester is effective (*71, 72*) although the sulfate ester of N-hydroxy-FAA is not a powerful carcinogen, possibly because it reacts rapidly with nonspecific targets.

The observation that continuous feeding of 2-FAA increases the urinary levels of N-hydroxy-2-FAA but markedly reduces sulfotransferase activity may make this ester less likely to be the ultimate carcinogen (*173*). In other tissues, the ultimate carcinogen is still in doubt, because sulfotransferase is not present (*93*). The phosphate (*16*), the acetate (*65, 66, 67*), N-nitroso-2-fluorene, 2-fluorenylhydroxylamine, the O-glucuronide of fluorenylhydroxylamine or N-hydroxy-2-FAA (*132*), and free radicals (*174*) were suggested as possible

Table V.　Carcinogenic Activity of

Compound	Species	Route[a]	Adequacy[b]
2-Fluorenamine	mouse	V	A
	rat	V	A
2-Fluorenylacetamide	mouse	V	A
	rat	V	A
	hamster	V	A
	guinea pig		
	rabbit	O	A
	cat	O	S
	dog	O	S
	monkey[d]		
	fish		S
	chicken		S
9-Hydroxy-2-fluorenylacetamide	rat	O	S
9-Oxo-2-fluorenylacetamide	rat	O	S
2-Fluorenyldimethylamine	rat	O	A
2-Fluorenyldiethylamine	rat	O	S
2-Fluorenylmonomethylamine	rat	O	A
N-Acetoxyfluorenylacetamide	rat	S.C.	S
N-Benzoyloxyfluorenylacetamide	rat	S.C.	S
2-Fluorenyldiacetamide	rat	O	A
2-Nitrofluorene	rat	O	S
N-Hydroxy-2-FAA	mouse	V	A
(Fluorenyl-2-acethydroxamic acid)	rat	V	A
	hamster	V	A
	rabbit	V	A
	guinea pig	V	A
2-Fluorenylhydroxylamine	rat	S.C.	S
2-Nitrosofluorene	rat	S.C.	S
N-Fluorenyl-2-benzamide	rat	I.P.	S
N-Fluorenyl-2-benzohydroxamic acid	rat	I.P.	S
N,2-Fluorenylformamide	rat	O	S
N-Fluorenyl-2-phthalimic acid	rat	O	S
N-Fluorenyl-2-benzenesulfonamide	rat	I.P.	S
N-Hydroxy-N-fluorenylbenzene-sulfonamide	rat	I.P.	S
N-2-Fluorenyl(2'-carboxybenz)amide	rat	O	A
N-2-Fluorenylsuccinamic acid	rat	O	S
N-2-Fluorenyl-p-toluenesulfonamide	rat	O	S
N-(2-Fluorenyl)-2,2,2-trifluoroacetamide	rat	O	S

2-Fluorenamine and Related Compounds

			Tumors Induced in[c]				
Local	Blad-der	Kid-ney	Liver	In-testine	Ear Duct	Breast	Other
−	?	−	+	−	−	−	−
−	−	−	+	+	+	+	lung
−	+	−	+	−	−	+	−
−	+	+	+	+	+	+	various
−	−	−	+	−	−	−	−
−	−	−	−	−	−	−	−
−	+	−	−	−	−	−	ureter
−	−	−	+	−	−	−	lung
−	+	−	+	−	−	−	−
−	−	−	−	−	−	−	−
−	−	−	+	−	−	−	−
−	−	+	+	−	−	−	fallopian tube, ovary
−	−	−	+	−	−	?	−
−	−	−	+	?	?	+	−
−	−	−	+	+	+	+	−
−	−	−	−	+	−	−	lung
−	−	−	+	−	+	+	lung
+	−	−	−	−	?	−	−
+	−	−	−	−	?	−	−
−	?	−	+	−	+	+	orbital and Harderian gland tumors
−	−	−	−	?	−	−	?
+	+	−	+	−	−	+	−
+	−	−	+	+	+	+	−
+	−	−	+	?	−	−	−
+	+	−	−	?	−	−	−
+	−	−	−	+	−	−	−
+	−	−	−	−	+	+	−
+	−	−	−	−	+	−	−
−	−	−	−	−	−	−	−
+	−	−	−	+ (small)	−	+	−
−	−	−	−	−	+	+	−
−	−	−	+	−	−	−	−
−	−	−	−	−	−	−	−
+	−	−	−	−	−	+	? lung
−	−	−	+	−	−	−	−
−	−	−	+	−	−	−	−
−	−	−	−	−	−	−	−
−	−	−	+	−	+	+	−

Table V.

Compound	Species	Route[a]	Adequacy[b]
N-3-Glycylaminofluorene	rat	O	S
1-Fluoro-2-FAA	rat	O	S
3-Fluoro-2-FAA	rat	O	S
4-Fluoro-2-FAA	rat	O	S
5-Fluoro-2-FAA	rat	O	S
6-Fluoro-2-FAA	rat	O	S
7-Fluoro-2-FAA	rat	O	A
8-Fluoro-2-FAA	rat	O	S
7-Fluoro-2-N-(fluorenyl)acethydroxamic acid	rat	O	S
7-Chloro-2-FAA	rat	O	A
3-Iodo-2-FAA	rat	O	S
7-Iodo-2-FAA	rat	O	S
1-Methoxy-2-FA	rat	O	A
3-Methoxy-2-FA	rat	O	A
1-Methoxy-2-FAA	rat	O	A
3-Methoxy-2-FAA	rat	O	A
7-Methoxy-2-FAA	rat	O	A
2,5-Dinitrofluorene	rat	O	S
2,7-Dinitrofluorene	rat	O	S
2,7-Fluorenyldiamine	rat	O	S
2,5-Fluorenylenebisacetamide	rat	O	S
2,7-Fluorenylbisacetamide	mouse	O	S
	rat	O	A
1-Fluorenylacetamide	rat	I.P.	A
1-Fluorenylacethydroxamic acid	rat	I.P.	S
3-Fluorenylacetamide	rat	I.P.	S
3-Fluorenylacethydroxamic acid	rat	I.P.	S

[a] O, oral; S.C., subcutaneous; I.P., intraperitoneal injection; V, various routes.
[b] A, tested in more than one institute; S, evidence less convincing.
[c] +, tumors reported; −, tumors not reported; ?, evidence equivocal.

carcinogens. The ultimate carcinogen may have to be determined in each tissue which responds to 2-FAA.

Synthetic N-Hydroxy Compounds. Certain substituents on the amino groups of FA are inimical to its enzymic N-hydroxylation. Thus, N-2-fluorenylbenzamide (33) is inactive whereas N-2-fluorenylbenzohydroxamic acid induces tumors locally, in the small intestine, and in the breast tissue on intraperitoneal injection (Table V). Similarly, N-hydroxy-N,2-fluorenylbenzenesulfonamide induces tumors at the injection site in the breast and in the lung, whereas the N-2-fluorenylbenzenesulfonamide is not active (33, 175). In sub-

Continued

Tumors Induced in[c]

Local	Blad-der	Kid-ney	Liver	In-testine	Ear Duct	Breast	Other
−	−	−	+	−	−	−	−
−	−	−	−	−	+	+	−
−	−	−	+	−	+	+	−
−	−	−	−	−	+	+	−
−	−	−	−	−	+	+	−
−	−	−	+	+	+	+	−
−	−	−	+	−	+	+	−
−	−	−	+	?	+	+	−
+	−	−	+	+	+	+	−
−	−	−	?	−	−	−	−
−	−	−	−	−	+	−	−
−	−	−	−	−	−	−	−
−	−	−	+	+	?	−	−
−	−	−	−	−	−	−	−
−	−	−	−	?	−	?	−
−	−	−	−	−	−	−	−
−	−	−	+	−	+	+	−
−	−	−	−	−	−	?	−
−	−	−	−	−	−	+	−
−	−	−	−	−	−	+	−
−	−	−	−	−	−	+	−
−	−	−	+	−	−	−	−
−	−	−	+	+	+	+	various, including jejunum, lung, glandular stomach
−	−	−	−	−	−	+	−
−	−	−	−	−	−	+	−
−	−	−	−	−	−	+	−

[d] In experiments with monkeys, there is doubt whether the chronic toxicity tests were terminated before tumors could have appeared.

sequent studies it was shown that N-hydroxy-N,2-fluorenylbenzenesulfonamide was converted to N-2-fluorenylhydroxylamine *in vivo* (*176*).

Esterification and Isomeric FAA's. The positional isomers of 2-FAA, namely 1-FAA (**72**) and 3-FAA (**73**) are carcinogenic, especially to the mammary glands of female Holtzman rats (*175*).

Recently, Yost and Gutmann (*177*) compared the carcinogenicity of 2-, 3-, and 4-fluorenylacethydroxamic acids and showed that the 2-isomer and 3-isomer had approximately equal carcinogenicities and that both were much more carcinogenic than the 4-isomer (the 1-isomer has an intermediate level

**Table VI.   Carcinogenicity of 2-Fluorenylacetamide in Mice.
Effect of Mouse Strain (*167*)**

			Mouse Strain		
	CBA	IF	R111	White Label	Strong A
Number of mice surviving 20 weeks (male and female)	18	20	21	24	25
Hepatomas %[a]	73	44	16	10	5
Bladder tumors %[a]	78	70	48	22	22

[a] Percent yields based on number of mice examined histologically.

of carcinogenicity (*175*). By examination of the reactivity of the *N*-acetoxy-fluorenylacetamides with methionine, *t*RNA, guanosine, and adenosine, they concluded that the carcinogenicity of the positional isomers could not be rationalized on the basis of the reactivity of the corresponding *N*-acetoxy-arenamides. Since most of the tumors in the carcinogenicity tests were in the mammary gland of female rats, this result, together with that already quoted (*93*), demonstrates that neither the *N*-acetoxy- nor the *O*-sulfate of 2-FAA is likely to be concerned in mammary carcinogenesis in the rat by derivatives of 2-FAA. A recent report indicates that an acetyl transferase may be the activating enzyme in this tissue (*68*).

The study of the covalent binding of 2-9[^{14}C]-FAA and 2-9[^{14}C]-fluorenylacethydroxamic acid to DNA, RNA, and protein *in vivo* throws further light on the nature of the reactive esters of 2-fluorenylacethydroxamic acid. Binding was first demonstrated by Williard and Irving (*178*) and Marroquin and Farber (*179*). The nature of the binding was established by Lotlikar *et al.* (*180*) who allowed *N*-acetoxy-FAA to react with glycylmethion-

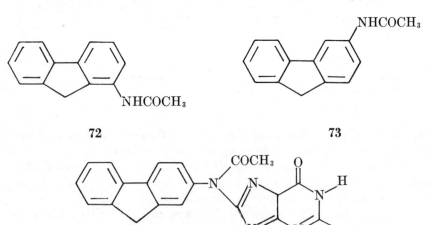

72   73

74

ine and methionine and deduced that a methiononium intermediate was formed which, in the former instance, split and rearranged to 3-methylmercapto-2-FAA and homoserine lactone in equimolar amounts. Kriek *et al.* (*181*), in the same way, mixed N-acetoxy-2-FAA with guanosine and obtained N-2-(8-guaninyl) FAA (**74**) after mild hydrolysis to remove the ribose.

Using 9-[^{14}C]-N-hydroxy-2(2′-[^3H]acetyl)FA, Irving *et al.* (*182*) demonstrated that the covalently bound adducts with DNA and RNA which were formed in rat liver *in vivo* did not carry as many acetyl groups as suggested by the number of bound fluorenes. This "loss" of bound acetyl was mimicked by the binding of the glucuronide of the doubly radiolabeled derivative to yeast *t*RNA at pH's of 7.0–9.5 *in vitro*. The greater the pH, the more acetyl was lost.

Kriek (*183*) separated the covalently bound derivatives of N-hydroxy-2-9 [^{14}C]-FAA and its corresponding tritiated acetyl derivative with nucleic acids in rat liver. Both N-(guanosin-8-yl)2-FAA and N-(guanosin-8-yl)2-FA were obtained. Much of the guanosine obtained from ribosomal RNA retained the acetyl group, whereas with DNA the deacetylated product predominated.

Kriek suggested that the deacetylated product might arise from deacetylation of 2-fluorenylacethydroxamic acid, as originally suggested by Irving (*184*), or from its glucuronide to give reactive arylhydroxylamine. In rat liver the sulfate ester might account for any acetylated fluorene product bound. The variety of possible reactive intermediates makes even this cautious suggestion possibly too simple.

Marroquin and Coyote (*60*) showed that with synthetic polyribonucleotides N-hydroxy-[9-^{14}C]-2-FAA bound to polyguanosine and polyadenosine in the ratio of 6:1. Nevertheless, Kriek and Reitsema (*185*) found that N-acetoxy-N-2-FAA reacted sluggishly with adenosine or its monophosphate. With polyadenosine the expected reaction rate was obtained, which indicates that the steric configuration of the bases is critically important for their reaction with N-acetoxy-N-2-FAA.

NAPHTHYLAMINES. In the 1930's, the growing realization that 2-naphthylamine (**4**) (2-NA) was a bladder carcinogen in workmen exposed as a result of their occupation led to intensive attempts to reproduce the human disease in laboratory animals. Hueper *et al.* (*13*) effectively demonstrated the susceptibility of the dog to this chemical in 1938. In their only report, an interim statement, appearing about 26 months after the experiment began, they reported that 13 out of 16 dogs developed bladder tumors after subcutaneous injection and later oral administration of 2-NA. Tumors were detected in two dogs at autopsy; the others were found by cystoscopy. This experiment involved the relatively impure commercial chemical, but in later tests (*15*) rigorously purified 2-NA gave similar results. More recent results showed that the tumor response depended on the dose of 2-NA (*39*).

The way in which different species respond to 2-NA is shown in Table VII. The hamster, when subjected to high levels of 2-NA, the dog, and the monkey all develop bladder tumors similar to those found in man. The mouse develops liver tumors, whereas other species fail to respond. The failure to induce

Table VII.   Carcinogenicity of Aromatic Amines and Their Anthracene,

Compound	Species	Route[a]	Adequacy[b]
1-Naphthylamine	mouse	O	S[d]
	hamster	O	S
	dog	O	S[d]
2-Naphthylamine	mouse	O	A
	rat	O	A
	hamster	O	S
	rabbit	O	S
	cat	O	S
	dog	O/S.C.	A
	monkey	O	S
1-Naphthylacetamide	mouse	O	S
1-Naphthylhydroxylamine	mouse	Skin	S
	rat	O	S
1-Naphthylacethydroxamic acid	rat	I.P./S.C.	S
2-Naphthylhydroxylamine	mouse	Skin	S
	rat	I.P.	A
1-Fluoro-2-naphthylamine	mouse	S.C.	S
1-Methoxy-2-naphthylamine	mouse	S.C.	S
3-Methyl-2-naphthylamine	rat	O/S.C.	
3-Nitro-2-naphthylamine	rat	O	S
N,N-Bis(2-chloroethyl)-2-naphthylamine	mouse	I.P.	S
1-Anthramine	rat	Top	S
2-Anthramine	mouse	S.C.	S
	rat	Top/S.C.	A
	hamster	Top	A
9-Anthramine	rat	S.C.	S
2-Anthranylacetamide	rat	S.C.	S
1-Phenanthrylamine	mouse	O	S
	rat	O	S
2-Phenanthrylamine	mouse	O	S
	rat	O	S
3-Phenanthrylamine	mouse	O	S
	rat	O	S
9-Phenanthrylamine	mouse	O	S
	rat	O	S
1-Phenanthrylacetamide	mouse	I.M.[e]	S
	rat	O[f]	S
9,10-Dihydro-2-phenanthramine	rat	O	A
2-Phenanthrylacetamide	mouse	I.M.	S
	rat	O	A
2-Phenanthrylacethydroxamic acid	rat	S.C.	S

Derivatives with Fused Aromatic Rings: Naphthalene, Phenanthrene etc.

Tumors Induced in[c]

Local	Bladder	Kidney	Liver	Intestine	Ear Duct	Breast	Other
−	−	−	?	−	−	−	−
−	−	−	−	−	−	−	−
−	?	−	−	−	−	−	−
−	−	−	+	−	−	−	−
−	−	−	−	−	−	−	−
−	+	−	−	−	−	−	−
−	−	−	−	−	−	−	−
−	+	−	−	−	−	−	−
−	+	−	−	−	−	−	−
+	−	−	−	−	−	−	−
+	−	−	+	−	−	−	−
−	−	−	−	−	−	−	−
+	−	−	−	−	−	−	−
+	−	−	−	−	−	−	−
−	−	−	−	−	−	−	−
−	−	−	−	+	−	−	−
+	−	?	−	+	−	+	skin
−	−	−	−	−	?	−	skin
−	−	−	−	−	−	−	lung
−	−	−	−	−	−	−	−
−	−	−	+	−	−	−	−
+ (skin)	−	−	−	−	−	+	−
+	−	−	−	−	−	−	−
−	−	−	−	−	−	−	−
−	−	−	−	−	−	−	−
−	−	−	−	−	−	+[g]	−
−	−	−	−	−	−	+[g]	−
−	−	−	−	−	−	+[g]	−
−	−	−	−	−	−	+[g]	−
−	−	−	−	−	−	−	−
−	−	−	−	+	+	+	−
−	−	−	−	+	+	+	leukemia
+	−	−	−	−	−	+	−

Table VII.

Compound	Species	Route[a]	Adequacy[b]
9-Phenanthrylacetamide	mouse	I.M.[f]	S
	rat	O[e]	A
N-Acetoxy-4-phenanthrylacetamide	rat	S.C.	S

[a] O, oral; S.C., subcutaneous injection; I.P., intraperitoneal injection; Top, topical; I.M., intramuscular injection.
[b] A, tested in more than one institute; S, evidence less convincing; S*, preliminary communication or abstract.
[c] +, tumors reported; −, tumors not reported; ?, evidence equivocal.

significant incidences of tumors in rats and rabbits given 2-NA was demonstrated in several independent experiments.

Commercial 1-naphthylamine (1-NA) (5), in the United Kingdom at least, contained 4–10% of 2-NA. In about 1950, using the analytical methods of Butt and Strafford (186), one of us (DBC) found 3.5% 2-NA in a purified sample of 1-NA. Because of this contamination the earlier attempts to induce tumors with 1-NA, which sometimes gave positive results, are not emphasized. For example, Gehrmann et al. (187) fed five dogs five times weekly with 300–350 mg 1-NA without inducing bladder tumors; Bonser (188) reported a bladder papilloma in one of two surviving dogs fed 500 mg 1-NA three times weekly for life. In the young adult mouse, Clayson and Ashton (189) fed 1-NA (free from 2-NA) in the drinking water at a level of 0.01% for 70 weeks and obtained a just significant incidence of hepatomas in female but not in male mice. Newborn mice gave similar inconclusive results (40). The Syrian golden hamster was not affected by 1-NA at levels of 0.1 or 1.0% in the diet (190, 191). The most that can be said from these experiments is that 1-NA is a much less potent experimental carcinogen than 2-NA.

The first comparative experiments on the metabolism of 2-NA (192) showed that in four species—dog, rabbit, rat, and mouse—the proportion of a dose of amine converted to metabolites which gave 2-amino-1-naphthol on acid hydrolysis was proportional to the carcinogenicity of 2-NA in those species. 2-Amino-1-naphthol hydrochloride was carcinogenic on bladder implantation. It was suggested that 2-amino-1-naphthol and other o-aminophenols were the active intermediates determining the carcinogenicity of 2-NA and other aromatic amines (123). However, 1-amino-2-naphthol was carcinogenic by bladder implantation. Because it was present in large amounts in conjugated form in the urine of animals fed the questionably carcinogenic 1-NA, this idea was abandoned (189).

Boyland and his colleagues intensively studied the metabolism of 2-NA, particularly in the rat, and obtained nearly 30 different metabolites (193). These consisted of the free, or O-conjugated, derivatives of 1-hydroxy or 6-hydroxy-2-NA and 2-napthylacetamide (2-NAA). 2-NA-Sulfamate and

Continued

Tumors Induced in[c]

Local	Blad-der	Kid-ney	Liver	In-testine	Ear Duct	Breast	Other
—	—	—	—	—	—	—	? leukemia
—	—	—	—	—	—	—	—
+	—	—	—	—	—	—	—

[d] Earlier results not included because 1-isomer was often contaminated with 2-naphthylamine.
[e] One dose only.
[f] Two doses only.
[g] Three doses.
[h] Possibly due to physico-chemical properties of the drug.

glucuronide were also present. A number of derivatives of 2-NA-5,6-epoxide *viz.*, the 5,6-dihydrodiol and its glucuronide conjugate, the corresponding mercapturic acid, and 5-*O*-sulfato-6-hydroxy-NA (**75**) were also detected. One unusual metabolite of 2-NA to be isolated was 1-*O*-sulfato-2-naphthyl-formamide (*194*) (**76**). Troll and colleagues (*195*) discovered bis(2-amino-1-naphthyl)phosphate (**77**) in dog urine. Although several of these metabolites appeared to be carcinogenic using the bladder implant technique, none induced tumors in more conventional tests, and these metabolites appear therefore to be detoxication products. The discovery of the importance of the *N*-hydroxyla-tion of aromatic amines for their carcinogenicity led to the search for similar products among the metabolites of 2-NA.

In the case of 1-NA, the following urinary metabolites were demonstrated by paper chromatography—the *N*-sulfate, glucuronide, glucoside and the 1- and 4-hydroxylated derivatives conjugated with sulfate and glucuronide (*189*).

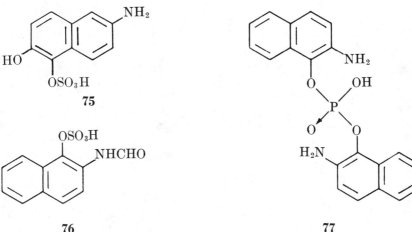

75

76

77

Since dogs are the most sensitive species to the carcinogenic action of 2-NA, they have been important in elucidating the way in which this substance exerts its effect. Dogs differ from other laboratory animals because they are unable to acetylate aromatic amines. Therefore, metabolites like N-hydroxy-2-NAA are unlikely to be involved in the metabolic activation of 2-NA in the dog.

Boyland and his colleagues (196) and Troll and Nelson (197) demonstrated the presence of 2-naphthylhydroxylamine in the urine of dogs fed 2-NA. The former group showed it to induce local sarcomas on intraperitoneal injection. Nevertheless, despite the fact that nearly all dogs develop bladder cancer when fed 2-NA, not all dogs excreted 2-NA in their urine as 2-naphthylhydroxylamine (198). This discrepancy was explained by demonstrating 2-nitrosonaphthalene as a metabolite (199). In a similar study of the metabolism of 1-NA in dogs, Deichmann and Radomski (41) stated that although 1-naphthylhydroxylamine was present, they could not detect 1-nitrosonaphthalene. At the time they thought that this indicated that the nitrosonaphthalene was the ultimate carcinogen, but it has since been realized that these two metabolites are easily interconverted by reduction—oxidation in tissues:

$$\mathrm{RNHOH} \overset{+2\mathrm{H}}{\underset{-2\mathrm{H}}{\rightleftharpoons}} \mathrm{RNO}$$

The nitroso and hydroxylamino-derivatives of 1-NA and 2-NA were tested for carcinogenicity by intravesical instillation in dogs, i.e., the transfer of a dimethylsulfoxide solution of the test substance by catheter into the bladder lumen. These substances were also tested by subcutaneous injection in newborn mice within the first 24 hours and on the third and fifth day after birth or by intraperitoneal injection in rats. In dogs no tumors were formed after instillation of 2-NA, but 2-naphthylhydroxylamine induced three cases of bladder carcinoma in four dogs (40). In mice an excessive incidence of hepatomas and pulmonary adenomas was found after administering 1- and 2-naphthylhydroxylamine and, in male mice only, after 1- and 2-nitrosonaphthalene. Rats were susceptible only to 1-naphthylhydroxylamine and 1-nitrosonaphthalene. Quantitative experiments involving gas chromatography of 1- and 2-naphthylhydroxylamine and 1- and 2-nitrosonaphthalene from the urine of dogs fed a single dose of the respective amines showed that (38, 40) after 5 mg/kg 2-NA, 0.2% was converted into the specific oxidation products whereas only traces were converted after the same dose of 1-NA. With larger doses (70 mg/kg) administration of 2-NA led to far more of these oxidation products than did the same amount of 1-NA. Furthermore, 4-BPA, which is a more potent bladder carcinogen in dogs than 1-NA or 2-NA, led to more of these oxidation products than either of the naphthylamines (200). For this limited series of only three compounds, there is a quantitative correlation between their carcinogenicity to the dog bladder and the combined excretion of nitrosoarene and arylhydroxylamine.

An interesting derivative of 2-NA (Table VII), 2-naphthylamine mustard (78) (2-bis(-2′-chloroethyl)aminonaphthalene) was marketed under the name chlornaphazin. It was originally intended for patients with leukemia and Hodgkin's disease, both of which had a poor prognosis at that time. Unfortunately it found favor in Scandinavia for treating polycythemia vera, a disease involving overproduction of red blood cells and for which there is a more favorable prognosis. In a series of 61 patients, of whom 27 survived (*9*), 10 so far have bladder cancer and 5 more have abnormal cells in their urine suggestive of a developing bladder tumor (*i.e.*, abnormal urinary cytology). Polycythemia alone does not predispose to bladder cancer, nor does the ^{32}P administered to most of these patients concomitantly with the chlornaphazin. The dose required to induce abnormal urinary cytology or tumors ranged from 2–350 g; the mean latent period of the tumors was 5.5 (range (2.5–11) years —a much shorter period than that associated with industrial bladder cancer. This alkylating drug induces lung adenomas in mice (*201*). It probably derives its carcinogenic action by being converted to derivatives of 2-naphthylamine. Thus Boyland and Manson (*202*) showed that in the rat it was converted to 2-amino-1-naphthyl hydrogen sulfate and 2-acetamidonaphthalene hydrogen sulfate.

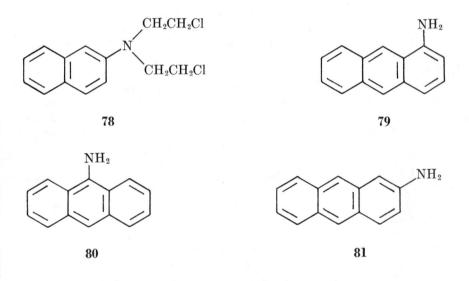

78

79

80

81

ANTHRAMINES. 1-Anthramine (**79**) and 9-anthramine (**80**) have not induced tumors in limited tests in rats (Table VII). 2-Anthramine (**81**), however, is unusual since it is one of the few aromatic amines which leads to skin tumors when painted on to the skin of rats or hamsters (*203, 204*). These tumors resemble the range of tumors found in human skin and were used for pathological studies (*205*). No evidence has been reported on the metabolic activation of 2-anthramine in skin.

PHENANTHRAMINES. Most of the phenanthrene derivatives recorded in Table VII were investigated only in the Huggins' system in which one, two, or three large doses of a carcinogen are given by intubation to fifty-day old female Sprague–Dawley rats, and the incidence of breast tumors is used as an index of carcinogenicity (*205*).

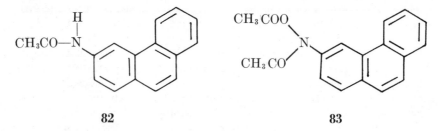

82   **83**

2-Phenanthrylacetamide (2-PAA) (**82**), which is carcinogenic (*55*), has been studied in more detail to provide a firmer base for the general theory of aromatic amine activation (*32*). Small quantities of *N*-hydroxy-2-PAA were found in the urine of 2-PAA-treated rats, and the synthetic compound induced mammary adenocarcinomas in female Holtzmann rats (*32*).

In kinetic experiments it was shown that *N*-acetoxy-2-PAA (**83**) like most other *N*-acetoxyarylacetamides but unlike *N*-acetoxy-2-FAA, decomposed relatively slowly in water. Also, *N*-acetoxy-2-PAA reacted more slowly than the fluorene analog with methionine and guanosine; the effect of this was that *N*-acetoxy-PAA formed adducts with adenosine and guanosine with almost equal affinity. As a result of molecular orbital calculations and studies of the reaction of some *N*-acetoxyarylacetamides with the free radical trapping agent, 2,2-diphenyl-1-picrylhydrazyl, it was found that *N*-acetoxy-2-PAA decolorized the reagent more slowly than *N*-acetoxy-2-FAA. It was concluded that *N*-acetoxy-2-FAA might react by a free radical mechanism, but probably formed an intermediate nitrenium ion (*62*). It must be emphasized that the application of the principles derived from kinetic and chemical experiments may not be directly relevant to the situation *in vivo*, especially since part of the guanosine-bound FAA was deacetylated—an observation not explained by this work (*173*).

OTHER ARYLAMINES. Higher arylamines, e.g., 7-benz[*a*]anthramine, have been recorded in the carcinogenesis literature. These are not discussed here because there is no adequate work on their carcinogenicity or mechanisms of action.

Aminoazo Compounds and Related Azodyes. This group of carcinogens is so large that it is more convenient to consider it under three headings. First, there are those dyes which have an unsubstituted amino group, such as 4-(*o*-tolylazo)-*o*-toluidine (**84**). Secondly, there are dyes in which the amino group is methylated as with *N*,*N*-dimethyl-4-phenylazoaniline (**85**). Thirdly, there are various azodyes which have been tested for carcinogenicity because they are required for use in food, medicine, or other applications. These may not necessarily be aromatic amines, but in each example amines may be produced as a result of *in vivo* reduction.

DERIVATIVES OF 4-(PHENYLAZO) ANILINE. 4-Phenylazoaniline (4-aminoazobenzene) (AB) (**86**) was tested for carcinogenicity in several species. Generally, the data suggest that AB and 4-(phenylazo)acetanilide (AAB) are not carcinogenic. However, there are few experiments in which the maximum tolerated dose of chemical was given for the major part of the life span of a substantial number of animals. Kirby and Peacock (*207*) reported liver tumors in rats. They fed the highest tolerated dose of AB (0.2–0.3%) in the diet to 16 male rats on a low protein diet and induced two metastasizing liver cell carcinomas and five hepatomas. No liver tumors were reported in eight male and eight female control rats. Also, injection of AB into the kidney of frogs (*Rana pipiens*) leads to kidney tumors (*208*). Since the latent period of these tumors was as short as three weeks, they were probably induced by the Lucké virus, which is known to produce tumors in this species.

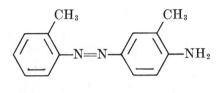

84

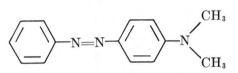

85

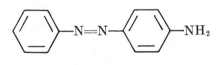

86

The oncogenicity of AB derivatives was compared by feeding them at a level equivalent, on a molar basis, to 0.057% N-methyl-AB for 54 weeks (*44*). This schedule adequately demonstrates whether or not these compounds are potently carcinogenic but does not exclude the possibility that they are weakly carcinogenic. No tumors were induced by N-hydroxy-4-phenylazoacetanilide (N-hydroxy-AAB) or its cupric chelate, N-hydroxy-AB, AB, AAB, or N-acetoxy-AAB. It was also shown that AAB, N-hydroxy-AAB, 3-hydroxy-AAB, and 4′-hydroxy-AAB were all present (often in relatively small amounts) in the urine of rats fed AAB, N-hydroxy-AAB, AB, N-methyl-AB (MAB), N,N-dimethyl-AB (DAB), or N-hydroxy-AB. These metabolic data confirm previous observations on these compounds (*209*).

On the other hand there is no doubt about the carcinogenicity of 4-(o-tolylazo)-o-toluidine (o-aminoazotoluene) (Table VIII). Historically, this was the first carcinogenic azo compound to be discovered. Yoshida reported that it induced hepatomas in rats in 1932 (*210*). It is more carcinogenic in mice than in rats, leading to hepatomas, pulmonary adenomas, and hemangioendotheliomas in several tissues, and, from only one report, to bladder tumors. It is also carcinogenic in hamsters, dogs, and possibly in rabbits (Table VIII). It appears to be N-hydroxylated *in vivo* because 4,4'-bis(o-tolylazo)-2,2'-dimethylazobenzene (**87**) has been isolated from the liver of

Table VIII. Carcinogenicity of

Compound	Species	Route[b]	Adequacy[c]
4-(Phenylazo)aniline	rat	Top/O	A
	frog	intrarenal	S
4-(Phenylazo)acetanilide	rat	O	A
4-(Phenylazo)diacetanilide	rat	O	S
4-(Phenylazo)-N-phenylhydroxylamine	rat	S.C.	S
4-(Phenylazo)-N-phenylacethydroxamic acid	rat	O/I.P.	S
4-(Phenylazo)-o-anisidine	rat	O/Top	A
4[(p-Methoxyphenyl)azo]-o-anisidine	rat	O	S
4-(m-Tolylazo)aniline	rat	O	S
4-(m-Tolylazo)acetanilide	rat	O	S
4(o-Tolylazo)-o-toluidine	mouse		A
	rat		A
	rabbit		A
	hamster		S
	dog		S
2(p-Tolylazo)-p-toluidine	mouse	O	S
	rat	O	A
4(o-Tolylazo)-m-toluidine	rat	O	S
2(o-Tolylazo)-p-toluidine	mouse	O	S
	rat	O	S
4-(m-Tolylazo)-m-toluidine	mouse	O	
	rat	O	
4-(p-Tolylazo)-m-toluidine	mouse	O	
	rat	O	
4-(p-Tolylazo)-o-toluidine	mouse	O	
	rat	O	
4-(o-Tolylazoxy)-o-toluidine	rat	O	S
1-[4(o-Tolylazo)-o-tolylazo]-2-naphthol (Scarlet Red)	Abnormal proliferative lesions only		
4'-Fluoro-p-phenylaniline	rat	O	S
1-(Phenylazo)-2-naphthylamine	rat	O/S.C.	A
1-(o-Tolylazo)-2-naphthylamine	mouse	O	S
	rat	O/S.C.	A
	dog	O	S

[a] Excluding N,N-dimethyl derivatives.
[b] O, oral; Top, topical; S.C., subcutaneous injection; I.P., intraperitoneal injection.
[c] A, tested in more than one institute; S, evidence less convincing.

mice treated with 4-(*o*-tolylazo)-*o*-toluidine (*210*). This metabolic activation is confirmed indirectly by the demonstration that 4-(*o*-tolylazo)-*o*-toluidine interacts *in vivo* with DNA, RNA, and protein (*212, 213, 214*).

Five positional isomers of 4-(*o*-tolylazo)-*o*-toluidine were tested for

Derivatives of 4-Phenylazoaniline[a]

			Tumors Induced in[d]				
Local	Blad-der	Kid-ney	Liver	In-testine	Ear Duct	Breast	Other
+skin	−	−	−[e]	−	−	−	−
−	−	+	−	−	−	−	−
−	−	−	−	−	−	−	−
−	−	−	−	−	−	−	−
−	−	−	−	−	−	−	−
−	−	−	−	−	−	−	−
+skin (Top)	−	−	+	?	+	−	skin (O)
−	−	−	+	+	?	−	−
−	−	−	−	−	−	−	−
−	+[f]	−	+	−	−	−	lung, hemangio-endothelioma
−	−	−	+	−	−	−	−
−	?	−	−	−	−	−	−
−	+	−	+	−	−	+	−
−	+	−	?	−	−	−	gall bladder
−	−	−	−	−	−	−	−
−	−	−	+	−	−	−	−
−	−	−	+	−	−	−	−
−	−	−	−	−	−	−	−
−	−	−	+	−	−	−	−
−	−	−	−	−	−	−	−
−	−	−	−	−	−	−	−
−	−	−	−	−	−	−	−
			Abnormal proliferative lesions only				
−	−	−	−	−	−	−	−
−	−	−	−	−	−	−	−
−	−	−	−	−	−	−	−
−	−	−	−	−	−	−	−

[d] +, tumors reported; −, tumors not reported; ?, evidence equivocal.
[e] One author claims to have induced hepatomas (*see* text).
[f] Possibly on rice diet (*86*).

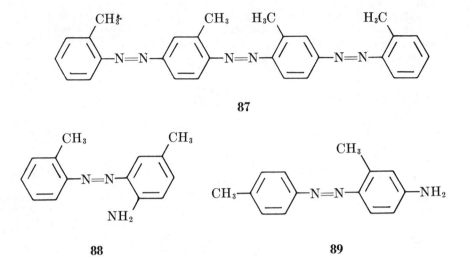

87

88   **89**

carcinogenicity in groups of 17–27 rats and 11–15 mice (*215*). Only 2-(*o*-tolylazo)-*p*-toluidine (**88**) was carcinogenic to the liver of both species while 4-(*p*-tolylazo)-*m*-toluidine (**89**) gave hepatomas in mice.

N-Methyl- and *N*,*N*-dimethyl-4-(phenylazo)-*o*-anisidine are unusual among the derivatives of *N*,*N*-dimethyl-4-(phenylazo)aniline in so far as they induce extrahepatic tumors, *i.e.*, ear duct, intestinal, and skin carcinomas. 2-Methoxy-AB behaves similarly (*216*). Fare and his colleagues first used these compounds to elucidate the possible protective effect of dietary copper acetate on hepatocarcinogenesis. This treatment apparently protected the liver from tumors but not the skin or ear duct (*217*). *N*,*N*-Dimethyl-4-(phenylazo)-*o*-anisidine induced keratinitis and a variety of skin tumors by direct painting on rat skin (*218*). Ear duct carcinomas were the only other tumor to be induced. Finally, Fare (*219*) demonstrated that painting AB, *N*-methyl-AB, *N*,*N*-dimethyl-AB, and the 3-methoxy derivatives of these compounds on the skin of male rats gave a range of skin tumors, although a similar experiment in mice was not successful.

These results could be important in a number of ways. The fact that AB is definitely carcinogenic on painting but is, at the most, weakly carcinogenic on feeding seemingly contraindicates the idea that some of the compound travels to the liver to be metabolically activated and that the active metabolite is then "liberated" in the skin, although the ability of *N*,*N*-dimethyl-4-(phenylazo)-*o*-anisidine to induce skin tumors, whether fed or painted, seemingly supports it. Possibly rat skin contains *N*-hydroxylating enzymes and therefore activates these compounds. Alternatively, there may be another pathway for the activation of these azodyes. These observations demonstrate the need for skin painting in addition to feeding studies for aromatic amines and for a more detailed study of the transport mechanisms and the enzyme distribution which activate these carcinogens.

The tumors induced by these azo compounds and by 2-anthramine (*see* page 411) closely resembled those observed in human skin. They included keratoacanthoma, squamous carcinoma, basal carcinoma, anaplastic carcinoma, and several miscellaneous tumors.

DERIVATIVES OF *N,N*-DIMETHYL-4-PHENYLAZOANILINE. *N,N*-Dimethyl-4-phenylazoaniline, often known as 4-dimethylaminoazobenzene (DAB) or butter yellow, was used to give a yellow color to hair creams in Scandinavia (*220*) as well as in many other technical applications. This group of carcinogens induces liver tumors in rats when the compounds are fed continuously in the diet. DAB itself was tested in several species and led to invasive bladder tumors in two dogs fed 20 mg/kg body weight/day for three to four years (*220*). One-fourth part of this dose was ineffective. The chemical induced liver tumors in mice with a latent period of more than one year, but negative results were obtained with squirrels, chickens, guinea pigs, hamsters, chipmunks, and cotton rats. Some of these negative results may have resulted more from the inadequate early carcinogenicity protocols than from the resistance of the species. The work on derivatives of DAB, described in Tables IX and X, is almost entirely confined to changes in the rat liver in tests which are usually relatively short. This means that compounds reported as without carcinogenic activity in these tests may prove to be carcinogenic if fed for a longer period or at higher levels.

The azo group in DAB is essential to the carcinogenic action of the chemical. Kensler and his colleagues (*222*) postulated that the split products, in which the azo group is reduced to two amino groups, might be carcinogenic. Nevertheless, feeding rats with mixtures of the hydrochlorides of aniline and *N,N*-dimethyl- or *N*-methyl-4-phenylenediamine (**90**) or of *m*-toluidine with *N,N*-dimethyl-4-phenylenediamine (**91**), failed to induce tumors (*223, 224, 225, 226*). Furthermore, riboflavin in the diet protects

Table IX.   Effect of Substituents on the Carcinogenic Activity of *N,N*-Dimethyl-*p*-phenylazoaniline

Substituent	2	3	2'	3'	4'	2,3'	2,4'	2,6	3',4'	3',5'	2',4',6'
$-CH_3$	−	+	+	+	+	−	−		+	−	
$-C_2H_5$			−	+	+				+		
$-CF_3$			−	−	−						
$-F$	+	+	+	+	+				−	+	+
$-Cl$			+	+	+					+	
$-Br$			−								
$-OH$	−	−	−	−	−						
$-OCH_3$	±	+[a]	+	+	+						
$-OC_2H_5$							±				
$-NO_2$				+	+	−					
$-NH_2$							−				
$-SO_3H$						−					
$-CO_2H$				±[b]	±	−					

[a] Ear duct, skin, and intestinal tumors but no hepatomas.
[b] Bladder papillomas, hepatomas possibly induced (*see* text).

Table X.   Liver Carcinogenicity of

Positive

N,N-Dimethyl-4(4′-benzimidazolylazo)aniline
N,N-Dimethyl-4(6′-benzthiazolylazo)aniline
N,N-Dimethyl-4(7′-benzthiazolylazo)aniline
N,N-Dimethyl-4[4′(2′,6′-dimethylpyridyl-1′-oxide)azo]aniline
N,N-Dimethyl-4(6′-*IH*-indazylazo)aniline
N,N-Dimethyl-4(4′-isoquinolinylazo)aniline
N,N-Dimethyl-4(5′-isoquinolinylazo)aniline
N,N-Dimethyl-4(7′-isoquinolinylazo)aniline
N,N-Dimethyl-4(5′-isoquinolyl-2′-oxide)azoaniline
N,N-Dimethyl-4[4′-(2′,5′-lutidyl)azo]aniline
N,N-Dimethyl-4[4′-(2′,6′-lutidyl-1′-oxide)azo]aniline
N,N-Dimethyl-4[3′,5′-lutidyl-1′-oxide)azo]aniline
N,N-Dimethyl-4[4′(2′-methylpyridyl)azo]aniline
N,N-Dimethyl-4[2′-methylpyridyl-1′-oxide)azo]aniline
N,N-Dimethyl-4[4′-(3′-methylpyridyl-1′-oxide)azo]aniline
N,N-Dimethyl-4[4′(3′-methylpyridyl-1′-oxide)azo]aniline
N,N-Dimethyl-4[4′(2′-methylpyridyl-1′-oxide)azo]aniline
N,N-Dimethyl-4[4′(2′-methylpyridyl-1′-oxide)azo]*o*-toluidine
N,N-Dimethyl-4[5′(3′-methylquinolyl)azo]aniline
N,N-Dimethyl-4[5′(6′-methylquinolyl)azo]aniline
N,N-Dimethyl-4[5′(7′-methylquinolyl)azo]aniline
N,N-Dimethyl-4[5′(8′-methylquinolyl)azo]aniline
N,N-Dimethyl-4(2′-naphthylazo)aniline
N,N-Dimethyl-4[3′-picolyl-1′-oxide)azo]-*o*-toluidine
N,N-Dimethyl-4[3′-picolyl-1′-oxide)azo]-*m*-toluidine
N,N-Dimethyl-4[4′-pyridyl-1′-oxide)azo]-2,3-xylidine
N,N-Dimethyl-4[(4′-pyridyl-1′-oxide)azo]-2,5-xylidine
N,N-Dimethyl-4[(4′-pyridyl-1′-oxide)azo]-3,5-xylidine
N,N-Dimethyl-4(3′-pyridylazo)aniline
N,N-Dimethyl-4[4′-pyridyl-1′-oxide)azo]aniline
N,N-Dimethyl-4(5′-quinaldylazo)aniline
N,N-Dimethyl-4(3′-quinolylazo)aniline
N,N-Dimethyl-4(4′-quinolylazo)aniline
N,N-Dimethyl-4(5′-quinolylazo)aniline
N,N-Dimethyl-4(6′-quinolylazo)aniline
N,N-Dimethyl-4[(4′-quinolyl-1′-oxide)azo]aniline
N,N-Dimethyl-4[(5′-quinolyl-1′-oxide)azo]aniline
N,N-Dimethyl-4[(6′-quinolyl-1′-oxide)azo]aniline
N,N-Dimethyl-4(5′-quinolylazo)-*m*-toluidine
N,N-Dimethyl-4(2′-quinoxalylazo)aniline
N,N-Dimethyl-4(5′-quinoxalylazo)aniline
N,N-Dimethyl-4(6′-quinoxalylazo)aniline

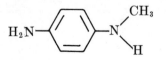

90

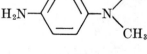

91

N,N-Dimethyl-p-phenylazoanilines in Rats

Negative

2-Dimethylamino-5(phenylazo)pyridine
N,N-Dimethyl-4(5'-benzimidazolylazo)aniline
N,N-Dimethyl-4(2'-dibenzofuranylazo)aniline
N,N-Dimethyl-4(1'-dibenzothienylazo)aniline
N,N-Dimethyl-4(2'-dibenzothienylazo)aniline
N,N-Dimethyl-4(3'-dibenzothienylazo)aniline
N,N-Dimethyl-4(3-dibenzothienylazo)aniline
N,N-Dimethyl-4(4'-benzthiazylazo)aniline
N,N-Dimethyl-4(5'-benzthiazylazo)aniline
N,N-Dimethyl-4(2-fluorenylazo)aniline
N,N-Dimethyl-4(3'-IH-indazylazo)aniline
N,N-Dimethyl-4(4'-IH-indazylazo)aniline
N,N-Dimethyl-4(5'-IH-indazylazo)aniline
N,N-Dimethyl-4(7'-IH-indazylazo)aniline
N,N-Dimethyl-4[2'-(4'-methylpyridyl)azo]aniline
N,N-Dimethyl-4[2'-(6'-methylpyridyl)azo]aniline
N,N-Dimethyl-4-(7'-quinolylazo)aniline
N,N-Dimethyl-4-(8'-quinolylazo)aniline
N,N-Dimethyl-4[2'-quinolyl-1'-oxide)azo]aniline
N,N-Dimethyl-4[3'-quinolyl-1'-oxide)azo]aniline
N,N-Dimethyl-4[7'-quinolyl-1'-oxide)azo]aniline
N,N-Dimethyl-4[8'-quinolyl-1'-oxide)azo]aniline
N,N-Dimethyl-4[2'-(4'-methylpyridyl-1'-oxide)azo]aniline
N,N-Dimethyl-4[2'-(6'-methylpyridyl-1'-oxide)azo]aniline

against DAB carcinogenesis in rat liver. Riboflavin is a component of a flavine adenine dinucleotide which acts as an essential cofactor for the enzyme azo reductase (227). The azo group could be lost also by reduction to a hydrazine and conversion in an acid medium to benzidines or semidines. These could be carcinogenic (*see* page 392). This hypothesis was shown to

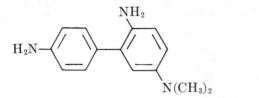

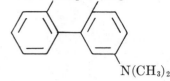

92 *   93 *

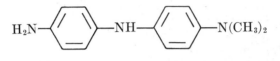

94 *

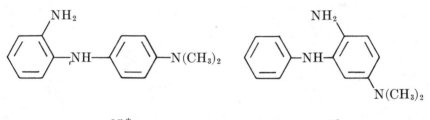

95 *   96

be unlikely by the synthesis of four of the five possible derivatives (**92***, **93***, **94***, **95***, **96**), which are shown above, and then demonstrating that they were not carcinogenic to rats (*228*). Since $2',4',6'$-trifluoro DAB is a more potent carcinogen than DAB itself and since the C-F bond is unlikely to be broken in the mild conditions of a benzidine transformation, the formulae marked by an asterisk are unlikely to participate in the carcinogenicity of DAB.

N-Methylaminoazobenzenes are, in most cases, equipotent to the corresponding DAB derivatives whereas AB itself is apparently noncarcinogenic. on feeding. Thus, at least one methyl group seems to be essential for carcinogenicity to rat liver. This is confirmed by considering the carcinogenic activity of a series of *N,N*-dialkyl-AB derivatives and a further series of *N*-alkyl-*N*-methyl derivatives. Although DAB is carcinogenic, none of the following derivatives gives tumors on feeding to rats—*N,N*-diethyl-AB, *N,N*-di-*n*-propyl-AB, *N,N*-di-*n*-butyl-AB, and *N,N*-di-*n*-amyl-AB or 4-(phenylazo)formanilide. On the other hand, *N*-ethyl-*N*-methyl-AB and *N*-methyl-4-(phenylazo)formanilide are both potent carcinogens. This rule of thumb may not apply to all de-

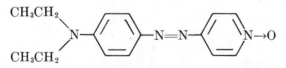

97

rivatives of DAB since 4-[4-(diethylamino)phenylazo]pyridine-1-oxide (**97**), for example, is carcinogenic to rat liver. However, examples of this nature need not be regarded as contraindicating the significance of the *N*-methyl group since the exceptions may induce cancer by mechanisms different from those to be described for other derivatives of DAB.

DAB derivatives which were tested for carcinogenicity are given in Tables IX and X. A similar but smaller table could be drawn up for derivatives of *N*-monomethyl-4-phenylazoaniline (MAB), but the carcinogenicity of each MAB derivative would not differ appreciably from that of the DAB derivative.

The number of DAB derivatives, which were tested by feeding to rats, is large and probably reflects their ease of synthesis and testing rather than their importance to man's environment or to the development of theories of carcinogenesis. To help to quantify this data, Miller and Miller (*228*) introduced the concept of an "index of relative activity" of carcinogenic azo dyes, defined as:

$$\text{Relative activity} = \frac{6 \times \text{months feeding DAB} \times \text{percent tumors with test chemical}}{\text{months feeding test chemical} \times \text{percent tumors with DAB}}$$

While DAB itself has a relative activity of 6, other derivatives vary from 0 to 200 or more. If not too much emphasis is placed on the absolute figures, this index can be used to grade carcinogens according to activity.

The carcinogenic derivatives of DAB usually induce hepatomas in rats, the only species to be tested. 3-Methoxy-DAB, as previously described, leads to skin, ear duct, and intestinal tumors (*see* page 416), while 2'-carboxy-DAB (*229*) (methyl red) was reported to yield bladder papillomas and hepatomas. This result, however, must be regarded with caution since a subsequent study (*230*) failed to confirm the finding while a third experiment led to only a single hepatoma (*231*). The DAB derivatives in which the prime ring is replaced by a heterocyclic ring system may be hepatocarcinogenic. For example, 6-[(*p*-dimethylamino)phenylazo]quinoxaline (**98**) at 0.3% in

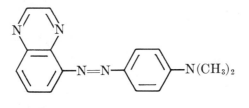

98

the diet led to 10 histologically confirmed hepatomas in 10 rats by two months, whereas the 2-isomer (**99**) was inactive at eight months after feeding at the same level in the diet (*232*). Nevertheless, heterocyclic derivatives are not necessarily the most potently carcinogenic because *N*,*N*-dimethyl-4-(2,3-

xylylazo)aniline (**100**) fed in the diet at a level of 0.06% gave 10 histologically confirmed hepatomas in 10 rats by the end of one month (*233*).

The metabolism of DAB has been studied extensively. The major reactions are stepwise demethylation, acetylation, C-hydroxylation, and reductive splitting of the azo linkage (Figure 4). Azo reduction has already been referred to as a detoxication mechanism (*see* page 417), as has the second demethylation step (*see* page 420). The study of the demethylation step was facilitated by the development of a quantitative method for the separation of DAB, MAB, and AB (*234*). Using N,N-dimethyl-4-(*m*-tolylazo)aniline, which is resistant to C-hydroxylation and reduction of the azo group, it was shown that fortified rat liver brei *in vitro* quantitatively removed the N-methyl group as formaldehyde, which was trapped as the semicarbazone (*228*). In the earlier literature, it was stated that DAB and MAB were interconvertible *in vivo*. This has subsequently been found to be incorrect. The earlier analytic method was unable to separate DAB from N-methyl-4-phenyl-azo-2-(methylthio)aniline (**101**).

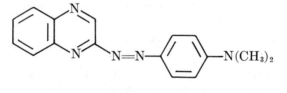

99

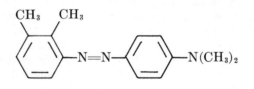

100

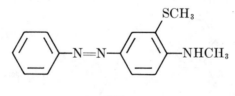

101

Gas chromatography achieved this separation and indicated that DAB and MAB probably resemble other aromatic amines insofar as they are converted to a highly reactive intermediate which reacts with methionine and its derivatives to give the methylthioether (*42, 235*).

Miller and Miller reported in 1947 that DAB and MAB reacted with rat liver cell protein *in vivo* (*236*). This was the first conclusive demonstra-

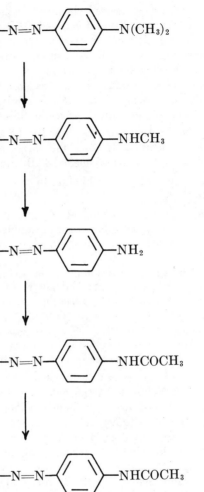

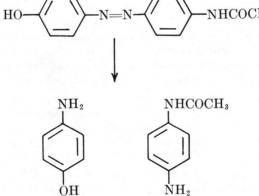

Figure 4.   Major routes of metabolism of DAB

tion that a carcinogen reacted chemically with tissue macromolecules. Protein from the perfused liver of rats fed DAB was pink in acidic media and yellow at a higher pH whereas untreated liver was colorless. The color could not be extracted by continuous solvent extraction. Degradation of the protein–dye complex by trypsinization or, more effectively, by ethanolic–alkaline hydrolysis liberated the dye as nonpolar and polar fractions. The nonpolar dye was identified in 1947 as a mixture of DAB, MAB, and AB; the former probably contained the methyl thioether (**101**).

The polar fraction was later found to be a mixture containing 3-(homocystein-S-yl)-N-methyl-4AB (*42*), the corresponding S-oxide, N-(3-tyrosyl)-N-methyl-4AB, 3(3-tyrosyl)-N-methyl-4AB, and other components (*237, 238*).

The relevance of protein binding to carcinogenesis was demonstrated by the facts that

1. the concentration of bound dye was higher in liver, the target tissue, than in any of the seven other tissues examined; only red blood cells, which cannot proliferate, had an approximately equivalent level of bound dye to that in liver;

2. there was more dye bound to the perfused liver of DAB-fed rats than to liver of other species which did not readily develop hepatomas, such as cotton rats, chickens, rabbits, guinea pigs, or mice;

3. the study of the level of DAB binding to rat liver during carcinogenesis demonstrated that the level of dye rose to a maximum at three to four weeks and then progressively fell until the bound dye could not be detected in the tumor, despite the presence of free dye in the circulating blood plasma.

The study of a series of C-methylated DAB derivatives, including the noncarcinogenic N,N-dimethyl-4-(phenylazo)-m-toluidine and N,N-dimethyl-4-(p-tolylazo)aniline, showed that both carcinogenic and noncarcinogenic azo dyes bound to protein (*239*). The carcinogenic dyes attained their maximum binding more rapidly than their inactive counterparts. For example, the active dyes N,N-dimethyl-4-(m-tolylazo)aniline and DAB achieved their maximum binding in 2 and 3–4 weeks, respectively whereas the inactive compounds took more than 12 weeks. In this study equimolar levels of dye were fed because the time taken to reach maximum binding depends on the level of dye in the diet. The further development of this work, using both labeled and unlabeled dyes showed that these dyes bound covalently with most, if not all, constituents of rat liver cells, including nucleic acids and proteins (*240*).

Much effort was expended in the study of those proteins which bind DAB and its derivatives most effectively. Sorof and his colleagues found that electrophoresis of soluble cell proteins from the liver of rats treated with DAB or its derivatives caused most of the bound dye to be concentrated in a specific band, the so-called "h" protein (*241*). 2-FAA also bound to the same protein (*242*), as did the carcinogenic polycyclic hydrocarbons with mouse epithelial cell protein (*243, 244*). The most slowly sedimenting class of these soluble non-particulate proteins was then separated by preparative ultracentrifugation and shown to contain the bound dye. This centrifuged fraction split on electrophoresis into two components, one of which was the "h" protein (*245*).

Finally, zonal electrophoresis showed that carcinogenic azo dyes bound more to the slowly moving fraction (slow h_2) than did the noncarcinogens (*246*).

Ketterer and his colleagues (*247*) isolated three dye binding proteins by a combination of electrophoretic and other techniques. One protein was characterized as a basic protein (molecular weight 45,000; isoelectric point 8.4). The other two proteins had a molecular weight of near 13,800 and isoelectric points near pH 7. It was shown that the lower molecular weight proteins bound azo dyes through a methionyl group (*248*). However, the use of $8M$ urea, which breaks down the tertiary structure of proteins, released some of the azo dye as a very low molecular weight entity while the rest remained bound to protein. The liberated fraction was suggested to be a glutathione conjugate which binds extremely tightly by physical forces to the protein (*249*). A further paper then gave strong evidence for the identity of the azo dye binding protein (molecular weight 45,000 by gel filtration) and the proteins which bound a wide range of other bioorganic and organic molecules. Carcinogen binding was covalent while noncarcinogens bound noncovalently. This protein, with the trivial name of ligandin, is present in adult liver cell sap at a level of 4%. It is also present in kidney and small intestine but not in the other tissues examined. The protein is a major determinant of the hepatic uptake of small molecules (*250*). Its function in azo dye carcinogenesis is not understood, but despite all the work described above, it is possible that protein binding represents a further detoxication mechanism responsible for the partial removal of the activated metabolite.

The details of the mechanism by which the azo dyes induce cancer have not been fully worked out. Attempts to prepare *N*-hydroxy-MAB were unsuccessful because of its instability, although *N*-benzoyloxy-MAB (**27**) is a potent carcinogen and reacts with nucleic acids and proteins to give the same products as obtained from rat liver nucleic acids and protein after treatment with DAB or MAB *in vivo* (*62*). An alternative suggestion that *N,N*-dimethyl-4-(phenylazo)aniline-*N*-oxide (**102**) might be the metabolically activated product seems unlikely to be true since it is only about as carcinogenic as DAB and is considerably less carcinogenic than *N*-benzoyloxy MAB (*251*).

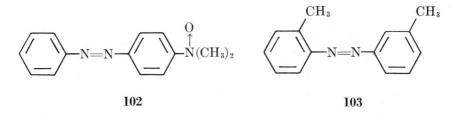

102   **103**

o-TOLYLAZO-*m*-TOLUENE. *o*-Tolylazo-*m*-toluene (**103**) and 4(*o*-tolylazo)-2-methylbenzoic acid methylcarbonate (**104**) induce bladder papillomas when fed at a level of 0.1–0.3% to rats in the food (*252, 253*). Strömbeck (*254*) at first failed to confirm the result with *o*-tolylazo-*m*-toluene. However, when he used a polished rice diet, as favored by the earlier Japanese workers, he obtained bladder papillomas which were often accompanied by bladder stones.

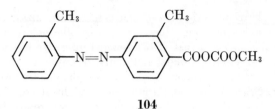

104

Because neither of these earlier experiments was properly controlled, Ström-beck and Ekman (*255*) and Ekman and Strömbeck (*256, 257*) administered the azo dye, *o*-toluidine, *p*-aminophenol, *o*-aminobenzoic acid, aniline, and 2-FAA, separately to groups of rats on semisynthetic diets and obtained a number of bladder papillomas. Similar tumors were obtained without any added chemical. Urinary calculi were recorded at necropsy in about 50% of the animals with bladder tumors. The difficulties in interpreting the significance of bladder tumors in the presence of bladder stones were summarized (*86*).

PHENYLAZONAPHTHOL DYES. Derivatives of phenylazonaphthol are important as dyes in food, etc. Several derivatives have led to bladder tumors after bladder implantation in mice (*258, 259*). However, the significance of these observations is difficult to assess.

Substances intended for use as food dyes, which include derivatives of 1-phenylazo-2-naphthol, should be assayed for carcinogenic activity by oral administration and preferably by inclusion in the diet. This is important for reasons other than mimicking the route of human exposure. First, the gut flora reductively degrades the azo group (*260*). In the case of tartrazine and other water soluble azo dyes, bacterial reduction is more important to the overall reduction of the dye than the hepatic azoreductase (*261, 262, 263*). The reaction was studied *in vitro*, and the relevant enzyme isolated (*264, 266*). Second, parenteral administration, especially by subcutaneous injection, leads to problems with non-chemically induced sarcomas (*267, 268*). This is particularly well illustrated by Patent Blue V, a triphenylmethane dye, which gave no tumors on feeding at the maximum tolerated level. The sodium salt of Patent Blue V gave sarcomas on injection whereas the calcium salt did not (*269*). Golberg and his colleagues showed that sarcomas at the injection site did not depend on the chemical structure of the test substance but on the physical properties of the solution. Surfactant solutions, for example, led to sarcomas (*268, 270*). For these reasons oral administration of derivatives of 1-phenylazo-2-naphthol will be emphasized.

There have been few attempts to assess the carcinogenicity of the "oil soluble" derivatives of 1-phenylazo-2-naphthol (**105**) by conventional methods. Injection of 1-phenylazo-2-naphthol into the subcutaneous tissue of stock mice led to seven hepatomas in 24 animals surviving for 15 months, the males being more sensitive than the females. No proper controls were kept. There were only five hepatomas in 449 similar mice used in other experiments (*270*). Bonser was unable to confirm this observation in CBA mice although two bladder papillomas were induced in rabbits. 1-*o*-Tolylazo-2-naphthol (**106**) induced tumors of the ileo-caecal junction in mice fed or injected with this compound (*136*). Thirteen untreated mice of this stock, which is no longer available, developed one papilloma of the ileo-caecal region. Citrus Red No. 2, *i.e.*, 1-(2,5-dimethoxyphenylazo)-2-naphthol (**107**) led to bladder epithelial hyperplasia and a low incidence of bladder papillomas and carcinomas in each species on feeding to rats and mice (*272*). The carcinogenicity associated with each of these compounds must be regarded as equivocal. Sharratt (*273*) confirmed the carcinogenicity of Citrus Red No. 2 in female, but not male mice.

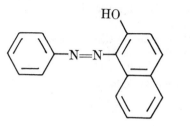

105

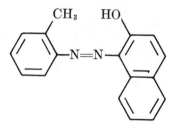

106

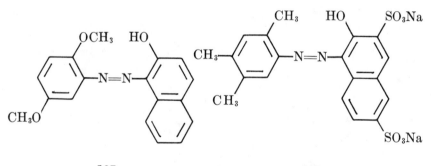

107   108

Grice *et al.* (*274*) fed 0.3, 1.0, and 5.0% Ponceau 3R (Food Red No. 6) ; disodium salt of 1-[(2,4,5-trimethylphenyl)azo]-2-hydroxy-3,6-naphthalene-disulfonic acid) (**108**) to groups of 30 rats for 65 weeks. Although there was a dose-related incidence of trabecular cell carcinomas of the liver (0, 7, and 24%), the result was not statistically significant. In another experiment 5.0, 2.0, 1.0, and 0.5% of the dye was fed to large groups of weanling Osborn Mendel rats of both sexes, and it was demonstrated unequivocably that the substance was a liver carcinogen in rats (*275*). Unfinished experiments in mice feeding levels of 2.0, 1.0, and 0.5% dye also suggested that Ponceau 3R was hepatocarcinogenic. Mannell (*276*) provided further corroborative information and, by examining the trimethylaniline after reduction of the azo group, demonstrated the gross lack of specificity in structure of the food dye.

A similar substance, Ponceau MX (disodium salt of 1-[(2-4-xylyl)azo]-2-hydroxy-3,6-naphthalenedisulfonic acid) (**109**), fed to rats at levels of 0.27,

1, and 3%, led to a dose-related incidence of liver changes (*277*). The original workers diagnosed these lesions as tumors, but this was disputed (*278*). A further large experiment led to the induction of similar lesions also with a disputed diagnosis (*279, 280*). Similar lesions were found in mice (*281*). Prudence suggests that this substance is unsuitable for addition to food.

Similar compounds were shown not to induce tumors in large scale feeding experiments including D and C Red No. 10 (monosodium salt of 1-[2-(1-naphthalenesulfonic acid)azo]-2-naphthol (**110**) in rats (*274*), Ponceau SX (disodium salt of 4-hydroxy-3-[(5-sulfo-2,4-xylyl)azo]-1-naphthalenesulfonic acid (**111**) in rats and mice (*282*), Chocolate Brown FB (the coupling product of diazotized naphthionic acid and a mixture of 2',3',4',6,7-pentahydroxyflavone and pentahydroxybenzophenone) in rats and mice (*283*), and Black PH (tetrasodium salt of 2-(7-sulfo-4-*p*-phenylsulfonylazo-1-naphthylazo)-1-naphthol-3,5-disulfonic acid (**112**) in rats (*284*). Other compounds were reported to be inactive in less extensive tests.

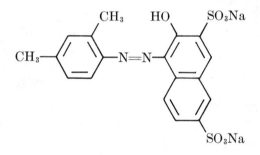

109

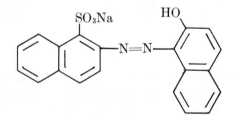

110

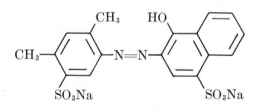

111

Trypan Blue (tetrasodium salt of 3,3'-[(3,3'-dimethyl-4,4'-biphenylene) bis(azo)]bis[5-amino-4-hydroxy-2,7-naphthalenedisulfonic   acid]）   (**113**) after injection into pregnant rats, induces abnormalities in the fetuses which closely resemble those seen in human pregnancies and   is used as a model teratogen for experimental studies. Trypan Blue, when repeatedly injected into normal rats, results in the dye being absorbed by serum albumin and taken up by the reticulo-endothelial system. Malignant tumors of this tissue appeared after as little as 100 days (*285, 286*).

The structural features necessary for the carcinogenicity of Trypan Blue were examined. Although Evans Blue (tetrasodium salt of 3,3'-[(3,3'-dimethyl-4,4'-biphenylene)bis(azo)]bis(5-amino-4-hydroxy-6,8-naphthalenedisulfonic acid) (**114**) is active, Vital Red (tetrasodium salt of 1,1'[(3,3'-dimethyl-4,4'-biphenylene)bis(azo)]bis(2-amino-3,6-naphthalenedisulfonic acid) (**115**) and benzopurpurin 4B (disodium salt of 2,2'-[3,3'-dimethyl-4,4'-biphenylene) bis(azo)]bis[1-amino-4-naphthalenesulfonic acid] (**116**) are without carcino-

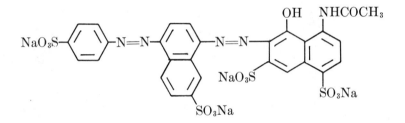

112

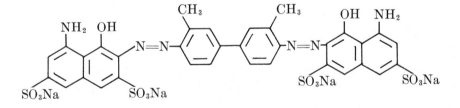

113

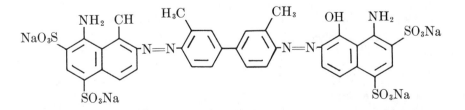

114

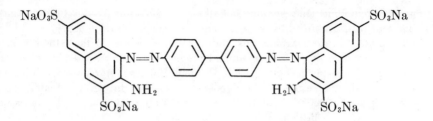

115

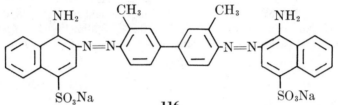

116

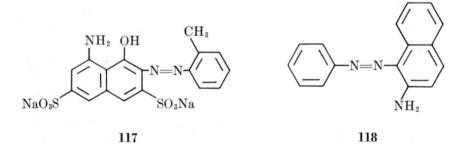

117   **118**

genic activity (*288*). Semi-Trypan Blue (2-[(*o*-tolyl)azo]-4-hydroxy-8-amino-3,6-naphthalenedisulfonic acid) (**117**) is also without activity (*289*).

Limited metabolism studies on the phenylazonaphthols gave little indication of their metabolic activation (*290*). The simple suggestion that reduction of the azo group leads to liberation of a carcinogenic aromatic amine could explain the results obtained with the oil soluble derivatives, Ponceau 3R and Ponceau MX, from which analogs of the known but weak carcinogen *o*-toluidine are liberated (*see* page 397). Nevertheless, the fact that Trypan Blue induces histiocytic or Kupfer cell tumors of the liver whereas the aromatic amine derived from it, *o*-tolidine, does not induce liver tumors (Table II) seemingly contraindicates this idea.

OTHER AZO COMPOUNDS. Other technically important azo compounds were tested for carcinogenicity under more or less adequate conditions. Substances such as 1-phenylazo-2-naphthylamine (**118**) and 1-*o*-tolylazo-2-naphthylamine (F, D, and C Yellow No. 4) (**119**) failed to induce tumors in several tests. Despite this, unless great care is taken to ensure that each batch is free from 2-naphthylamine residues, an absence of tumors could be grossly misleading as an index of safety to man.

A number of azo compounds whose structures have not been discussed are commercially important. They include the food dyes amaranth (*291*) (**120**) and tartrazine (*292*) (**121**) which are apparently noncarcinogenic.

Heterocyclic Compounds. 4-NITROQUINOLINE-1-OXIDE AND ITS DERIVA-TIVES. The present state of knowledge of the carcinogenicity of 4-nitroquino-line-1-oxide (**34**) and its analogs was summarized by Endo *et al.* (*49*). NQO has a low degree of electrophilic reactivity. The nitro group can be replaced *in vitro* by halogens, alkoxyl, aryloxyl, mercapto, hydroxyl, and amino acids, *e.g.*:

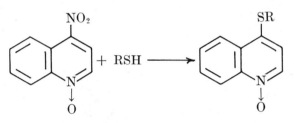

Although it was first thought that NQO might react directly with DNA, RNA, and protein *in vivo* to induce carcinogenic transformation, it was found that the reduction product, 4-hydroxylaminoquinoline-1-oxide (HAQO), is more likely to be the proximate carcinogen.

The carcinogenicity of NQO, HAQO, and their analogs is set out in Tables XI and XII. Both NQO and HAQO act locally on skin painting, subcutaneous injection, gastric intubation, or esophageal infusion, thus demonstrating that many tissues probably possess the enzymes required to activate these compounds. NQO is also carcinogenic in a range of animal species including mouse, rat, lovebird, guinea pig, and hamster.

Table XII indicates the molecular specificity necessary for the carcinogenic activity of NQO. Loss of the nitro group, the 1-oxide, or the second benzene ring (as in 4-nitropyridine-1-oxide) leads to inactive compounds. Addition of a further benzene ring, as in 9-nitroacridine-1-oxide, likewise

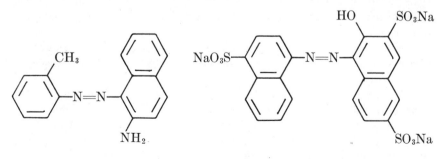

119   120

Table XI.   Substituted 4-Nitroquinoline-1-oxide and 4-Hydroxylaminoquinoline-1-oxide Derivatives Tested for Carcinogenic Activity in Mice

R = *Position* =	2	3	5	6	7	8	6,7di	6,8di
4-Nitro								
Fluoro			+		+		+	
Chloro			+	+	+		+	−
Bromo			+	+	+	+		
Methoxy	+	−	+	+				
Methyl	+	−	+	+	+	+	+	
Ethyl	−							
Nitro				−	+	−	−	
Carboxylic acid				+				
Cyclohexyl				−				
n-hexyl				+				
n-butyl				−				
4-Hydroxylamino								
Chloro			+	+	+		+	
Methoxy	−							
Methyl	+	+	+	+	+	+		
Nitro				+	+			
Carboxylic acid				+				
Cyclohexyl				−				
n-butyl				+				
tert-butyl				−				

gives an inactive compound. Similarly, the positional isomers, 3- and 5-nitro-quinoline-1-oxide are not carcinogenic. 4-Aminoquinoline-1-oxide has not been proved to induce tumors. On the other hand, many substituted derivatives of NQO are potent carcinogens (Table XI).

NQO does not react covalently with DNA *in vitro*; nevertheless, it may intercalate in, and certainly physically binds to, the macromolecule. The magnitude of physical binding between NQO and various polynucleotides decreased in the order native DNA > poly-A > apyrimidinic acid > denatured DNA > apurinic acid. This indicates that NQO physically binds to purine rather than to pyrimidine bases (*293*). As most bound NQO may be recovered from the polynucleotides by solvent extraction, this binding is not chemical.

When NQO or its derivatives were injected into rats bearing transplantable hepatoma cells in an ascites form and the DNA from these cells were subsequently isolated, fluorescence was found in the DNA at a maximum of 465–475 nm (*294*). The DNA from untreated cells did not fluoresce in this region nor did that from cells growing in rats treated with noncarcinogenic compounds. The fluorescence could not be removed from the DNA either by making it single-stranded to destroy intercalation or by solvent extraction, and it was still bound to nucleosides after enzymic digestion. The level of fluorescence indicated that, depending on the dose of NQO, 0.5–1.5 molecules of

NQO were bound per 1000 nucleotides. Thus, NQO requires metabolic activation to enable it to "bind" with DNA in the covalent sense.

The overall evidence suggests that the metabolic activation of NQO to HAQO is important. The failure of 3-methyl- and 3-methoxy-NQO to give tumors in animals may be because it is difficult to convert these NQO derivatives to HAQO derivatives enzymically. Whereas NT-diaphorase can readily reduce 2-methyl-, 6-chloro-, 6,7-dichloro-, or 8-methyl-NQO in the presence of reduced pyridine nucleotide, 3-methyl-, 3-methoxy-, 3-chloro-, and 3-bromo-NQO are only slightly reduced. Of the latter compounds, 3-methyl-, 3-chloro-, and 3-methoxy-NQO are not carcinogenic, whereas the 3-bromo-derivative may be hydrolyzed before reduction *in vivo* (*295*).

In general, NQO is devoid of activity in systems where it cannot be reduced to HAQO. For example, the inactivation of transforming DNA of *Bacillus subtilis* (*296*), the inactivation of T4 phage (*297*), and the mutation of T4 phage were brought about by HAQO but not by NQO.

O-Acetyl-HAQO (**122**), a possible esterified product of HAQO, did not induce tumors in the one reported series of tests (*298*). The reactions of HAQO indicate that a free radical may be formed under oxidizing conditions. In aqueous solution, at pH 7.5 and in the presence of oxygen, hydrogen peroxide is produced (*299*). This did not occur with either NQO or 4-amino-quinoline-1-oxide. The formation of this radical explains why HAQO acts as a catalyst in the reduction of cytochrome C by glutathione and the formation of 4,4'-azoxyquinoline-1,1'-dioxide in aqueous solution in the presence of oxygen (*297*). This also could explain the carcinogenicity of HAQO (*300*). The production of the azoxy compound is as follows:

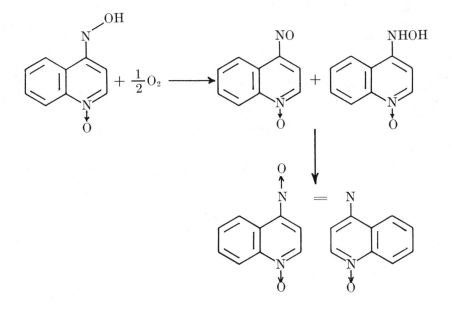

Table XII.   Carcinogenic Activity of

Compound	Species	Route[a]	Adequacy[b]
4-Nitroquinoline-1-oxide (NQO)	rabbit	S.C.	A
	guinea pig	Top	S
	hamster	Top	S
	rat	V	A
	mouse	V	A
4-Aminoquinoline-1-oxide	rat	S.C.	A
	mouse	S.C.	S
Quinoline-1-oxide	mouse	S.C.	S
4-Hydroxylaminoquinoline-1-oxide	rat	O	A
	mouse	S.C./O	A
3-Hydroxylaminoquinoline-1-oxide	rat	S.C.	S
	mouse	S.C.	S
5-Hydroxylaminoquinoline-1-oxide	rat	S.C.	S
	mouse	S.C.	S
4-Nitropyridine-1-oxide	rat	S.C.	S
	mouse	S.C.	S
4-Hydroxylaminopyridine-1-oxide	rat	S.C.	S
	mouse	S.C.	S
9-Nitroacridine-9-oxide	mouse	S.C.	S

[a] O, oral; S.C., subcutaneous injection; Top, topical; V, various routes.
[b] A, tested in more than one institute; S, evidence less convincing.

Enomoto *et al.* showed that the *N,O*-diacetyl-4-hydroxylaminoquinoline-1-oxide (*69, 301*) reacts covalently with DNA, RNA, and polynucleotides to a greater extent than HAQO. It also reacts with methionine. This substance would therefore appear to be a candidate for the ultimate carcinogenic form

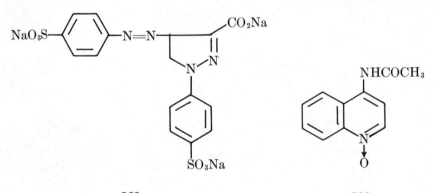

121   122

Analogs of 4-Nitroquinoline-1-oxide

Tumors Induced in[c]

Local	Bladder	Kidney	Liver	Intestine	Ear Duct	Breast	Other
+	−	−	−	−	−	−	lung
+	−	−	−	−	−	−	−
+	−	−	−	−	−	−	lung
+	−	−	−	−	−	−	lung adenomas, leukemia
−	−	−	−	−	−	−	−
−	−	−	−	−	−	−	−
−	−	−	−	−	−	−	−
+	−	−	−	−	−	+	lung, glandular stomach
+	−	−	−	−	−	−	glandular stomach, lung
−	−	−	−	−	−	−	−
−	−	−	−	−	−	−	−
−	−	−	−	−	−	−	−
−	−	−	−	−	−	−	−
−	−	−	−	−	−	−	−
−	−	−	−	−	−	−	−
−	−	−	−	−	−	−	−

[c] +, tumors reported; −, tumors not reported.

of NQO if it or *O*-acetyl HAQO was found *in vivo*. However, carcinogenicity studies using this compound showed it to be less active than NQO, possibly because of its ready action with noncritical nucleophiles (*301*). The salient feature of the 4-nitroquinoline-1-oxides is their conversion to derivatives of HAQO which can react with DNA and phage without further activation. Therefore, HAQO might be the reactive form in contrast to *N*-hydroxy-FAA which requires further activation, although as discussed earlier, further activation might occur through the phosphate ester.

PURINE OXIDES. The demonstration that the subcutaneous injection of unspecified "oxides" of xanthine and purine gave rise to local sarcomas in rats (*302*) has led to another example where *N*-hydroxylation is a determining factor in carcinogenesis. It was shown that 3-hydroxyxanthine and 3-hydroxyguanine were effective, but 3-hydroxyadenine was not. The carcinogenicity of various derivatives is given in Table XIII (*303*).

8-Methylmercaptoxanthine and 8-methylmercaptoguanine were present as metabolites of the carcinogenic 3-acetoxypurines (*303*) which, with the information gathered from a study of the chemistry of these compounds (*304*), led to the following proposed mechanisms for metabolic activation:

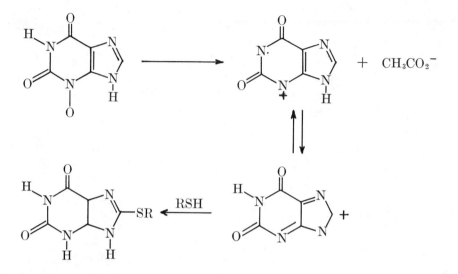

The 7-, 8-, or 9-methyl derivatives of the 3-hydroxypurines are not carcinogenically active because the methyl interferes with the activation of the 8 position.

Formation of a sulfate ester is unlikely to be the final activating step for these oxides. Incubation *in vitro* of a cell extract containing sulfotransferase

Table XIII.   Carcinogenicity of Hydroxypurine Derivatives by Subcutaneous Injection in Rats

Compound	*Activity*[a]
3-Hydroxyxanthine	+++
3-Acetoxyxanthine	++
3-Hydroxy-1-methylxanthine	+++
3-Hydroxy-7-methylxanthine	O
3-Hydroxy-8-methylxanthine	O
3-Hydroxy-9-methylxanthine	O
3-Hydroxy-8-azaxanthine	O
3-Hydroxy-7,9-dimethylxanthine	O
3-Hydroxyguanine	++
3-Hydroxy-1-methylguanine	++
3-Hydroxy-7-methylguanine	O
3-Hydroxy-8-methylguanine	O
3-Hydroxy-9-methylguanine	O
1-Hydroxyxanthine	O
7-Hydroxyxanthine	O
Hypoxanthine-3-oxide	++
Adenine-1-oxide	+
Purine-3-oxide	++

[a] +++, highly carcinogenic; ++, carcinogenic; +, moderately carcinogenic; O, not carcinogenic.

and 3'-phosphoadenylsulfate-[^{35}S] was performed with each 3-hydroxypurine derivative which had been tested for carcinogenicity. The liberated sulfate measured as free [^{35}S]-SO$_4$ produced by the sulfation of the 3-hydroxy groups and their subsequent rapid reaction with nucleophiles did not correspond with the carcinogenicity of the purine used (*305*). Acetoxy derivatives of these purines, on the other hand, inactivate and mutate *B. subtilis* transforming DNA (*306*).

There has been much speculation on the possibility of endogenous carcinogenesis—*i.e.*, the production of carcinogens within the body which may be responsible for cancer of "natural" or unknown origin. To the best of our knowledge there is no evidence for the production of 3-hydroxypurines *in vivo*.

AMINO- AND NITRO-DERIVATIVES OF FIVE-MEMBERED HETEROCYCLIC RING COMPOUNDS. Furan (**123**), pyrrole (**124**), thiophene (**125**), and several other heterocyclic five-membered ring systems are aromatic because they have two unsaturated bonds and a hetero-atom which contributes a "lone pair" of electrons to make up an aromatic sextet. Their nitro and amino derivatives therefore belong to this chapter.

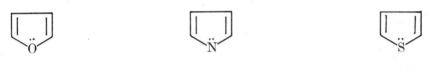

123   **124**   **125**

Compounds of this nature play an important role in human and veterinary medicine. The observation that some of these derivatives are carcinogenic has placed a further obstacle in the way of development of efficient drugs.

The first observations on 2-nitro-5-furyl derivatives were carried out by Price and his group (*307*) and Stein and his colleagues (*308*). The demonstration that *N*-[4-(5-nitro-2-furyl)-2-thiazolyl]formamide (**36**) was an exceedingly potent bladder carcinogen in mice, dogs, and hamsters established interest in the group (*54, 55, 309, 310*). This compound is one of the most potent bladder carcinogens known in the rat (*311*).

A related compound *N*-[4-(5-nitro-2-furyl)-2-thiazolyl]acetamide (**126**) was used pharmaceutically in some countries against human infectious disease. It was tested in female rats, and, unlike the formamide, led to mammary gland adenocarcinomas, renal pelvic tumors, lung adenocarcinoma, and salivary gland adenocarcinoma. In dogs and hamsters the formamide and acetamide induced similar tumor types while in mice the acetamide led to leukemia and tumors of the forestomach (*55, 310, 312, 313*). The other compound of this series which has been tested with equal thoroughness is formic acid 2-[4-(5-nitro-2-furyl)-2-thiazolyl]hydrazide (**127**). It is one of a series of drugs whose routine testing for carcinogenicity led to the discovery of this series of compounds. In rats the hydrazide led to tumors of the renal pelvis, tubular epithelium, and renal stroma (*314*). In mice there were stomach, lung, and mammary tumors while urinary tract tumors predominated in hamsters (*310, 315*).

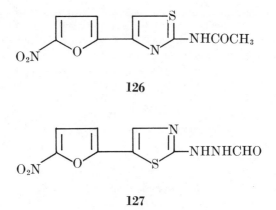

126

127

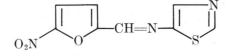

128

The remainder of the 5-nitro-2-furyl compounds were tested in rats and occasionally in mice. They show the structural features necessary for carcinogenic activity. In general, compounds containing two directly joined heterocyclic rings are among the most active. This proximity of two rings with aromatic character makes these compounds similar to aromatic amines of the biphenylamine and benzidine series—a hypothesis which is confirmed by the demonstration that 2-hydrazino-4-(4-aminophenyl)thiazole and 2-hydrazino-4(4-nitrophenyl)thiazole are active in rats (*316*). A second carcinogenic structure helps to demonstrate the variety of systems which may be involved (**128**). In the heterocyclic series, linkage by the –CH=N–bond produces carcinogenic derivatives, in contrast to observations in the carbocyclic series with stilbenamine analogs where the –CH=N group between two carbocyclic aromatic rings does not lead to carcinogenic compounds.

Single-ring 2-nitro-5-furyl and other nitroheterocyclic compounds present some interesting problems. 5-Nitro-2-furanidoxime and 5-nitro-2-furnanoethanediol diacetate are inactive while 5-nitro-2-furaldehyde semicarbazone induced only fibromas of the rat mammary gland. Mammary fibromas are considered benign by many pathologists, but Bryan and his colleagues (*316*) believe them to be malignant because they were transplantable into untreated rats. This is one of the classical properties associated with malignancy, but with the increasing use of pure line and other relatively inbred animals, its significance has been undermined. The standing of the mammary fibroma in carcinogenicity tests is important since the possible carcinogenicity of some valuable substances depends on it including 5-nitro-2-furaldehyde semicarbazone, an important antiseptic for the urinary tract known as Furadantin or nitrofurantoin and 1,2-dimethyl-5-nitroimidazole, a veterinary medicine (*317*). 1-)2-Hydroxymethyl)-3-methyl-5-nitroimidazole, used in the treatment of leprosy and known as Flagyl or Metronidazole, was tested in mice and shown to induce an excess of lymphomas and lung tumors (*318*). In our view, the carcinogenicity of the single aromatic five-membered ring heterocyclics has many similarities to the derivatives of single ring carbocyclic aromatic amines. They are either inactive or only show their carcinogenicity at higher dose levels or in special cases.

The metabolic activation of these compounds has not been reported. It appears that the active moiety is probably 5-nitro-2-furyl which can be activated by biological reduction of the nitro to a hydroxylamino group. Nevertheless, in several examples (Table XIV) the second heterocyclic ring carried an amino, hydrazino, or nitro group which are equally available for activation. There is a diversity of chemical structures leading to carcinogenicity including the imidazole and triazole structures. 3-Aminotriazole is a goitrogen, but unlike the other goitrogens it apparently induces tumors of the rat liver. We therefore prefer to relate the carcinogenicity of this class of compounds to an amino or nitro group attached to a suitable heterocycle than merely to the possession of a 2-nitrofuryl group.

TRYPTOPHAN AND INDOLE. The essential amino acid, tryptophan, and two related compounds, indole and indoleacetic acid, enhance the incidence of bladder cancer in certain closely defined situations. Dunning and her coworkers (*319, 320*) showed that rats fed 2-FAA in the diet with 1.4 or 4.9% DL-tryptophan (**129**), 0.8 or 1.6% indole (**130**), or 1.0% indoleacetic acid (**131**) developed bladder tumors whereas those fed 2-FAA alone did not. This experiment has been repeated although attempts to substitute other aromatic amines such as benzidine or 2-naphthylamine for 2-FAA (*321*) or to use DL-tryptophan and 3-aminodibenzofuran in female IF x C57 mice did not lead to bladder tumors (*321a*). In hamsters, indole or DL-tryptophan and 2-FAA gave slightly more bladder tumors than did 2-FAA by itself (*322, 323*). Feeding 2-FAA with a vitamin B_6 deficient diet also enhanced bladder tumor induction (*324*).

A possible explanation for these results is that the additive protects the liver against tumorigenesis. In a study in which the two strains of rat used did not develop bladder cancer after feeding with 2-FAA and excess DL-tryptophan, the most noteworthy result was a reduced incidence of liver tumors (*325*). This was confirmed and extended to show that rats on 2-FAA alone induced aggressive trabecular cell carcinomas of the liver after a few months, whereas,

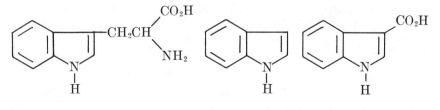

129   130   131

Table XIV.   Carcinogenicity of 2-Nitrofuryl

Compound	Species	Route[a]	Adequacy[b]
2-(2,2-Dimethylhydrazino)-4-(5-nitro-2-furyl)thiazole	rat	O	A
	mouse	O	S
Formic acid, 2-[4-(5-nitro-2-furyl)-2-thiazolyl]hydrazide	rat	O	S
	hamster	O	S
	mouse	O	S
2-Hydrazino-4-(5-nitro-2-furyl)thiazole	rat	O	S
	mouse	O	S
2-Hydrazino-4-(4-nitrophenyl)thiazole	rat	O	S
	mouse	O	S
N-[4-(5-Nitro-2-furyl)-2-thiazolyl] formamide	dog	O	S
	rat	O	A
	hamster		S
	mouse	O	S
5-Acetamido-3-(5-nitro-2-furyl)-6H-1,2,4-oxadiazine	rat	O	S
5-Nitro-2-furaldehyde semicarbazone	rat	O	S
N-[4-(5-Nitro-2-furyl)-2-thiazolyl] acetamide	rat		S
	hamster		S
	mouse		S
1-(5-Nitro-2-furylidene)amino hydantoin	rat	O	
4-Methyl-1-[5-nitrofurylido)amino]-2-imidazolidinone	rat	O	S
1-5-Morpholinomethyl-3-[(5-nitro-2-furylidene)amino]-2-oxazolidine	rat	O	S
1-(2-Hydroxyethyl)-3-[5-nitrofurylidene)amino]-2-imidazolidine	rat	O	S
1-[(5-Nitrofurylidene)amino]-2-imidazolidinone	rat	O	S
5-Nitro-2-furamidoxime	rat	O	S
4,6-Diamino-2-(5-nitro-2-furyl)-s-triazine	rat	O	S
N,N'-[6-(5-Nitro-2-furyl)-s-triazine-2,4-diyl]-bisacetamide	rat	O	S
Hexamethylmelamine	rat	O	S
2-Hydrazino-4-phenylthiazole	rat	O	S
D-(−)-Threo-1-(p-nitrophenyl)-2-dichloracetamido-1,3-propanediol	rat	O	S

Compounds and Related Substances

			Tumors Induced in [c]				
Local	Blad-der	Kid-ney	Liver	In-testine	Ear Duct	Breast	Other
−	−	−	−	−	−	+	salivary gland, various other tissues
−	?	?	−	−	−	−	stomach
−	−	+	?	−	−	+	lung? skin? stomach
−	+	−	−	−	−	−	stomach?
−	−	−	−	−	−	+	lung?
−	−	?	−	−	−	+	stomach?
−	−	−	−	−	−	+	stomach?
−	−	−	−	−	−	+	skin? salivary gland?
−	−	−	−	−	−	−	stomach?
−	+	−	−	−	−	+	gall bladder
−	+	+	−	−	−	+	−
−	+	−	−	−	−	−	stomach
−	+	−	−	−	−	−	lung? leukemia?
−	−	−	+	−	−	−	lung, mesentery (hemangio-endothelio-sarcomas)
−	−	−	−	−	−	?	−
−	−	+	−	−	−	+	lung, salivary gland
−	+	−	−	−	−	−	−
−	−	−	−	−	−	−	leukemia, stomach
−	−	−	−	−	−	−	−
−	−	−	−	−	−	+	−
−	−	−	−	−	−	+	lymphoma
−	−	−	−	−	−	+	−
−	−	−	−	−	−	+	lymphoma
−	−	−	−	−	−	−	−
−	−	−	−	−	−	+	−
−	−	−	−	−	−	+	−
−	−	?	−	−	−	?	−
−	−	−	−	−	−	−	−
−	−	−	−	−	−	−	−

Table XIV.

Compound	Species	Route[a]	Adequacy[b]
1-(2-Hydroxyethyl)-2-methyl- 5-nitroimidazole	rat	O	S
1,2-Dimethyl-5-nitroimidazole	rat	O	S
2-Amino-5-phenyl-2-oxazolin- 4-one + Mg(OH)$_2$	rat	O	S
3-Aminotriazole	rat	O	A
	mouse	O	A
1-(2-Hydroxy)ethyl-2-methyl- 5-nitroimidazole	mouse	O	S

[a] O, oral.
[b] A, tested in more than one institute; S, evidence less than convincing.

when there was a dietary supplement, these early tumors did not develop; instead relatively benign cystic tumors of the liver appeared at a later date. The latent period of the bladder tumors was such that they were induced later than the trabecular cell tumors. The experiments in hamsters (*323*) suggested that DL-tryptophan or indole protected against cholangiofibrosis and cholangio-sarcoma. DL-Tryptophan was without effect on the induction of bladder tumors by *N*-nitrosodibutylamine in rats, but it inhibited liver induction by the nitrosamine (*326*).

Boyland (*327*) noted that those metabolites of tryptophan which lie on the niacin pathway were *o*-aminophenol derivatives and, as *o*-aminophenols, were postulated to be active metabolites of the aromatic amines at the time; he tested some of them for carcinogenicity by bladder implantation. 3-Hydroxykynurenine (**46**), 3-hydroxyanthranilic acid (**47**) (in a cholesterol but not a paraffin wax pellet), and 2-amino-3-hydroxyacetophenone (**132**) were carcinogenic. The fact that these *o*-aminophenols were carcinogenic when suspended in cholesterol but not paraffin wax was further established in other experiments (*328, 329*). Many reservations have been expressed about the meaning of tumors produced by bladder implantation. The pellet is believed to participate in tumor formation. This was demonstrated by Bryan and Springberg (*86*) who showed that bladder implanted xanthurenic acid-8-methyl ether gave bladder tumors in mice whereas the same chemical was ineffective when injected, unless there was a cholesterol pellet in the bladder

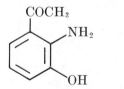

132

Continued

Tumors Induced in [c]

Local	Blad-der	Kid-ney	Liver	In-testine	Ear Duct	Breast	Other
—	—	—	—	—	—	+	—
—	—	—	—	—	—	+	—
—	—	—	—	—	—	?	—
—	—	—	+	—	—	—	thyroid
—	—	—	+	—	—	—	thyroid
—	—	—	—	—	—	—	lymphoma, lung

[c] +, tumors reported; —, tumors not reported; ?, evidence equivocal.

lumen. This compound led to an increased incidence of lymphoreticular tumors in rats injected three times weekly with 1 mg for about 600 days (*330*). To the best of our knowledge, no other suspect tryptophan metabolite has been shown to induce tumors as a result of testing by a conventional feeding or injection experiment. Therefore, the significance of these bladder implantation results are in question.

Price and his colleagues (*331*) reasoned that since aromatic amines were the only known causes of human bladder cancer, the spontaneous disease might be induced by endogenous aromatic amines. The only naturally occurring aromatic amines in human urine were metabolites of tryptophan. They therefore developed methods for quantitation of the metabolites. Patients with bladder cancer excreted significantly more kynurenic acid, acetylkynurenine, kynurenine, and 3-hydroxykynurenine after ingesting a loading dose of L-tryptophan than did control subjects with no known disease. Half of the patients with nonindustrial bladder cancer excreted an excess of these metabolites after a loading dose of L-tryptophan, but 10 industrial bladder cancer patients did not (*332*). Conflicting results were obtained in other centers (*333, 334, 335, 336*), possibly because of the technical difficulty of the analysis. An attempt by the original authors to repeat their observations using patients from the greater Boston area instead of from Wisconsin gave unconvincing results (*337*). To explain these differences, it was suggested that tryptophan had a relatively weak influence on the development of bladder cancer which was easily overlaid by other factors such as traces of bladder carcinogens in urban environments.

Abnormal tryptophan metabolism is not specific to bladder cancer patients. It was reported in patients with nonmalignant genitourinary tract disease (*336*), other forms of cancer (*338*), neurological conditions (*339*), scleroderma (*340*), rheumatoid arthritis (*341*), and pregnancy (*342*). Thus, although abnormal tryptophan metabolism may be found in some patients with bladder cancer, the significance of this observation to the natural history of the disease is obscure.

Some progress towards determining the effect of tryptophan and its metabolites has been published recently. Radomski *et al.* (*89*) fed dogs seven times the normal dietary concentration of DL-tryptophan for seven years and demonstrated that there was hyperplasia of the bladder epithelium but no tumors between three months and seven years. Similarly, Yoshida (*343*) found transitional cell hyperplasia, and increased proliferation which was demonstrated radioautographically after the injection of tritiated thymidine in rats given a tryptophan supplement. In our view these two papers constitute the only direct evidence for the interaction of the bladder epithelium with tryptophan or its metabolites. Indirect evidence of bladder cancer induction by tryptophan or its metabolites was adduced in experiments on the effect of dietary modification on spontaneous tumor incidence (*344*). The incidence of most spontaneous tumors was reduced in rats fed a high protein (51.0% casein) diet compared with that in rats receiving 22.0 and 10.0% casein, despite increased longevity in the high protein group. Benign bladder papillomatosis and tumors of the lymphoid tissue, however, were more frequent in the high protein groups. Since the protein is the main source of the essential amino acid tryptophan, it is possible but not proved that tryptophan is involved in the formation of these tumors. The solution to the problem may lie in the synthesis of the *N*-hydroxy derivatives of tryptophan and its metabolites and their specific identification in the urine of patients and animals receiving high doses of DL-tryptophan.

OTHER HETEROCYCLIC AROMATIC AMINES. The remaining compounds are analogs of two- or, generally, three-ringed carbocyclic aromatic amines

Table XV.   Carcinogenicity of Other

Compound	Species	Route[a]	Adequacy[b]
2-Carbazolylacetamide	rat	O	S
3-Carbazolylacetamide	rat	O	S
3-Dibenzofuranylacetamide	rat	O	S
3-Dibenzofuranylamine	mouse	O	S
2-Dibenzothiophenylacetamide	rat	O	S
3-Dibenzothiophenylacetamide	rat	O	S
2-Methoxy-3-benzofuranylamine	rat	O	S
S-Oxydibenzothiophenyl-2-acetamide	rat	O	S
6-[(1-Methyl-4-nitroimidazol-5-yl)thio]purine (Azathioprine)	mouse	I.M.	S
	rat	O	S
3,6-Bisdimethylaminoacridine HCl (Acridine orange)	mouse	Top/S.C.	S
	rat	O	S

[a] O, oral; S.C., subcutaneous injection; I.M., intramuscular injection.
[b] A, tested in more than one institute; S, evidence less convincing.

with one or more oxygen, nitrogen, or sulfur atoms replacing –CH– in the ring system. Most of the compounds recorded in Table XV are analogs of FA or FAA (*120, 155, 345*). Little work has been carried out to determine the mode of action of these compounds. They further indicate the range of aromatic ring systems which, when substituted with an amino group, are carcinogenic in animals.

Modification of Aromatic Amine Carcinogenesis

The complete and quantitative analysis of the way in which aromatic amine carcinogenesis may be modified requires an understanding of the pharmacokinetics of the action of each agent—*i.e.*, of the concentrations of an aromatic amine and its metabolites in each of the body compartments (blood, urine, bile, etc.) and of the activity of each of the metabolizing enzymes (*346*). The laborious nature of such investigations was illustrated in the stilbenamine series (*347*). The information considered here is more fragmentary.

During metabolism the extent to which all the metabolizing enzymes act on a foreign compound is determined by the available concentrations of the compound and its metabolites, the activity of the enzymes, and their affinity for each substrate. If a specific detoxifying enzyme is affected by a modifying agent, the concentration of carcinogen and its time of availability to the tissues may be altered, and consequently, the number and severity of the induced tumors may be different from that obtained in the absence of the modifying agent. This was the case when riboflavin concentration in the diet was shown to be inversely related to the carcinogenicity of DAB to rat liver. The concentration of riboflavin determined the concentration of a

Heterocyclic Aromatic Amines and Their Analogs

				Tumors Induced in[c]			
Local	Blad-der	Kid-ney	Liver	In-testine	Ear Duct	Breast	Other
−	−	−	−	−	−	?	−
−	−	−	−	−	−	−	−
−	−	−	−	−	+	+	−
−	+	−	+	−	−	−	−
−	−	−	−	+	+	+	−
−	−	−	−	+	+	+	−
−	+	+	−	−	+	+	−
−	−	−	−	−	+	?	−
−	+[d]	+[d]	−	−	−	−	+[d]
−	−	−	−	−	+	−	thymoma
−	−	−	?	−	−	−	−
−	−	−	+	−	−	−	−

[c] +, tumors reported; −, tumors not reported; ?, evidence equivocal.
[d] In NZB × NZW strain.

flavin-adenine cofactor which in turn determined the activity of the enzyme azo-reductase. This enzyme detoxified DAB, so the lower its activity the more DAB was available for conversion to the proximate carcinogen (228). Nevertheless, 2'- and 3'-methyl-DAB were unaffected by higher levels of dietary riboflavin because of the reduced ability of the liver to store riboflavin during the feeding of these compounds (228). Other vitamins, which do not contribute to cofactors essential for these metabolizing enzymes, have no effect.

One form of modification is enzyme induction, in which the modifying agent increases the synthesis of some microsomal metabolizing enzymes. Enzyme-inducing agents consist of a spectrum of different chemical structures such as polycyclic aromatic hydrocarbons and quinones, barbiturates, steroids, certain chlorocarbons, and so on (348). Enzyme induction and carcinogenicity may be, but are not necessarily, properties of the same molecule.

3-Methylcholanthrene is an enzyme-inducing agent as well as a carcinogen. Feeding 3-methylcholanthrene and the potent hepatocarcinogen, 3'-methyl-DAB, in the diet to rats inhibited the appearance of liver tumors until after 25 weeks whereas 3'-methyl-DAB alone gave a 98% tumor yield in 15–29 weeks (349, 350). The route of administration of the hydrocarbon was immaterial , as inhibition followed intravaginal, oral, subcutaneous, or intraperitoneal administration, but the greatest inhibition occurred when both compounds were given in the diet. This observation was repeated many times with different derivatives of DAB; inhibition was produced if 3-methylcholanthrene feeding were started no later than six weeks after the beginning of azo dye feeding (351). 3-Methylcholanthrene may be successfully replaced by benzo(a)pyrene, dibenz(a,h)anthracene, benzo(a)anthracene, dibenz(a,h)anthracene-7,14-quinone, and dibenz(a,h)anthracene-5,6-quinone (352, 353, 354). The level of protein binding was also inhibited by the enzyme-inducing agent, indicating that the amount of metabolically activated carcinogen was reduced (352). The levels of azo-reductase and N-demethylase measured in vitro were increased several-fold as a result of treatment by the enzyme-inducing agents (353).

2-FAA-induced hepatocarcinogenesis in rats was also inhibited by the use of dietary 3-methylcholanthrene as an enzyme-inducing agent (353). In an extension of these findings it was shown that feeding 3-methylcholanthrene with 2-FAA to rats resulted in a reduced urinary excretion of N-hydroxy-2-FAA (36). To circumvent the problem of the exact nature of the active ester of 2-FAA, Irving and his associates (355) studied in vivo the binding to rat liver nucleic acids of 9-[^{14}C]-2-FAA and N-hydroxy-9-[^{14}C]-2-FAA. If 3-methylcholanthrene were pre-fed before dietary 2-FAA to induce the metabolizing enzymes, the binding level was lower in the hydrocarbon-plus-2-FAA-treated rat livers than in those using 2-FAA alone. The hydrocarbon did not affect the level of binding when the hydroxamic acid was used. This clearly indicates that the hydrocarbon-mediated enzyme induction was concerned with the hydroxylation step of 2-FAA activation. If higher levels of the hydrocarbon were injected prior to a single dose of 2-FAA or N-hydroxy FAA, both amine and hydroxylamine binding levels were reduced, demonstrating that enzyme induction inhibited both N-hydroxylation and esterification under these conditions. The position is further complicated by changes in the excretion of hydroxamic acid derivatives during continuous feeding of 2-FAA. Rats excreted about 20% of a single dose of 2-FAA in the bile as the glucuronide of N-hydroxy-2-FAA and 1% of this metabolite in the urine. Moreover, when the glucuronide was administered, it was excreted unchanged in the rat bile, but in a variously metabolized form in rat urine (356). Irving (355) suggested that the increased urinary excretion of N-hydroxylated 2-FAA with time of feeding was the result of impaired biliary excretion of the N-glucuronide in the rat. This was consistent with the observed impairment of biliary secretion in 2-FAA fed rats (357) and with electron microscopic demonstration of changes at the borders of the bile ducts (358). It also explained why feeding 3-methylcholanthrene with 4-BPAA failed to affect the tumor incidence in rats (34). The absence of liver injury when BPA was fed meant that there was no change in the excretion pattern of N-hydroxy-4-BPAA. The concept that liver injury may affect the proportion of N-hydroxy-2-FAA derivatives produced from 2-FAA and excreted in the urine is further supported by studies concerning the feeding of the hepatotoxins 2-FAA, 3'-methyl-DAB, thioacetamide, thermally oxidized oils, and also from surgical or chemical (carbon tetrachloride-induced) partial hepatectomy (359, 360, 361).

Despite the inhibition of 2-FAA tumorigenesis brought about by inducing hydrocarbons *in vivo*, hydrocarbon induction of rat liver raises the levels of the microsomal N-hydroxylating enzymes measured *in vitro* several fold (362). It is the balance of the effective activities of all the metabolizing enzymes which is relevant *in vivo*.

Phenobarbital as an inducing agent increased the excretion of N-hydroxy-2-FAA glucuronide by rats (363, 364). It modified the carcinogenicity of 2-FAA in two ways (365). When it was fed simultaneously with 2-FAA, it reduced the incidence of hepatomas, because, as suggested by Weisburger and Weisburger (366), it induced N-glucuronyltransferase to a high level so that the glucuronide was readily cleared in the bile. If phenobarbital were given after feeding 2-FAA for 11–26 days, the incidence of hepatomas significantly increased. The phenobarbital-increased proliferation rate returned to normal values in hepatocytes and littoral cells in less than 70 days. The mechanisms of this action are not known, but, as stated by the authors, it is not likely to be caused by immunosuppression since azothioprine, an immunosuppressant, did not increase the carcinogenicity of N-hydroxy-2-FAA to rats (367). Possibly the phenobarbital-induced proliferation locks in 2-FAA-induced malignant transformation. Butylated hydroxytoluene, an antioxidant, also led to more of a dose of 2-FAA being excreted as the glucuronide of N-hydroxy-2-FAA (368).

Enzyme-induction studies using 3-methylcholanthrene were conducted in species other than the rat. The proportion of the dose excreted as N-hydroxy-2-FAA derivatives was increased by feeding 3-methylcholanthrene to rabbits (29) and hamsters (36, 369). In contrast to the rat, the rabbit excretes all but a trace of the N-glucuronide of N-hydroxy-2-FAA produced from 2-FAA in the urine (370). In the hamster the incidence of tumors induced by 2-FAA was increased by 3-methylcholanthrene (369). Mice maintained a similar level of N-hydroxy-2-FAA derivatives with or without hydrocarbon induction (*366*).

Feeding a 40-molar excess of acetanilide with 2-FAA to rats inhibited the appearance of hepatomas that would have been expected with 2-FAA alone (*371*). The hepatotoxic effects of 2-FAA were also inhibited, and this suggested that acetanilide might be interfering with the metabolism and possibly the N-hydroxylation of 2-FAA. The experiment was confirmed, and *m*-acetotoluidide and *m*-aminobenzoic acid, but not the *o*- and *p*-isomers of these chemicals, were shown to mimic acetanilide. N-Hydroxy-2-FAA carcinogenicity, however, was also inhibited by acetanilide, demonstrating that the N-hydroxylation step was not necessarily affected. As predicted (*16*), the *p*-hydroxyacetanilide formed from acetanilide competed with N-hydroxy-2-FAA for sulfate ion. Feeding excess sulfate overrode the inhibition induced by acetanilide on N-hydroxy-2-FAA, but not 2-FAA, and led to liver tumors (*73*). Since the liver tumors with added sulfate were not as advanced, nor were the toxic effects as pronounced as with 2-FAA alone, further experiments with higher levels of sulfate were conducted. All surviving animals had large multiple hepatomas (*73*). 8-Hydroxyquinoline also inhibited 2-FAA hepatocarcinogenesis and may act by the same mechanism as acetanilide (*372*).

Thus, many compounds are likely to affect some aspect of the metabolism of the aromatic amines and thereby alter their toxic or carcinogenic response. Matsushima and Weisburger (*373*) in addition to the substances already discussed, examined the effect of pre-feeding for four weeks with chloramphenicol, indole, L-tryptophan, L-methionine, L-tyrosine, guanosine, and inosine on N-hydroxy-FAA-induced alterations to body and liver weight, binding to DNA and other fractions, and tumorigenicity. Chloramphenicol and indole (*see* page 440) decreased N-hydroxy-FAA binding to liver nuclear DNA and were inhibitors of hepatocarcinogenesis. Chloramphenicol increased the proportion of N-2-fluorenyldiacetamide excreted as the N-hydroxy glucuronide (which is readily excreted in the bile) and probably decreased the amount available for esterification to the ultimate carcinogen (*374*). Blunck (*375*) showed that pre-feeding chloramphenicol for from 7–20 days also inhibited 3′-methyl DAB hepatocarcinogenesis. She then demonstrated that the protein binding of 3′-methyl DAB was not significantly changed by chloramphenicol (*376, 377*). Nevertheless, the livers were grossly enlarged between 4 and 20 days, and the RNA–DNA ratio was elevated in chloramphenicol-fed animals. Azo-reductase, normally suppressed by 3′-methyl DAB, was returned to more normal levels. Unfortunately, DNA-to-dye binding was not measured in these experiments.

Hormonal changes brought about by endocrine ablation and/or injection of appropriate hormones affect the metabolism of aromatic amines and thereby their carcinogenicity (*377*). For example, the male rat liver is more susceptible than the female rat liver to carcinogenesis by 2-FAA and N-hydroxy-2-FAA. The esterification step is of overriding importance since male rat liver has much higher levels of sulfotransferase than female rat liver (*72*). Castration alone or followed by the injection of testosterone propionate had little effect on the sulfotransferase activity in the liver of either sex. On the other hand, injection of 17β-estradiol into castrated animals of either sex resulted in at least a 50% depression in sulfotransferase activity 14 weeks after the operation (*72, 378*).

Adrenalectomy inhibited hepatocarcinogenesis in 2-FAA treated rats as first demonstrated by Symeonidis *et al* (*379*). It inhibited the N-hydroxylation of 2-FAA but had little effect on sulfotransferase activity (*377*). Replacement therapy with cortisone and deoxycorticosterone restored N-hydroxylation to near normal levels (*378*). Hypophysectomy inhibited both N-hydroxylation and sulfotransferase levels. Adrenocorticotrophic hormone restored N-hydroxylation and carcinogenicity (*72, 378, 381*). Surgical thyroidectomy has an inhibiting effect on sulfotransferase activity but not on N-hydroxylation and inhibits 2-FAA carcinogenesis (*382, 383*). Similar studies have been reported for other carcinogens, especially the amino azo dyes (*384–389*).

Certain lessons must be drawn from this brief discussion of exogenous and endogenous modifiers of carcinogenesis. First, the two-stage activation of 2-FAA and related compounds leads to a variety of effects—changes in N-hydroxylation or sulfotransferase or both. If some of the postulated second activation steps other than sulfate esterification are effective, as appears to be the case with certain extra-hepatic tumors, further types of modification may be found. Second, *in vitro* studies are only of limited use in this area. The amount of the compound which is metabolically activated depends on the relative activities of the activating and detoxifying enzymes and the concentrations of their substrates. *In vivo*, these concentrations vary with time. Third, exogenous and endogenous factors may have variable effects. Fourth, although some of the modifying agents might be able to reduce the carcinogenicity of an agent to man over a short period, there is as yet nothing acceptable to inhibit carcinogenesis on a long-term basis. The information given in this section may imply that the effectiveness of a potential inhibitor of carcinogenesis would have to be evaluated directly in man.

Finally, mention must be made of an experiment in which 2-FAA was fed and croton oil painted concurrently on to the skin. Skin papillomas were induced showing that 2-FAA is not only a carcinogen at many sites but "initiates" tumor cells in the skin and possibly elsewhere (*390*).

Conclusions

There is strong evidence that N-hydroxylation is the primary stage in conversion of aromatic amines to their ultimate carcinogenic form. With certain compounds there is also sound evidence that a further activation step is necessary. This has only been defined with certainty in the single case of 2-FAA carcinogenesis in (rat) liver which depends on the formation of the sulfate ester of N-hydroxy-2-FAA.

The evidence reviewed here suggests that aromatic amine carcinogenesis is the result of bioactivation to the ultimate carcinogenic form (**133**) and then dissociation of the reactive species to give a positively charged ion (**134**).

Unfortunately, the present evidence is not sufficient to distinguish in detail between the effect of different aromatic structures, alkyl or aryl groups,

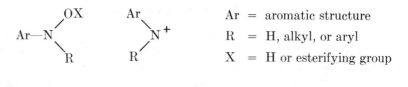

133   134

or different esters on the biosynthetic and dissociation stages. Nevertheless, a few generalizations can be drawn from the extensive literature.

1. Potent carcinogenicity is associated with aromatic groups consisting of two or more conjugated or fused aromatic rings. Single aromatic or non-conjugated ring systems may be carcinogenic in some cases, but, on the evidence now available, it appears that much higher doses are required [e.g., o-toluidine, 4,4′-methylene bis(2-chloroaniline)]. Aromatic rings in which the group para to the amino group is substituted are generally more carcinogenic than those in which the para position is unsubstituted.

2. The aryl or alkyl group on the amino nitrogen can modify the carcinogenicity of a carbocyclic aromatic amine by interfering with N-hydroxylation. The effect of R (134) on carcinogenicity becomes progressively less activating in the order: $OX > OH[NO] > H$, $COCH_3$, CH_3, $(NO_2) > COA > A > COPh > SO_2Ph$ (where X = esterifying group, A = alkyl other than methyl, Ph = aromatic ring, [NO] represents arylnitrosamine, [NO_2] represents nitroarene). More evidence is required before it can be determined whether heterocyclic aromatic amines will resemble the carbocyclic compounds in this respect.

3. The effect of certain substitutions in the aryl ring on the carcinogenicity of the compound is fairly constant. For example, substitution of methyl or methoxy ortho to the aromatic amino group often enhances reactivity whereas sulfonic acid derivatives are often without activity. As far as we can ascertain, these are useful guidelines but are not invariably true.

4. The ester group X (134) may be concerned in aromatic amine carcinogenesis but still requires further investigation.

The aromatic amines are one of the few classes of chemical carcinogens for which there is convincing evidence that some members induce cancer in man. Therefore, there are convincing reasons why, with these compounds, animal tests must be taken as having a particular relevance to man, who is able to N-hydroxylate. Nevertheless, the single-ring aromatic amines which need to be fed in large quantities if tumors are to be induced pose more difficult questions. To the best of our knowledge, o-toluidine has never been convincingly demonstrated to induce bladder or other tumors in man despite the fact that it was used as a basic industrial chemical for many decades. Our present qualitative approach to carcinogenesis prevents us from answering questions of this nature without extensive and expensive epidemiological investigations, probably made more than a generation after the original large scale use of the substance under consideration.

To overcome the problem of the long time lag between exposure to a carcinogen and the appearance of cancer, so that future workers need not be exposed to hazardous chemicals, a number of short term tests are being developed. These tests, which rely on the biological detection of activated metabolites, often with microorganisms, mean that it may be possible to screen compounds for carcinogenicity in a matter of days.

What questions should be asked quantitatively to understand the differences between man and animal in response to a carcinogen? The first series of questions should surely concern the relative exposures by all routes of the test and the human species. The second series of questions concerns genetic factors which are now slowly being dissected into single phenomena. The questions of enzymic activation and detoxication of aromatic amine carcinogens and the effects of induction and other modifying effects upon them were discussed at length in this chapter. Other factors, such as the ability to repair genetic and tissue damage or the competence of the immune system to remove precancerous cells, are intrinsic to the biology of the host but no less important if carcinogenesis is to be put on a quantitative footing, especially in relation to apparently weak carcinogenic stimuli.

Addendum

Since this chapter was written (June 1974) there have been inevitably a number of advances in the field. In particular mention should be made of the mechanism of activation of NQO. There is evidence that HAQO is not the ultimate carcinogenic form; its reaction with DNA in a buffer solution is thought to proceed through a free radical mechanism giving rise to DNA products different from those found with enzyme-activated NQO *in vivo*. It has been suggested that seryl *t*RNA synthetase could be the activating enzyme, it aminoacylating HAQO to give a reactive ester species (*391*). Similar activating mechanisms using seryl *t*RNA synthetase or other *t*RNA synthetases could be found for other *N*-hydroxy compounds.

Two papers have appeared also reporting the synthesis of *N*-hydroxy-MAB and the identification of this compound as a liver microsomal metabolite of MAB (*392, 393*). *N*-Hydroxy MAB is rather unstable but readily reacts with proteins and to a much lesser extent with DNA.

N-Hydroxylation as an initial activation step has also been suggested for benzidine and its analogs. Structure–activity studies on the microsomal activation of a group of benzidine derivatives to bacterial mutagens have shown that mutagenicity is dependent on the ease of oxidation of the amino group (*394*).

Acknowledgment and Apologia

We thank the Yorkshire Council of the Cancer Research Campaign for financial support while writing this chapter. We also warmly thank Margaret Davis for typing the manuscript.

In compressing the vast amount of information in the aromatic amine field, even to the generous length which the editor allotted us, we have had to select ruthlessly. We wholeheartedly apologize to those authors who feel we have ignored or have paid too little attention to their work.

Literature Cited

1. Rehn, L., *Arch. Klin. Chir.* (1895) **50**, 588.
2. Hueper, W. C., "Occupational Tumors and Allied Diseases," Thomas, Springfield, 1942.
3. Case, R. A. M., Hosker, M. E., McDonald, D. B., Pearson, J. T., *Br. J. Ind. Med.* (1954) **11**, 75.
4. Case, R. A. M., Pearson, J. T., *Br. J. Ind. Med.* (1954) **11**, 213.
5. Case, R. A. M., Hosker, M. E., *Br. J. Prev. Soc. Med.* (1954) **8**, 39.
6. Davies, J., *Lancet* (1965) **ii**, 143.
7. Annotation, *Lancet* (1966) **ii**, 1183.
8. Anthony, H. M., Thomas, G. M., *J. Natl. Cancer Inst.* (1971) **45**, 879.
9. Thiede, T., Christensen, B. C., *Acta Med. Scand.* (1969) **185**, 133.
10. Melick, W. F., Escue, H. M., Naryka, J. J., Mezera, R. A., Wheeler, E. P., *J. Urol.* (1955) **74**, 760.
11. Melick, W. F., Naryka, J. J., Kelly, R. E., *J. Urol.* (1971) **106**, 220.
12. *I.A.R.C. Monographs* (1972) **1**, 74.
13. Hueper, W. C., Wiley, F. H., Wolfe, H. D., *J. Ind. Hyg.* (1938) **20**, 46.
14. Bonser, G. M., *J. Pathol. Bacteriol.* (1943) **55**, 1.
15. Bonser, G. M., Clayson, D. B., Jull, J. W., Pyrah, L. N., *Br. J. Cancer* (1956) **10**, 533.
16. Miller, J. A., *Cancer Res.* (1970) **30**, 559.
17. Weisburger, E. K., Weisburger, J. H., *Adv. Cancer Res.* (1958) **5**, 331.
18. Miller, E. C., Miller, J. A., *Pharmacol. Rev.* (1966) **18**, 805.
19. Miller, J. A., Miller, E. C., *Jerusalem Symp. Quantum Chem. Biochem.* (1969) **I**.
20. Cramer, J. W., Miller, J. A., Miller, E. C., *J. Biol. Chem.* (1960) **235**, 885.
21. Kiese, M., Uehleke, H., *Naunyn-Schmiedeberg's Arch. Exp. Pathol. Pharmakol.* (1961) **242**, 117.
22. Heubner, W., *Naunyn-Schmiedeberg's Arch. Exp. Pathol. Pharmakol.* (1913) **72**, 241.
23. Brodie, B. B., Axelrod, J., *J. Pharmacol. Exp. Ther.* (1948) **94**, 29.
24. Uehleke, H., *Proc. Int. Pharmacol. Meet., 1st* (1962) **6**, 31.
25. Smith, P. A. S., "The Chemistry of Open Chain Nitrogen Compounds," Vol. 1, Chap. 3, p. 85, Benjamin Inc., New York, 1965.
26. Schultzen, O., Naunyn, B., *Arch. Anat. Physiol.* (1867) 349.
27. Uehleke, H., *Biochem. Pharmacol.* (1963) **12**, 219.
28. Irving, C. C., *Biochim. Biophys. Acta* (1962) **65**, 564.
29. Irving, C. C., *Cancer Res.* (1962) **22**, 867.
30. Kiese, M., *Pharmacol. Rev.* (1966) **18**, 1091.
31. Miller, J. A., Cramer, J. W., Miller, E. C., *Cancer Res.* (1960) **20**, 950.
32. Miller, E. C., Lotlikar, P. D., Pitot, H. C., Fletcher, T. L., Miller, J. A., *Cancer Res.* (1966) **26**, 2239.
33. Gutmann, H. R., Galitski, S. B., Foley, W. A., *Cancer Res.* (1967) **27**, 1443.
34. Miller, J. A., Wyatt, C. S., Miller, E. C., Hartmann, H. A., *Cancer Res.* (1961) **21**, 1465.
35. Andersen, R. A., Enomoto, M., Miller, E. C., Miller, J. A., *Cancer Res.* (1964) **24**, 128.
36. Lotlikar, P. D., Enomoto, M., Miller, J. A., Miller, E. C., *Proc. Soc. Exp. Biol. Med.* (1967) **125**, 341.
37. Clayson, D. B., "Chemical Carcinogenesis," J. and A. Churchill, London, 1962.
38. Radomski, J. L., Brill, E., *Arch. Toxikol.* (1971) **28**, 159.
39. Conzelman, G. M., Moulton, J. E., *J. Natl. Cancer Inst.* (1972) **49**, 193.
40. Radomski, J. L., Brill, E., Deichmann, W. B., Glass, E. M., *Cancer Res.* (1971) **31**, 1461.
41. Deichmann, W. B., Radomski, J. L., *J. Natl. Cancer Inst.* (1969) **43**, 263.

42. Scribner, J. D., Miller, J. A., Miller, E. C., *Biochem. Biophys. Res. Commun.* (1963) **20,** 560.
43. Bebawi, G. M., Kim, Y. S., Lambooy, J. P., *Cancer Res.* (1970) **30,** 1520.
44. Sato, K., Poirier, L. A., Miller, J. A., Miller, E. C., *Cancer Res.* (1966) **26,** 1678.
45. Lotlikar, P. D., Miller, E. C., Miller, J. A., Margreth, A., *Cancer Res.* (1965) **25,** 1743.
46. Ames, B. N., Gurney, E. G., Miller, J. A., Bartsch, H., *Proc. Natl. Acad. Sci. (U.S.)* (1972) **69,** 3128.
47. Miller, J. A., Miller, E. C., *Prog. Exp. Tumor Res.* (1969) **11,** 273.
48. Fukuda, S., Yamamoto, N., *Cancer Res.* (1972) **32,** 435.
49. "Chemistry and Biological Actions of 4-Nitroquinoline-1-Oxide," H. Endo, T. Ono, T. Sugimura, Eds., p. 101, Springer-Verlag, Hamburg, 1971.
50. Shirasu, Y., *Gann* (1963) **54,** 487.
51. Endo, H., Kume, F., *Gann* (1965) **56,** 261.
52. Yamamoto, N., Fukuda, S., Takebe, H., *Cancer Res.* (1970) **30,** 2532.
53. Kato, R., Takahashi, A., Oshima, T., *Biochem. Pharmacol.* (1970) **19,** 45.
54. Ertürk, E., Price, J. M., Morris, J. E., Cohen, S., Leith, R. S., von Esch, A. M., Crovetti, A. J., *Cancer Res.* (1967) **27,** 1998.
55. Ertürk, E., Atassi, S. A., Yoshida, O., Cohen, S. M., Price, J. M., Bryan, G. T., *J. Natl. Cancer Inst.* (1970) **45,** 535.
56. Akao, M., Kuroda, K., Miyaki, K., *Biochem. Pharmacol.* (1971) **20,** 3091.
57. Feller, D. R., Morita, M., Gillette, J. R., *Proc. Soc. Exp. Biol. Med.* (1971) **137,** 433.
58. Miller, E. C., Miller, J. A., Hartman, H. A., *Cancer Res.* (1961) **21,** 815.
59. Miller, E. C., Miller, J. A., Enomoto, M., *Cancer Res.* (1964) **24,** 2018.
60. Marroquin, F., Coyote, N., *Chem. Biol. Interact.* (1970) **2,** 151.
61. Irving, C. C., Veazey, R. A., Hill, J. T., *Biochim. Biophys. Acta* (1969) **179,** 189.
62. Poirier, L. A., Miller, J. A., Miller, E. C., Sato, K., *Cancer Res.* (1967) **27,** 1600.
63. Scribner, J. D., Miller, J. A., Miller, E. C., *Cancer Res.* (1970) **30,** 1570.
64. Lotlikar, P. D., Luha, L., *Mol. Pharmacol.* (1971) **7,** 381.
65. Bartsch, H., Traut, M., Hecker, E., *Biochim. Biophys. Acta* (1971) **237,** 556.
66. Bartsch, H., Miller, J. A., Miller, E. C., *Biochim. Biophys. Acta* (1972) **273,** 40.
67. Bartsch, H., Dworkin, M., Miller, J. A., Miller, E. C., *Biochim. Biophys. Acta* (1972) **286,** 272.
68. Bartsch, H., Dworkin, C., Miller, E. C., Miller, J. A., *Biochim. Biophys. Acta* (1973) **304,** 42.
69. Enomoto, M., Miller, E. C., Miller, J. A., *Proc. Soc. Exp. Biol. Med.* (1971) **136,** 1206.
70. King, C. M., Phillips, B., *Science* (1968) **159,** 1351.
71. De Baun, J. R., Rowley, J. Y., Miller, E. C., Miller, J. A., *Proc. Soc. Exp. Biol. Med.* (1968) **129,** 268.
72. De Baun, J. R., Miller, E. C., Miller, J. A., *Cancer Res.* (1970) **30,** 577.
73. Weisburger, J. H., Yamamoto, R. S., Williams, G. M., Grantham, P. H., Matsushima, T., Weisburger, E. K., *Cancer Res.* (1972) **32,** 491.
74. De Baun, J. R., Smith, J. Y. R., Miller, E. C., Miller, J. A., *Science* (1970) **167,** 184.
75. Lotlikar, P. D., Luha, L., *Biochem. J.* (1971) **124,** 69.
76. Lotlikar, P. D., Wasserman, M. B., *Biochem. J.* (1970) **120,** 661.
77. Tada, M., Tada, M., *Biochem. Biophys. Res. Commun.* (1972) **46,** 1025.
78. Irving, C. C., Veazey, R. A., Hill, J. T., *Biochim. Biophys. Acta* (1969) **179,** 189.
79. Irving, C. C., Wiseman, R., *Cancer Res.* (1971) **31,** 1645.

80. Maher, V. M., Miller, E. C., Miller, J. A., Szybalski, W., *Mol. Pharmacol.* (1968) **4**, 411.
81. Irving, C. C., Russell, L. T., *Biochemistry* (1970) **9**, 2471.
82. Maher, V. M., Reuter, M., *Proc. Am. Ass. Cancer Res.* (1971) **12**, 72.
83. Bonser, G. M., Jull, J. W., *J. Pathol. Bacteriol.* (1956) **72**, 489.
84. Clayson, D. B., Pringle, J. A. S., *Br. J. Cancer* (1961) **20**, 564.
85. Clayson, D. B., Cooper, E. H., *Adv. Cancer Res.* (1970) **13**, 271.
86. Clayson, D. B., *J. Natl. Cancer Inst.* (1974) **52**, 1685.
87. Bryan, G. T., Springberg, P. D., *Cancer Res.* (1966) **26**, 105.
88. Manson, D., *Chem. Biol. Interact.* (1972) **5**, 47.
89. Radomski, J. L., Glass, E. M., Deichmann, W. B., *Cancer Res.* (1971) **31**, 1690.
90. Gutmann, H. R., Erickson, R. R., *J. Biol. Chem.* (1972) **247**, 660.
91. Grantham, P. H., Weisburger, E. K., Weisburger, J. H., *Biochim. Biophys. Acta* (1965) **107**, 414.
92. Järvinen, M., Santti, R. S. S., Hopsu-Havu, V. K., *Biochem. Pharmacol.* (1971) **20**, 2971.
93. Irving, C. C., Janss, D. H., Russell, L. T., *Cancer Res.* (1971) **31**, 387.
94. Conzelman, G. M., Flanders, L. E., *Proc. West. Pharmacol. Soc.* (1972) **15**, 96.
95. Hartwell, J. L., "Survey of compounds which have been tested for carcinogenic activity," U.S. Pub. Health Service Publication No. **149**, Govt. Printing Office, Washington, D.C., 1951.
96. Shubik, P., Hartwell, J. L., "Survey of compounds which have been tested for carcinogenic activity," U.S. Pub. Health Service Publication No. **149**, Supp. 1, Govt. Printing Office, Washington, D.C., 1957.
97. *Ibid.*, Supp. 2, 1969.
98. *Ibid.*, 1961-7.
99. *Ibid.*, 1968-9.
100. *Ibid.*, 1970-71.
101. Bonser, G. M., *Br. Med. Bull.* (1947) **4**, 379.
102. Bengksston, U., Angervall, L., Ekman, H., Lehmann, L., *Scand. J. Urol. Neph.* (1968) **2**, 145.
103. Begley, M., Chadwick, J. M., Jepson, R. P., *Med. J. Aust.* (1970) **ii**, 1133.
104. Mannion, R. A., Susmano, D., *J. Urol.* (1971) **106**, 692.
105. Morris, H. P., Lombard, L. S., Wagner, B. P., Weisburger, J. H., *Proc. Am. Ass. Cancer Res.* (1957) **2**, 234.
106. Yamamoto, R. S., Frankel, H. M., Weisburger, J. H., *Toxicol. Appl. Pharmacol.* (1970) **17**, 98.
107. Homburger, F., Friedell, G. H., Weisburger, E. K., Weisburger, J. H., *Toxicol. Appl. Pharmacol.* (1972) **22**, 280.
108. Russfield, A. B., Homburger, F., Weisburger, E. K., Weisburger, J. H., *Toxicol. Appl. Pharmacol.* (1973) **25**, 446.
109. Clark, R., Thompson, R. P. H., Borirakchanyavat, V., Widdop, B., Davidson, A. R., Goulding, R., Williams, R., *Lancet* (1973) **i**, 66.
110. Prescott, L. F., Newton, R. W., Swainson, C. P., Wright, N., Forrest, A. R. W., Matthew, H., *Lancet* (1974) **i**, 588.
111. Mitchell, J. R., Jollow, D. J., Potter, W. Z., Davis, D. C., Gillette, J. R., Brodie, B. B., *J. Pharmacol. Exp. Ther.* (1973) **187**, 185.
112. Potter, W. Z., Davis, D. C., Mitchell, J. R., Jollow, D. J., Gillette, J. R., Brodie, B. B., *J. Pharmacol. Exp. Ther.* (1973) **187**, 203.
113. Walpole, A. L., Williams, M. H. C., Roberts, D. C., *Br. J. Ind. Med.* (1954) **11**, 105.
114. *Ibid.* (1952) **9**, 255.
115. Deichmann, W. B., Radomski, J. L., Anderson, W. A. D., Coplan, M. M., Woods, F. M., *Ind. Med. Surg.* (1958) **27**, 25.

116. Deichmann, W. B., Radomski, J. L., Anderson, W. A. D., Coplan, M. M., Glass, E., Woods, F. M., *Ind. Med. Surg.* (1965) **34,** 640.
117. Deichmann, W. B., McDonald, W. E., *Food Cosmet. Toxicol.* (1968) **6,** 143.
118. Deichmann, W. B., McDonald, W. M., Coplan, M. M., Woods, F. M., Anderson, W. A. D., *Ind. Med. Surg.* (1958) **27,** 634.
119. Clayson, D. B., Lawson, T. A., Santana, S., Bonser, G. M., *Br. J. Cancer* (1965) **19,** 297.
120. Clayson, D. B., Lawson, T. A., Pringle, J. A. S., *Br. J. Cancer* (1967) **21,** 755.
121. Bonser, G. M., "Precancerous changes in the urinary bladder," "The Morphological Precursors of Cancer," L. Severi, Ed., p. 435, Perugia, 1962.
122. Miller, E. C., Sandin, R. B., Miller, J. A., Rusch, H. P., *Cancer Res.* (1956) **16,** 525.
123. Clayson, D. B., *Br. J. Cancer* (1953) **7,** 460.
124. Cleveland, J. C., Cole, J. W., *Surg. Forum* (1966) **17,** 314.
125. Walpole, A. L., Williams, M. H. C., Roberts, D. C., *Br. J. Cancer* (1955) **9,** 170.
126. Walpole, A. L., Williams, M. H. C., *Br. Med. Bull.* (1958) **14,** 141.
127. King, E. S. J., Varasdi, G., *Aust. N. Z. J. Surg.* (1959) **29,** 38.
128. Hendry, J. A., Matthews, J. J., Walpole, A. L., Williams, M. H. C., *Nature (Lond.)* (1955) **175,** 1131.
129. Matthews, J. J., Walpole, A. L., *Br. J. Cancer* (1958) **12,** 234.
130. Bonser, G. M., Bradshaw, L., Clayson, D. B., Jull, J. W., *Br. J. Cancer* (1956) **10,** 539.
131. Gorrod, J. W., Carter, R. L., Roe, F. J. C., *J. Natl. Cancer Inst.* (1968)**41,** 403.
132. Irving, C. C., *Xenobiotica* (1971) **1,** 387.
133. Radomski, J. L., Rey, A. A., Brill, E., *Cancer Res.* (1973) **33,** 1284.
134. Goldwater, L. J., Rosso, A. J., Kleinfeld, M., *Arch. Environ. Health* (1965) **11,** 814.
135. Spitz, S., Maguigan, W. H., Dobriner, K., *Cancer* (1950) **3,** 789.
136. Bonser, G. M., Clayson, D. B., Jull, J. W., *Br. J. Cancer* (1956) **10,** 653.
137. Pliss, G. B., *Acta Unio Int. Contra Cancrum* (1963) **19,** 499.
138. Pliss, G. B., *Gig. Tr. Prof. Zabol.* (1965) **9,** 18.
139. Pliss, G. B., *Vop. Onkol.* (1959) **5,** 524.
140. Pliss, G. B., Zabezhinsky, M. A., *J. Natl. Cancer Inst.* (1970) **45,** 283.
141. Stula, E. F., Sherman, H., Zapp, J. A., Clayton, J. W., *Toxicol. Appl. Pharmacol.* (1975) **31,** 159.
142. Clayson, D. B., *Acta Unio Int. Contra Cancrum* (1959) **15,** 581.
143. Meigs, J. W., Sciarini, L. J., Van Sandt, W. A., *Arch. Indust. Hyg.* (1954) **9,** 122.
144. "IARC Monographs on the evaluation of carcinogenic risk of chemicals to Man," Vol. 4, p. 79, 1974.
145. *Ibid.,* 72.
146. *Ibid.,* 78.
147. Kopelman, H., Robertson, M. H., Sanders, P. G., Ash, I., *Br. Med. J.* (1966) **i,** 514.
148. Munn, A., "Bladder Cancer—A Symposium," Deichmann and Lampe, Eds., p. 187, Aesculapius, Birmingham, 1967.
149. Steinhoff, D., Grundmann, E., *Naturwissenschaften* (1971) **58,** 578.
150. Russfield, A. B., Homburger, F., Boger, E., Weisburger, E. K., Weisburger, J. H., *Toxicol. Appl. Pharmacol.* (1975) **31,** 4.
151. Stula, E. F., Sherman, H., Zapp, J. A., Clayton, J. W., *Toxicol. Appl. Pharmacol.* (1975) **31,** 159.
152. Linch, A. L., O'Connor, G. B., Barnes, J. R., Killian, A. S., Neeld, W. E., *Am. Ind. Hyg. Assoc. J.* (1971) **32,** 802.
153. Williams, M. H. C., Bonser, G. M., *Br. J. Cancer* (1962) **16,** 87.

154. Walpole, A. L., *Acta Unio Int. Contra Cancrum* (1963) **19,** 483.
155. Miller, J. A., Sandin, R. B., Miller, E. C., Rusch, H. P., *Cancer Res.* (1955) **15,** 188.
156. Haddow, A., Harris, R. J. C., Kon, G. A. R., Roe, E. M. F., *Phil. Trans. Roy. Soc.* (Lond.) (1941) **A241,** 167.
157. Druckrey, H., Ciba Foundation Symposium: "Carcinogenesis: Mechanisms of Action," Wolstenholme and O'Connor, Eds., p. 110, Churchill, London, 1959.
158. Baldwin, R. W., Smith, W. R. D., *Br. J. Cancer* (1965) **19,** 433.
159. Watabe, T., Akamatsu, K., *Biochem. Pharmacol.* (1974) **23,** 1845.
160. Wilson, R. H., DeEds, F., Cox, A. J., *Cancer Res.* (1941) **1,** 595.
161. *Ibid.* (1947a) **7,** 444.
162. *Ibid.* (1947b) **7,** 450.
163. *Ibid.* (1947c) **7,** 453.
164. Cox, A. J., Wilson, R. H., DeEds, F., *Cancer Res.* (1947) **7,** 647.
165. Bielschowsky, F., *Br. J. Exp. Path.* (1944) **25,** 1.
166. *Ibid.* (1946) **27,** 135.
167. Armstrong, E. C., Bonser, G. M., *J. Pathol. Bacteriol.* (1947) **59,** 19.
168. Littlefield, N. A., Ceuto, C., Davis, A. K., Medlock, K., *Proc. Soc. Toxicol.* (1974) 63.
169. Frith, C. H., Jaques, W. E., *Proc. Soc. Toxicol.* (1974) 63.
170. Morris, H. P., *Adv. Cancer Res.* (1965) **9,** 227.
171. Weber, G., "Liver Cancer," *Proc. Work. Conf., 1969* (1971) **1,** 69.
172. Miller, J. A., Enomoto, M., Miller, E. C., *Cancer Res.* (1962) **22,** 1381.
173. Irving, C. C., Veazey, R. A., *Cancer Res.* (1971) **31,** 19.
174. Scribner, J. D., Naimy, N. K., *Cancer Res.* (1973) **33,** 1159.
175. Gutmann, H. R., Leaf, D. S., Yost, Y., Rydell, R. E., Chen, C. C., *Cancer Res.* (1970) **30,** 1485.
176. Malejka-Giganti, D., Gutmann, H. R., Rydell, R. E., Yost, Y., *Cancer Res.* (1971) **31,** 778.
177. Yost, Y., Gutmann, H. R., *Proc. Am. Cancer Res.* (1974) **15,** 21.
178. Willard, R. F., Irving, C. C., *Fed. Proc. Fed. Am. Soc. Exp. Biol.* (1964) **23,** 167.
179. Marroquin, F., Farber, E., *Cancer Res.* (1965) **25,** 1262.
180. Lotlikar, P. D., Scribner, J. D., Miller, J. A., Miller, E. C., *Life Sci.* (1966) **5,** 1263.
181. Kriek, E., Miller, J. A., Juhl, U., Miller, E. C., *Biochemistry* (1967) **6,** 177.
182. Irving, C. C., Veazey, R. A., Russell, L. T., *Chem. Biol. Interact.* (1969) **1,** 19.
183. Kriek, E., *Chem. Biol. Interact.* (1969) **1,** 3.
184. Irving, C. C., *Cancer Res.* (1966) **26,** 1390.
185. Kriek, E., Reitsema, J., *Chem. Biol. Interact.* (1971) **3,** 397.
186. Butt, L. T., Strafford, N., *J. Appl. Chem.* (1956) **6,** 525.
187. Gehrmann, G. H., Foulger, J. H., Fleming, A. J., *Proc. Int. Congr. Ind. Med., 9th* (1948), 472.
188. Bonser, G. M., Clayson, D. B., Jull, J. W., *Br. Med. Bull.* (1958) **14,** 146.
189. Clayson, D. B., Ashton, M. J., *Acta Unio Int. Contra Cancrum* (1963) **19,** 539.
190. Saffiotti, U., Cefis, F., Montesano, R., Sellakumar, A. R., "Bladder Cancer—A Symposium," Deichmann and Lampe, Eds., p. 129, Aesculapius, Birmingham, 1967.
191. Sellakumar, A. R., Montesano, R., Saffiotti, U., *Proc. Am. Ass. Cancer Research* (1969) **10,** 78.
192. Bonser, G. M., Clayson, D. B., Jull, J. W., *Lancet* (1951) **ii,** 286.
193. Boyland, E., "The Biochemistry of Bladder Cancer," p. 34, Thomas, Springfield, Ill., 1963.
194. Boyland, E., Manson, D., *Biochem. J.* (1966) **99,** 189.
195. Troll, W., Belman, S., Nelson, N., *Proc. Soc. Exp. Biol.* (1959) **100,** 121.

196. Boyland, E., Dukes, C. E., Grover, P. L., *Br. J. Cancer* (1963) **17,** 79.
197. Troll, W., Nelson, N., *Fed. Proc. Fed. Am. Soc. Exp. Biol.* (1961) **20,** 41.
198. Brill, E., Radomski, J. L., "Bladder Cancer—A Symposium," Deichmann and Lampe, Eds., p. 90, Aesculapius, Birmingham, 1967.
199. Boyland, E., Manson, D., *Biochem. J.* (1966) **101,** 84.
200. Deichmann, W. B., Scotti, T., Radomski, J. H., Bernal, E., Coplan, M., Wood, F., *Toxicol. Appl. Pharmacol.* (1965) **7,** 657.
201. Shimkin, M. B., Weisburger, J. H., Weisburger, E. K., Gubareff, N., Suntzeff, V., *J. Natl. Cancer Inst.* (1966) **36,** 915.
202. Boyland, E., Manson, D., *A. R., Br. Emp. Cancer Campaign* (1963) **41,** 69.
203. Bielschowsky, F., *Br. J. Exper. Pathol.* (1946) **27,** 54.
204. Shubik, P., Pietra, G., Della Porta, G., *Cancer Res.* (1960) **20,** 100.
205. Lennox, B., *Br. J. Cancer* (1955) **9,** 631.
206. Dannenberg, H., Huggins, C., *Z. Krebsforsch.* (1969) **72,** 321.
207. Kirby, A. H. M., Peacock, P. R., *J. Pathol. Bacteriol.* (1947) **59,** 1.
208. Strauss, E., Mateyko, G. M., *Cancer Res.* (1964) **24,** 1969.
209. Ishidate, M., Tamura, Z., Nakajima, T., Samejima, K., *Chem. Pharm. Bull. (Tokyo)* (1962) **10,** 75.
210. Yoshida, T., *J. Proc. Imp. Acad. Japan* (1932) **8,** 464.
211. Matsumoto, M., Terayama, H., *Gann* (1965) **56,** 339.
212. Lawson, T. A., *Biochem. J.* (1968) **109,** 917.
213. Lawson, T. A., *Chem. Biol. Interact.* (1970) **2,** 9.
214. Lawson, T. A., Dzhioev, F. K., *Chem. Biol. Interact.* (1970) **2,** 165.
215. Crabtree, H. G., *Br. J. Cancer* (1949) **3,** 387.
216. Miller, J. A., Miller, E. C., *Cancer Res.* (1961) **21,** 1068.
217. Fare, G., Howell, J. S., *Cancer Res.* (1964) **24,** 1279.
218. Fare, G., Orr, J. W., *Cancer Res.* (1965) **25,** 1784.
219. Fare, G., *Cancer Res.* (1966) **26,** 2406.
220. Williams, M. H. C., *Acta Unio Int. Contra Cancrum* (1962) **18,** 676.
221. Nelson, A. A., Woodard, G., *J. Natl. Cancer Inst.* (1953) **13,** 1497.
222. Kensler, C. J., Dexter, S. O., Rhoads, C. P., *Cancer Res.* (1942) **2,** 1.
223. Miller, J. A., Miller, E. C., *J. Exp. Med.* (1948) **87,** 139.
224. Kinosita, R., *Yale J. Biol. Med.* (1940) **12,** 287.
225. Sugiura, K., Halter, C. R., Kensler, C. J., Rhoads, C. P., *Cancer Res.* (1945) **5,** 235.
226. White, F. T., White, J., *J. Natl. Cancer Inst.* (1946) **7,** 99.
227. Mueller, G. C., Miller, J. A., *J. Biol. Chem.* (1950) **185,** 145.
228. Miller, J. A., Miller, E. C., *Adv. Cancer Res.* (1953) **1,** 339.
229. Kinosita, R., *Gann* (1936) **30,** 423.
230. Kinosita, R., *Trans. Jap. Pathol. Soc.* (1937) **27,** 665.
231. Crabtree, H. G., *Br. J. Cancer* (1955) **9,** 310.
232. Brown, E. V., Fisher, W. M., *J. Med. Chem.* (1969) **12,** 1113.
233. Brown, E. V., *J. Med. Chem.* (1968) **11,** 1234.
234. Miller, J. A., Mueller, G. C., *J. Biol. Chem.* (1953) **202,** 579.
235. Lin, J. K., Miller, J. A., Miller, E. C., *Biochem. Biophys. Res. Commun.* (1967) **28,** 1040.
236. Miller, E. C., Miller, J. A., *Cancer Res.* (1947) **7,** 468.
237. Lin, J. K., Miller, J. A., Miller, E. C., *Biochemistry* (1968) **7,** 1889.
238. *Ibid.* (1969) **8,** 1573.
239. Miller, E. C., Miller, J. A., Sapp, R. W., Weber, G. M., *Cancer Res.* (1949) **9,** 336.
240. Salzberg, D. A., Hane, S., Griffin, A. C., *Cancer Res.* (1951) **11,** 276.
241. Sorof, S., Cohen, P. P., Miller, E. C., Miller, J. A., *Cancer Res.* (1951) **11,** 383.
242. Sorof, S., Young, E. M., Ott, M. G., *Cancer Res.* (1958) **18,** 33.
243. Heidelberger, C., Weiss, S. M., *Cancer Res.* (1951) **11,** 885.
244. Miller, E. C., *Cancer Res.* (1951) **11,** 100.

245. Sorof, S., Golder, R. H., Ott, M. G., *Cancer Res.* (1954) **14,** 190.
246. Sorof, S., Young, E. M., McCue, M. M., Fetterman, P. L., *Cancer Res.* (1963) **23,** 864.
247. Ketterer, B., Ross-Mansell, P., Whitehead, J. K., *Biochem. J.* (1967) **103,** 316.
248. Ketterer, B., Christodoulides, L., *Chem. Biol. Interact.* (1969) **1,** 173.
249. Ketterer, B., Beale, D., Litwack, G., Hackney, J. F., *Chem. Biol. Interact.* (1971) **3,** 285.
250. Litwack, G., Ketterer, B., Arias, I. M., *Nature* (London) (1971) **234,** 466.
251. Terayama, H., Orii, H., *Gann* (1963) **54,** 455.
252. Otsuka, I., Nagao, N., *Gann* (1936) **30,** 561.
253. Nagao, N., Hashimoto, T., *Gann* (1939) **33,** 196.
254. Strömbeck, J. P., *J. Pathol. Bacteriol.* (1946) **58,** 275.
255. Strömbeck, J. P., Ekman, B., *Acta Pathol. Microbiol. Scand.* (1949) **26,** 480.
256. Ekman, B., Strömbeck, J. P., *Acta Pathol. Microbiol. Scand.* (1949) **26,** 447.
257. *Ibid.,* 472.
258. Clayson, D. B., Jull, J. W., Bonser, G. M., *Br. J. Cancer* (1958) **12,** 222.
259. Bonser, G. M., Boyland, E., Busby, E. R., Clayson, D. B., Grover, P. L., Jull, J. W., *Br. J. Cancer* (1963) **17,** 127.
260. Childs, I. J., Nakajima, C., Clayson, D. B., *Biochem. Pharmacol.* (1967) **16,** 1555.
261. Jones, R., Ryan, A. J., Wright, S. E., *Food Cosmet. Toxicol.* (1966) **4,** 213.
262. Roxon, J. J., Ryan, A. J., Wright, S. E., *Food Cosmet. Toxicol.* (1966) **4,** 419.
263. Daniel, J. W., *Food Cosmet. Toxicol.* (1967) **5,** 533.
264. Roxon, J. J., Ryan, A. J., Welling, P. G., Wright, S. E., *Food Cosmet. Toxicol.* (1966) **4,** 419.
265. Roxon, J. J., Ryan, A. J., Wright, S. E., *Food Cosmet. Toxicol.* (1967) **5,** 645.
266. Grasso, P., Golberg, L., *Food Cosmet. Toxicol.* (1966) **4,** 297.
267. *Ibid.,* 269.
268. Gangolli, S. D., Grasso, P., Golberg, L., *Food Cosmet. Toxicol.* (1967) **5,** 601.
269. Truhaut, R., *Bull. Soc. Sci. Hyg. Ailment.* (1962) **50,** 77.
270. Grasso, P., Gangolli, S. D., Gaunt, I. F., *Food Cosmet. Toxicol.* (1971) **9,** 1.
271. Kirby, A. H. M., Peacock, P. R., *Glasgow Med. J.* (1949) **30,** 364.
272. Dacre, J. C., *Proc. Univ. Otago Med. School* (1965) **43,** 31.
273. Sharratt, M., Frazer, A. C., Paranjoti, I. S., *Food Cosmet. Toxicol.* (1966) **4,** 493.
274. Grice, H. C., Mannell, W. A., Allmark, M. G., *Toxicol. Appl. Pharmacol.* (1961) **3,** 509.
275. Hansen, W. H., Davis, K. J., Fitzhugh, O. G., Nelson, A. A., *Toxicol. Appl. Pharmacol.* (1963) **5,** 105.
276. Mannell, W. A., *Food Cosmet. Toxicol.* (1964) **2,** 169.
277. Ikeda, Y., Horiuchi, S., Furuya, T., Omori, Y., *Food Cosmet. Toxicol.* (1966) **4,** 485.
278. Grasso, P., *Food Cosmet. Toxicol.* (1968) **6,** 821.
279. Grasso, P., Lansdown, A. B. G., Kiss, I. S., Gaunt, I. F., Gangolli, S. D., *Food Cosmet. Toxicol.* (1969) **7,** 425.
280. Bonser, G. M., Roe, F. J. C., *Food Cosmet. Toxicol.* (1970) **8,** 477.
281. Ikeda, Y., Horiuchi, S., Kobayashi, K., Furaja, T., Kohgo, K., *Food Cosmet. Toxicol.* (1968) **6,** 591.
282. Davis, K. J., Nelson, A. A., Zwickey, R. E., Hansen, W. H., Fitzhugh, O. G., *Toxicol. Appl. Pharmacol.* (1966) **8,** 306.
283. Gaunt, I. F., Brantom, P. G., Grasso, P., Creasey, M., Gangolli, S. D., *Food Cosmet. Toxicol.* (1972) **10,** 3.
284. Gaunt, I. F., Corpanini, F. M. B., Grasso, P., Kiss, I. S., Gangolli, S. D., *Food Cosmet. Toxicol.* (1972) **10,** 17.
285. Gillman, J., Gillman, T., Gilbert, C., *S. Afr. J. Med. Sci.* (1949) **14,** 21.
286. Gillman, J., Gillman, T., *Cancer* (1952) **5,** 792.

287. Brown, D. V., Norlind, L. M., *Arch. Pathol.* (1961) **72**, 251.
288. Marshall, A. H. E., *Acta Pathol. Microbiol. Scand.* (1953) **33**, 1.
289. Fujita, K., Iwase, S., Matusubara, T., Ischiguro, I., Matsui, H., Mizuno, T., Arai, T., Takayanagi, T., Sugiyama, Y., Shirafuji, K., *Gann* (1956) **47**, 181.
290. Childs, J. J., Clayson, D. B., *Biochem. Pharmacol.* (1966) **15**, 1247.
291. Rubenchik, B. L., *Vop. Pitan* (1962) **21**, 72.
292. Davis, K. J., Fitzhugh, O. G., Nelson, A. A., *Toxicol. Appl. Pharmacol.* (1964) **6**, 621.
293. Nagata, C., Kodama, M., Tagashira, Y., Imamura, A., *Biopolymers* (1966) **4**, 409.
294. Matsushima, T., Kobuna, I., Sugimura, T., *Nature* (1967) **216**, 508.
295. Kawazoe, Y., Tachibana, M., Aoki, K., Nakahara, W., *Biol. Pharmacol.* (1967) **16**, 631.
296. Ono, T., *Tampakushitsu Kakusan Koso* (1964) **9**, 112.
297. Ishikawa, M., Endo, H., *Biochem. Pharmacol.* (1967) **16**, 637.
298. Shirazu, Y., *Gann* (1963) **54**, 487.
299. Hozumi, *Gann* (1969) **60**, 83.
300. Nagata, C., Imamura, A., Fukui, K., Saito, H., *Gann* (1963) **54**, 401.
301. Enomoto, M., Sato, K., Miller, E. C., Miller, J. A., *Life Sci.* (1968) **7**, 1025.
302. Brown, G. B., Sugiura, K., Cresswell, R. M., *Cancer Res.* (1965) **25**, 986.
303. Brown, G. B., Teller, M. N., Smullgan, I., Birdsall, N. J. M., Lee, T. C., Parham, J. C., Stöhrer, G., *Cancer* (1973) **33**, 1113.
304. Birdsall, N. J. M., Parham, J. C., Wölcke, U., Brown, G. B., *Tetrahedron* (1972) **28**, 3.
305. McDonald, J. J., Stöhrer, G., Brown, G. B., *Cancer Res.* (1973) **33**, 3319.
306. McCuen, R. W., Stöhrer, G., Sirotno, F. M., *Cancer Res.* (1974) **34**, 378.
307. Price, J. M., Morris, J. E., Lalich, J. J., *Fed. Proc. Fed. Am. Soc. Exp. Biol.* (1966) **25**, 419.
308. Stein, R. J., Yost, D., Petroliunas, F., Von Esch, A., *Fed. Proc. Fed. Am. Soc. Exp. Biol.* (1966) **25**, 291.
309. Ertürk, E., Cohen, S. M., Bryan, G. T., *Cancer Res.* (1970) **30**, 1309.
310. Croft, W. A., Bryan, G. T., *J. Natl. Cancer Inst.* (1973) **51**, 941.
311. Ertürk, E., Cohen, S. M., Price, J. M., Bryan, G. T., *Cancer Res.* (1969) **29**, 2219.
312. Cohen, S. M., Ertürk, E., Bryan, G. T., *Cancer Res.* (1970) **30**, 2320.
313. Ertürk, E., Cohen, S. M., Bryan, G. T., *Cancer Res.* (1970) **30**, 936.
314. *Ibid.*, 2098.
315. Cohen, S. M., Ertürk, E., Bryan, G. T., *Cancer Res.* (1970) **30**, 906.
316. Cohen, S. M., Ertürk, E., Von Esch, A. M., Crovetti, A. J., Bryan, G. T., *J. Natl. Cancer Inst.* (1973) **51**, 403.
317. Morris, J. E., Price, J. M., Lalich, J. J., Stein, R. J., *Cancer Res.* (1973) **29**, 2145.
318. Rustia, M., Shubik, P., *J. Natl. Cancer Inst.* (1972) **48**, 721.
319. Dunning, W. F., Curtis, M. R., Maun, M. E., *Cancer Res.* (1950) **10**, 454.
320. Dunning, W. F., Curtis, M. R., *Proc. Soc. Exp. Biol. N.Y.* (1958) **99**, 91.
321. Boyland, E., Harris, J., Horning, E. S., *Br. J. Cancer* (1954) **8**, 647.
321a. Lawson and Clayson, unpublished data.
322. Oyasu, R., Sumie, H., Burg, H. E., *J. Natl. Cancer Inst.* (1970) **45**, 853.
323. Oyasu, R., Kitajima, T., Hopp, M. L., Sumie, H., *Cancer Res.* (1972) **32**, 2027.
324. Morris, H. P., Sidransky, H., Wagner, B. P., *Proc. Am. Ass. Cancer Res.* (1960) **3**, 136.
325. Dunning, W. F., Curtis, M. R., *Cancer Res.* (1954) **14**, 299.
326. Okajima, E., Hiramatsu, T., Motomiya, Y., Iraya, K., Ijuin, M., Ito, N., *Gann* (1971) **62**, 163.
327. Allen, M. J., Boyland, E., Dukes, C. E., Horning, E. S., Watson, J. G. *Br. J. Cancer* (1957) **11**, 212.

328. Bryan, G. T., Brown, R. R., Price, J. M., *Cancer Res.* (1964) **24,** 582.
329. *Ibid.* (1964) **24,** 596.
330. Bryan, G. T., *Cancer Res.* (1968) **28,** 183.
331. Price, J. M., *Can. Cancer Conf.* (1966) **6,** 224.
332. Price, J. M., Brown, R. R., *Acta Unio Int. Contra Cancrum* (1962) **18,** 684.
333. Abul-Fadl, M. A. M., Khalafallah, A. S., *Br. J. Cancer* (1961) **15,** 479.
334. Trout, G. E., Gillman, J., Prates, M. D., *Acta Unio Int. Contra Cancrum* (1962) **18,** 575.
335. Quagliariello, E., Tancredi, F., Fedele, L., Saccone, C., *Br. J. Cancer* (1961) **15,** 367.
336. Benassi, C. A., Perissinotto, B., Allegri, G., *Clin. Chem. Acta* (1963) **8,** 822.
337. Brown, R. R., Price, J. M., Friedell, G. H., Burney, S. W., *J. Natl. Cancer Inst.* (1969) **43,** 295.
338. Leppänen, V. V. E., Oka, M., *Ann. Med. Exp. Biol. Fenn.* (1963) **41,** 123.
339. Price, J. M., Brown, R. R., Peters, H. A., *Neurology* (1959) **9,** 456.
340. Price, J. M., Brown, R. R., Rukavina, J. G., Mendelson, C., Johnson, S. A. M., *J. Invest. Dermatol.* (1957) **29,** 289.
341. Flinn, J. H., Price, J. M., Yess, N., Brown, R. R., *Arthritis Rheum.* (1964) **7,** 201.
342. Brown, R. R., Thornton, M. J., Price, J. M., *J. Clin. Invest.* (1961) **40,** 617.
343. Miyakawa, M., Yoshida, O., *Gann* (1973) **64,** 411.
344. Ross, M. H., Bras, G., *J. Nutr.* (1973) **103,** 944.
345. Radomski, J. L., Brill, E., Glass, E. M., *J. Natl. Cancer Inst.* (1967) **39,** 1069.
346. Weisburger, J. H., Grantham, P. H., Weisburger, E. K., *Jerusalem Symp. Quantum Chem. Biochem.* (1969) **I,** 262.
347. Groth, U., Neumann, H. G., *Chem. Biol. Interact.* (1971) **4,** 409.
348. Conney, A. H., *Pharm. Rev.* (1967) **19,** 317.
349. Richardson, H. L., Stier, A. R., Borsos-Nachtnebel, E., *Cancer Res.* (1952) **12,** 356.
350. Miyaji, T., Moszkowski, L. I., Senoo, T., Ogata, M., Oda, T., Kawai, K., Sayama, Y., Ishida, H., Matsuo, H., *Gann* (1953) **44,** 281.
351. Meechan, R. J., McCafferty, D. E., Jones, R. S., *Cancer Res.* (1953) **13,** 802.
352. Miller, E. C., Miller, J. A., Brown, R. R., MacDonald, J. C., *Cancer Res.* (1958) **18,** 469.
353. Conney, A. H., Miller, E. C., Miller, J. A., *Cancer Res.* (1956) **16,** 450.
354. Arcos, J. C., Conney, A. H., Buu-Hoi, N. G., *J. Biol. Chem.* (1961) **236,** 1291.
355. Irving, C. C., Peeler, T. C., Veazey, R. A., Wiseman, R., *Cancer Res.* (1971) **31,** 1468.
356. Irving, C. C., Wiseman, R., Hill, J. T., *Cancer Res.* (1967) **27,** 2309.
357. Morris, H. P., Wagner, B. P., Lombard, L. S., *J. Natl. Cancer Inst.* (1958) **20,** 1.
358. Mikata, A., Luse, S. A., *Am. J. Pathol.* (1964) **44,** 455.
359. Sugai, M., Witting, L. A., Tsuchiyama, H., Kummerow, F. A., *Cancer Res.* (1962) **22,** 510.
360. Weisburger, J. H., Weisburger, E. K., *Acta Unio Int. Contra Cancrum* (1963) **19,** 513.
361. Magreth, A., Lotlikar, P. D., Miller, E. C., Miller, J. A., *Cancer Res.* (1964) **24,** 920.
362. Lotlikar, P. D., Wasserman, M. B., Luka, L., *Proc. Soc. Exp. Biol. Med.* (1973) **144,** 445.
363. Wyatt, P. L., Cramer, J. W., *Cancer Res.* (1970) **11,** 83.
364. Matsushima, T., Grantham, P. H., Weisburger, E. K., Weisburger, J. H., *Biochem. Pharmacol.* (1972) **21,** 2043.
365. Peraino, C., Fry, R. J. M., Staffeldt, E., *Cancer Res.* (1971) **31,** 1506.
366. Weisburger, J. H., Weisburger, E. K., *Pharmacol. Rev.* (1973) **25,** 1.
367. Frankel, H. H., Yamamoto, R. S., Weisburger, E. K., Weisburger, J. H., *Toxicol. Appl. Pharmacol.* (1970) **17,** 462.

368. Ulland, B. M., Weisburger, J. H., Yamamoto, R. S., Weisburger, E. K., *Toxicol. Appl. Pharmacol.* (1972) **22,** 281.
369. Enomoto, M., Miyake, M., Sato, K., *Gann* (1968) **59,** 177.
370. Irving, C. C., Wiseman, R., Hill, J. T., *Cancer Res.* (1967) **27,** 2309.
371. Yamamoto, R. S., Glass, R. M., Frankel, H. H., Weisburger, E. K., Weisburger, J. H., *Toxicol. Appl. Pharmacol.* (1968) **13,** 108.
372. Yamamoto, R. S., Williams, G. M., Frankel, H. H., Weisburger, J. H., *Toxicol. Appl. Pharmacol.* (1971) **19,** 687.
373. Matsushima, T., Weisburger, J. H., *Chem. Biol. Interact.* (1969–70) **1,** 211.
374. Weisburger, J. H., Shirasu, Y., Grantham, P. H., Weisburger, E. K., *J. Biol. Chem.* (1967) **242,** 372.
375. Blunck, J. M., *Pathology* (1971) **3,** 99.
376. Blunck, J. M., *Chem. Biol. Interact.* (1970) **2,** 217.
377. Blunck, J. M., Leeds, B. J., Masden, N. P., *Chem. Biol. Interact.* (1971–2) **4,** 219.
378. Lotlikar, P. D., Enomoto, M., Miller, E. C., Miller, J. A., *Cancer Res.* (1964) **24,** 1835.
379. Weisburger, E. K., Grantham, P. H., Weisburger, J. H., *Biochemistry* (1964) **3,** 808.
380. Symeonidis, A., Mulay, A. S., Burgoyne, F. H., *J. Natl. Cancer Inst.* (1954) **14,** 805.
381. O'Neal, M. A., Hoffman, H. E., Dodge, B. G., Griffin, A. C., *J. Natl. Cancer Inst.* (1958) **21,** 1161.
382. Reuber, M. D., *Fed. Proc. Fed. Am. Soc. Exp. Biol.* (1964) **23,** 336.
383. Bielschowsky, F., Hall, W. H., *Br. J. Cancer* (1953) **7,** 358.
384. Griffin, A. C., Richardson, H. L., Robertson, C. H., O'Neal, M. A., Spain, J. D., *J. Natl. Cancer Inst.* (1955) **15,** 1623.
385. Ward, D. N., Spain, J. D., *Cancer Res.* (1957) **17,** 623.
386. Fujita, K., Iwase, S., Ito, T., Arai, T., Takayanagi, T., Sugiyama, Y., Matsuyama, M., Takagi, C., Ohmae, T., Mine, T., *Gann* (1957) **48,** 277.
387. Spain, J. D., Clayton, C. C., *Cancer Res.* (1958) **18,** 155.
388. Takashi, M., Iwase, S., *Nature* (1958) **181,** 1211.
389. Mulay, A. S., O'Gara, R. W., *Proc. Soc. Exp. Biol. Med.* (1959) **100,** 320.
390. Ritchie, A. C., Saffiotti, U., *Cancer Res.* (1955) **15,** 84.
391. Tada and Tada, *Nature* (1975) **255,** 510.
392. Hashimoto and Degawa, *Gann* (1975) **66,** 215.
393. Kadlubar, Miller, and Miller, *Cancer Res.* (1976) **36,** 1196.
394. Garner, Walpole, and Rose, *Cancer Lett.* (1975) **1,** 39.

Chapter

9

The Epidemiology of the Aromatic Amine Cancers

H. G. Parkes, British Rubber Manufacturers' Association Ltd., Health Research Unit, Scala House, Holloway Circus, Birmingham B1 1EQ, England

THE ROLE OF THE epidemiologist is to study the interaction of man and his environment. He is concerned with the statistical analysis of the incidence of different diseases but only insofar as it may enable him to relate that incidence to an expected frequency. If he can establish that a selected population has experienced a significantly excessive incidence of a particular disease, he is entitled to draw the conclusion that some environmental factor is or has been in operation to create the excess. The detection and identification of such environmental causes of disease are the main aims of all epidemiological studies.

The chemical induction of cancer has been the subject of intensive study since 1932 when Cook *et al.* (*1*) first reported the experimental production of cancer in mice by dibenz(*a,h*)anthracene, but the involvement of chemical substances in the etiology of certain types of cancer was established by the epidemiologist many years earlier. By the end of the last century the carcinogenic properties of soot, tar, pitch, and shale oil were already appreciated. In 1895 the first report linking bladder cancer with a group of chemical workers soon led to the incrimination of certain aromatic amines.

Since the discovery of aniline in 1826, the commercial potential of the aromatic amino and nitro compounds has been progressively explored by chemists. It is now understood that the theoretical number of such compounds—if one includes primary, secondary, and tertiary derivatives—is almost infinite. Today they represent a large and still expanding group of commercially important compounds extensively used in industrial processes.

The toxicity of the aromatic amines—which is closely linked with the toxicity of the related nitro compounds—has been recognized since the early industrial use of aniline when the clinical picture of "anilism" was first seen. Cystitis, hematuria, methemoglobinemia, and dermatitis were the principal manifestations of this toxicity, but such symptoms and signs were in most cases speedily resolved by removal from exposure.

Aromatic amino and nitro compounds share, in their ability to induce methemoglobinemia, what may prove to be a highly significant toxicological property. In recent investigations of the mechanisms of chemical carcinogenesis, Radomski (2) observed that the methemoglobin producing capabilities of the aromatic amines appear to be directly related to their carcinogenic potential. This finding could render the further study of the aromatic nitro compounds equally as important as the present intensive investigation of the corresponding amino derivatives.

When attention was first drawn to the possibility of a carcinogenic effect resulting from exposure to the aromatic amines, it is hardly surprising that aniline came at first under suspicion. The tumors that were found were bladder tumors and were thought to result from the hemorrhagic cystitis associated with aniline exposure. They were therefore described originally as aniline tumors, and the misnomer persisted in medical textbooks until recent times. In fact, the experimental evidence which finally incriminated other aromatic amines and cleared aniline of suspicion was not reported until 1938 when Hueper *et al.* (3) successfully induced bladder tumors in female dogs after prolonged oral administration of commercial 2-naphthylamine. It was then realized that earlier attempts to demonstrate the carcinogenic activity of 2-naphthylamine had failed because the compound had been tested in the wrong animal species and because there had been insufficient understanding of the lengthy latent period of tumor induction. The experimental carcinogenicity of 2-naphthylamine in dogs was confirmed by the experiments of Bonser in 1943 (4).

With the accumulation of the experimental evidence to indicate the potent carcinogenicity of 2-naphthylamine, workers made an intensive survey of related chemical compounds. From 1950 onwards, a growing list of the aromatic amines were carefully investigated. Very few in the event proved to have the carcinogenic potency of 2-naphthylamine, but a number were nevertheless revealed as carcinogens. Furthermore, although the experiments with dogs had established the bladder as the principal target organ, tests with other species provided evidence of cancer induction in many different sites. As a result of this valuable work, for which much of the credit must go to Bonser *et al.* (5) at Leeds University, it became possible to formulate the currently accepted theories regarding the mode of action of the aromatic amines in the carcinogenic process. These are discussed in detail in Chapters 8 and 16.

The practical importance of these studies is more readily appreciated when they are considered in the context of the industrial use of the aromatic amines. While their commercial origins are deeply rooted in the manufacture of dyestuffs, many of them have since been found to have important applications in other industries. They were used on a large scale in the rubber and cablemaking industries, in textile dyeing and printing, and in the manufacture of pigments, paints, and plastics. The most important members of the series from the standpoint of industrial epidemiology are 1- and 2-naphthylamine, benzidine, 4-biphenylamine, 4,4'-methylenebis(2-chloroaniline), 3,3'-dichlorobenzidine, and diphenylamine (Figure 1). Among these are amines which have proved responsible for almost all of the known incidence of industrial bladder cancer.

Aromatic Amines of Industrial Importance

1-Naphthylamine (α-Naphthylamine). 1-Naphthylamine was extensively used in industry in the manufacture of azo dyes and in the chemical construction of antioxidants for the rubber industry. It is not easily produced in pure form but usually contains a small proportion of 2-naphthylamine as an impurity. Within the U.S., it is believed that 1-naphthylamine manufactured after 1953 did not contain more than 0.5% 2-naphthylamine impurity, but certain grades of European origin probably contained up to 10% until 1-naphthylamine manufacture was finally abandoned. However, the carcinogenicity of pure 1-naphthylamine is still in doubt. Scott (6) records a total of 56 reported cases of bladder cancer attributed to 1-naphthylamine exposure and concludes that present evidence tends to incriminate 1-naphthylamine as a carcinogen. Nevertheless, the possibility that its carcinogenic effect is attributable to its 2-naphthylamine impurity cannot yet be discarded. Experimentally, pure 1-naphthylamine has thus far induced only one bladder tumor in the dog experiments carried out by Bonser *et al.* (7) after a prolonged exposure of nine years, so it would only seem to rank as a weak carcinogen.

2-Naphthylamine (β-Naphthylamine). The commercial uses of 2-naphthylamine have been similar to those of 1-naphthylamine, but its most significant use was probably in the large scale manufacture of rubber industry antioxidants. Although the carcinogenicity of 1-naphthylamine remains unproved, there is no doubt that 2-naphthylamine is one of the most potent industrial carcinogens ever encountered. It was the first aromatic amine to be conclusively established as an experimental carcinogen by Hueper in 1938 (8), and the epidemiological evidence, which is discussed below, has been overwhelming. Because of its commercial value and importance, attempts were made to devise safe procedures for its manufacture and use, but as these proved ineffectual, the industrial use of the compound diminished, and its manufacture was gradually abandoned. 2-Naphthylamine production ceased in Britain in 1949, but regrettably continued on a limited scale for many years thereafter in other parts of the world. The last U.S. plant which manufactured 2-naphthylamine was not shut down till 1970, and some production continued in Japan until as recently as 1972. Latest reports, however, seem to confirm that all commercial production has finally ceased.

Benzidine (4,4′-Diaminobiphenyl). Benzidine, which has been manufactured on an industrial scale for nearly 100 years, was mainly used in the dyestuffs industry as the starting point for the making of azo dyes. Unlike the naphthylamines, its use in the rubber industry was very limited, although it was also a hardener and a constituent of some adhesives and plastics. It had valuable properties which were used in the textile printing industry, it was used in the production of security paper, and it was, for many years, the essential chromogen in the standard hospital laboratory test for occult blood (Chapter 10). Although epidemiological evidence implicating benzidine was already accumulating (9), it was not until 1950 when Spitz *et al.* (10) published their report on the induction of bladder tumors in dogs that its carcinogenicity was experimentally confirmed. Unlike 2-naphthylamine its industrial use was not thereafter abandoned. Production ceased in Britain in October 1962, but it is still manufactured in substantial quantity in many parts of the world, chiefly in the form of dihydrochloride.

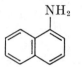

1-Naphthylamine

NH₂

2-Naphthylamine

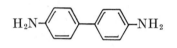

Benzidine

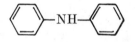

4-Biphenylamine

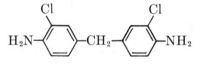

4,4'-Methylenebis(2-chloroaniline)

3,3'-Dichlorobenzidine

4,4'-Methylenedianiline

Diphenylamine

Figure 1.   Aromatic amines of industrial importance

4-Biphenylamine (4-Aminobiphenyl; Xenylamine; BPA). The history of the industrial use of BPA differs in some important respects from that of the naphthylamines and of benzidine. Unlike these compounds, which had their major application in the dystuffs industry at the turn of the century, BPA manufacture was not started until 1935 when it was used in the rubber industry as an antioxidant. It was then produced only in the U.S., and production continued for 19 years before evidence of its carcinogenic potential was revealed in the reports of Melick *et al.* (*11*) who found 19 cases of bladder tumor in a population of 171 men. The fact that no fewer than 11% of those exposed developed tumors within such a short space of time was evidence enough of the highly carcinogenic nature of the compound. In a more recent study (*12*) Melick has reported 53 cases in a population of 315 men. In Britain a similar tragedy was averted by the foresight of Williams *et al.* (*13*) who published in 1952 the first experimental proof of its carcinogenicity. In

1954 they confirmed their work with dog experiments and warned that the compound could be expected to cause bladder tumors in exposed workmen. For this reason, manufacture of BPA in Britain was never started, although limited amounts of the imported material were used for a time in the British rubber industry. Existing experimental and epidemiological evidence seems to indicate now that the carcinogenic potency of BPA is at least equal to, and is possibly even greater than, that of 2-naphthylamine.

4,4'-Methylenebis(2-chloroaniline) (MBOCA; DACPM). This relative newcomer to the aromatic amine series of industrially important compounds has only been produced in quantity for approximately 15 years, and its most significant industrial application is as a curing agent for polyurethane elastomers. It is, however, an extremely versatile and efficient compound in this role, and there has been a heavy demand to stimulate production. It is synthesized by reacting formaldehyde with o-chloroaniline.

Routine testing of MBOCA for carcinogenicity showed that the compound is certainly carcinogenic on both oral and subcutaneous administration in rats, giving rise to a variety of malignant tumors including lung and liver carcinomas (*14, 15*).

There is at present insufficient epidemiological evidence to justify any reliable assessment of this compound's human carcinogenicity, but because of the strong suspicions aroused by the experimental evidence, many British manufacturers, on the recommendation of the British Rubber Manufacturers' Association, have refrained from its use. In the U.S., MBOCA is listed as subject to a Permanent Standard (*16*) under an order made by the Occupational Safety and Health Administration, Department of Labor. In effect this order requires American producers and users of MBOCA to regulate their handling of the compound to ensure that their manufacturing operations do not permit any significant exposure to MBOCA. (At the time of writing this order stands temporarily in abeyance on a technical point arising out of an appeal against the implementation of the standard. It is, however, to be expected that in due course a new standard will be promulgated with similar provisions).

3,3'-Dichlorobenzidine (DCB). 3,3'-Dichlorobenzidine has been commercially produced for approximately 40 years and has been substantially used as an intermediate in the dyestuffs industry. More recently it has come to be used as a curing agent for polyurethane elastomers. It is, however, less generally effective for this purpose than MBOCA.

Under experimental conditions the compound appears to have potent carcinogenic activity when administered to a variety of different animals by different routes. It induced tumors of the skin, Zymbal gland, mammary gland, and intestines in rats (*17*).

It is uncertain whether DCB should be accepted as a human carcinogen. As its production is frequently associated with the production of benzidine, it is difficult to separate the possible carcinogenic effects of exposure to each of these compounds. It is highly probable that DCB has significant human carcinogenic potential.

In the United Kingdom, DCB is a controlled substance under the U.K. Carcinogenic Substances Regulations 1967—Statutory Instrument No. 879 (*18*). Like MBOCA, it is subject in the U.S. to a Permanent Standard of the Department of Labor.

4,4'-Methylenedianiline (4,4'-Diaminodiphenylmethane; MDA). MDA, which is usually made by the reaction of formaldehyde with aniline, has been manufactured and used on a commercial scale for more than 50 years. The compound has found a variety of applications, such as a laboratory analytical agent in tungsten determination, a corrosion inhibitor, and an intermediate in nylon yarn production. Today it is chiefly used as an important curing agent for polyurethane elastomers and epoxy resins. For some applications, it is considered a useful substitute for MBOCA which increasingly is suspected as a possible human carcinogen.

MDA itself has never attracted serious suspicion as a human carcinogen although there is animal experimental data which provided some evidence that the incidence of liver tumors in rats injected with MDA was significantly higher than in a group of control animals (*19*).

The chief epidemiological interest of the compound relates to the so-called Epping jaundice outbreak in 1966 (*20*). This occurred in England following the accidental contamination of a sack of flour with MDA. Bread baked from this flour in an Epping bakery was subsequently identified as the source of the outbreak which affected some 84 persons. There were fortunately no deaths reported, but some of the victims experienced a severe hepatotoxic effect. The hepatotoxicity of this compound has been amply confirmed by animal experimentation (*21*).

Diphenylamine. The inclusion of diphenylamine in a short list of industrially important aromatic amines would not be justified solely on the grounds of its possible carcinogenicity. Indeed there is no evidence of substance, either experimental or epidemiological, upon which it can at present be indicated. There are, however, two features connected with this compound which give grounds for some concern. First, it was observed that commercial diphenylamine usually contains a small amount of 4-biphenylamine as an impurity, and second, the industrial use of diphenylamine is rapidly expanding. Although its original use in the early years of this century was largely confined to the dyestuffs industry, it has been extensively used for the past 20 years in the manufacture of rubber industry antioxidants. This last application may once again be greatly expanded. Many rubber manufacturers, confronted with the medical and legal problems connected with the use of antioxidants containing trace quantities of 2-naphthylamine, have now abandoned these in favor of others against which this criticism cannot be made, and they are turning for their alternatives to the condensation products of acetone and diphenylamine. If this trend continues, then the manufacture and use of diphenylamine is certain to be dramatically increased, and Scott (*6*) points to the urgent need to maintain a careful watch on what may yet prove to be a dangerous manufacture.

Table I.   Bladder Cancer (Male) Ranked with other Sitings in England and Wales, 1970[a]

Cancer Site	Crude Death Rates/Million
Lung and bronchus	1,045
Stomach	305
Colon	172
Prostate	164
Rectum	130
→Bladder	113
Pancreas	111
Esophagus	71
Brain	42
Other urinary organs	38

[a] Data from Registrar General's Statistical Review, p. 205, Table 17A.

Epidemiology of Bladder Cancer

From what has been said so far, it is apparent that the epidemiology of the aromatic amine cancers is, for all practical purposes, synonymous with the epidemiology of industrial bladder cancer. Before this is considered further, it is helpful to refer briefly to the epidemiology of bladder cancer in a general way without special reference to the question of its industrial etiology.

In the U.S., figures published in 1970 (22) and drawn from four regional cancer registries situated in California, Connecticut, Nevada, and Texas illustrate the major differences in bladder cancer incidence which can be seen within a large national population. In Texas, for example, morbidity is as low as 44 bladder cancer cases per million male population per annum, but in Connecticut it is 235 per million. Nevertheless, in all four states bladder cancer ranks as the fourth commonest malignancy affecting the white male population.

Within a more compact population such as that of England and Wales, we find that bladder cancer currently ranks as the sixth commonest cause of all male cancer deaths (see Table I) and produces an annual morbidity (as opposed to mortality) in the different geographic regions ranging from 140–195 per million population.

Table II.   Bladder Cancer: Crude Death Rates/Million in England and Wales, 1950–1970[a]

	1950	1952	1954	1956	1958	1960	1962	1964	1966	1968	1970
Males	79	89	87	93	92	97	102	103	107	110	113
Females	34	32	37	37	37	39	39	40	41	44	45

[a] Figures for years 1950–60 are from Registrar General's Statistical Review (1960), Table 8. They are based on the reporting of deaths for I.C.D. No. 181, which includes all deaths attributable to malignant neoplasm of the bladder and other urinary organs. Figures shown for 1962–70 are drawn from Registrar General's Statistical Review (1970), Table 8 and are based on I.C.D. No. 188, which includes only deaths attributable to malignant neoplasm of the bladder, and excludes other urinary organs. (Figures for I.C.D. No. 188 were not published prior to 1962).

More interesting, however, is the observation that world bladder cancer mortality rates have been steadily rising. This can be seen in Table II which sets out the crude death rates per million population for England and Wales from 1950–1970.

A number of theories have been advanced to explain this increased incidence, but all that we can say with reasonable certainty is that there is no single or dominating etiologic factor. Evidence is accumulating to show a positive correlation with cigarette smoking, especially in males, and the disease has also been associated with abnormal tryptophan metabolism (*23, 24*). Apart from these two findings, there is little to indicate what other factors might be influencing the overall rate increase. For this reason interest is now chiefly centered upon the more readily definable area of industrial exposure to chemical carcinogens.

Industrial Bladder Cancer

Although it is convenient here to consider industrial bladder cancer as if it were a distinctive condition, it should be clearly understood that we are concerned only with a different manifestation of the same disease. This creates a problem for those who seek to determine what proportion of all bladder tumors can rightly be attributed to industrial exposure and makes it desirable to consider by what means the industrial tumor may be identified. Although attempts have been made to do so, it has thus far proved impossible to detect any significant pathological, biochemical, or immunological differences between those tumors which are of industrial origin and those which are not. The presenting features, clinical course, and prognosis are likewise identical. It is therefore necessary to take into account evidence which is non-specific and largely circumstantial. In this context, it should be said that the most important piece of evidence—namely that of industrial exposure to aromatic amines—is not infrequently missed, either as a result of inadequate history taking or of a failure to realize that exposure may occur in occupations other than those within the chemical and rubber industries.

The other important factor which may provide a clue to an industrial etiology is the age of the patient. Although cancer of the bladder is among the 10 most frequent forms of malignant disease, its impact is chiefly upon those between 65 and 74 years old (Table III). Since it is rare below the age of 45, bladder cancer in a man aged 50 or less should arouse instant suspicion of an industrial etiology and provoke a detailed enquiry into his work history. With the lack of any absolute distinguishing features, it is hardly surprising that there are widely differing estimates of the frequency of occupational tumors. While many would concede that environmental and social factors (including cigarette smoking) probably play an important part in the etiology of all bladder cancers, there is agreement that tumors attributable directly to aromatic amine exposure constitute no more than 5% of the total.

Epidemiology of Industrial Bladder Cancer

That the aromatic amines are deeply involved in the epidemiology of industrial bladder cancer is today a matter of historical record. It was, how-

Table III.   Deaths from Malignant Bladder Neoplasms

Numbers

Ages	All Ages	0–1	1–4	5–9	10–14	15–19	20–24	25–29	30–34
Male	2763	2	—	—	—	—	—	—	3
Female	1107	—	—	—	—	—	—	—	—

Rates (per Million Living)

Ages	All Ages	0–1	1–4	5–14	15–24	25–34
Male	116	2	1	—	—	1
Female	44	—	—	—	—	—

^a I.C.D.＝International Classification of Diseases, published by the World Health Organization.

ever, more than 50 years before the full implications of this involvement were properly understood and before Scott and Williams published in 1953 the first effective Code of Practice designed to protect workers against hazardous exposure to carcinogenic amines (25).

The starting point of this lengthy epidemiological investigation can be accurately placed in 1895, when a Congress of the German Surgical Society received a report from a Frankfurt surgeon, Rehn (26), on the effects of exposure of a group of chemical workers to certain aromatic amines. Rehn noted chiefly the frequency of cyanosis and hematuria but drew attention also to the unexpected finding of four cases of bladder tumor. All the men concerned had been working in the manufacture of fuchsin for periods of up to 20 years. At the time Rehn suggested that all these observed effects probably resulted from aniline exposure, but his conclusion were contested by some of his contemporaries who asserted that aniline would not cause bladder tumors. In 1898 Leichtenstern (27) suggested, for the first time, that exposure to "naphthylamines" could cause bladder tumors. During the next few years evidence to support this conclusion was gradually accumulated and in 1906 Rehn (28) reported 38 cases of bladder tumor and suggested the possible involvement of naphthylamine and benzidine. By this time interest in the industrial etiology of bladder tumors was aroused in other European countries, and in 1912 Leuenberger (29) reported an extended series of cases among aniline dye workers in Basle, Switzerland. By a comparison of his findings with data obtained from the general population, he showed that the male dye worker experienced 33 times the risk of other industrial employees. At this point the chain of investigation was unfortunately broken by the First World War. Although the existing evidence and state of knowledge were extensively reviewed in an I.L.O. Report in 1921 (30), interest had waned to a point which allowed the establishment of the developing dyestuffs industries of Britain, France, Italy, and the U.S. without any real appreciation or understanding of the hazards being introduced.

The first reference to industrial bladder cancer in Britain was made by Wignall in 1929 (31) when he referred to the discovery of 14 cases of tumor

(I.C.D. 188.0)[a] in Great Britain, 1971 (24a)

Numbers

35–39	40–44	45–49	50–54	55–59	60–64	65–69	70–74	75–79	80–84	85+
2	23	42	102	221	382	521	553	449	301	162
2	8	21	37	73	92	148	185	201	187	153

Rates (per Million Living)

35–44	45–54	55–64	65–74	75–84	85+
9	49	219	620	1238	1511
4	19	54	138	318	489

Registrar General's Statistical Review

among 1-naphthylamine and benzidine workers. Undoubtedly, however, it was the reports of Goldblatt in 1947 (*32*) and 1949 (*33*) which first drew attention to the gravity of the problem. These reviewed in detail the evidence which had accumulated during the years of the Second World War and established beyond doubt the existence of a major health hazard in the British industry. His findings provided the compelling reasons for the appointment in 1948 of Case as a research fellow charged with conducting a full epidemiological investigation of the dyestuffs industry.

In the meantime, cases of industrial bladder cancer appeared elsewhere in the world. Gehrmann in 1934 (*34*) reported 27 cases in the U.S., and in 1949 Gehrmann *et al.* (*35*) jointly attributed those tumors to 2-naphthylamine exposure. Concurrently, in 1949 di Maio (*36*) and Barsotti and Vigliani (*37*) reported cases from Italy and Billiard-Duchesne (*38*) from France.

Thus, a great mass of evidence, both experimental and epidemiological, had accumulated by the late 1940's to support the conclusion that exposure to certain aromatic amines, notably 2-naphthylamine, benzidine, and 1-naphthylamine, would inevitably constitute a serious bladder cancer hazard. It fell to the lot of one man to provide the ultimate proof and to reveal the risk involving as yet unsuspected groups of industrial workers. This was achieved by one of the most careful and comprehensive epidemiological studies ever carried out, which even today stands as a model.

The Work of R. A. M. Case

The classic study of Case and his colleagues followed his appointment as a research fellow at the Chester Beatty Research Institute in London to carry out an investigation of the incidence and causes of industrial bladder cancer for the Association of British Chemical Manufacturers. Case's first task was to construct, from factory records, a nominal roll of all those men who had been employed in the dyestuffs industry and had been in contact with one or more of the suspect carcinogens for longer than six months. It was possible to trace 4,622 names of men meeting these criteria. Steps were then taken to identify, within this population, all those who had either died as a result of or who had been treated for bladder tumors. In the "at risk" population, 341 such cases were found. Case then conducted a careful search of all local hospital records and examined mortality data provided by the Registrar General to establish the number of males in the area population dying between 1921 and 1949 who were known to have had bladder tumors. He then analyzed these data by "comparative composite cohort analysis." Case describes this as "a technique whereby the actual occurrence of an event in a population defined by individual name and working environment, with the age and date of entry into the environment, is observed, and the result compared with what would be expected from a general population, or population not exposed to a specific risk of the event, observed for the same length of time. Thus the unit of the analysis is the cohort which is defined by two or more characteristics, each defining a sub-cohort, e.g., age, environment, and date of entry into environment. These sub-cohorts are later combined by summation of the expected frequency of the event introducing the composite elements."

Case points out that the particular advantage of this type of analysis when applied to environmental problems is that much more data can be used than in alternative techniques, since withdrawal from the environment does not affect the method of estimation. The only difficulty is that it is essential for the successful application of this technique to secure the willing and un-stinted cooperation of the industry or manufacturers concerned in the investigation since free access to personnel records is an indispensable prerequisite.

Case's work greatly advanced existing knowledge of occupational bladder tumors. In addition to establishing the precise incidence of the disease, he showed that the risks of contracting it were 30 times as great for the exposed chemical worker as they were for the general population, and he also ranked the suspected chemicals in order of carcinogenic potency. He showed the relative potencies for 2-naphthylamine, benzidine, and 1-naphthylamine were in the ratios of 5, 1.7, and 1, while mixed exposures gave a result of 2.7. He could not find any evidence to incriminate aniline as a carcinogen. 2-Naph-thylamine, therefore, stood at last revealed—at least in the British dyestuffs industry—as the principal carcinogenic amine. Williams (39) later sub-stantiated this with the dramatic finding that the bladder tumor incidence among a small group of 18 men working for longer than five years on the distillation of benzidine and 2-naphthylamine had risen to 94%.

The application of Case's comprehensive analytical technique to the problems of the British dyestuffs industry allowed him to extend his original frame of reference and thereby greatly increase the value of his contribution. In particular, he devised a statistical method for the estimation of the expected number of cases of bladder tumor in both an exposed (40) and a non-exposed population (41). He showed that the availability of such information could be invaluable in detecting hitherto unsuspected hazards.

It should be noted here that much of the complexity of the epidemiological techniques such as those described by Case derives from the necessity to extend the time scale of the investigation retrospectively over many years. This is because of the lengthy induction period of occupational tumors, and those involved in the investigation of industrial bladder cancer have provided us with evidence about the length of this latent period. The latent period is, of course, defined as that interval of time which elapses between the date of first exposure to or contact with the industrial hazard and the date of the first established onset of disease. Among those who reported on this matter, there is a remarkable unanimity about the average duration of the latent period. Case's own calculation for the British Chemical Industry showed a figure of 18 years, and this is entirely consistent with the findings of others whose various estimates are confined to the range of 16–21 years. It must be fully understood, however, that while these are average figures, the overall range of induction times is very wide indeed. Some tumors have been reported within 12 months of exposure while others have only appeared more than 40 years after exposure.

There is one further element in Case's study which requires particular mention as it represents what was possibly his most important discovery. Until 1949 it was believed and generally accepted that the hazard of industrial bladder cancer resulting from exposure to the aromatic amines was confined within the chemical industry to the dyestuff manufacturers. Case was the first to show that the hazard extended beyond the confines of chemical manufacture and that it also involved other major manufacturing operations. Had it not been for the element of chance combined with the astute perception of the epidemiologist, this important discovery could well have been delayed many more years.

During the early days of his investigation in the chemical industry Case sought to establish a suitable control population to match his study population against. For this purpose he explored at first the possibility of establishing such a population within a large conurbation in a different geographical location. When he came to examine the incidence of bladder cancer within this control population, he was astonished to discover an incidence in excess of national expectation which seemed itself to merit further enquiry. He therefore proceeded to note the last recorded occupation of the bladder cancer cases in this area and immediately observed that a disproportionate number of them appeared to have occurred in men listed as rubber workers.

Following up this line of investigation, he soon discovered that many of these had been employed in a large tire factory situated in the area. From this point it was a relatively short step to the realization that the suspect carcinogen 2-naphthylamine was an important chemical component of a rubber antioxidant then in use and to the understanding that the existence of a major industrial health hazard was now likely to be uncovered in a considerable number of rubber factories spread throughout the country. In fact, it was not until 1957 that the full extent of this was really appreciated, and by that time Case's enquiry had already extended to other areas of manufacture in which the use of benzidine and 2-naphthylamine had been demonstrated. Laboratory workers, rodent exterminators, textile printers, makers of security paper, cobblers, and gas retort house workers all attracted early suspicion, and more recent epidemiological studies such as those of Anthony and Thomas (42) and Cole et al. (43) now indicate the possible extension of the hazard to include such diverse occupations as weavers, tailor's cutters, hairdressers, cooks, and kitchen workers. Nevertheless there can be little doubt that by far the major share of the hazard remains with the dyestuffs workers and with the rubber and cable manufacturers.

If the findings of the Case enquiry were important and dramatic, the consequences were hardly less so. Certainly the most important consequence of all was the decision which was taken by the British chemical manufacturers in 1949 promptly to abandon the further production of 2-naphthylamine. This was followed, on the advice of the chemical manufacturers, by the decision of the rubber manufacturers immediately to discontinue use of the suspect rubber antioxidants containing 2-naphthylamine and to return or destroy all existing stocks. As has already been noted, the production of benzidine continued until some years later, since it was thought that such production could be rendered entirely free from risk by the careful implementation of the Code of Practice described by Scott and Williams (25). Only when in 1962 that was finally thrown into question by the occurrence of a case of bladder cancer in a benzidine worker was the decision taken to cease production in Britain of benzidine. Other and remoter consequences, which will be discussed in greater detail later, included the provision of financial support by the manufacturers for the victims of industrial bladder cancer and the acceptance and recognition of the disease as being of industrial origin, so that in 1953 it became officially prescribed in Britain as "Industrial Disease No. 39" under the National Insurance (Industrial Injuries) Act (44). Many years later, under the British Carcinogenic Substances Regulations 1967 (45), the manufacture and use of the principal carcinogenic amines were specifically prohibited, subject only to certain exemptions.

These more recent developments have focused attention upon the grave hazards of industrial exposure to the carcinogenic amines, the manufacture and use of which have been generally abandoned during the past decade. The need, however, for continuing epidemiological study of industrial workers at risk has become increasingly apparent in order to establish that no unidentified carcinogens have remained in use. Only during the past few years, with the growing availability of more sophisticated analytical techniques, has it been recognized that a number of industrial chemicals in widespread use do in fact contain as impurities trace quantities of carcinogenic amines such as 2-naphthylamine. It has therefore been a matter of urgent concern to verify that the impurity level in such cases has not been sufficient to allow of any extension of the bladder cancer hazard. The most critical part of this investigation has been concerned with the industrial use of N-phenyl-2-naphthylamine. Some grades of this rubber antioxidant, which has been extensively used from about 1930 until the present time, contain approximately 50 ppm 2-naphthylamine as an impurity, but thus far no excess of bladder tumors has ever been associated with its use. An epidemiological study by Veys (46), supported by similar results obtained by Fox et al. (47), now confirm that, at least at these exposure levels, no risk of a bladder cancer hazard is incurred. These results are currently being more fully explored in a comprehensive epidemiological study of the British rubber industry now in progress.

Screening

While it may be seen that appropriate steps are now being implemented to achieve proper epidemiological control of industrial bladder cancer, it is clearly no less important that all possible measures should be taken to protect those known to have been at risk and to compensate those now suffering from bladder cancer as a result of industrial exposure. Unhappily, protection in this context is limited to the provision of adequate medical supervision and routine diagnostic screening procedures, as the fact of past exposure is clearly irreversible. Nevertheless, the implementation of cytodiagnostic screening programs do offer at least the opportunity for early treatment in a high proportion of cases and may thereby exert a favorable effect upon prognosis. Comprehensive cytological screening facilities of this nature have been generally available to all "at risk" workers in the British Chemical and Rubber Industries for over 15 years, cytodiagnostic facilities being provided first for chemical workers in 1951 and subsequently for rubber workers in 1957. To date, these services have detected more than 200 new cases of bladder cancer in an exposed-to-risk register of some 20,000 employees, and although there is evidence now to suggest that the incidence of new cases is beginning to decline, it is expected that the need for screening will continue for at least another decade.

Compensation

It is arguably impossible to compensate a victim of industrial bladder cancer adequately for the infliction of an injury which will in many cases cost him his life. Nevertheless, his entitlement at least to some relief from financial hardship must be recognized even though the scale and mode of obtaining such compensation will vary considerably according to custom and practice in different parts of the world. When the condition of occupational bladder cancer was prescribed in Britain as an industrial disease in 1953, it became possible under the relevant social security legislation for those affected to claim state benefits in respect of industrial injury. In addition to this, private schemes have been set up by a number of British chemical and rubber manufacturers which provide for additional *ex gratia* payments to be made, and it is the broad intention of such schemes to protect the affected worker against loss of earnings. From neither of these sources however can the victim expect to recover any substantial sum, and he may therefore seek to bring a common law action for damages against his employer in the courts. The possibility of a successful outcome to such litigation remained in doubt until recent times, when an important test case involving both a manufacturer and a user of carcinogenic aromatic amine compounds was successfully fought by the plaintiffs in the British High Court, the judgment of that court being subsequently upheld on appeal. The circumstances of this case are of wider than usual interest in that the judgment defines, and appears to establish, some important new legal principles concerned with an employer's liability.

Legal Liability

The High Court Action in the British Courts (48) was brought by two Dunlop workers suffering from industrial bladder cancer who claimed that they had contracted their disease through exposure to carcinogenic aromatic amines manufactured by Imperial Chemical Industries Ltd. (I.C.I.) and sold to Dunlop. They alleged negligence against I.C.I. on the grounds that the carcinogenic properties of the antioxidant Nonox S were recognized prior to 1949, when the compound was ultimately withdrawn, and against Dunlop on the ground that the company had failed to provide, at a sufficiently early date, cytodiagnostic screening facilities in accordance with recommendations generally accepted by the industry in 1957. Finding for the plaintiffs, the High Court judge awarded each plaintiff £1,000 against Dunlop and a total of £21,000 for the two plaintiffs against I.C.I. On appeal, I.C.I. submitted that at no time prior to 1949 could they have known that the free amines in their compound Nonox S would give rise to cases of bladder cancer among workers in Dunlop factories. Their Lordships concluded, however, that contemporaneous documentation showed that I.C.I. had known from 1942 onwards that very small amounts of the free amines could constitute a grave hazard to health and that appropriate steps had then been taken by I.C.I. to protect their own workers. They held that I.C.I. should then have given thought to the risks to Dunlop workers and should either have withdrawn the product or given due warning to Dunlop of the danger that existed. They held also that I.C.I. owed a duty to Dunlop employees in respect of Nonox S, the extent of that duty being to take all reasonable steps to satisfy themselves that Nonox S would be a safe product to use in the expected conditions of use.

On the face of it this judgment appears to extend very significantly the previously held view of common law liability, introducing the concept of strict liability for the safety of a product. It is apparent that the British courts are now prepared to hold, not only that a manufacturer must fully satisfy himself that his product will not constitute a hazard to his own employees in the production process, but also that it can be safely used by the purchaser. The implication of this is that he must also have knowledge of and give adequate consideration to those processes in which his product may subsequently be used. In setting out the duty of a manufacturer in respect to products which might constitute a health hazard, the appeal court stated that "If a manufacturer discovers that his product is unsafe or if he has reason to believe that it might be unsafe, his duty may be to cease forthwith to manufacture or supply the product in its unsafe form." In this context it becomes all-important to seek a satisfactory definition of what is to be regarded as an unsafe product. It is relevant to note the views of the trial judge Mr. Justice O'Connor who, in the High Court judgment, said:

"The duty of a manufacturer of chemical products can be simply stated. It is to take reasonable care that the product is safe in use. . . . If a manufacturer chooses to use a chemical which he knows to be a dangerous carcinogen in the manufacture of a product and knows or ought to know that the product contains a proportion of the carcinogen, and if he chooses to market the product without giving warning of the presence of the carcinogenic material, then I hold that the law imposes a very high duty indeed upon him to satisfy himself that the product will not prove dangerous when used for the purposes for which it is supplied. The discharge of the duty requires that he should inform himself of the circumstances in which the product will be used, the quantities in which it will be used and the possibilities of exposure to which men may be subjected. If in the state of knowledge at the time he cannot say positively that the proportion of carcinogen present in the product will be harmless, then I hold that he cannot market it without giving adequate warning of the presence of the carcinogenic material."

There is little comfort to be found in these words for either the manufacturer or the user of chemical compounds which may contain trace quantities of suspect carcinogens. Although it is evidently reasonable to postulate the existence of an exposure threshold below which contact with chemical carcinogens may be regarded as safe, in practice this is rarely if ever possible to determine. In the particular case of the aromatic amines it has not even been attempted. Furthermore, although it is indicated that complete withdrawal or abandonment of a potentially carcinogenic product may not necessarily be required and that an adequate warning of its dangerous properties may suffice, it is clear that the judge was in no doubt about the course which should have been adopted in this case. In a later passage from the judgment he states, "the alternative of giving an appropriate warning of its possible carcinogenicity is really an academic consideration because it is common ground that any such warning would have made it unsaleable."

We are left therefore with the conclusion that the recognized presence of any quantity of a suspect carcinogen in a manufacturer's product may force its withdrawal from the market. No doubt there will be exceptions to this generalization, *e.g.*, asbestos products, but the threatened application of the principle of strict legal liability will certainly influence future manufacturing and marketing policies.

Legislation

The influence which government action by legislation may have upon the manufacture and use of carcinogenic or suspect carcinogenic materials must be considered. Experience suggests that effective action in this field is likely to be impeded as much by the complexity of the problem as by ignorance of its full extent. There is, however, some precedent for legislative intervention and this, allied to increasing expression of popular concern, led in Britain to passage of the Carcinogenic Substances Regulations in 1967 (*18*) and in January 1974 in the U.S. to the publication by the Department of Labor (Occupational Safety and Health Administration—OSHA) of new Occupational Health and Safety Standards relating to the manufacture and use of certain carcinogens (*16*).

The effect of the British regulations, together wtih the Prohibition of Importation order (*45*) coming into operation on the same date, has been to prohibit the importation, manufacture, or use of the major carcinogens in the aromatic amine series, *e.g.*, 2-naphthylamine, benzidine, and 4-biphenylamine, and to impose strict controls upon others in the same series such as 1-naphthylamine, o-tolidine, dianisidine, 3,3'-dichlorobenzidine, auramine and magenta. There is some provision for exemption from the regulations in special circumstances, and they are stated not to apply in any case where all, or any one or more of the said compounds, is present as a by-product of a chemical reaction in any other substance in a total concentration not exceeding 1%. This last proviso has caused some confusion about the correct interpretation of the regulations. This also was a matter of some concern to the High Court, where it was suggested that the use of the antioxidant Nonox S would still be lawful since the 2-naphthylamine impurity would only be present in that compound as a by-product of a chemical reaction and would in any case be within the permitted 1%. This submission was not accepted by the judge who held that the 2-naphthylamine impurity was present not as a by-product but as an unreacted material part of the original constituents. He declined also to infer that the regulations implied that 1% 2-naphthylamine was harmless. On the contrary he stated that, "if any conclusion is to be drawn from the regulation it is the exact opposite."

In spite of such difficulties in construction and intepretation, there are few who would dispute today that the Carcinogenic Substances Regulations have probably made an important contribution to the final elimination from the industrial scene in Britain of bladder cancer attributable to aromatic amine exposure.

In the U.S., the more recently promulgated permanent OSHA standards relate to 14 different listed compounds which are either already accepted as being or are currently under suspicion of being important industrial carcinogens. The standard contains control measures and designated work practices designed to protect employees from industrial exposure to these compounds. There is a considerable variation in the degree of carcinogenic potential which is currently attributed to these listed carcinogens. At the one end of the scale are the potent and established carcinogens such as 2-naphthylamine and 4-biphenylamine whereas at the other end are such compounds at 4,4'-methylenebis(2-chloroaniline) and ethyleneimine. The case for including all these compounds together in the same listing rests upon acceptance of the view that it would be improper to afford a lesser degree of protection to workers exposed to substances found only to be carcinogenic in experimental animals and that it is not possible in the present state of knowledge to establish a safe level of exposure to any of the 14 listed compounds. This view of the situation would appear to correspond broadly with that expressed in the British High Court. In one important respect however the U.S. standard goes further than the British regulation, insofar as it requires employers to provide for the indoctrination and training of their employees in the nature of carcinogenic hazards which may exist in the establishment. Information relating to the training and education which may be required is specified in each of the standards for each individual chemical compound.

Legislation of this character, intended to protect workers who may be in a risk situation as a result of potential exposure at work to carcinogenic chemicals, is of course not confined only to the U.S. and U.K. Similar steps are being or have already been taken in many Western European and other countries, and in the future regulatory control of known or suspected occupational hazards will be greatly intensified.

Finally, it is hoped that some profit may be gained from our past experience of dealing with a major chemical cancer hazard. We have learned much about the mechanisms of chemical carcinogenesis and the techniques of epidemiological investigation. This knowledge, properly applied, should enable us to anticipate, or at least detect in its early stages, any similar threat which may emerge in the future (*49*).

Literature Cited

1. Cook, J. W., Hieger, I., Kennaway, E. L., Mayneord, W. V., *Proc. Roy. Soc. London, Ser. B* (1932) **111,** 455.
2. Radomski, J. L., Brill, E., *Science* (1970) **167,** 992.
3. Hueper, W. C., Wiley, F. H., Wolfe, H. D., *J. Ind. Hyg.* (1938) **20,** 46.
4. Bonser, G. M., *J. Pathol. Bacteriol.* (1943) **55,** 1.
5. Bonser, G. M., Clayson, D. B., Jull, J. W., Pyrah, L. N., *Br. J. Cancer* (1952) **6,** 412.
6. Scott, T. S., "Carcinogenic and chronic toxic hazards of aromatic amines," Elsevier, Amsterdam and New York, 1962.
7. Bonser, G. M., Clayson, D. B., Jull, J. W., *Br. Med. Bull.* (1958) **14,** 147.
8. Hueper, W. C., *Arch. Pathol.* (1938) **25,** 856.
9. Hueper, W. C., "Occupational tumors and allied diseases," Thomas, Springfield, 1942.
10. Spitz, S., Maguigan, W. H., Dobriner, K., *Cancer* (1950) **3,** 789.
11. Melick, W. F., Escue, H. M., Naryka, J. J., Mezera, R. A., Wheeler, E. P., *J. Urol.* (1955) **74,** 760.
12. Melick, W. F., Naryka, J. J., Kelly, R. E., *J. Urol.* (Baltimore) (1971) **106,** 220.
13. Walpole, A. L., Williams, M. H. C., Roberts, D. C., *Br. J. Ind. Med.* (1952) **9,** 255.
14. Stula, E. F., Sherman, H., Zapp, J. A., "Experimental neoplasia in ChR–CD rats with the oral administration of 3,3'-dichlorobenzidine, 4,4'-methylenebis(2-chloroaniline), and 4,4'-methylenebis(2-methylaniline)," p. 39, *Soc. Toxicol. 10th Ann. Meet.,* Washington, 1971.
15. Steinhoff, D., Grundmann, E., *Naturwissenschaften* (1971) **58,** 578.
16. U.S. Government, Dept. of Labor, Occupational Safety and Health Standards, *U.S. Federal Register* (1974) **39,** 20.
17. Stula, E. F., Sherman, H., Zapp, J. A., *Toxicol. Appl. Pharmacol.* (1971) **19,** 380.
18. U.K. Government, *Carcinogenic Substances Regulations 1967*, Statutory Instrument No. 879, Her Majesty's Stationery Office, London.
19. Steinhoff, D., Grundmann, E., *Naturwissenschaften* (1970) **57,** 247.
20. Kopelman, H., Robertson, M. H., Sanders, P. G., Ash, I., *Br. Med. J.* (1966) **1,** 514.
21. Munn, A., "Occupational bladder tumours and carcinogens: recent developments in Britain," in "Bladder Cancer," p. 187, K. F. Lampe, Aesculapius, Birmingham, 1967.
22. Doll, R., Muir, C., Waterhouse, J. A. H., "Cancer Incidence in Five Continents," U.I.C.C., Springer–Verlag, Berlin, New York, 1970.
23. Price, J. M., Brown, R. R., *Acta Un. Int. Cancr.* (1962) **18,** 684.
24. Boyland, E., "The Biochemistry of Bladder Cancer," Thomas, Springfield, 1963.
24a. Registrar General's Statistical Review, Table 17.
25. Scott, T. S., Williams, M. H. C., *Br. J. Ind. Med.* (1957) **14,** 150.

26. Rehn, L., *Arch. Klin. Chir.* (1895) **50**, 588.
27. Leichtenstern, O., *Dtsch. Med. Wochenschr.* (1898) **24**, 709.
28. Rehn, L., *Verh. Dtsch. Ges. Chir.* (1906) **35**, 313.
29. Leuenberger, S. C., *Beitr. Klin. Chir.* (1912) **80**, 208.
30. International Labour Office, Studies and Reports, Series F., No. **1**, p. 6, 1921.
31. Wignall, T. H., *Br. Med. J.* (1929) **2**, 258.
32. Goldblatt, M. W., *Br. Med. Bull.* (1947) **4**, 405.
33. Goldblatt, M. W., *Br. J. Ind. Med.* (1949) **6**, 65.
34. Gehrman, G. H., *J. Urol.* (1934) **31**, 126.
35. Gehrman, G. H., Foulger, J. H., Fleming, A. J., "Proceedings IXth International Congress of Industrial Medicine, 1949," p. 472, Wright, London, Bristol.
36. Maio, G. di, *Proc. Int. Congr. Ind. Med., 9th, 1948* (1949), 476.
37. Barsotti, M., Vigliani, E. C., *Med. d. Lavaro* (1949) **40**, 129.
38. Billiard-Duchesne, J. F., *Proc. Int. Congr. Ind. Med., 9th, 1948* (1949), 507.
39. Williams, M. H. C., "Cancer," R. W. Raven, Ed., Vol. **3**, p. 377, Butterworth, London, 1958.
40. Case, R. A. M., Hosker, M. E., McDonald, D. B., Pearson, J. T., *Br. J. Ind. Med.* (1954) **11**, 75.
41 Case, R. A. M., *Br. J. Prev. Soc. Med.* (1953) **7**, 14.
42. Anthony, H. M., Thomas, G. M., *J. Nat. Cancer Inst.* (1970) **45**, 879.
43. Cole, P. T., Hoover, R., Friedell, G. H., *Cancer* (1972) **29**, 1250.
44. U.K. Government, National Insurance (Industrial Injuries) Act, Her Majesty's Stationery Office, London, 1946.
45. U.K. Government, *Carcinogenic Substances (Prohibition of Importation) Order*, Statutory Instrument No. 1675, Her Majesty's Stationery Office, London, 1967.
46. Veys, C. A., M.D. Thesis, University of Liverpool, 1973.
47. Fox, A. J., Lindars, D. C., Owen, R., *Br. J. Ind. Med.* (1974) **31**, 140.
48. "The Times" Newspaper, London, Law Report November 1st, 1972. Cassidy v Imperial Chemical Industries Ltd., Wright v Same. Before Lord Justice Sachs, Lord Justice Megaw, and Lord Justice Lawton.
49. Parkes, H. G., *Practitioner* (1975) **214**, 80.

Chapter

10

Chemical Carcinogens as Laboratory Hazards

W. H. S. George, Department of Chemical Pathology, City Hospital,
Derby, DE3 3NE, England

C. E. Searle, Department of Cancer Studies, University of Birmingham,
Birmingham B15 2TJ England

Epidemiological Aspects

IN THE 1930's AND 1940's when almost the only known chemical carcinogens were benzo(*a*)pyrene and some related polycyclic aromatic hydrocarbons, there was little reason for concern about carcinogenic hazards to laboratory workers except, of course, in laboratories using these unusual chemicals in cancer research. This situation was changed completely in the years after the Second World War by Case's extensive epidemiological investigations into the causes of occupational bladder cancer in British factory workers. It then became clear that some aromatic amines, particularly the naphthylamines and benzidine, were potent causes of bladder cancer in man under the conditions of manufacturing industry. This work and its far-reaching implications were discussed by Case in his Michael Williams Lecture (*1*) (*see also* Chapter 9).

Unlike the polycyclic aromatic hydrocarbon carcinogens, some of the carcinogenic aromatic amines are common chemicals with widespread uses in many types of laboratories as well as in manufacture, and the industrial findings thus showed that laboratory workers in many fields could be subjected to some degree of carcinogenic hazard. Moreover, since then the list of recognized carcinogens has enlarged to include chemicals of many other classes, especially the *N*-nitroso carcinogens, also with important implications for safety in the laboratory as well as in the factory and the environment.

As laboratory work is concerned with chemicals on a generally small scale in comparison with industry, it seems reasonable to suppose that the risks of handling carcinogens are correspondingly less, but epidemiological evidence of actual risks is, however, very scanty. Clinical impression led

481

Case to the view that some urinary tract tumors in laboratory workers were caused by exposure to aromatic amines (2, 3). In their study of the occupations of 1030 patients with papilloma and cancer of the bladder in the Leeds area of England during 1959–1967, Anthony and Thomas reported an increased risk of bladder cancer in medical workers, particularly in nurses and laboratory technicians (4). Williams had earlier suggested that nurses might be at risk through their use of benzidine in testing for the presence of occult blood in urine and feces (5).

The first serious attempt to study the mortality of chemists was made by Li et al. (6), who determined the causes of death of 3637 members of the American Chemical Society who died between 1948 and 1967. Most were males, who were studied in two groups. The 2152 dying between the ages of 20 and 64 were compared with 9957 U.S. professional men dying between the same ages, but in 1950 only. The 1370 chemists dying over the age of 64 were compared with all U.S. males who died over 64 years of age in 1959. There were only 112 female ACS members in the study, and these were compared with the U.S. white females dying in 1959.

Both groups of male chemists showed a significantly increased mortality from cancers, particularly the younger age group with 444 observed deaths compared with the 354 expected. The individual malignancies which showed significant increases were malignant lymphomas and cancer of the pancreas and not cancer of the bladder, lungs, or skin as might have been expected. Deaths from respiratory diseases and cirrhosis of the liver were significantly reduced. The chief findings in the females were a doubling of breast cancer mortality, probably associated more with the relatively large proportion of unmarried women and higher socioeconomic status than with chemical exposure, and a fivefold raised rate of suicide.

The authors were well aware of the disparities in the years of comparison and several other weaknesses which they could not avoid in this study, but they nevertheless considered that the increased mortalities from certain cancers, which were seen in both male age groups, were unlikely to be due to chance. This view received some support from reports of an increased incidence of lymphomas in anesthesiologists and in patients on certain types of drug and from scanty evidence of increased pancreatic cancer associated with exposure to carcinogenic aromatic amines and with heavy smoking and drinking. It is therefore unfortunate that important studies of this type were not pursued further in the U.S. or elsewhere. There would be great interest and value in a really sound study of mortality (or better, of disease incidence) in practicing chemists, perhaps in comparison with physicists and biologists, as well as with those in nonscientific professional occupations. The health of laboratory workers in general, including those exposed to hazards such as bacteria and viruses as well as chemicals, is a field of special interest to the TUC Centenary Institute of Occupational Health at the London School of Hygiene and Tropical Medicine. A study, financed by the Department of Health and Social Security, into the health of workers in Health Service laboratories was recently completed here.

Carcinogenic Chemicals in Hospital and Other Laboratories

The aromatic amine carcinogens probably remain the most important, though by no means the only, carcinogens considered as hazards to laboratory personnel. Nowhere have these hazards been of more concern than in clinical chemistry laboratories, where a number of important tests formerly relied on the use of benzidine, o-tolidine, or o-dianisidine as chromagens. Various other methods have now been devised as replacements for potentially hazardous procedures or in the course of normal development. It is presumed that methods which avoid the use of the carcinogenic amines are at least much safer than the former methods, although this cannot be proven in the absence of comprehensive biological testing of the replacement reagents.

Fecal Occult Blood. The detection of gastro-intestinal bleeding is of major importance to both clinician and patient. The blood may be present as intact erythrocytes or as hemoglobin. A suitable test should be such that a blood loss of more than 4.5 ml/day can be detected (7).

The order of sensitivity of the chromagens used has been o-tolidine > benzidine > phenolphthalein > guaiac (8). Owing to the carcinogenicity of benzidine and o-tolidine, the choice now lies between phenolphthalein, guaiac, or one of the more recent methods. One such method marketed in the U.S. utilizes the method of Hoerr et al. (9), in which the specimen of urine or feces under test is placed on a piece of guaiac-impregnated electrophoresis paper. A drop or two of hydrogen peroxide is added; the extent and rapidity of appearance of a blue ring indicates the quantity of blood present. A British company markets an adaptation of the method of Clark and Timms (10) for blood glucose determination as subsequently modified by Deadman and Timms (11) for occult blood in feces. This uses 2,6-dichlorophenolindophenol as chromagen. In Varley's reduced phenolphthalein method (12) a pink coloration forms in the aqueous phase when phenolphthalein and hydrogen peroxide are added to an ethanol extract of feces.

3,3',5,5'-Tetramethylbenzidine, now being advertised as a sensitive substitute for benzidine in the detection of blood, has produced no tumors specifically attributable to it when injected subcutaneously into rats in doses greater than those in which benzidine and o-tolidine cause a high yield of neoplasms (13). In view of its close relationship to these carcinogens, however, more comprehensive biological tests seem desirable before it is accepted as safe for widespread laboratory use.

Blood Glucose. An extensive bibliography has grown up around blood glucose determinations (14, 15, 16). One recent method uses 2,2'-diazobis(3-ethylbenzothiazoline-6-sulfonic acid) as chromagen (17) while others use the hexokinase method (15). Auto analyzer methodologies using ferricyanide or neocuprein are available for automated laboratories. The various methods available and the factors which may invalidate them are discussed by Chernoff (16). Unfortunately o-tolidine, with its carcinogenic hazard, has many advantages and gives values approximating closely to "true" glucose.

Haptoglobin Demonstration. The method described by Ratcliff and Hardwicke (18) for estimation of haptoglobins on Sephadex G100 columns gives a simple, reproducible method which correlates well with the comparison method and obviates the use of benzidine or o-tolidine as chromagen. Immunological methods for haptoglobin estimation are also available.

Preparation of Protein Aggregates. Bis-diazotized dapsone (4,4'-diaminodiphenylsulfone) was used satisfactorily to cross-link gamma globulin in the formation of soluble aggregates in place of bis-diazotized benzidine (19).

Other Analyses Using Carcinogenic Amines. The use of benzidine and related compounds in analysis has been widespread because of the ease of their oxidation to colored quinonoid products. Feigl and Anger stated in 1966 (20) that benzidine was then used in some 60 spot-test procedures. Following a warning by the Society for Analytical Chemistry against the use of benzidine (21), these authors reported the replacement of benzidine by copper ethylacetoacetate and tetra base, bis(4-dimethylaminophenyl)methane, as spot-test reagents for cyanide and cyanogen (20). Other methods for cyanide determination use pyridine in conjunction with p-phenylenediamine (22) or with 3-methyl-1-phenyl-5-pyrazolone (23).

Important analyses which depended on the use of benzidine and o-tolidine included the analysis of chlorine in water at water supply undertakings or swimming pools. The DPD methods of Palin (24), which use N,N-diethyl-p-phenylenediamine, are however well established for this determination, also for chlorite, bromine, iodine, and ozone in water. Similarly, 1-naphthylamine has been replaced by Cleve's acid (8-aminonaphthalene-2-sulfonic acid) in the determination of nitrites in water (25).

In one of a series of papers on laboratory safety, George (26) recommended that the use of liquid reagents containing carcinogens was no longer justified and also raised the question of the legal position of the head of a department where potential carcinogens had not been eliminated if a laboratory worker develops a bladder tumor. Collier has more recently discussed the health hazards of o-tolidine and o-dianisidine to laboratory workers (27) and pointed out the absence of information on carcinogens even in some recent practical textbooks and chemical catalogs.

Carcinogens in Cancer Research Laboratories. Reference was made previously to the use of polycyclic aromatic hydrocarbons in laboratories engaged in cancer research. Countless experiments have been made in which carcinogens, especially benzo(a)pyrene and related polycyclic compounds, were applied repeatedly in a solvent to the skin of experimental animals, usually mice. Contamination of the experimenter's skin by the polycyclics can occur through rubber gloves and is readily detectable by their strong fluorescence in ultraviolet light. Darlow et al. (28) investigated the extent to which carcinogens might also be dispersed into the laboratory atmosphere during such experiments. They simulated the application of a carcinogen by the use of an acetone suspension of Bacillus globigii, the spores of which could subsequently be detected on culture plates by the pigmentation of the resultant colonies. Very high air and surface counts were obtained for 6 hr after a single application to the skin of 30 mice. Counts then fell sharply, but rose again many days later when the animals' hair was clipped, their bedding was changed, or the floor was swept.

Even if one has doubts about how faithfully the use of a bacillus reproduces the effects of a carcinogen which may become bound to the skin, absorbed, or licked off, the work drew attention to the possibilities of such dispersal, with consequent risks to personnel and to other experiments carried out in the vicinity. Darlow *et al.* (*28*) listed many factors besides carcinogenic potency that are important in relation to the actual degree of hazard in such tests. These include the compound's solubility, its volatility, ease of absorption into the body, the vehicle used to administer it, and a variety of factors in the methods of housing the animals, changing their bedding, and the size, ventilation, and methods of cleaning the room in which they are housed.

Because of the nature of the work carried on in cancer research laboratories, their personnel may be exposed to a much greater range of chemical carcinogens than elsewhere, without the possibility of replacing them by innocuous materials. However, these are also the laboratories where there should now be the greatest awareness of carcinogenic properties and of the precautions which the use of carcinogens demands.

The Volatility of Chemical Carcinogens

Volatility is a factor of outstanding importance in determining the degree of hazard posed by a carcinogen, wherever it is encountered. The volatility of the carcinogenic aromatic amines, for example, has played an important part in their dangers in industry. The recently recognized industrial carcinogens, mustard gas (bis(2-chloroethyl) sulfide) and bis(chloromethyl) ether, are volatile liquids and vinyl chloride monomer, a gas. However, 1,3-propane sultone, a compound of industrial interest which is carcinogenic in animals, has very low volatility and would be expected to be correspondingly less hazardous on this account.

The volatile liquid carcinogen N-nitrosodimethylamine (dimethylnitrosamine) was investigated by Barnes and Magee (*29*) after it had caused liver injury to two out of three men who had used it as a solvent in an industrial research laboratory. After confirming the hepatotoxicity of the nitrosamine in animals (*29*), they discovered its strong carcinogenicity (*30*) and thus initiated the tremendous amount of research on the N-nitroso carcinogens which has since been carried out. Apart from its outstanding importance to cancer research (Chapter 11), this has clearly demonstrated the great hazards which widespread industrial or laboratory use of these chemicals would involve. The volatility of N-nitrosodimethylamine under experimental conditions was strikingly demonstrated by Huberman *et al.* (*31*) in the course of experiments on carcinogenesis *in vitro*. Up to 25% of the carcinogen added to culture medium in petri dishes in an incubator was lost, and its presence could be demonstrated in dishes to which it had not been added.

Laboratory Precautions

The great importance of laboratory procedures based on the use of some carcinogenic aromatic amines necessitated their continued use for some time after their hazards had been recognized, and it was essential that they should be used with stringent precautions to minimize risks to laboratory workers. With this need in mind, a code of practice was drawn up by the Harlow Industrial Health Service for the guidance of laboratory staff in factories. This code was published in 1966 with modifications and widely distributed by the Chester Beatty Research Institute in London (32).

Substances listed as hazardous in this booklet are the naphthylamines, benzidine, o-tolidine, o-dianisidine, 4-biphenylamine, 4-nitrobiphenyl, nitrosamines, nitrosophenols, nitronaphthalenes, and 1-naphthylthiourea (which may be contaminated with naphthylamines). Attention was drawn to possibilities of exposure from inhalation of dusts or vapors, absorption through the skin, and from contaminated hands, clothing, benches, floors, or apparatus. Personnel were instructed to take precautions in the use of closed containers, avoidance of skin contact, use of protective clothing and impervious bench surfaces, and the use of copious cold water for removing contamination. Some statements can usefully be quoted verbatim:

"Protective measures are thus intended to prevent any contact with the chemical through the lungs, mouth, or skin. Other chemicals should be used whenever possible, and young persons should not be asked to use the carcinogenic substances. . . . Under laboratory conditions the risk is less (than for industrial workers), but we do not feel that we can recommend any precautions less thorough than the ones suggested above. The risk of absorption into the body is much greater than with most (though not all) toxic chemicals, the effect is long-term, and may be delayed until many years after exposure has ceased, and the carcinomatous process, once commenced, is irreversible. Effective protection is therefore the only prevention."

In the following year the Carcinogenic Substances Regulations 1967 came into force in Britain (33). These imposed a complete ban on the manufacture and use of 2-naphthylamine, benzidine, 4-biphenylamine, and 4-nitrobiphenyl, and controls on the use of other materials including 3,3'-dichlorobenzidine and o-tolidine. Since these Regulations only applied to the industrial scene, use of the chemicals remained legal in hospital and educational laboratories.

Obviously, carcinogenicity is only one sort of toxic reaction which may be encountered in a chemical, but in many important instances it is a property of chemicals which had long been regarded as substantially harmless. The highly irritant nature of carcinogens such as mustard gas and bis(chloromethyl) ether should ensure that they are handled with precautions to avoid exposure. The methylating agent diazomethane is potentially explosive and also so toxic that its carcinogenicity, demonstrated in animals, is of minor importance, but it should be prepared from N-methyl-N-nitroso-p-toluenesulfonamide and not from the carcinogenic N-methyl-N-nitrosourea or the still more dangerous N-methyl-N-nitrosourethane! In contrast, the carcinogenic aromatic amines are free enough of short-term toxic effects for them to have been used in huge quantities for many years before their great long-term dangers to health became clear (Chapter 9).

Moreover, chemical laboratories contain many potential hazards apart from those caused by chemical toxicity—risks of fire or explosion due to gas, from damaged gas cylinders or broken glassware, to mention but a few. Education in all matters concerning laboratory safety and high standards of technique and discipline in the laboratory are so important that understandably little attention has been paid to carcinogenic hazards, which are long-term and relatively recently recognized. As with laboratory safety in general, many of the problems arise through failures of communication. It is regrettable that, although a few accounts of chemical carcinogens have appeared in chemical journals (*34, 35, 36, 37*), information on carcinogens has in the past found its way so slowly from the world of cancer research into chemical textbooks, particularly where these are practical textbooks recommending experiments we now recognize to be hazardous. The great interest and concern aroused by the carcinogenicity of vinyl chloride since its recognition in 1973 perhaps indicates a new awareness of carcinogenic hazards in general in the chemical fraternity.

Some textbooks on laboratory safety have, however, devoted some attention to carcinogens. Pieters (*38*) described carcinogens of a variety of types, including polycyclic hydrocarbons, aromatic amines, and inorganic and radioactive substances, but this account is probably not very helpful now in evaluating their risks under laboratory conditions. The very comprehensive textbook on laboratory safety edited by Steere is not concerned only with chemical laboratories, but its table of the hazards of nearly 1100 chemicals (*39*) mentions the carcinogenicity of a number of classes including nitrosamines. A British safety handbook for chemical laboratories only (*40*) gives more accessible data on toxicity, fire hazards, and disposal of a smaller range of industrial materials but with no mention of carcinogenicity outside the range of aromatic amines.

Hospital laboratories face special problems because, with a constantly increasing work load, they have to carry out various analyses on patient specimens which may carry tuberculosis, infective or serum hepatitis, or other infections. The precautions needed to protect personnel against infection from specimens are so important that a writer in this field (*41*) may perhaps be excused for omitting reference to the carcinogenicity of certain reagents mentioned above.

Carcinogens in Teaching Laboratories

What appears to have been the first realization that even school chemistry teaching might present carcinogenic hazards occurred with the discovery of a recently purchased bottle of benzidine in the chemical store of an English Midlands school in 1966. By that time benzidine was labeled "carcinogenic," so the bottle had not been opened, but its suspected original purpose was as a chromatographic spray, surely one of the most hazardous uses to which such a chemical could be put.

The risks of school children handling carcinogens were then brought to the attention of educational authorities in the Midlands, and in Birmingham the Education Department carried out a survey of carcinogen stocks in the stores of schools under its jurisdiction. While most schools had none, sufficient stocks of benzidine and naphthylamines came to light to make it clear that some action was needed on a national scale (*42, 43*). The information about carcinogen hazards was then sent to schools, teacher training colleges, and further education establishments in England and Wales from the Department of Education and Science in London (*44*). Similar steps were taken by authorities in Scotland and Northern Ireland, and teachers also received information directly through the publication of the Association for Science Education (*45*). The journal *Education in Chemistry* pointed out the carcinogenicity of some aromatic amines and the high toxicity of nitrobenzene and aniline (*46*) and concluded: "for the chemistry teacher, the safest precaution is, presumably, to ban experiments with aromatic amines. After all, are any of them really necessary to an understanding of chemistry?"

A convincing demonstration of the need for such action was the publication in a teachers' journal of a suggested experiment for schoolchildren in which benzidine was to be prepared, converted to a dye with an unspecified naphthalene derivative, and the dye used for dyeing cotton. This appeared in 1967, the year in which use of benzidine in British factories became illegal. The following issue carried a warning that benzidine was carcinogenic and must not be used in schools.

Doubts have sometimes been raised about the safety of using magenta and diphenylamine in teaching. The manufacture of magenta has carried a carcinogenic hazard to workmen, and the process is thus controlled under the Carcinogenic Substances Regulations 1967 (*33*), but there appears to be no firm evidence that magenta itself is carcinogenic. Diphenylamine should not be hazardous provided it is pure, but impure material may be contaminated with the very potent carcinogen 4-biphenylamine (Chapter 9).

Great care should be exercised that the efforts to increase the value and interest of school science teaching do not introduce new hazards. Very recently, for example, a school experiment involving heating small pieces of lithium has been reported to carry a risk of explosion (*47*). A teacher, aware of the high toxicity of benzene, might decide to substitute an experiment with naphthalene for demonstrating nitration and reduction (*46*), unless he had been made aware of the carcinogenic hazards of the nitronaphthalenes and naphthylamines. Possibly this was the origin of a small sample of nitronaphthalene found in one school store.

Probably few would dispute the view (*1, 46*) that schools should not make or use chemicals such as the naphthylamines and benzidine. Not only are the pupils very inexperienced in handling any chemicals, but carcinogenic hazards need to be taken especially seriously in young people with a long life expectancy. As one passes up the educational scale, the problems of carcinogen usage have less clear-cut answers. Naphthylamines and benzidine have long figured in traditional courses of practical organic chemistry, and alternative experiments should be introduced in courses where this has not already been done. Dialkylnitrosamines may also be prepared in such courses, and this is at least as undesirable. At some stage, however, a chemist has to learn to handle chemicals which are hazardous in one way or another without danger to himself or others. If in a given situation a chemical hazard is to be accepted, there must be no doubt that those concerned fully understand the situation. With carcinogens, it also has to be remembered that acceptance of a carcinogenic risk may involve similar risks to others in a factory making the chemical or after its disposal.

Sensible and responsible decisions in such matters can only be made on the basis of sound information. In 1965 Haddow (*48*) suggested that an introduction to chemical carcinogenesis might well form part of the education of chemists, and 10 years later one can only reinforce this view.

Literature Cited

1. Case, R. A. M., *Proc. Roy. Soc. Med.* (1969) **62,** 1061.
2. Case, R. A. M., *Ann. Rep. Br. Empire Cancer Campaign* (1966) **44,** 56.
3. *Ibid.* (1967) **45,** 90.
4. Anthony, H. M., Thomas, G. M., *J. Nat. Cancer Inst.* (1970) **45,** 879.
5. Williams, M. H. C., "Cancer," R. Raven, Ed., Vol. 3, p. 337, Butterworths, London, 1957.
6. Li, F. P., Fraumeni, J. F., Jr., Mantel, N., Miller, R. W., *J. Nat. Cancer Inst.* (1969) **43,** 1159.
7. Ebaugh, F. J., Becker, W. L., *J. Lab. Clin. Med.* (1959) **53,** 777.
8. Huntsman, R. G., Liddell, J., *J. Clin. Pathol.* (1961) **14,** 436.
9. Hoerr, S. O., Bliss, W. R., Kauffman, J., *J. Am. Med. Ass.* (1949) **141,** 1213.
10. Clark, A., Timms, B. G., *Clin. Chim. Acta* (1968) **20,** 352.
11. Deadman, N. M., Timms, B. G., *Clin. Chim. Acta* (1969) **26,** 3691.
12. Varley, H., "Practical Clinical Biochemistry," 2nd ed., p. 275, Heinemann, London; Interscience, New York, 1962.
13. Holland, V. R., Saunders, B. C., Rose, F. L., Walpole, A. L., *Tetrahedron* (1974) **30,** 3299.
14. Henry, R. J., "Clinical Chemistry: Principles and Techniques," p. 780, Hoeber, New York, 1964.
15. Richterich, R., "Clinical Chemistry: Theory and Practice," p. 229, S. Karger, Basel, New York, 1969.
16. Chernoff, H. N., "Monographs on Proficiency Testing," National Communicable Diseases Center, Department of Health, Education and Welfare, Atlanta, Ga., 1970.
17. Werner, W., Rey, H. G., Wielinger, H., *Fresenius Z. Anal. Chem.* (1970) **252,** 224.
18. Ratcliff, A. P., Hardwicke, J., *J. Clin. Pathol.* (1964) **17,** 676.
19. Stanworth, D. R., Coombes, E., personal communication, 1972.
20. Feigl, F., Anger, V., *Analyst* (1966) **91,** 282.
21. *Proc. Soc. Anal. Chem.* (1965) **2,** 69.
22. Bark, L. S., Higson, H. G., *Talanta* (1964) **11,** 621.
23. "Standard Methods for the Examination of Water and Wastewater," 11th ed., American Public Health Association, New York, 1965.
24. Palin, A. T., *J. Inst. Water Eng.* (1967) **21,** 537.
25. Bunton, N. G., Crosby, N. T., Patterson, S. J., *Analyst* (1969) **94,** 585.
26. George, W. H. S., *Ann. Clin. Biochem.* (1971) **8,** 130.
27. Collier, H. B., *Clin. Biochem.* (1974) **7,** 3.
28. Darlow, H. M., Simmons, D. J. C., Roe, F. J. C., *Arch. Environ. Health* (1969) **18,** 883.
29. Barnes, J. M., Magee, P. N., *Br. J. Ind. Med.* (1954) **11,** 167.
30. Magee, P. N., Barnes, J. M., *Br J. Cancer* (1956) **10,** 114.
31. Huberman, E., Traut, M., Sachs, L., *J. Natl. Cancer Inst.* (1970) **44,** 395.

32. "Precautions for Laboratory Workers Who Handle Carcinogenic Aromatic Amines," Chester Beatty Research Institute, London, 1966; reprinted with notes, 1971.
33. "The Carcinogenic Substances Regulations 1967 No. 879," H.M. Stationery Office, London, 1967.
34. Sampey, J. R., *J. Chem. Educ.* (1955) **32**, 448.
35. Weisburger, J. H., Weisburger, E. K., *Chem. Eng. News* (1966) **44**, 124.
36. Searle, C. E., *Chem. Br.* (1970) **6**, 5.
37. Searle, C. E., *Chem. Ind.* (1972) 111.
38. Pieters, H. A., "Safety in Chemical Laboratories," 2nd ed., p. 65, Butterworths, London, 1957.
39. "Handbook of Laboratory Safety," N. V. Steere, Ed., p. 442, Chemical Rubber Co., Cleveland, Ohio, 1967.
40. "Hazards in the Chemical Laboratory," G. D. Muir, Ed., 2nd ed., Royal Institute of Chemistry, London, 1977.
41. Luxon, S. G., in "Hazards in the Chemical Laboratory," G. D. Muir, Ed., p. 241, Royal Institute of Chemistry, London, 1971.
42. Machin, E. J., personal communication, 1968.
43. Searle, C. E., *Ann. Rep. Br. Empire Cancer Campaign* (1968) **46**, 247.
44. Department of Education and Science, 'Avoidance of Carcinogenic Aromatic Amines in Schools and Other Educational Establishments," Administrative Memorandum no. **3/70**, 1970.
45. Searle, C. E., *Sch. Sci. Rev.* (1969) **51**, 282.
46. *Educ. Chem.* (1969) **6**, 163.
47. Bullock, A., *Chem. Br.* (1975) **11**, 115.
48. Haddow, A., *New Sci.* (1965) **25**, 348.

Chapter

11

N-Nitroso Compounds and Related Carcinogens

P. N. Magee, Courtauld Institute of Biochemistry, Middlesex Hospital Medical
School, London, England

R. Montesano, International Agency for Research on Cancer, Lyon, France

R. Preussmann, Deutsches Krebsforschungszentrum, Heidelberg, Federal
Republic of Germany

THE CURRENT INTEREST in the carcinogenic and other biological actions of
N-nitroso compounds arose following the reports of the hepatotoxicity (*1*)
and carcinogenicity (*2*) of the simplest nitrosamine, *N*-nitrosodimethylamine
(dimethylnitrosamine), and the subsequent observations of Schoental (*3*) and
Druckrey *et al.* (*4*) on the carcinogenic action of the nitrosamides *N*-methyl-
N-nitrosourethane and *N*-methyl-*N*-nitrosourea. About 100 *N*-nitroso compounds are now known to be carcinogenic in experimental animals, largely
because of the extensive studies of Druckrey, Preussmann, Schmähl, Ivankovic,
and their colleagues. These and other studies were discussed in several previous reviews (*5, 6, 7*).

The hepatotoxic action of *N*-nitrosodimethylamine in man was, however,
clearly recognized and reported some years previously by Freund (*8*), who
described the clinical and autopsy findings in two chemists accidentally
poisoned with *N*-nitrosodimethylamine. In addition to their toxic and carcinogenic properties, many *N*-nitroso compounds are mutagenic, and some
are teratogenic in experimental animals. These latter topics were discussed
previously (*6*) and are only briefly considered here.

Some relevant aspects of the chemistry of *N*-nitroso compounds are
described, followed by a short account of their toxicity, mutagenicity, and
teratogenic action. The carcinogenic action of the compounds is discussed in
greater detail, and an account of some aspects of their metabolism is given.
Recent work on the formation of carcinogenic nitrosamines in the body from
nitrites and amine precursors is briefly reviewed, and possible environmental
hazards from nitrosamines are discussed.

Chemistry of N-Nitroso Compounds

Although N-nitroso compounds have been known almost from the beginning of organic chemistry, little research on such compounds was done until recently. Since the chemistry of nitrosamines (9)—the synthesis of nitrosamines and nitrosamides (10) and the group of acyl aryl nitrosamides (11)—was recently reviewed, only some new aspects are mentioned below.

Nitrosating Agents and Synthesis of N-Nitroso Compounds (9). It is believed that nitrosation is effected by agents related to nitrous acid having the structure ONX, where X = OAlk, NO_2, NO_3, halogen, tetrafluoroborate, hydrogen sulfate, or $^+OH_2$. Depending on the experimental conditions, any member of this series may become the main nitrosating agent. The nitrosonium cation is present at high concentrations only at high acidities. In the presence of an active nucleophilic agent (*e.g.*, hydroxide ions) the nitrosonium cation is converted into nitrous acid and further into nitrite ions:

$$ON^+ + OH^- \rightleftarrows HNO_2 \rightleftarrows H^+ + NO_2^-$$

At pH $\geq$ 7 the equilibrium in the reaction is completely displaced to the right.

In its simplest form the nitrosation of amines includes electrophilic attack by the nitrosating species on the lone pairs of electrons of the nitrogen atom and subsequent deprotonation of the alkylnitrosammonium cation:

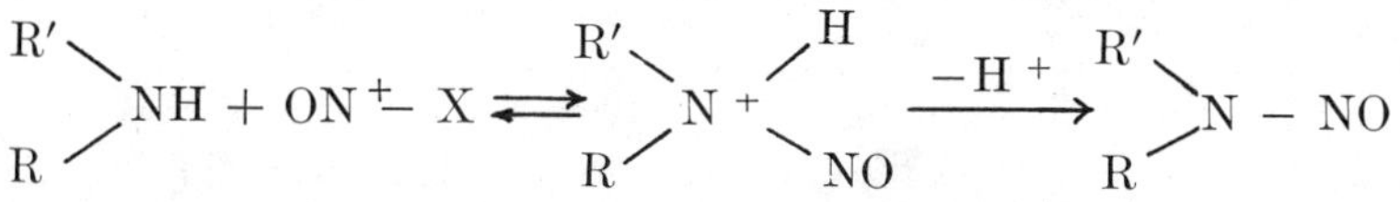

The reaction of primary amines with aldehydes in the presence of alcohols and nitrite under mildly acidic reaction conditions forms nitrosamines bearing an ether group in the α-position (12).

Chemical Properties of N-Nitroso Compounds. The reactions of aliphatic nitrosamines are varied because the nitrosamino group has four lone pairs of electrons, which make nitrosamines potential Lewis bases (9). The occurrence of p-π conjugations, with the withdrawal of the electron cloud towards the oxygen atom, is responsible for many interesting reactions of nitrosamines.

REACTION WITH INORGANIC ACIDS; THE FISCHER–HEPP REARRANGEMENT. N-Nitrosodialkylamines decompose on heating with hydrochloric acid into dialkylamine hydrochloride ($13, 14, 15, 16, 17$):

$$R_1R_2N\text{—}N{=}O \underset{H_2O}{\overset{HCl}{\rightleftarrows}} R_1R_2NH \cdot HCl + HNO_2$$

Hydrogen chloride has a more pronounced denitrosating activity ($9, 18, 19$). The carbonyl group has also a significant influence on the results of the denitrosation (20).

The study of the acid cleavage of alpihatic nitrosamines led to the hypothesis that an equilibrium between nitrosamine and its protonated form is established before separation of the nitroso group:

$$R'RN\!-\!N\!=\!O + H^+ \; \rightleftarrows \; R'R\overset{+}{H}N\!-\!N\!=\!O \; \overset{slow}{\rightleftarrows} \; R'RNH + NO^+$$

The denitrosation takes place more readily in hydrochloric acid than in sulfuric or perchloric acid. The authors explain this by the following nucleophilic reaction (*9*):

$$\underset{/}{\overset{\backslash}{>}}{}^+NH - N = O \xrightarrow{Cl^-} \underset{/}{\overset{\backslash}{>}}{}^+ NH - N\underset{O^-}{\overset{Cl}{<}} \longrightarrow \underset{/}{\overset{\backslash}{>}}NH + NOCl$$

Fridman *et al.* (*9*), however, believe that a more correct mechanism of the denitrosation of aliphatic nitrosamines involves electrophilic attack on the oxygen atom of the nitroso group. The latter is readily eliminated as a result of the generation of partial positive charges at the nitrogen atom (*21*):

$$\underset{/}{\overset{\backslash}{>}}\overset{\zeta+}{N}\cdots\cdots\overset{\zeta+}{N}\cdots\cdots\overset{\zeta-}{O}\cdots\cdots H \xrightarrow{HA} \underset{/}{\overset{\backslash}{>}}NH \cdot HA + NO^+$$

Complete denitrosation by acids can be performed very smoothly under mild conditions in an anhydrous medium; for example, HBr in acetic acid (*22*). The rearrangement of aromatic nitrosamines on treatment with acids to give ring-substituted isomers is known as the Fischer–Hepp rearrangement. Its mechanism was recently studied (*23*).

REDUCTION AND OXIDATION. The reduction and oxidation of nitrosamines were recently reviewed in detail by Fridman *et al.* (*9*) and therefore are mentioned here only briefly. The possible reduction of the nitroso group of nitrosamines to the amino group to yield hydrazines was discovered by Fischer (*24*). The reducing agent was zinc dust in acetic acid. Apart from the hydrazines, ammonia and amines were isolated. By reducing *N*-nitroso-diethylamine with zinc and acetic acid, tetraethyltetrazene together with diethylhydrazine was formed (*25*). In the catalytic reduction of *N*-nitroso-diethylamine with hydrogen a similar reaction was noted (*26*):

$$2(C_2H_5)_2\!=\!N\!-\!N\!=\!O + 2H_2 \rightarrow (C_2H_5)\!=\!N\!-\!N\!=\!N\!-\!N\!=\!(C_2H_5)_2 + 2\,H_2O$$

As well as zinc and acetic acid, sodium amalgam (*27, 28*), tin and hydro-chloric acid (*28*), lithium aluminum hydride (*29, 30*), zinc and aluminum in the presence of mercury salts, zinc in hydrochloric acid, and other reduction processes have been used (*31*).

Nitrosamines can also be reduced electrochemically (32) to the corresponding hydrazines or amines with the elimination of one nitrogen atom as ammonia:

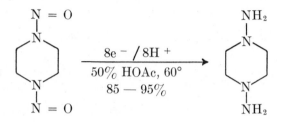

On treatment with lithium in liquid ammonia nitrosamines undergo far-reaching cleavage (Overberger–Lombardino reaction) (33, 34):

$$(RCH_2)_2N\!-\!N\!=\!O \xrightarrow{\ Li/H_3N\ }$$

$$(RCH_2)_2N\!-\!NHOH \rightarrow (RCH_2)_2\, N\!-\!N\!- \xrightarrow{\ -N_2\ } (RCH_2)_2$$

Best oxidation results in preparing secondary nitramines are obtained when nitric acid mixed with ammonium persulfate or trifluoroperacetic acid (35) is used as the oxidizing agent:

$$R_2N\!-\!N\!=\!O \xrightarrow{\ CF_3COOOH\ } R_2N\!-\!NO_2$$

DEVELOPMENTS IN DIAZOALKANE CHEMISTRY (36). Diazoalkanes can be prepared by direct diazotization with aqueous nitrous acid only when the amine possesses a strongly electron-withdrawing substituent on the α-carbon atom (37) (e.g., aminoacetic ester (38)):

$$C_2H_5O\!\cdot\!CO\!\cdot\!CH_2NH_2 \xrightarrow[H_2O]{HONO} C_2H_5OCO\!\cdot\!CH_2N^+{}_2 \xrightarrow{-H^+} C_2N_5OCO\!\cdot\!CH\!=\!N_2$$

The trifluoromethyl group has an inductive effect similar to that of the ester group in aminoacetic ester, and preparations of 2,2,2-trifluorodiazoethane (39), 2,2,3,3,4,4,4-heptafluorodiazo-n-butane (39), and 1,1,1-trifluoro-2-diazopropane (40) by diazotization of the corresponding amines were recently reported. Unstabilized diazoalkanes cannot be prepared from simple alkylamines by this method since the intermediate diazonium species decomposes faster with loss of N_2 than deprotonation and isolation of the diazoalkane can occur. The classical methods for preparing diazoalkanes involve treatment of a nitroso compound (general formula $RCH_2N(NO)X$) with a suitable base to yield the diazoalkane, $RCH\!=\!N_2$. Diazomethane thus is readily prepared by treating either N-methyl-N-nitrosourea or N-methyl-N-nitrosourethane with alkali (37, 41, 42, 43):

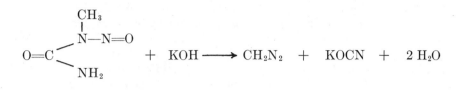

Some new stable crystalline intermediates for preparing diazomethane are *N*-nitroso-3-(methylamino) sulfolane *(44)*, *N*-methyl-*N*-nitrosotoluene-*p*-sulfonamide *(45)*, and *NN'*-dinitroso-*NN'*-dimethyloxamide *(46)*.

A displacement on the carbonyl carbon was proposed for the mechanism of the diazoalkane formation from nitrosoureas with base *(47, 48)*:

$$R_2CH-\overset{\overset{\displaystyle N=O}{|}}{\underset{\underset{\displaystyle O=C-NH_2}{|}}{N}} \quad + \quad {}^-OEt \longrightarrow R_2CH-N=N-O^- + C_2H_5Et\overset{\overset{\displaystyle O}{||}}{O}C-NH_2$$

$$\xrightarrow{R'OH} R_2CH-N=N-OH \xrightarrow{-H_2O} R_2CN_2$$

However, it was shown more recently that the conversion of nitrosoureas to diazoalkanes proceeds instead by addition of ethoxide ion to the nitroso nitrogen:

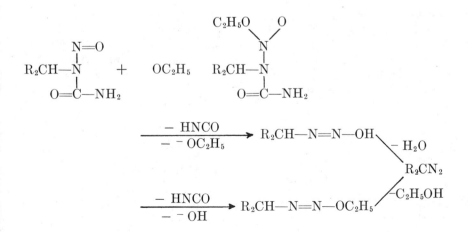

On the other hand, N-alkyl-N-nitrosourethanes and N-alkyl-N-nitrosoamides appear to undergo competitive reaction at the nitroso nitrogen and the carbonyl carbon. The competitive processes are sensitive to the alkyl group, the group attached to the carbonyl carbon atom, the solvent, and the nature of the base. Both mechanisms have a common latter stage which has been investigated in detail (49). Depending upon the nature of the alkyl group, formation of diazoalkane or decomposition of the diazotic acid to carbonium ion (50) products occurs:

$$
\begin{array}{c}
\xrightarrow{\ -N_2,\ -OH^-\ } \quad R_2-CH^+ \longrightarrow \text{Products}\\[1em]
R_2CH-N=N-OH \\[0.5em]
\xrightarrow[\ +H_2O\ ]{\ -H^+,\ -OH^-\ } R_2CN_2
\end{array}
$$

Recently it was reported that arylamines can be diazotized with amyl nitrite in benzene to give biaryls. Thus it was expected that aliphatic amines could react similarly with alkyl nitrites in an aprotic diazotization to generate the corresponding diazoalkane, water, and alcohol. In effect, this would constitute a direct preparation of diazoalkanes from amines (51):

$$RCH_2NH_2 + R'ONO \longrightarrow RCH_2\overset{+}{N}H_2NO + R'O^- \xrightarrow{\ -R'OH\ }$$

$$RCH_2NHNO \longrightarrow RCH_2N=NOH \longrightarrow RCH=N_2 + H_2O$$

One of the standard methods for effecting the diazoalkane ring enlargement of cycloalkanones involves the *in situ* generation of diazoalkane by the action of a base on nitroso compounds of the general structure $R-\overset{\overset{\textstyle N=O}{|}}{N}-R$ where $R = COOC_2H_5$, $COCH_3$, $CONH_2$, and so forth.

UNSATURATED CARBENES BY ALKALINE TREATMENT OF N-NITROSO-OXAZO-LIDONES. Unsaturated carbenes (A) or vinyl cations (B) have been suggested as intermediates in the basic decomposition of 5,5-dialkyl-3-nitrosooxazolidones $(52, 53, 54, 55, 56)$.

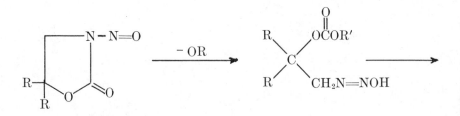

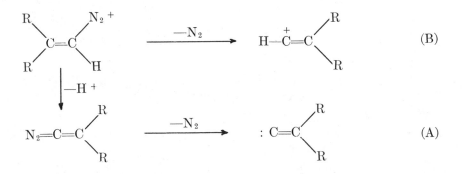

From the experience to date apparently unsaturated ions (B) are involved in protic solvents, but unsaturated carbenes (A) are involved in aprotic media.

A NEW METHOD FOR THE DEAMINATION OF ALIPHATIC AMINES *via* N-ALKYL N-NITROSAMIDES. The only method previously available for converting aliphatic amines into alcohols or their derivatives, the deamination with nitrous acid, furnishes low yields. A new method for this conversion is based on the facile elimination of nitrogen from the N-alkyl-N-nitrosamides (57). The steps are acylation of the amine, nitrosation of the amide, and thermal elimination of nitrogen from the resulting N-alkylnitrosamide.

$$
RNH_2 \rightarrow R\!-\!NH\!-\!\overset{\displaystyle O}{\overset{\|}{C}}\!-\!R' \rightarrow R\!-\!\overset{\displaystyle N=O}{\underset{\displaystyle \underset{\|}{O}}{N}}\!-\!\overset{}{C}\!-\!R' \xrightarrow{\triangle}
\begin{array}{l}
RO\!-\!\overset{\displaystyle O}{\overset{\|}{C}}\!-\!R' + N_2 \\
\text{and} \\
N_2 + R'COOH + \text{olefins} \\
\text{(corresponding to R).}
\end{array}
$$

DIAZENES AND ALKOXY-DIAZENIUM SALTS. *Diazenes.* The alkaline reduction of N-nitroso compounds with dithionite (58) yields 1,1-substituted diazenes and finally hydrazenes. The diazenes tend to fragment (59), rearrange (60, 61, 62), and dimerize (63).

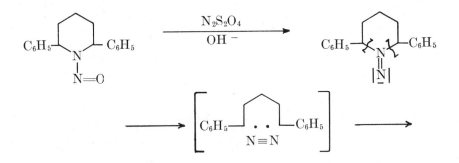

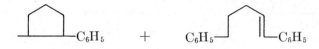

Alkoxydiazenium Salts. Alkoxydiazenium salts can be prepared easily by alkylation of nitrosamines with trialkyloxonium salts or a $AgClO_4/RX$ system (*63–73*).

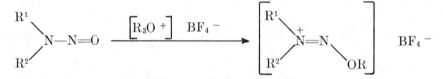

The most important reaction of the alkoxydiazenium salts is their easy irreversible deprotonation if R^1 or R^2 have a primary alkyl group:

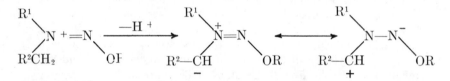

Especially interesting are the 1,3-dipolar cycloadditions of this species to various multiple bond systems to yield five-membered heterocyclic compounds:

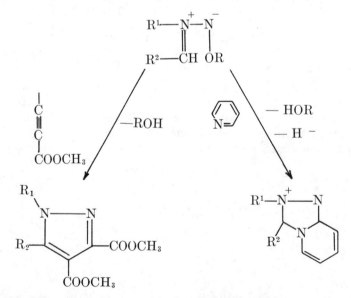

Physical Properties and Spectra of *N*-Nitroso Compounds. NMR SPECTRA (*74, 75, 76, 77*). One has to distinguish between restricted rotation caused by steric hindrance and by partial double bonds. In the first case steric hindrance (*78*) of the rotation about the aryl–N bonding is the reason for the nonequivalence of the marked protons in the NMR resonance:

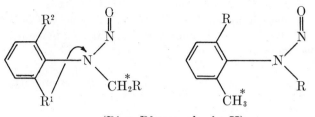

(R¹ or R² may also be H)

In the second case the nonequivalence of the protons arises from the restricted rotation caused by a partial double bond (*79*):

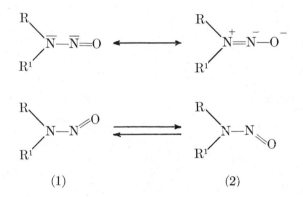

With suitable substituents, (R), the rotamers, (1) and (2), are stable enough to be separated by thin layer chromatography. The anisotropy effect (*80*) of the NO group is shown in the following heterocyclic *N*-nitrosamine:

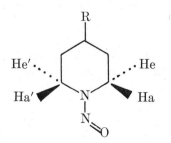

The signals of the equatorial protons He and He′ which are coplanar with the C—N—N—O plane appear close together at low field, those of the axial protons Ha and Ha′ at higher field. Because the proton Ha is situated in the semicircular deshielding zone of the N-nitroso group, its NMR signal is shifted far more to a higher field than the signal of the proton Ha'.

IR SPECTRA (9). The nitrosamines show three relatively intense bands in the infrared region of 7.1–7.4, 7.6–8.6, and 9.15–9.55 μm. The first two were assigned to the vibrations of the N=O bond and the last to the vibrations of the N–N bond. Table I summarizes the principal literature data on the infrared spectra of nitrosamines (R_2N—N=O).

Table I.   Infrared Spectral Data of Nitrosamines in Carbon Tetrachloride

R	$\nu_{N=O}$, cm^{-1}	ν_{N-N}, cm^{-1}
CH_3	1460	1041
C_2H_5	1459	1061
$n-C_3H_7$	1460	1067
$i-C_3H_7$	1438	1139
$n-C_5H_{11}$	—	1082
$C_6H_5CH_2$	1463	1120
C_6H_{13}	—	1085
CF_3CH_2	1528	1046

UV SPECTRA (9, 81). The ultraviolet spectra of nitrosamines show two absorption bands at 230–235 and 332–374 nm in water. The first maximum is more distinct than the second. The positions of the bands in the uv spectra depend greatly on the nature of the substituents and the solvent.

MS SPECTRA (9, 82, 83). Accurate mass measurements on different compounds indicate that the M-17 and M-30 peaks result from molecular ion losses of OH and NO, respectively. The loss of OH was rationalized in terms of a McLafferty-type rearrangement (84, 85):

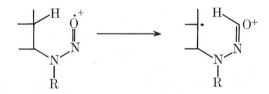

The mass spectra of most simple dialkylnitrosamines are quite normal, but a series of dibenzyl-N-nitrosamines fragment upon electron impact with a profound skeletal rearrangement (86):

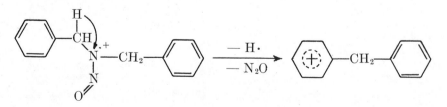

Toxic, Teratogenic, and Mutagenic Effects

The toxic actions of the dialkylnitrosamines are clearly different from those of the nitrosamides. These differences may be related to the relative chemical stability of the nitrosamines under physiological conditions and the varying degrees of nitrosamide instability (*see* sections on chemistry and metabolism). The main acute action of the dialkyl and cyclic nitrosamines is on the liver, resulting in hemorrhagic centrilobular necrosis (*1, 6*). Other organs are much less severely affected; the main features are peritoneal and sometimes pleural exudates which may contain a high proportion of blood and a tendency to hemorrhage into the lungs and other organs. In protein-deficient rats there may be detectable necrosis of some renal tubules (*87*) and of the testes (*88*) following treatment with *N*-nitrosodimethylamine. Chronic administration of many nitrosamines induces tumors of the liver and other organs (*see* section on carcinogenic effects). The livers of rats and other species chronically exposed to nitrosamines show various pathological changes, including biliary hyperplasia, fibrosis, nodular prenchymal hyperplasia, and the formation of enlarged hepatic parenchymal cells with very big nuclei. Subacute and chronic liver changes induced by *N*-nitrosomorpholine were described in detail by Bannasch (*89*).

In contrast to the nitrosamines, the nitrosamides have relatively little damaging action on the liver, and necrosis, when it occurs, is periportal rather than centrilobular (*90*). Unlike the nitrosamines, the nitrosamides cause severe tissue injury at the application site. The degree of local damage varies and may be related to the rate at which the compound decomposes at the site. Severe damage to the stomach, the skin, or the subcutaneous tissue may follow application by the intragastric, topical, or subcutaneous routes. The systemic targets of the nitrosamides, for example, *N*-methyl-*N*-nitrosourea (*91*), are mainly the organs of rapid cell turnover, including the bone marrow, crypt cells of the small intestine, and the lymphoid tissues. The action of such nitrosamides is of the so-called "radiomimetic" type. The relative degrees of local and systemic damage by the nitrosamides may be related to their decomposition rate in the body since the tissue damage is probably caused by a breakdown product rather than by the compound itself.

The nitrosamides include some of the most powerful known chemical mutagens, for example *N*-methyl-*N'*-nitrosoguanidine. This topic was briefly discussed by Magee and Barnes (*6*). As with acute toxicity, there is a clear distinction between the mutagenic actions of the nitrosamines and of the nitrosamides. The latter compounds are powerfully mutagenic in all the usual microbial test systems and in *Drosophila*, but the nitrosamines are active only in the insect. This difference seems to be related to the lack of nitrosamine metabolism in the microorganisms and the probable capacity of *Drosophila* to perform the enzyme-catalyzed reactions necessary for their biological activation. This conclusion is supported by the demonstration that *N*-nitrosodimethylamine is mutagenic when incubated with bacteria in the presence of rat liver microsomes (*92*) and the fact that several nitrosamines are actively mutagenic when tested by the host-mediated assay (*93*). In the host-mediated assay for mutagenesis, test organisms are placed in the peritoneal cavity or elsewhere in the body, and the suspected mutagenic chemical is injected by another route. The test shows mutagenic activity in compounds which require metabolic acivation in the body but which are inactive when applied directly to the test organism.

The teratogenic actions of the nitroso compounds have been much less extensively investigated. As with transplacental carcinogenesis, the nitrosamides are active while the nitrosamines are not except when administered late in pregnancy (94). This is probably related to the capacity for direct action of the former compounds and the lack of sufficient amounts of the activating enzymes in the fetus until the last.few days of pregnancy. The teratogenicity of the nitroso compounds is discussed briefly in the review by Magee and Barnes (6). The induction of deformities in pig fetuses by intravenous administration of N-ethyl-N-nitrosourea was recently reported (95).

Carcinogenic Effects

The Hepatobiliary System. Liver tumors were induced by different N-nitroso compounds in various animal species (see Table II). Rats developed liver tumors after treatment with dialkylnitrosamines, cyclic nitrosamines, and nitrosamines with functional groups. Among the 1-aryl-3,3-dialkyltriazenes and the azo- and axoxy alkanes, liver tumors were only reported after chronic treatment with 1-phenyl-3,3-diethyltriazene and azoethane, but no liver tumors were induced with acyl alkyl nitrosamides. These tumors are generally induced after continuous administrations of fractionated small doses over long periods, except in a few experimental conditions.

Druckrey et al. (147) administered N-nitrosodiethylamine in the drinking water to rats at nine dose levels, ranging from 14.2 to 0.075 mg/kg/day and obtained liver carcinomas even with the lowest dose. This corresponds to 1/4000 parts of the acute LD_{50} in the five rats which survived more than 800 days of the treatment, and suggests that no indication of a sub-threshold dose could be found. Similar results were obtained with other N-nitroso compounds as well as other carcinogens selectively producing tumors in organs apart from the liver (370). Terracini et al. (105) found that in rats fed for their lifespan with a diet containing as little as 2 or 5 ppm of N-nitrosodimethylamine there were no morphological changes in the liver other than tumors which provide a sensitive exposure index to this carcinogen. Similar conclusions were reached by Svoboda and Higginson (152) who examined the chronic ultrastructural changes in rat liver cells caused by N-nitrosodimethyl- and diethylamine.

Attempts to induce liver tumors with a single dose of N-nitroso compounds have been described. A single dose of N-nitrosodimethylamine administered to newborn rats induced a relatively high incidence of hepatocellular carcinomas (104, 106), but in adult rats liver tumors developed very rarely after a single dose of nitrosamines (371, 372). Craddock (371, 373) induced liver tumors after administering a single dose of N-nitrosodimethylamine,

N-nitrosodiethylamine, or *N*-methyl-*N'*-nitro-*N*-nitrosoguanidine to adult partially hepatectomized rats, suggesting that replicating cells are especially sensitive to the carcinogenic action. Similar findings were reported by Pound *et al.* (*372*) who observed an increase of liver tumors in rats treated with a single dose of *N*-nitrosodimethylamine 42 or 60 hr after a single dose of carbon tetrachloride. However, chronic administrations of *N*-nitrosodimethyl- or *N*-nitrosodiethylamine to partially hepatectomized rats did not change the incidence of liver tumors compared to the intact rats receiving the nitrosamines (*150, 373*). A single dose of *N*-methyl-*N*-nitrosourea failed to induce liver tumors in newborn and adult rats (*273*), even after intraportal injection (*267*).

The tumors in rats were described as hepatomas and hepatocellular carcinomas with a varying degree of differentiation and anaplasia (*2, 7, 105, 145, 374*), cholangiomas and cholangiocarcinomas (*151, 238, 253*), fibrosarcomas (*112, 145, 151, 256, 257*), and angiosarcomas (*375, 376*).

Liver tumors developed in mice and rats following chronic treatment with a variety of *N*-nitroso compounds. In the 11 strains of adult mice in which *N*-nitrosodimethylamine was tested, hemangiomatous tumors (hemangioma, hemangiosarcoma, hemangioendothelioma, and hemangioendothelialsarcoma) are the most frequent liver tumors, and parenchymal cell tumors developed less frequently. *N*-Nitrosodiethylamine induced mainly parenchymal cell tumors in the seven strains tested except in the Balb/c and NMRI strains where hemangiosarcomas and hemangioendotheliomas were predominant (*119, 162*). Newborn and young adult mice appear more likely to develop parenchymal liver cell tumors (*115, 116, 117, 121, 122, 161, 164, 200*). Both types of tumors were induced with other nitrosamines such as *N*-nitrosodibutylamine, *N*-nitrosopiperidine, di-*N*-nitrosopiperazine, *N*-nitrosomorpholine, and a single dose of *N*-methyl-*N*-nitrosourea produced parenchymal cell tumors in newborn BC3 F_1 mice but not in adults (*273*).

Different authors have attributed a varying degree of malignancy to the parenchymal cell tumors induced in mice by nitrosamines. Malignant hepatocellular carcinomas were described (*114, 115, 377*) according to the criteria of altered morphology, invasiveness, and metastases. The morphology and histogenesis of hemangioendothelial sarcomas after chronic exposure to *N*-nitrosodimethylamine (*114, 124, 378*) showed that these tumors seem to arise from the proliferation of sinusoidal endothelial cells. No cholangiomatous tumors were reported in mice.

N-Nitrosodiethylamine given to Syrian golden hamsters either by intragastric, interaperitoneal, or intradermal routes produced hepatocelluar carcinomas which metastasized and were transplantable (*167, 168*). Cholangiocarcinomas were also induced following continuous oral administration of *N*-nitrosodiethylamine (*132*). The incidence of liver tumors after oral administration of *N*-nitrosodiethylamine was much higher than with other routes. Multiple or single subcutaneous injections to adult or newborn hamsters induced mainly respiratory tumors and very few liver tumors (*172, 173*). In contrast, the incidence of liver tumors was much higher following treatment

(text continued on page 558)

Table II.   Carcinogenic Activity of *N*-Nitroso

Compounds	*Species*

Symmetrical Dialkyl (aryl) nitrosamines

N-Nitrosodimethylamine,   rat
   Dimethylnitrosamine,
   Nitrosodimethylamine,
   DMN, DMNA

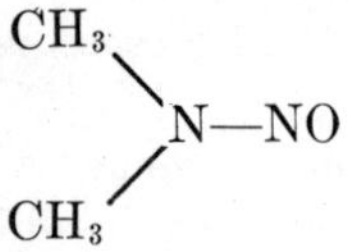

                                            mouse
                                            S.G. hamster

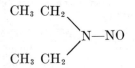

rabbit
mastomys
   (*Praomys natalensis*)
guinea pig
trout (Rainbow)
newt (*Triturus helveticus*)
aquarium fish
   (*Lebistes reticulatus*)
mink
European hamster

N-Nitrosodiethylamine,   rat
   Diethylnitrosamine,   African white-tailed rat
   DEN, DENA   mouse

                                            S.G. hamster
Chineses hamster
European hamster
guinea pig
rabbit
dog
pig
trout
Brachydanio rerio
grass parakeet
monkey

N-Nitrosodi-*n*-propylamine,   rat
   Di-*n*-propylnitrosamine

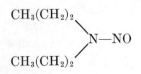

Compounds and Related Substances (2)

Principal Organs Affected	References
liver, kidney, nasal cavities	*2, 7, 87, 96, 97, 98, 99, 101–112, 145*
liver, lung, kidney	*113–128*
liver, nasal cavities	*129, 130, 131, 132, 133*
liver	*134*
liver	*135*
liver	*136*
liver	*137*
liver	*138*
liver	*139, 140*
liver	*141*
liver, kidney	*142*
liver, esophagus, nasal cavities, kidney	*7, 143–153*
liver	*154*
liver, lung, forestomach, esophagus, nasal cavities	*114, 119, 123, 155–164*
trachea, larynx, nasal cavities, lung, liver	*165–173*
esophagus, forestomach, liver	*174, 175,*
nasal cavities, trachea, bronchi, larynx	*176*
liver	*177–182*
liver	*183, 184*
liver	*185*
liver	*186, 187*
liver	*188*
liver	*189*
liver	*190*
liver	*191, 192*
liver, esophagus, tongue	*7, 193*

Table II.

Compounds   *Species*

Symmetrical Dialkyl (aryl) nitrosamines *(continued)*

N-Nitrosodiisopropylamine,   rat
Diisopropylnitrosamine

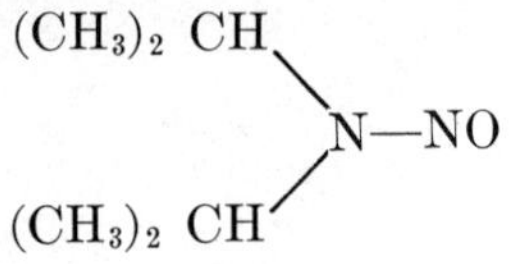

$(CH_3)_2$ CH
$\qquad\qquad$ N—NO
$(CH_3)_2$ CH

N-Nitrosodiallylamine,   rat
Diallylnitrosamine

$H_2C{=}CHCH_2$
$\qquad\qquad$ N—NO
$H_2C{=}CHCH_2$

N-Nitrosodi-n-butylamine,   rat
Di-n-butylnitrosamine,
DBN, DBNA
$\qquad\qquad\qquad\qquad\qquad$ mouse

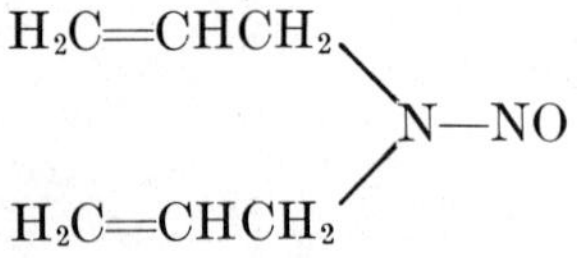

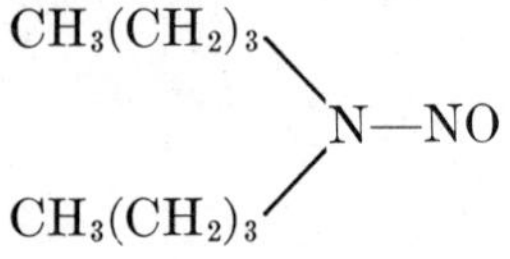

$CH_3(CH_2)_3$
$\qquad\qquad$ N—NO   S.G. hamster
$\qquad\qquad$ Chinese hamster
$CH_3(CH_2)_3$ guinea pig

N-Nitrosodiisopropanolamine   S.G. hamster

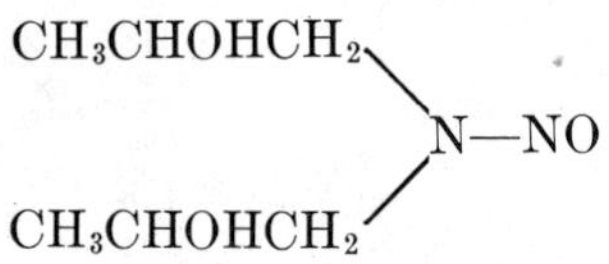

$CH_3CHOHCH_2$
$\qquad\qquad$ N—NO
$CH_3CHOHCH_2$

N-Nitrosodi-n-pentylamine,   rat
Di-n-pentylnitrosamine,
Di-n-amylnitrosamine

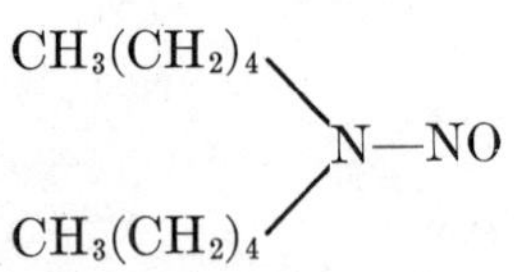

$CH_3(CH_2)_4$
$\qquad\qquad$ N—NO
$CH_3(CH_2)_4$

Continued

Principal Organs Affected	*References*
liver	*7*
—	*7*
bladder, esophagus, liver	*7, 193–198*
esophagus, bladder, liver, forestomach, tongue, lung	*112, 123, 199, 200*
bladder, trachea, lung, forestomach	*201, 202, 203*
forestomach, bladder	*201, 202*
liver, bladder	*204*
pancreas, respiratory tract, liver, kidney	*205*
liver, lung	*7, 193, 206*

Table II.

Compounds   *Species*

Symmetrical Dialkyl (aryl) nitrosamines (*continued*)

N-Nitrosodicyclohexylamine,   rat
  Dicyclohexylnitrosamine

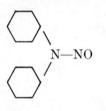

N-Nitrosodiphenylamine,   rat
  Diphenylnitrosamine

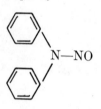

N-Nitrosodibenzylamine,   rat
  Dibenzylnitrosamine

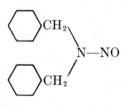

Asymmetrical Dialkylnitrosamines

  N-Nitrosomethylethylamine,   rat
  Ethylmethylnitrosamine

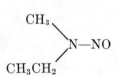

Continued

Principal Organs Affected	References
—	*7*
—	*7, 145, 193, 207*
—	*7*
liver	*7*

Table II.

Compounds	*Species*

Asymmetrical Dialkylnitrosamines (*continued*)

N-Nitrosomethylvinylamine,   rat
Methylvinylnitrosamine

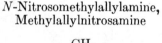
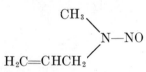

N-Nitrosomethylallylamine,   rat
Methylallylnitrosamine

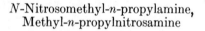
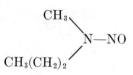

N-Nitrosomethyl-n-propylamine,   S.G. hamster
Methyl-n-propylnitrosamine

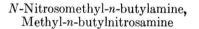
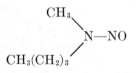

N-Nitrosomethyl-n-butylamine,   rat
Methyl-n-butylnitrosamine

                                                        mouse
                                                        S.G. hamster

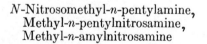

N-Nitrosomethyl-n-pentylamine,   rat
Methyl-n-pentylnitrosamine,
Methyl-n-amylnitrosamine

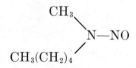

Continued

Principal Organs Affected	*References*
esophagus, pharynx, tongue, nasal cavities	7, 148, 208
esophagus, kidney, nasal cavities, liver	7, 208, 209
nasal cavities, trachea, lung, liver	210
esophagus, nasal cavities, liver	211, 212, 213
eyelid, nasal cavities	214
trachea, lung	215
esophagus	7

Table II.

Compounds   *Species*

Asymmetrical Dialkylnitrosamines (*continued*)

N-Nitroso-N-(2-hydroxypropyl)-   S.G. hamster
n-propylamine,
2-Hydroxypropyl-n-propylnitrosamine

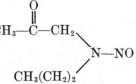

N-Nitroso-N-propyl-2-oxopropylamine   rat

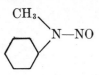

N-Nitrosomethylcyclohexylamine,   rat
Methylcyclohexylnitrosamine

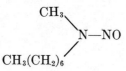

N-Nitrosomethyl-n-heptylamine,   rat
Methyl-n-heptylnitrosamine

CH$_3$
       N—NO
CH$_3$(CH$_2$)$_6$

N-Nitroso-N-methylaniline,   rat
N-Nitroso-N-methylphenylamine,
Methylphenylnitrosamine
                                                         mouse
CH$_3$
       N—NO

Continued

Principal Organs Affected	*References*
nasal cavities, trachea, lung, liver	*216*
liver	*217*
esophagus, pharynx, lung	*7, 218*
—	*7*
esophagus, pharynx, forestomach	*7, 218, 219, 220, 221*
lung	*222*

Table II.

Compounds	*Species*

Asymmetrical Dialkylnitrosamines (*continued*)

N-Nitrosomethylbenzylamine,   rat
  Methylbenzylnitrosamine

mouse

$$CH_3$$
$$N—NO$$
$$CH_2$$

N-Nitrosomethyl-(2-phenylethyl)amine,   rat
  Methyl-(2-phenylethyl)nitrosamine

$$CH_3$$
$$N—NO$$
$$(CH_2)_2$$

N-Nitroso-4-methylaminoazobenzene   rat

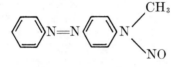

$$N{=}N$$ $$N$$ $$CH_3$$ $$NO$$

N,N'-Dinitroso-*N,N'*-dimethyl-   rat
  ethylenediamine

$$CH_3—N—(CH_2)_2—N—CH_3$$
$$\quad\ \ NO \qquad\qquad NO$$

N,N'-Dinitroso-*N,N'*-dimethyl-1,   rat
  3-propanediamine

$$CH_3—N—(CH_2)_3—N—CH_3$$
$$\quad\ \ NO \qquad\qquad NO$$

Continued

Principal Organs Affected	*References*
esophagus	*7, 223*
esophagus, forestomach	*224*
esophagus	*7*
—	*7, 225*
esophagus, pharynx	*7, 223, 226*
esophagus, pharynx, tongue, forestomach	*227*

Table II.

Compounds	*Species*

Asymmetrical Dialkylnitrosamines (*continued*)

N-Nitroso-*N*-ethylvinylamine,   rat
Ethylvinylnitrosamine
                                       guinea pig

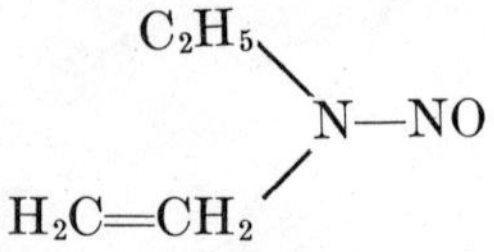

$$\begin{array}{c} C_2H_5 \\ \diagdown \\ N\!-\!NO \\ \diagup \\ H_2C\!=\!CH_2 \end{array}$$

N,*N*'-Dinitroso-*N*,*N*'-diethyl-   rat
ethylenediamine

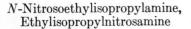
$$\underset{\displaystyle NO \qquad\quad NO}{C_2H_5\!-\!N\!-\!(CH_2)_2\!-\!N\!-\!C_2H_5}$$

N-Nitroso-*n*-butyl-*n*-pentylamine,   rat
n-Butyl-*n*-pentylnitrosamine

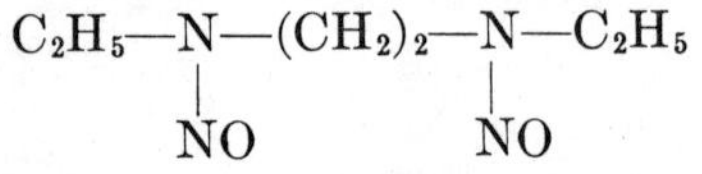

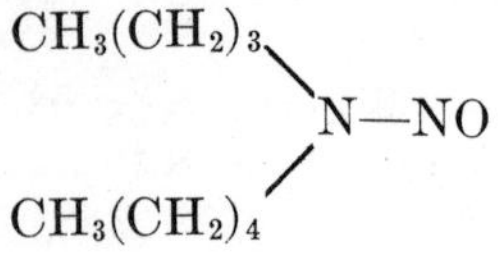

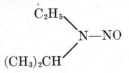
$$\begin{array}{c} CH_3(CH_2)_3 \\ \diagdown \\ N\!-\!NO \\ \diagup \\ CH_3(CH_2)_4 \end{array}$$

N-Nitrosoethylisopropylamine,   rat
Ethylisopropylnitrosamine

$$\begin{array}{c} \overset{.}{C}_2H_5 \\ \diagdown \\ N\!-\!NO \\ \diagup \\ (CH_3)_2CH \end{array}$$

N-Nitrosoethyl-*n*-butylamine,   rat
Ethyl-*n*-butylnitrosamine
                                       mouse

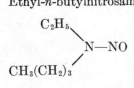
$$\begin{array}{c} C_2H_5 \\ \diagdown \\ N\!-\!NO \\ \diagup \\ CH_3(CH_2)_3 \end{array}$$

Continued

Principal Organs Affected	References
esophagus, phàrynx, forestomach, nasal cavities	*7, 223*
esophagus	*7*
esophagus, pharynx, tongue, forestomach	*227*
liver	*7*
esophagus, liver	*7*
esophagus, liver, kidney	*7, 148, 223*
forestomach	*228*

Table II.

Compounds	*Species*

Asymmetrical Dialkylnitrosamines *(continued)*

N-Nitrosoethyl-*tert*-butylamine,   rat
Ethyl-*tert*-butylnitrosamine

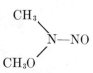

Nitrosamines with Functional Groups

N-Nitrosomethylaminosulfolane,   rat
Tetrahydro-N-methyl-N-nitroso-
3-thiophenamine-1,1-dioxide

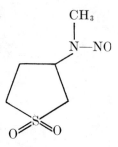

N-Nitroso-N-methyl-O-methyl-   rat
hydroxylamine

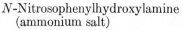

N-Nitrosophenylhydroxylamine   rat
(ammonium salt)

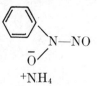

Continued

	Principal Organs Affected	*References*
	—	*7*
	esophagus	*7*
	—	*7*
	—	*7*

Table II.

Compounds   *Species*

Nitrosamines with Functional Groups (*continued*)

N-Nitroso-N,N',N'-trimethylhydrazine   rat

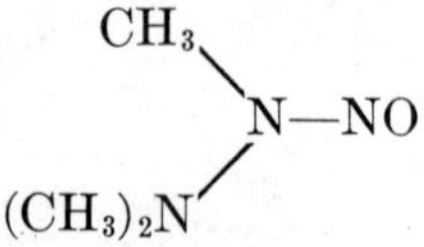

$$
\begin{array}{c}
CH_3 \\
\diagdown \\
\quad N\!-\!NO \\
\diagup \\
(CH_3)_2N
\end{array}
$$

N-Nitrosoethyl-2-hydroxyethylamine   rat

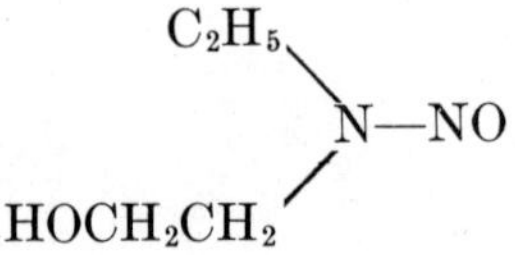

$$
\begin{array}{c}
C_2H_5 \\
\diagdown \\
\quad N\!-\!NO \\
\diagup \\
HOCH_2CH_2
\end{array}
$$

N-Nitrosodiethanolamine   rat

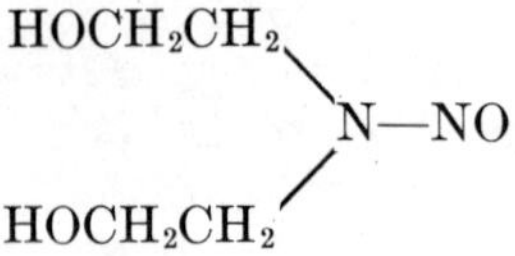

$$
\begin{array}{c}
HOCH_2CH_2 \\
\diagdown \\
\quad N\!-\!NO \\
\diagup \\
HOCH_2CH_2
\end{array}
$$

N-Nitrosobis(acetoxyethyl)amine   rat

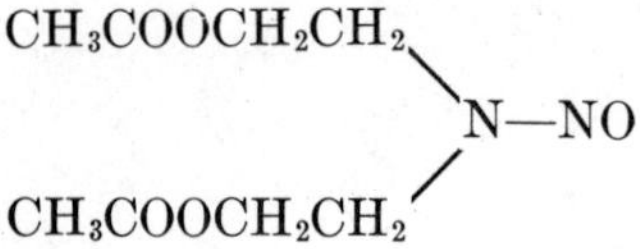

$$
\begin{array}{c}
CH_3COOCH_2CH_2 \\
\diagdown \\
\quad N\!-\!NO \\
\diagup \\
CH_3COOCH_2CH_2
\end{array}
$$

N-Nitroso-n-butyl-(4-hydroxybutyl)amine,   rat
4-n-Butylnitrosamino-1-butanol,
n-Butyl-(4-hydroxybutyl)nitrosamine   mouse

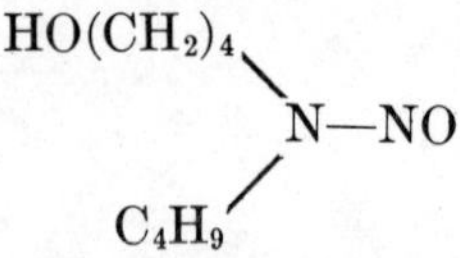

$$
\begin{array}{c}
HO(CH_2)_4 \\
\diagdown \\
\quad N\!-\!NO \\
\diagup \\
C_4H_9
\end{array}
$$

Continued

Principal Organs Affected	*References*
liver, kidney	7
liver, esophagus, kidney	7, *148, 223*
liver	7
liver	7
bladder, pelvis	7, *195, 229–233*
bladder	*232, 234*

Table II.

Compounds	*Species*

Nitrosamines with Functional Groups (*continued*)

N-Nitroso-*n*-butyl-(3-carboxypropyl)amine   rat

$$\begin{array}{c} CH_3(CH_2)_3 \\ \diagdown \\ \diagup \\ HO—OC(CH_2)_2 \end{array} N—NO$$

N-Nitroso·*n*-butyl-(3-hydroxypropyl)amine   rat

$$\begin{array}{c} CH_3(CH_2)_3 \\ \diagdown \\ \diagup \\ HOCH_2(CH_2)_2 \end{array} N—NO$$

N-Nitroso-*n*-propyl-(4-hydroxybutyl)amine   rat

$$\begin{array}{c} CH_3(CH_2)_2 \\ \diagdown \\ \diagup \\ HOCH_2(CH_2)_3 \end{array} N—NO$$

N-Nitroso-(2-hydroxyethyl)-*n*-butylamine   rat

$$\begin{array}{c} CH_3(CH_2)_3 \\ \diagdown \\ \diagup \\ HOCH_2CH_2 \end{array} N—NO$$

N-Nitroso-(2-oxopropyl)-*n*-butylamine   rat

$$\begin{array}{c} CH_3(CH_2)_3 \\ \diagdown \\ \diagup \\ CH_3COCH_2 \end{array} N—NO$$

N-Nitrosomethyl-2-chloroethylamine   rat

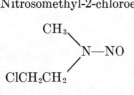

$$\begin{array}{c} CH_3 \\ \diagdown \\ \diagup \\ ClCH_2CH_2 \end{array} N—NO$$

Continued

	Principal Organs Affected	*References*
bladder		*233, 235*
—		*236*
bladder		*236*
liver, esophagus		*236*
liver		*236*
liver		*7*

Table II.

Compounds   *Species*

Nitrosamines with Functional Groups (*continued*)

N-Nitrosomethylaminoacetonitrile   rat

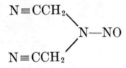

N-Nitrosodiacetonitrile   rat

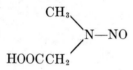

N-Nitrososarcosine   rat

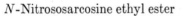

N-Nitrososarcosine ethyl ester   rat

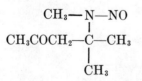

N-Nitroso-*N*-(1,1-dimethyl-3-oxobutyl)-   rat
  methylamine

$$CH_3-N-NO$$
$$\mid$$
$$CH_3COCH_2-C-CH_3$$
$$\mid$$
$$CH_3$$

Continued

	Principal Organs Affected	*References*
liver		*7*
liver, nasal cavities		*7*
esophagus		*7, 223*
esophagus		*7, 223, 237*
—		*7*

Table II.

| *Compounds* | *Species* |

Nitrosamines with Functional Groups (*continued*)

N-Nitroso-4-methylaminobenzaldehyde   rat

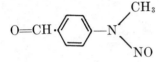

N-Nitrosoethyl-4-picolylamine,   rat
4[(Ethylnitrosamino)methyl]pyridine

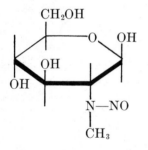

N-Methyl-*N*-nitroso-β-D-glucosamine   rat

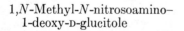

1,*N*-Methyl-*N*-nitrosoamino–   rat
1-deoxy-D-glucitole

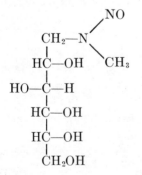

Continued

Principal Organs Affected	*References*
—	*7*
esophagus, lung, nasal cavities	
forestomach, liver	*238*
forestomach, liver, larynx, pharynx, esophagus	*238*

Table II.

Compounds   *Species*

Nitrosamines with Functional Groups (*continued*)

N-Methyl-N-nitroso–β-D-galactosamine   rat

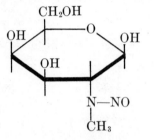

1-N-Methyl-N-nitrosoamino–   rat
    1-deoxy-D-galactitole

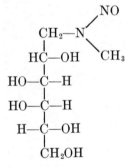

Cyclic Nitrosoamines

N-Nitrosoazetidine,   rat
    N-Nitrosotrimethyleneimine

                                         mouse
                                         S.G. hamster

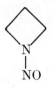

N-Nitrosopyrrolidine   rat
                                         mouse
                                         S.G. hamster

Continued

Principal Organs Affected	*References*
—	*238*
—	*238*
lung, liver, kidney	*239*
lung, liver	*239*
—	*240*
liver, nasal cavities, testis	*7, 241, 242*
lung	*243*
trachea, lung	*215*

Table II.

Compounds	*Species*

Cyclic Nitrosamines (*continued*)

N-Nitroso-L-proline   mouse

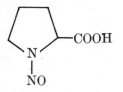

N-Nitroso-L-prolineethyl ester   rat

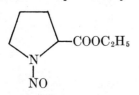

N-Nitrosopiperidine,   rat
   1-Nitrosopiperidine

                                                        mouse
                                                        S.G. hamster,
                                                        monkey

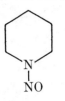

$S(+)$-N-Nitroso-2-methylpiperidine,   rat
   $S(+)$-N-Nitroso-d-pipecoline

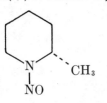

$R(-)$-N-Nitroso-2-methylpiperidine,   rat
   $R(-)$-N-Nitroso-d-pipecoline

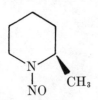

Continued

Principal Organs Affected	*References*
—	*243*
—	*7*
esophagus, liver, nasal cavities, larynx, trachea	*7, 193, 208, 220, 241, 244*
forestomach, liver, lung, esophagus	*123, 242, 245*
trachea, lung, larynx	*146, 246*
liver	*247*
peripheral nervous system, liver, nasal cavities	*248*
peripheral nervous system	*248*

Table II.

Compounds	Species

Cyclic Nitrosamines (continued)

N-Nitrosopiperazine   rat

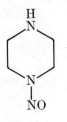

N,*N*′-Dinitrosopiperazine,   rat
1,4-Dinitrosopiperazine
                                                  mouse

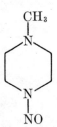

N-Nitroso-*N*′-methylpiperazine   rat

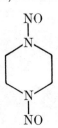

N-Nitroso-*N*′-carbethoxypiperazine   rat

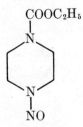

Continued

Principal Organs Affected	*References*
nasal cavities	*249*
esophagus, liver, nasal cavities, forestomach	*7, 208, 227, 241*
lung, liver	*222, 250*
nasal cavities	*7*
liver, nasal cavities	*7*

Table II.

Compounds	Species

Cyclic Nitrosamines (*continued*)

Tri-*N*-nitrosohexahydro-1,3,5-triazine,   rat
    Trinitrosotrimethylenetriamine

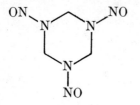

N-Nitrosoindoline   rat

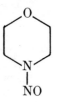

N-Nitrosomorpholine,   rat
    4-Nitrosomorpholine

                                                            mouse
                                                            S.G. hamster

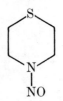

N-Nitrosothiomorpholine   rat

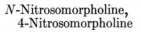

N-Nitroso-3,6-dihydro-1,2-oxazin   rat

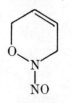

Continued

Principal Organs Affected	References
—	*7*
—	*7*
liver, nasal cavities, kidney, esophagus, ovary	*7, 148, 193, 208, 241, 251, 252, 253*
liver, lung	*222, 251, 254*
trachea, larynx, bronchi	*146, 246*
esophagus, tongue, nasal cavities	*249*
S.C. (site of injection)	*255*

Table II.

| *Compounds* | *Species* |

Cyclic Nitrosamines (*continued*)

N-Nitrosotetrahydro-1,2-oxazin   rat

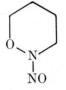

N-Nitrosoanabasine,   rat
  1-Nitrosoanabasine,
  N-Nitroso-2-(3′-pyridyl)piperidine

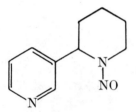

N-Nitrosohexamethyleneimine,   rat
  N-Nitrosoperhydroazepine,
  Hexahydro-1-nitroso-1,*H*-azepine

                                                   mouse
                                                   S.G. hamster

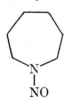

N-Nitrosoheptamethyleneimine,   rat
  Octahydro-1-nitrosoazocine
                                                   S.G. hamster

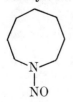

Continued

Principal Organs Affected	References
lung	*255*
esophagus	*220*
liver, nasal cavities, esophagus, tongue	*256, 257*
lung	*258*
trachea	*258*
lung, esophagus, tongue, trachea	*241, 259*
esophagus, pharynx, forestomach, trachea, nasal cavities	*240*

Table II.

Compounds	*Species*

Cyclic Nitrosamines (*continued*)

N-Nitrosooctamethyleneimine,   rat
    Octahydro-1-nitroso-1,*H*-azonine

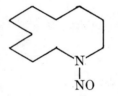

N-Nitrosodecamethyleneimine   mouse

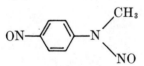

N,4-Dinitroso-*N*-methylaniline (Elastopax),   rat
    N-Methyl-*N*,*p*,-dinitrosoaniline,
    N-Methyl-*N*,4-dinitrosoaniline   mouse

ON—⟨benzene⟩—N⟨$^{CH_3}_{NO}$⟩

N,*N*'-Dinitrosopentamethylenetetramine,   rat
    3,7-Dinitroso-1,3,5,7-tetra-
    azabicyclo-(3,3,1)-nonane

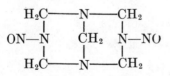

Continued

Principal Organs Affected	References
lung, esophagus, tongue, trachea	*259*
liver, glandular stomach	*260*
liver, mammary glands, peritoneal cavity (site of injection)	*207, 227*
—	*207*
—	*207, 227*

Table II.

Compounds   *Species*

Cyclic Nitrosamines *(continued)*

1-Nitroso-2,2,4-trimethyl-   rat
 1,2-dihydroquinoline,
   Polymer (Curetard)

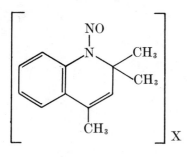

1-(4-*N*-Methyl-*N*-nitrosamino-   rat
   benzylidene)indene

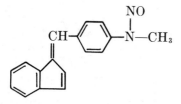

4-(4-*N*-Methyl-*N*-nitrosamino-   rat
   styryl)quinoline

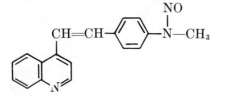

Continued

Principal Organs Affected	*References*

peritoneal cavity (site of injection)
   S.C. (site of injection)   *207, 261*

liver, ear duct   *262*

liver, ear duct   *262*

Table II.

<table>
<tr><td>Compounds</td><td>Species</td></tr>
</table>

Acylalkylnitrosamines

N-Methyl-*N*-nitrosourea,   rat
   Methylnitrosourea (MNU),
   Nitrosomethylurea (NMU)

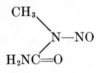
                                  mouse

                                  S.G. hamster

                                  European hamster
                                  guinea pig
                                  rabbit
                                  dog

N-Ethylnitrosourea,   rat
   Ethylnitrosourea (ENU)

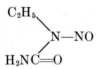
                                  mouse

N-Methyl-*N*-nitrosourethane,   rat
   N-Methyl-*N*-nitrosocarbamic acid,
     ethylester

                                  mouse
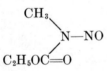
                                  S.G. hamster
                                  guinea pig

N-Ethyl-*N*-nitrosourethane,   rat
   N-Ethyl-*N*-nitrosocarbamic acid,
     ethylester

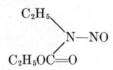

Continued

| *Principal Organs Affected* | *References* |

central and peripheral nervous system,
  intestine, kidney, forestomach,
  glandular stomach, skin and annexes,
  jaw, bladder, uterus, vagina   *4, 7, 91, 148 263–280*
lung, hematopoietic system, forestomach,
  kidney, skin, liver (only in newborn),
  central nervous system   *122, 125, 273, 281–288*
intestine, pharynx, esophagus, trachea,
  bronchi, oral cavity, skin and annexes,
  and S.C. (site of injection)   *266, 289, 290, 291, 292*
S.C. (site of injection)   *142*
stomach, pancreas, ear ducts   *293*
central nervous system, intestine, skin   *294, 295, 296, 297*
central and peripheral nervous system   *298, 299*

central and peripheral nervous system,
  kidney, hematopoietic system, skin,
  intestine, ovary, uterus   *7, 276, 278, 300, 301*
hematopoietic system, lung, central and
  peripheral nervous system, kidney   *302–307*

forestomach, lung, esophagus, intestine,
  kidney, ovary   *3, 4, 7, 90, 193, 308, 309*

lung, forestomach   *122, 310, 311*
esophagus, forestomach   *312*
pancreas, S.C. (site of injection)   *7, 293*

forestomach, intestine   *7, 308, 313*

Table II.

Compounds	*Species*

Acylalkylnitrosamines (*continued*)

2-Chloroethyl-*N*-nitrosourethane   rat

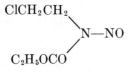

$ClCH_2CH_2$

N—NO

C_2H_5OCO

N,N′-Dinitrosodimethyloxamide   rat
(unstable substance)

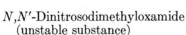

CH_3—N—CO—CO—N—CH_3
         | |
        NO   NO

N-Methyl-*N*-nitrosoacetamide   rat

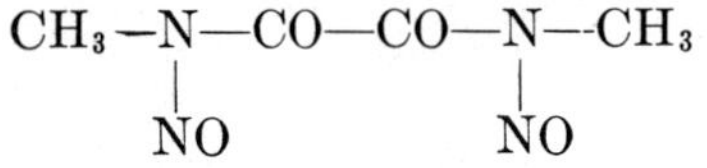

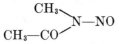

CH_3

N—NO

CH_3—CO

1,3-Dimethyl-*N*-nitrosourea   rat
                                                           mouse

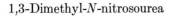

CH_3

N—NO

$CH_3NH \cdot C{=}O$

N-Nitrosotrimethylurea   rat

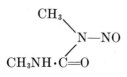

CH_3

N—NO

$(CH_3)_2NC{=}O$

N-n-Butyl-*N*-nitrosourea   rat

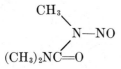

C_4H_9

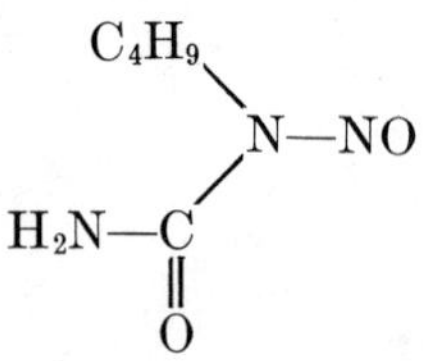

N—NO   mouse
                                                           S.G. hamster

H_2N—C
        ‖
        O

Continued

Principal Organs Affected	References
forestomach, glandular stomach, esophagus	*314*
liver	*7*
forestomach	*7*
central and peripheral nervous system, kidney hematopoietic system	*7* *315*
central and peripheral nervous system, kidney, skin	*7, 316*
hematopoietic system, mammary glands, central nervous system, esophagus, forestomach, ear ducts hematopoietic system peripheral nervous system	*7, 317–322* *319* *323*

Table II.

Compounds	*Species*

Acylalkylnitrosamines (*continued*)

N-Nitrosophenylurea   rat

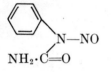

Streptozotocin   rat
   N-ᴅ-Glucosyl-(2)-
   N′-nitrosomethylurea   Chinese hamster

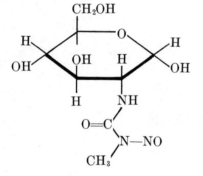

Hydrazodicarboxybis-   rat
   (methylnitrosamide)

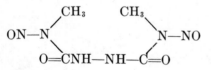

N-Methyl-*N*′-nitro-*N*-nitrosoguanidine   rat
   (MNNG)

                                       mouse
                                       S.G. hamster
                                       rabbit
                                       dog

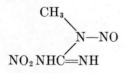

Continued

Principal Organs Affected	*References*
S.C. (site of injection)	*324*
kidney	*363, 364*
liver	*365*
S.C. (site of injection)	*7, 317*
glandular stomach, forestomach, intestine, S.C. (site of injection)	*7, 325–334*
intestine, forestomach, skin (site of injection)	*328, 335*
glandular stomach, intestine	*336, 337*
lung	*336*
stomach, intestine	*338, 339*

Table II.

Compounds	*Species*

Acylalkylnitrosamines (*continued*)

N-Ethyl-N'-nitro-N-nitrosoguanidine (ENNG)

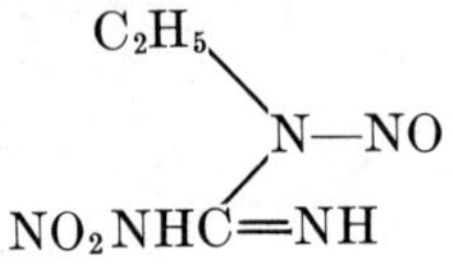

rat

mouse
S.G. hamster
dog

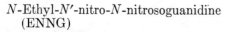

N-Nitrosoimidazolidone

rat

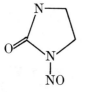

Toluene-p-sulfonylmethylnitrosamide

rat
mouse

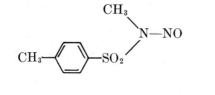

N,N'-Dinitroso-N,N'-dimethylphthalamide

rat

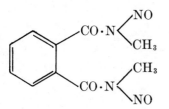

N-Methyl-N-nitrosobiuret

rat

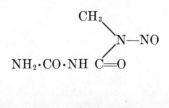

Continued

Principal Organs Affected	References
forestomach, intestine	*328*
skin (site of injection) esophagus, intestine	*328, 335, 340*
glandular stomach, duodenum	*341*
stomach	*342*
S.C. (site of injection)	*7, 317*
—	*7*
lung	*122*
—	*100, 227*
forestomach, glandular stomach, central nervous system, kidney, peripheral nervous system	*213*

Table II.

Compounds	*Species*

Acylalkylnitrosamines (*continued*)

N-Ethyl-*N*-nitrosobiuret   rat

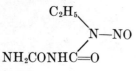

N-Methyl-*N*-nitroso-*N'*-acetylurea   rat

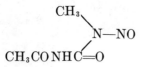

N-Nitroso-*N*-methyl-*N'*-   rat
 (2-benzothiazolyl)urea,
 N-(2-Benzothiazolyl)-*N'*-methyl-
 N'-nitrosourea

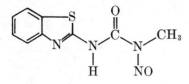

Hydrazo-, Azo-, Azoxyalkanes

1,2-Dimethylhydrazine,   rat
 sym-Dimethylhydrazine,
 Hydrazomethane

    CH₃—NH—NH—CH₃   mouse
                                                     S.G. hamster

1,1-Dimethylhydrazine,   rat
 unsym-Dimethylhydrazine
                                                     mouse

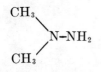

Continued

Principal Organs Affected	References

forestomach, glandular stomach, central
  and peripheral nervous system   *343*

glandular stomach, central and peripheral
  nervous system   *344*

forestomach, kidney   *345*

intestine, kidney, liver   *346, 347, 348, 349, 350*

intestine, blood vessels, lung   *351, 352, 353, 354, 355*
intestine, liver, blood vessels, stomach   *356, 357, 358*

liver   *7, 145, 193*

lung, blood vessels, kidney, liver   *351, 359, 360*

Table II.

| *Compounds* | *Species* |

Hydrazo-, Azo-, Azoxyalkanes (*continued*)

1,2-Diethylhydrazine,   rat
  sym-Diethylhydrazine,
  Hydroazoethane

$$C_2H_5—NH—NH—C_2H_5$$

1-Methyl-2-*n*-butylhydrazine   rat

$$CH_3—NH—NH—(CH_2)_3—CH_3$$

1-Methyl-2-benzylhydrazine   rat

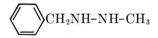

Azoethane   rat
$$C_2H_5—N{=}N—C_2H_5$$

Azoxymethane   rat

$$CH_3N{=}N—CH_3$$
$$\downarrow$$
$$O$$

Azoxyethane   rat

$$C_2H_5\ N{=}N—C_2H_5$$
$$\downarrow$$
$$O$$

Methylazoxybutane   rat

$$CH_3(CH_2)_3N{=}N—CH_3$$
$$\downarrow$$
$$O$$

Elaiomycin   rat

$$
\begin{array}{ccc}
 & O & CH_2OCH_3 \\
 & \uparrow & | \\
n—C_6H_{13}—CH{=}CH—N{=}N—CH \\
 & & | \\
 & & CHOH \\
 & & | \\
 & & CH_3
\end{array}
$$

Continued

Principal Organs Affected	*References*
mammary glands, nasal cavities, hematopoietic system, central nervous system	*361*
intestine, nasal cavities	*347*
central and peripheral nervous system, nasal cavities	*347*
liver, hematopoietic system, mammary glands, nasal cavities, central nervous system	*362*
intestine, liver, kidney	*347*
S.C. (site of injection)	*362*
intestine, liver, skin	*347*
kidney, liver, intestine, central nervous system	*366*

Table II.

Compounds	*Species*

1-Aryl-3,3-dialkyltriazenes

1-Phenyl-3,3-dimethyltriazene   rat

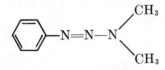

1-Phenyl-3-methyl-3-hydroxytriazene   rat

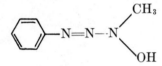

1-Phenyl-3-methyl-3-(2-hydroxy-
  ethyl)triazene   rat

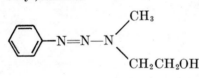

1-Phenyl-3-methyl-3-(2-sulfoethyl)triazene   rat
  (sodium salt)

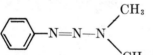

1-Phenyl-3,3-diethyltriazene   rat

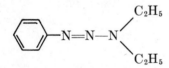

1-(2-Methylphenyl)-3,3-dimethyltriazene   rat

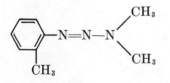
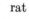

Continued

Principal Organs Affected	*References*
central and peripheral nervous system, kidney, uterus, ovary, heart, S.C. (site of injection)	*367, 368*
S.C. (site of injection), skin, forestomach	*368*
S.C. (site of injection), kidney	*368*
S.C. (site of injection)	*368*
liver, kidney, skin, central nervous system, hematopoietic system, uterus, ovary	*368*
kidney, central and peripheral nervous system, S.C. (site of injection)	*368*

Table II.

Compounds	*Species*

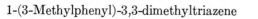

1-Aryl-3,3-dialkyltriazenes (*continued*)

1-(3-Methylphenyl)-3,3-dimethyltriazene rat

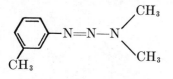

1-(4-Methyloxyphenyl)-3,3-dimethyltriazene rat

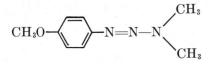

1-(4-Chlorophenyl)-3,3-dimethyltriazene rat

1-(4-Nitrophenyl)-3,3-dimethyltriazene rat

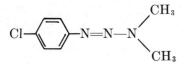

1-(Pyridyl-3)-3,3-dimethyltriazene rat

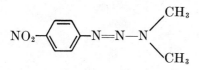

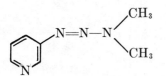

Continued

Principal Organs Affected	*References*
kidney, heart, mammary glands, central nervous system	*368*
S.C. (site of injection), kidney	*368*
central nervous system, skin, kidney	*368*
cental and peripheral nervous system, skin	*368*
central and peripheral nervous system, kidney, hematopoietic system, mammary glands	*368*

Table II.

Compounds   *Species*

1-Aryl-3,3-dialkyltriazenes (*continued*)

1-(Pyridyl-3)-3,3-diethyltriazene   rat

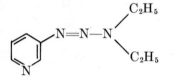

1-(Pyridyl-3-*N*-oxide)-3,3-dimethyltriazene   rat

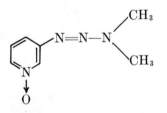

by various routes with *N*-nitrosodimethylamine which induced hepatocellular carcinomas, cholangiocarcinomas, and hemangioendotheliomas (*129, 131, 132*). In this species, liver tumors were induced in adult animals by a single oral dose of *N*-nitrosodimethylamine (*130*). Herrold (*131*) investigated the histogenesis of these liver tumors induced by *N*-nitrosodimethylamine and claimed that hemangioendotheliomas and cholangiocarcinomas arise from the sinusoidal endothelial cells and intraephatic bile ducts and not from hepatic cells. Liver tumors of various histological types were also induced in this species with other nitrosamines (*210, 216, 379*).

An example of species specificity by *N*-nitroso compounds is the cyclic nitrosamine, *N*-nitrosoazetidine, which induced tumors of the liver and other organs in rats and mice (*239*) but did not have any carcinogenic effect in hamsters (*240*).

The livers of many other animal species, including subhuman primates, were susceptible to the carcinogenic action of *N*-nitroso dimethyl- or -diethyl-amine. Benign and malignant parenchymal cell tumors were induced most frequently although other tumor types were observed in some species, such as leiomyosarcomas in dogs, reticulosarcomas in pigs, and cholangiomatous tumors in guinea pigs, *Mastomys*, and fish.

The Urinary System. KIDNEY. In adult rats kidney tumors developed after treatment with dialkyl and cyclic nitrosamines and with acyl alkyl nitrosamides (*see* Table II). These tumors were induced mainly with single or repeated high doses over a short time. An incidence of 85–100% of kidney tumors was obtained after six successive daily doses of 5–10 mg/kg of

Continued

Principal Organs Affected	*References*
central and peripheral nervous system, heart, hematopoietic system, mammary glands	*368, 369*
mammary glands, central and peripheral nervous system, hematopoietic system, ear duct	*368*

British Journal of Cancer

N-nitrosodimethylamine (*101, 380*). A single dose of 30 mg/kg induced renal tumors in 20% of the surviving rats (*97*). Although this is true for most of the *N*-nitroso compounds, a high incidence of renal tumors was reported following chronic administration of 17 mg/kg for 210 days (*110*). Newborn rats developed kidney tumors after a single injection of *N*-nitrosodimethyl amine or *N*-methyl-*N*-nitrosourea (*104, 106, 273*). Various 1-aryl-3-3-dialkyltriazenes administered either as single or repeated doses produced kidney tumors (*368*). *N*-Nitrosodiethylamine induced adenomas of the kidney in rats at doses as low as 1.25 or 2.5 mg/kg (*153*).

It was shown recently that rats on a protein-deficient diet at the time of administration of a single intraperitoneal dose of 60 mg/kg of *N*-nitrosodimethylamine are protected against its lethal acute effects and that kidney tumors developed in all surviving rats after 8–11 months (*381, 382*).

There are two types of tumors produced in the kidney of adult and newborn rats—epithelial and anaplastic (undifferentiated) cell tumors. The epithelial tumors have been described as adenomas, clear cell, and dark cell carcinomas. They appear as multiple growths, with tubular papillary or solid structure, localized in the cortical region. Their morphology has been well described by light and/or electron microscopy (*87, 97, 108, 383, 384, 385, 386, 387*). Various authors agree that adenomas and clear cell carcinomas originate from the epithelium of the proximal convoluted tubules (*87, 97, 103, 387, 388*), but the dark cell carcinomas may arise from both tubular epithelial cells and metanephrogenic tissue cells (*385*). The epithelial cell tumors seem to occur more frequently in male rats and the mesenchymal type in females, suggesting some hormonal influence on the development of these tumors (380).

The second tumor type usually appears as a large growth with a tendency to necrosis and hemorrhage and in some instances to invade the perirenal tissues. Histologically, it is composed of a multiplicity of structures and tissue types and has been referred to as anaplastic (97), nephroblastoma (101, 110, 380, 389), Wilm's tumor (145), anaplastic epithelial tumor (99), renal sarcoma (390), embryonal cell tumor and hemangioendothelioma (385, 391), stromal nephroma 103), and mesenchymal tumor (87, 383, 392).

The histogenesis of these tumors induced by N-nitrosodimethylamine was investigated extensively by light and electron microscopy by Hard and Butler (393, 394). They suggest that the neoplasms originate from interstitial mesenchymal cells within the renal cortex, probably of vascular origin, which show signs of intracellular injury after 24 hr of carcinogenic treatment and after three to six weeks give rise to differentiated cell forms characteristic of the tumor. Moreover, the authors claimed, as did Riopelle and Jasmin (103), that the epithelial tumors, which sometimes developed together with the mesenchymal tumors, are histogenetically a different tumor type originating from the tubular epithelial cells. In contrast, other authors (110, 385, 389) concluded that both types of neoplasms arise from the metanephrogenic tissue or the remains of the metanephrogenic cells in the interstitial areas of the kidney capable of bipotential differentiation into epithelial as well as mesenchymal tumors and that the hemangioendotheliomas derived from the blood capillaries. The mesenchymal tumors have been successfully transpalnted (395).

In some strains of mice, adenomas and adenocarcinomas of the kidney have been induced with N-nitrosodimethylamine (114, 117), N-methyl-N-nitrosourea (273), and N-ethyl-N-nitrosourea (303, 307). In Syrian golden hamsters only one adenoma of the kidney was induced with N-nitrosodimethylamine (130). N-Nitrosodiethylamine induced hyperplasic lesions but not tumors of this organ (167).

BLADDER. Bladder tumors have been induced in rats, mice, golden and Chinese hamsters, and guinea pigs by N-nitrosodibutylamine (see Table II). Variations in administration route, dose, and species lead to significant changes in its carcinogenic action.

In rats, oral administration of N-nitrosodibutylamine induced liver and esophageal tumors, but a higher incidence of bladder tumors was observed after subcutaneous injection (194, 195). The same is true for mice (200) and hamsters (202). A metabolite of N-nitrosodibutylamine, which has been identified as N-nitrosobutyl-4-hydroxybutylamine, induced only bladder tumors (195, 229). Another metabolite (N-nitrosobutyl-3-carboxypropylamine) is a potent and selective bladder carcinogen in the rat (235). These two substances were also carcinogenic for rat bladders following their direct application into the bladder (233). The fact that in ICR mice bladder tumors were not induced (396) was attributed to the low dose level of N-nitrosodibutylamine used (199). In C57Bl/6 mice an interesting sex difference was observed in the induction of bladder tumors. The male was more susceptible than the female, and a hormonal influence or difference in metabolic detoxification could be responsible for this response (*199*).

Morphologically, the tumors in the various species are papillomas, transitional and squamous cell carcinomas of multifocal origin with invasive pattern resembling human bladder tumors. The histogenesis of these tumors in rats was examined by various authors (*196, 197, 229*) who showed that hyperplasia and papilloma of the urinary bladder epithelium are precursors of bladder cancer. Cells of a transitional cell carcinoma induced by *N*-nitroso-butyl-4-hydroxybutylamine were successfully maintained in culture for 71 passages and, when injected subcutaneously into rats, grew and appeared morphologically similar to the original bladder tumor (*397*). A tumor line from a transitional cell carcinoma induced in mice by *N*-nitrosodibutylamine was also established (*398*).

Papillomas and transitional cell carcinomas of the pelvis and ureters were occasionally seen after treatment with *N*-nitrosobutyl-4-hydroxybutylamine (*231*), and their incidence could be greatly increased after one ureter was ligated (*399*), suggesting that concentration of the carcinogen is important in inducing tumors in the urinary system. Recently, Hicks and Wakefield (*275*) successfully produced a high incidence of transitional cell carcinomas of the bladder in rats after 30 weeks with four doses of 1.5 mg of *N*-methyl-*N*-nitroso-urea administered over six weeks by direct intravesicular instillation through a urethral catheter.

Nasal Cavities. *N*-Nitroso compounds and some related compounds, given by various administration routes, induce malignant tumors of the nasal cavities in mice, rats, and hamsters (*see* Table II).

Skin application or subcutaneous injection of *N*-nitrosodiethylamine or *N*-nitrosobutylamine induced squamous cell carcinomas of the nasal cavities in mice (*157, 158, 163, 214*). Rats and hamsters, after treatment with numerous *N*-nitroso compounds, developed different histological tumors—squamous cell papillomas, squamous cell carcinomas, or adenocarcinomas—which were mainly localized in the anterior or respiratory regions. Neuroepithelial tumors developed in the posterior or ethmoid region and were considered to be of neural origin. The pathology of these tumors is well described in rats (*107*) and hamsters (*169, 170, 172*). Macroscopically, they showed in some instances a marked swelling of the nasal and orbital regions, invading the surrounding tissues and infiltrating the olfactory bulbs and the frontal lobes of the brain.

The nasal cavities are particularly susceptible to these groups of carcinogens, and tumors of this site were induced in rats by a single dose of various nitrosamines (*148*) or after chronic inhalations of *N*-nitrosobutylmethylamine at a dose as low as 0.05 ppm (*213*). A single injection of 11 mg/kg of *N*-nitrosodiethylamine to newborn hamsters induced malignant tumors of the nasal cavities (*173*). A particular organotropism within this organ has been observed with *N*-nitrosodimethylamine which induced in hamsters only tumors of the posterior region (esthesioneuroepitheliomas) and not of the anterior or respiratory region of the nasal cavities (*131*). In comparison, N-nitroso-diethylamine induced tumors of both the olfactory and respiratory epithelium (*168*).

Respiratory Tract. The susceptibility of the respiratory tract to carcinogenic N-nitroso compounds was reported in various strains of mice, rats, and hamsters (*see* Table II) (*401*). Lung tumors were produced in practically all strains of mice tested with various N-nitroso compounds; however, there are some interesting variations in response among various strains and different N-nitroso compounds. Takayama and Oota (*114*) compared the carcinogenicity of N-nitrosodimethyl– and diethylamine in different strains of mice and found that the former compound was more potent than the latter in inducing lung tumors and that the ddN and ICR strains were more susceptible than the C3H. In Balb/c mice, Clapp *et al.* (*119*) reported 50% incidence of lung tumors with N-nitrosodimethylamine while N-nitrosodiethylamine was only slightly effective. In contrast, high incidence of lung tumors was induced in RF mice with both carcinogens. The tumors were solitary or multiple adenomas and/or adenocarcinomas localized usually in the periphery of the lung and showing local invasiveness and metastases (*114*).

Respiratory tumors of various histological types (squamous cell carcinoma, alveolar cell carcinoma, and adenocarcinoma) were induced in rats after systemic administration of N-nitrosodipentylamine and N-methyl-N-nitrosourethane (*7*). Oral administration of some cyclic nitrosamines (N-nitrosoazetidine, N-nitrosohepta- and N-nitrosooctamethyleneamine) produced a high incidence of respiratory tumors in a short period, and most of the tumors were squamous cell carcinoma (*239, 259*). In comparison, another cyclic nitrosamine, N-nitrosohexamethyleneamine gives rise to esophageal and liver tumors but does not have a carcinogenic effect in the lung (*256*).

The respiratory tract of the Syrian golden hamster seems particularly susceptible to the carcinogenic action of N-nitroso compounds (*see* Table II). In this species, the nitrosamine most extensively investigated was N-nitroso-diethylamine (*165, 166, 167, 168, 172, 173*). The carcinogenic response in adult and newborn hamsters to this nitrosamine followed a distinct pattern for the different segments of the respiratory system; the upper part (trachea and larynx) showed the highest tumor yield whereas the tumor response in the lower respiratory tract remained very low (*172*). This organ specificity was not influenced by the route of administration (*168*). Tumors of the trachea and larynx were multiple and often obstructed the lumen. Histologically they were papillary growths lined either by cuboidal mucus-secreting cells or squamous cells with patches of cells with anaplastic features. Although no signs of invasion or metastases were present, successful transplantation of these tumors was reported (*168*). Tumors of the lung parenchyma were of different histological type with a varying degree of malignancy. In addition, atypical hyperplasia and squamous metaplasia were observed. In adult hamsters, a positive dose response correlation for tumor induction in the upper respiratory tract was demonstrated following multiple injections of N-nitroso-diethylamine (*172*). Single subcutaneous doses of the same compound, rang-

ing from 40 to 0.3 mg/kg were tested by Mohr *et al.* (*171*), and tracheal
tumors were observed with doses as low as 7.5 mg/kg. The hamsters were
killed at 25 weeks of age, and the tumor incidence varied from 20 to 80%.
A smaller dose of *N*-nitrosodiethylamine (4 mg/kg) induced a 10% incidence
of tracheal papillomas in hamsters followed for their life span (*215*). In newborn hamsters a high yield of respiratory tumors was induced with a single
dose as low as 5.5 mg/kg of *N*-nitrosodiethylamine (*173*).

Other dialkyl and cyclic nitrosamines were carcinogenic in the respiratory tract of hamsters (*see* Table II). *N*-Nitrosodimethylamine is inactive in
the induction of hyperplastic or neoplastic changes of the respiratory epithelium of this species (*129, 130, 131, 132, 133*), showing the specificity of the
carcinogenic effect of these compounds for certain organs and type of
epithelium.

Alimentary Tract. ESOPHAGUS. Neoplasms of the esophagus are one
of the most common types of tumor to occur after treatment with *N*-nitroso
compound. These are squamous cell papillomas and carcinomas which mainly
occur at the site of physiological contractures of the organ and show keratini-
zation and horny pearls. Their morphology and histogenesis were described
in detail by Napalkov and Pozharisski (*221*), Gibel (*402*), and Ito *et al.*
(*403*), indicating that hyperplastic changes and papilloma are the precursors
of the squamous cell carcinomas. Some of the hyperplastic and papillomatous
changes, which appear as early as four weeks after oral administration of
N-nitrosopiperidine, apparently regress once treatment ceases, suggesting that
these lesions are reversible, as observed in the skin (*403*). In some instances,
tumors of the pharynx, tongue, and soft palate are reported in addition to the
esophageal tumors.

The administration route does not seem to be important in the induction
of esophageal tumors, which are mainly observed after oral administration
but also after intravenous and subcutaneous injection (*7*). The schedule of
administration does, however, appear important when determining the tumor
yield. For example, dialkyl and cyclic nitrosamines (*147, 256, 404*), induced
a higher incidence of esophageal tumors when administered at low doses for
a longer period than at high doses over short periods. Although this change
in incidence pattern is not understood, the reversibility of some precancerous
lesions following the interruption of treatment may explain it.

STOMACH. Various *N*-nitroso compounds induce tumors of the forestomach in rats, mice, and hamsters. The acyl alkyl nitrosamides are the
most effective. These tumors developed after oral administration and intravenous or intraperitoneal injections with, for example, *N*-methyl-*N*-nitrosourea
in rats (*7, 148, 273*). Single doses were also effective, as shown with *N*-methyl-
N-nitrosobiuret which produced a high incidence of forestomach tumors as
well as other tumors with oral doses ranging from 25 to 400 mg/kg (*405*).
Morphologically, these tumors were squamous cell papillomas and carcinomas
and have been described by Schoental and Magee (*90*) and Toledo (*406*) in
rats treated with *N*-methyl-*N*-nitrosourethane.

Recently, tumors of the glandular stomach were reported in many animal species with various acyl alkyl nitrosamides (*see* Table II). *N*–Acetyl-*N'*-methyl-*N'*-nitrosourea administered in the drinking water to rats at 2 mg/kg induced exclusively adenocarcinomas of the glandular stomach in all treated rats with an average induction time of 74 weeks (*344*). In guinea pigs, neoplasms of the stomach (which is only glandular as in man) were induced with *N*-methyl-*N*-nitrosourea and *N*-methyl–*N*-nitrosourethane (*293, 407*). Another compound, *N*-methyl-*N'*-nitro-*N*-nitrososoguanidine, was extensively tested and induced tumors of the stomach in rats, hamsters, and dogs, mostly localized in the pyloric region of the glandular stomach (*336*). The influence of the administration schedule of this carcinogen on the type of tumor induced and its location within the stomach was also extensively investigated in rats and hamsters. Administration in the drinking water of *N*-methyl-*N'*-nitro-*N*-nitrosoguanidine at a low concentration for a short period produced mainly adenocarcinomas of the glandular stomach in rats whereas a high concentration or a longer period of treatment induced mainly tumors of the forestomach and small intestine. These differences were attributed to the fact that adenocarcinomas of the glandular stomach develop later in life, and higher doses of the carcinogen are necessary to produce tumors of the forestomach or small intestine (*331, 332*). Schoental and Bensted (*328*) obtained tumors of the forestomach and not of the glandular stomach by oral administration. Sugimura *et al.* (*336*) suggested that these discrepancies may be explained by the fact that *N*-methyl-*N'*-nitro-*N*-nitrosoguanidine given in the drinking water directly reaches the pylorus region of the glandular stomach where it exerts its carcinogenic action. This was also confirmed by the finding of greater radioactivity in the glandular stomach than in the forestomach in an experiment using ^{14}C-labeled *N*-methyl-*N'*-nitro-*N*-nitrosoguanidine. In hamsters, high doses induced fibrosarcomas of the glandular stomach which appear relatively early in life whereas lower concentrations and a shorter exposure allowed, in addition, the development of adenocarcinomas (*332, 336*). Mice appear more resistant to the induction of stomach tumors, although atypical hyperplastic changes were reported in mice receiving continuous administration of 125 μg/ml of *N*-methyl-*N'*-nitro-*N*-nitrosoguanidine (*336*).

The morphological changes of the glandular stomach of rats receiving continuous treatment with *N*-methyl-*N'*-nitro-*N*-nitrosoguanidine in the drinking water were examined by Saito *et al.* (*408*). After atrophy and erosion of the mucosa a regenerative glandular hyperplasia developed within the first five weeks followed by an atypical adenomatoid hyperplasia at 20 weeks. Adenocarcinomas, showing in some instances areas of squamous, osseous, and cartilaginous metaplasia, appeared at 30 weeks and progressively invaded the submucosa, the muscularis mucosa, and the serosa.

INTESTINE. Tumors of this organ are induced by relatively few *N*-nitroso compounds, and the dialkyl-, cyclic nitrosamines, and the nitrosamines with a functional group are noncarcinogenic for the intestine. In contrast, some acylalkylnitrosamides (*see* Table II) were shown to induce intestinal neoplasms. *N*-Methyl-*N*-nitrosourea administered either orally or systemically induced tumors mainly of the large intestine and to a lesser degree of the

small intestine, and single high doses were more effective than fractionated
small doses (*91, 148, 267, 273*). The hamster and the rabbit, but not the
mouse, also developed intestinal tumors with the same compound (*291, 296*).
Intestinal tumors were observed in rats following intraperitoneal injections of
N-methyl- or *N*-ethylnitrosourethane (*303*). Some related carcinogens, including *N*-methyl-*N*'-nitro-*N*-nitrosoguanidine and *N*-ethyl-*N*'-nitro-*N*-nitrosoguani-
dine, produced tumors of the small and large intestine (*see* Table II).

Some 1,2-dialkylhydrazines, azo- and azoxy alkanes are selective intestinal
carcinogens. In rats, 1,2-dimethylhydrazine administered at weekly intervals
either subcutaneously (7–21 mg/kg) or orally (21 mg/kg) yielded a 100%
incidence of malignant adenocarcinomas of the intestine, most of which were
localized in the colon and rectum (*346, 347*). A single subcutaneous dose
(200 mg/kg) of the same compounds also induced tumors of the colon as well
as kidney tumors whereas a low dose (3 mg/kg) administered continuously in
the drinking water resulted in the induction of liver tumors only (*347*). Similarly, intestinal tumors were induced in mice and hamsters with 1,2-dimethyl-
hydrazine (*352, 353, 356, 357*). Azoxymethane is also effective in producing
malignant tumors of the colon and rectum in rats following weekly subcutaneous injections (2–12 mg/kg) or a single oral injection (16–30 mg/kg) (*347*).
The carcinogenic effect in the intestine appears less pronounced with 1-methyl-
2-butylhydrazine and methylazoxybutane (*347*). The fact that the ethyl compounds (1,2-diethylhydrazine, azo, and azoxyethane) induce tumors of other
organs but never intestinal tumors emphasizes the striking organotropism of
these carcinogens, as observed with the *N*-nitroso compounds (*361, 362*).

Nervous System. Among the various *N*-nitroso compounds, tumors of
the brain, the spinal cord, and the cranial and peripheral nerves were induced
only with the acyl alkyl nitrosamides in different animal species. In addition,
the related compounds (1-aryl-3,3-dialkyltriazenes, hydrazo-, azo-, and azoxy
alkanes appear very powerful carcinogens for the nervous system (*see* Table
II). The incidence and distribution of tumors within the nervous system
depend upon the dose, administration route, and chemical structure of the acyl
alkyl nitrosamides and upon the age of the animals. Single intravenous injections of 60–90 mg/kg of *N*-methyl-*N*-nitrosourea to adult rats resulted in
tumor production in the surviving rats after 305–380 days, with a low incidence in the nervous system (*7, 148*). The same compound given intravenously as fractionated smaller doses induced neurogenic tumors in more than
90% of the rats (*265, 267, 277*). Oral administration of *N*-methyl–*N*-nitroso-
urea gave less or even no tumors of the nervous system, but extraneural tumors,
mainly of the gastrointestinal tract, were induced (*91, 269, 271*). Druckrey
et al. (*300*) showed that a single subcutaneous injection of 20 mg/kg to newborn or 10-day-old rats resulted in an almost 100% incidence of malignant
tumors of the nervous system whereas a lower incidence was observed in
30-day-old rats. These data and the transplacental carcinogenesis studies with
acyl alkyl nitrosamides and other substances indicate the high carcinogenic
susceptibility of the developing nervous system in this species. Similarly, the
toxic effects of acyl alkyl nitrosamides in the nervous system vary with the

age of the animals, depending on the absence or presence of actively proliferating matrices. The highest vulnerability is observed during the perinatal
period in which cell proliferation occurs in the various matrices (409). That
there is no effect of antilymphocyte serum on the neurotropic carcinogenic
activity of N-methyl-N-nitrosourea suggests that the cell susceptibility to neoplastic transformation is more important in determining the organotropism
than the immunological surveillance (410).

Differences in incidence and distribution of neurogenic tumors induced
by N-methyl- and N-ethyl-N-nitrosourea were described among different
strains of rats and between male and female rats (277, 411, 412).

Tumors of the nervous system were also reported in rabbits and dogs
after administration of N-methyl-N-nitrosourea (294–299), and in adult hamsters with N-butyl-N-nitrosourea (323). In mice, a single intravenous or
subcutaneous injection of N-ethyl-N-nitrosourea induced tumors of the central
and peripheral nervous systems (305, 306), some of which are medulloblas-
tomas of the cerebellum which are rarely observed in rats.

The tumors of the central nervous system are generally multiple and are
preferentially located in the periventricular regions of the lateral ventricles
and subcortical white matter, less often in the spinal cord, and very rarely
in the cerebellum. Tumors of the peripheral nervous system developed more
frequently from the trigeminal nerves and the brachial and lumbrosacral
plexuses (277, 413, 414).

Most of the tumors of the central nervous system were malignant gliomas
with varying degrees of differentiation and anaplasia, and they were often
classified as oligodendrogliomas, astrocytomas, ependymomas, and glioblasto-
mas. Tumors of neuronal origin appear rarely, if at all (271, 297, 415). The
tumors of the peripheral nervous system are mainly malignant neurinomas,
which have been successfully transplanted (416, 417, 418). In these tumors a
nervous tissue specific protein, S-100 protein, and a highly specific activity of
2′,3′-cyclic nucleotide-3′-phosphohydrolase have been identified, suggesting the
participation of neuroectodermal cells in the neoplastic process (417, 419).
The histopathology of these tumors, induced in adult animals and after transplacental exposure with various N-nitroso compounds, was described and reviewed by various authors (277, 412, 414, 420) who pointed out some striking
similarities between these experimental tumors and the human neoplasms of
the nervous system regarding the basic morphological features and location
sites.

Hematopoietic System. Tumors of the lymphoreticular system were
reported in mice treated with various acyl alkyl nitrosamides (see Table II),
and they are mainly malignant lymphomas of thymic origin. A relatively low
incidence of leukemia developed in rats with N-ethyl-N-nitrosourea (7, 301),
azoethane (362), and various 1-aryl-3,3-dialkyl triazenes (see Table II). Recently, however, incidences of up to 100% of leukemia were reported in various strains of rats following chronic oral treatment with N-butyl-N-nitrosourea
(318, 319, 320, 321, 322). In contrast to the mouse, the rat developed mainly
leukemias of erythroblastic and stem-cell type and less frequently myeloid

leukemia; lymphoblastic sarcoma of thymic origin is extremely rare. Recently
C-type virus particles were identified by electron microscopy in primary,
transplantable, and cultured leukemia induced by *N*-butyl–*N*-nitrosourea in
WKA/MK rats (*421*).

Other Organs. Tumors of the skin were induced with *N*-methyl-*N*-
nitrosourea in mice, rats, and hamsters by topical applications (*266, 281, 282*)
and also by oral or intravenous administration in rats and rabbits (*91, 297*).
N-Methyl- and *N*-ethyl-*N'*-nitro-*N*-nitrosoguanidine applied to the skin of mice
induced skin tumors (*335*). *N*-nitrosodiethylamine administered by various
routes including topical applications to mice or hamsters produced tumors of
other organs but not of the skin (*157, 158, 168*). *N*-Butyl-*N*-nitrosourea induced a high yield of adenocarcinoma of the mammary glands in rats (*319,
321, 322*).

Tumors of certain organs, which in the past were difficult to observe
experimentally, were successfully induced, for example, in the pancreas of
guinea pigs by *N*-methyl-*N*-nitrosourea and *N*-methyl-*N*-nitrosourethane (*293*),
and odontogenic tumors in hamsters (*290*) and neoplasms in the heart (*369*)
(Table II) by *N*-methyl-*N*-nitrosourea and various 1-aryl-3,3-dialkyl triazenes,
respectively. Tumors of the testis (four papillary mesotheliomas, two interstitial cell tumors, and one cavernous hemangioma) were observed in seven
out of 12 rats fed with *N*-nitrosopyrrolidine for 67 weeks (*242*).

Transplacental Carcinogenesis. Neoplasms of the offspring as a
result of prenatal exposure to various *N*-nitroso compounds and related substances were demonstrated in different animal species, namely the rat, mouse,
Syrian golden hamster, and pig (Table III) (*422*). The pregnant animals
were treated by various administration routes (subcutaneous, intraperitoneal,
intravenous, oral, and inhalation) which were equally effective. However, a
critical factor was the time of treatment during gestation. In the rat, these
substances generally induced an embryotoxic effect when administered between days 1 and 10, a teratogenic effect between days 8 and 10, and a carcinogenic effect from day 10 to delivery. The relationship between embryo-
toxicity, teratogenicity, and carcinogenicity produced by various *N*-nitroso
compounds in rats was discussed by Napalkov and Alexandrov (*423*), Napalkov (*424*), and Druckrey (*425*).

Since many of these substances appear to be metabolically activated to
exert their carcinogenic action, the lack of an adequate metabolic system during the first period of pregnancy may explain the failure to observe tumors
when the exposure was limited to this period. *N*-Nitrosodimethylamine, azoxy-
urethane, and 1-phenyl-3,3-dimethyltriazene induced tumors in the offspring
only when administered during the last days of pregnancy (*425, 426*). In
keeping with these findings are the data of Magee (*427*) who detected the
formation of 7-methylguanine in nucleic acids of fetal rat tissues following
treatment at the 21st day of pregnancy but not at the 15th day, with ^{14}C–*N*-
nitrosodimethylamine.

Moreover, a striking difference was observed by Druckrey (*425*) between
methyl and ethyl derivatives of hydrazo-, azo-, and azoxy alkanes and 1-aryl-

Table III.   N-Nitroso Compounds and Related Substances

Compound	Species
N-Nitrosodimethylamine	rat
	mouse
N-Nitrosodiethylamine	rat
	mouse
	S.G. hamster
N-Methyl-N-nitrosourea	rat
	mouse
N-Ethyl-N-nitrosourea	rat
	mouse
	S.G. hamster
	pig
Ethylurea + sodium nitrite	rat
N-Nitroso-N-n-propylurea	rat
N-Ethyl-N-nitrosobiuret	rat
N-Methyl-N-nitrosourethane	rat
Azoxymethane	rat
1,2-Diethylhydrazine	rat
1-Benzyl-2-methylhydrazine	rat
Azoethane	rat
Azoxyethane	rat
1-Phenyl-3,3-dimethyltriazene	rat
1-Phenyl-3,3-diethyltriazene	rat
1-Pyridyl-3,3-diethyltriazene	rat
N-Isopropyl-α-2-(methyl-hydrazino)-p-toluamide	rat

3,3-dialkyl triazenes in transplacental carcinogenesis in rats. The ethyl derivatives produced tumors of the offspring when administered at the 15th day of pregnancy, but the corresponding methyl derivatives were active only during the last day of pregnancy. Among the acyl alkyl nitrosamides, N-ethyl-N-nitrosourea is more potent than the corresponding methyl derivative (428, 429, 430). The localization of tumors in the offspring is similar to that in adult animals treated with the same N-nitroso compounds.

The sensitivity of the nervous system in the various stages of prenatal development was examined by Ivankovic and Druckrey (429) using N-ethyl-N-nitrosourea which was administered to BD rats as a single dose on every day of pregnancy. A high incidence was observed when this carcinogen was given on the 18th day or shortly before delivery, and no tumors developed when the carcinogen was administered before the 12th day. A positive dose response was obtained following exposure at the 15th day of pregnancy to single doses ranging from 5 to 80 mg/kg. The lowest dose level, which corresponds to 2% of the LD_{50}, still produced a 63% incidence of malignant

Inducing Tumors Following Transplacental Exposure

Principal Organs Affected in the Offspring	*References*
kidney	*426*
lung and liver	*437*
kidney, mammary glands, nasal cavities and thymus	*438, 439*
lung, liver, esophagus, and forestomach	*440, 441*
trachea	*442, 443*
kidney and nervous system	*280, 444*
lung and liver	*437*
nervous system and kidney	*411, 412, 429, 432*
	445, 446, 447
lung, liver, nervous system, and hematopoietic system	*288, 448, 449*
nervous system	*429*
sweat glands and skin	*450*
nervous system	*451, 452*
nervous system	*453*
nervous system	*343*
kidney, nervous system, ovary, liver, mammary glands	*424, 454*
kidney, nervous system	*425*
nervous system	*455*
nervous system and kidney	*425*
nervous system	*455*
nervous system	*455*
nervous system and kidney	*425*
nervous system	*425*
nervous system	*425*
nervous system	*456*

neurogenic tumors. A dose as low as 2 mg/kg, 0.8% of LD_{50}, was also sufficient to show a carcinogenic response in the nervous system. In comparison, a dose of 160 mg/kg of *N*-ethyl-*N*-nitrosourea was necessary to induce in adult rats a 50% incidence of neurogenic tumors, showing that the sensitivity of the nervous system during prenatal development is about 50 times higher than in adults (*431*). Similar results were obtained by Swenberg *et al.* (*432*) in Sprague–Dawley and Fisher rats using a dose as low as 1 mg/kg during the end of gestation. Some strain differences were observed in transplacental carcinogenesis studies with *N*-ethyl-*N*-nitrosourea, indicating that Sprague–Dawley and Long–Evans rats were more susceptible than BD rats (*412, 433*). Similar observations were made by Druckrey *et al.* (*411*) using 10 inbred strains of BD rats. The high sensitivity of the fetal nervous system has been demonstrated with other substances (Table III), and the importance of these findings in human neurooncology has been discussed (*414, 434*).

Mice appear less susceptible than rats to the induction of neurogenic tumors by *N*-methyl- or *N*-ethylnitrosourea (*288, 435*). A new and interesting finding was observed by Tomatis *et al.* (*436*) who detected tumors of the kidney and central nervous system not only in the offspring of rats treated with a single dose of *N*-methyl-*N*-nitrosourea at the 19th day of pregnancy, but also in the second generation. These findings suggest that the information for the neoplastic transformation is carried by the first generation to the second.

Carcinogenesis in Vitro. Huberman *et al.* (*457*) reported that treatment of normal hamster cells *in vitro* with *N*-nitrosodimethylamine increased cell proliferation and lifespan, followed at eight months by production of colonies in agar and formation of tumors after transplantation into syngeneic hosts. The biological transformation (tumor growth) was, however, attributed to secondary changes rather than to a direct effect of the carcinogen. An increase in cell proliferation was also observed in rat liver cells exposed *in vitro* to the same carcinogen (*458*). Morphological or biological transformation of Chinese hamster lung cells or Syrian hamster embryo cells was not observed with *N*-nitrosodimethyl- or diethylamine (*459, 460*). However, when *N*-nitrosodiethylamine was administered to pregnant hamsters on day 12 of gestation and the total embryo explants were cultured *in vitro* on day 14, morphological transformation frequently occurred (*460*). Recently rat epithelial-like liver cells treated *in vitro* with *N*-nitrosodimethylamine developed carcinomas following their injection into syngeneic rats (*461, 462*).

Malignant transformation *in vitro* was more often observed with acyl alkyl nitrosamides, such as *N*-methyl-*N*-nitrosourea and *N*-methyl-*N'*-nitro-*N*-nitrosoguanidine which do not seem to require metabolic activation (*460, 463, 464, 465*). The transformation *in vitro* is the result of sequential events in which increased plating efficiency of treated cells, often accompanied by morphological and behavioral changes, appears first, followed by the appearance of morphologically transformed colonies and finally by the ability of such cells to produce tumors after transplantation in a suitable host. Recently Di Mayorca *et al.* (*466*) reported that brief exposure of a suspension of BHK_{21} LC 13 cells to *N*-nitrosodimethylamine or *N*-methyl-*N*-nitrosourea resulted in malignant transformation as determined by plating in soft agar. In addition, they observed that the transformed phenotype of cell transformed by these compounds is temperature dependent. Recently, Borland and Hard (*467*) reported that kidney cells originating from rats treated *in vivo* with a single dose of *N*-nitrosodimethyamine appear to behave *in vitro* as transformed cells showing a prolonged lifespan, morphological transformation, increased mitotic index, colony production in soft agar, and agglutination by Concanavalin A.

The *in vitro* system was used to examine interactions between viral and chemical carcinogens, and Freeman *et al.* (*468*) observed morphological transformation of rat embryo cells treated simultaneously with *N*-nitrosodiethylamine and RLV or CF-1 murine leukemia virus but not with the nitrosamine or the virus alone. However, they failed to observe tumor growth in homologous strain rats inoculated with the transformed cells. Frei and Oliver (*463*) were unable to demonstrate by various tests (COMUL test, the density gradient isolation of ^{3}H-uridine-labeled virus, and the XC rat-cell line mixed culture cytopathogenicity test) a murine leukemia virus in malignant mouse embryo cells transformed with N-methyl-N-nitrosourea. *In vivo* N-nitrosodimethylamine had no apparent effect on the development of malignant lymphomas in AKR mice (*116*)—a species in which a virus has been identified and shown to play a role in this process (*469*).

Modifying Factors. The influence of hormones on carcinogenesis by N-nitroso compounds was investigated to a small extent compared with other carcinogens. Goodall (*470*) demonstrated that hypophysectomy in rats failed to inhibit liver carcinogenesis by N-nitrosodimethylamine, in contrast to the well known inhibitory action of this procedure on carcinogenesis by aflatoxin, N-2-fluoreylacetamide, and azo dyes. Similar levels of methylation of rat liver nucleic acid by N-nitrosodimethylamine were found in intact and hypophysectomized rats (*471*). Orchidectomy had no effect on the induction of neurogenic tumors by N-methyl-N-nitrosourea in rats (*472*). In some experimental conditions, however, a hormonal influence was suggested. Reuber and Lee (*151*) found that the incidence of liver tumors was higher in Buffalo rats in which the treatment with N-nitrosodiethylamine was started at four weeks of age and progressively decreased as the age of the rats at the start of treatment increased. The greatest incidence of liver carcinomas was observed in females of the younger age groups. A clearer sex difference was observed by Vesselinovich (*121*) in (C57B x C3H) F_1 hybrid mice treated with six injections of N-nitrosodimethylamine at three-day intervals starting at seven days of age, which developed liver tumors more frequently in males than in females. The observations of Ivankovic (*473*), who found a 40% incidence of malignant tumors of the ovaries, uterus, or vagina in rats treated during pregnancy while treatment of nonpregnant rats with this carcinogen rarely induced these tumors, strongly suggesting the importance of hormonal influences.

Takizawa and Yamasaki (*321*) showed that ovariectomy and orchidectomy inhibit the development of mammary tumors in W/Fu rats treated with N-butyl-N-nitrosourea. A supplementary treatment with progesterone and estrogen or with an ovarian graft restored mammary tumor development in the castrated males and, to a lesser degree, in ovariectomized female rats. The higher susceptibility of male compared with female C57B1/6 mice treated with N-nitrosodibutylamine or N-nitrosobutyl-4-hydroxybutylamine in the induction of bladder tumors was attributed to the sex hormonal status of the animal (*199, 234*).

The importance of metabolic activation in the toxic effects of nitrosamines is well documented, and the influence on nitrosamine carcinogenesis of various substances known to interfere with drug metabolizing enzymes was examined. Aminoacetonitrile prevents the toxic and carcinogenic effects of N-nitrosodimethylamine in rat liver (*375, 474*) and inhibits the metabolism of this carcinogen *in vivo* and *in vitro* (*475, 476*). Similar findings are reported with a protein-deficient diet, which protects rats against acute liver damage by N-nitrosodimethylamine but increases late carcinogenic action in the kidney (*382, 477*). This effect was associated with decreased metabolism of the carcinogens in the liver but not in other organs (*478*). An increased incidence of kidney tumors was observed following a single dose of *N*-nitrosodimethylamine given after a single dose of carbon tetrachloride, and this effect was related to the reduced metabolism in the liver (*372, 479*). However, no significant difference in tumor incidence was observed in rats treated with *N*-nitrosodiethylamine and restricted to a dietary intake poor in protein (*480, 481*). A decrease of liver tumors and an increase of stomach tumors were claimed by Kunz *et al.* (*162*) in mice treated simultaneously with *N*-nitrosodiethylamine and phenobarbitone. Apparently contradictory results were obtained with DL-tryptophan which definitely enhanced the incidence of liver tumors in rats induced by *N*-nitrosodiethylamine whereas a decrease was observed with *N*-nitrosodibutylamine (*198, 482*). Another substance, dibenamine, reduced the hepatocarcinogenicity in rats by *N*-nitrosodimethylamine, probably by interference in its metabolism (*483*). Further biological and biochemical studies on the effect of these agents which interfere with the detoxification system of the liver appear extremely important because they may represent a unique experimental model to differentiate toxicity from carcinogenicity of *N*-nitroso compounds and to explain their particular carcinogenic organotropism in extrahepatic tissues.

There have been several reports of additive or synergistic effects on nitrosamine carcinogenesis. Hoch-Ligeti *et al.* (*111*) suggested an additive effect in lung tumor induction in rats following combined feeding with 3-methylcholanthrene and *N*-nitrosodimethylamine, but the small number of rats used does not allow a proper evaluation. Recently an increased incidence of lung and kidney tumors was reported in mice treated with 3-methylcholanthrene and *N*-nitrosodimethylamine when compared with control groups (*484*). Dontenwill (*485*) and Wynder and Hoffmann (*486*) reported enhanced bronchial metaplasia and tracheal papilloma formation in *N*-nitrosodiethylamine-treated hamsters by subsequent exposure to cigarette smoke, volatile acids, aldehydes, and methyl nitrite. Montesano *et al.* (*487*) showed that preliminary systemic treatment of hamsters with a relatively low dose of *N*-nitrosodiethylamine (which by itself induces few lung tumors) prepares the lung parenchyma to respond with a high susceptibility to subsequent intratracheal instillations of benzo(*a*)pyrene and/or ferric oxide particles. The possibility that the lung tumors could result from mechanical transplantation into the lower respiratory tract of cells originating from the papillomas of the trachea that developed following *N*-nitrosodiethylamine was discussed by Feron *et al.* (*488*). However, these workers obtained similar results after simultaneous intratracheal instillations of *N*-nitrosodiethylamine and ferric oxide particles and claimed that electron microscopic studies of these lung tumors indicated that they originate from alveolar cells. Squamous cell carcinomas of the tracheobronchial tract were observed only in hamsters treated with a low effect dose schedule of benzo(*a*)pyrene plus ferric oxide given intratracheally followed by a low dose of *N*-nitrosodiethylamine given systemically. Administration of single carcinogens did not cause similar tumors (*489*). A significant increase of lung tumors was observed in mice infected with influenza viruses and treated with *N*-nitrosodiethylamine as compared with mice receiving the nitrosamine alone (*490*). Similar findings are reported by Schreiber *et al.* (*491*) who observed that, with *N*-nitrosoheptamethyleneimine, there was a higher tumor response in the lung of rats suffering from chronic murine pneumonia than in specific pathogen-free or germ-free rats.

Modifying effects in nitrosamine carcinogenesis were reported in a few other systems. Kowalewski and Todd (*132*) induced a 68% incidence of adenocarcinomas of the gall bladder in hamsters having implanted intracholecystic cholesterol pellets while only one gall bladder tumor was observed out of 16 control *N*-nitrosodimethylamine-treated animals. A higher incidence of liver tumors than in the control groups was observed in mice treated chronically with *N*-nitrosodiethylamine and infected with a hepatitis-causing virus (Motol virus) (*492*). No significant differences from the respective control groups were observed in the induction of liver and bladder tumors in Fisher strain rats treated simultaneously with *N*-2-fluorenylacetamide and *N*-nitrosodiethyl-, dipentyl-, or dibutylamine, probably because of the high doses used (*493*). Montesano *et al.* (*481*) reported an additive effect in the induction of kidney tumors in rats treated with a single dose of *N*-nitrosodimethylamine and ethyl methanesulfonate. Whole body radiation did not have any effect on bladder tumor production in rats treated with *N*-nitrosodibutylamine (*494*).

Toxicity and carcinogenicity of various alkylnitrosoureas increased when these substances were administered with copper, nickel, or cobalt ions (*495*, *496*). In another study, a similar incidence of hepatic tumors was observed in rats treated with *N*-nitrosodimethylamine and fed either a copper-deficient or an excess copper diet whereas kidney tumors occurred in 57% of the rats receiving the copper-deficient diet and no tumors occurred in the group receiving the excess copper diet and *N*-nitrosodimethylamine (*497*). Rogers *et al.* (*498*) examined the effect of a diet high in fat and marginally deficient in lipotropes on the carcinogenicity of various dialkylnitrosamines. They observed enhancement of liver tumors with *N*-nitrosodiethylamine and *N*-nitrosodibutylamine but not with *N*-nitrosodimethylamine.

Metabolism. Since the reviews by Magee and Barnes (*6*) and by Druckrey *et al.* (*7*), aspects of the metabolism and possible mechanisms of biological action of the nitrosamines were discussed by several authors (*500–508*). Relationships between the electronic structure of dialkylnitrosamines and the carcinogenic mechanisms were discussed by Nagata and Imamura (*509*), and the valuable articles by Miller (*510*) and by Miller and Miller (*511*) relate the nitrosamines to other chemical carcinogens. The published *Proceedings of the 2nd International Symposium of the Princess Takamatsu Cancer Research Fund* (*512*) contains a number of important papers on the metabolism and mechanism of action of carcinogenic *N*-nitroso compounds. No attempt is made to cover all the relevant literature here because of space limitations.

METABOLISM OF NITROSAMINES *in Vivo* and *in Vitro*. The nitrosamines are stable chemically when not exposed to uv light while the nitrosamides are unstable in alkaline media and some decompose quite rapidly at neutral pH under physiological conditions. Photochemical decomposition gives nitrite in stoichiometric yield (513). The products of photochemical decomposition of N-nitrosodiethylamine were tested for carcinogenic action with negative results (514).

The decomposition rates of the nitrosamides vary with the nature of the compound and wtih pH (7, 515, 516, 517). In general, decomposition to form an alkylating agent occurs more rapidly at higher pH; but with some compounds (e.g., N-methyl-N-nitrosourea) it may occur at an appreciable rate under physiological conditions. Cysteine and other thiol compounds increase the decomposition rate of some nitrosamides, e.g., N-methyl-N-nitrosourethane (518) and N-methyl-N'-nitro-N-nitrosoguanidine (519, 520) but have no such effect on others, e.g., N-methyl-N-nitrosourea (520). N-Methyl-N-nitroso-p-toluenesulfonamide reacts with cysteine to yield p-toluenesulfonamide and the S-nitroso derivative of cysteine which decomposes to give cysteine and nitrous oxide. N-Methyl-N'-nitro-N-nitrosoguanidine reacts to give a substantial yield of 2-nitramino-4-carboxythiazoline with lesser amounts of cystine, N-methyl-N'-nitroguanidine, and S-methylcysteine (519). The extent and rate of alkylation of nucleic acids by nitrosamides in vitro are also affected by the presence of thiol compounds and are discussed later.

As expected, methyl- and ethylnitrosourea decompose rapidly in the animal body. Their respective half-lives after intravenous injection are about 2 min following a dose of 100 mg/kg body weight and 5-6 min after 200 mg/kg body weight (521, 522). Whole body autoradiography of rats killed 2 min after intravenous administration revealed widespread and apparently uniform distribution of radioactivity which presumably represented mainly the undegraded compound (523). Kawachi et al. (524, 525) studied the metabolism of N-methyl-N'-nitro-N-nitrosoguanidine labeled with ^{14}C in the methyl and guanidino groups respectively in rats after oral administration. About 40 and 60% of the radioactivity of the methyl- and guanidino-labeled materials were excreted in the urine within 24 hr and less than 3% in the feces. The major urinary metabolites appeared to be N-methyl-N'-nitroguanidine and nitroguanidine, and about 24 and 3% of the radioactivity were expired as $^{14}CO_2$ within 48 hr after giving the methyl- and guanidino-labeled materials, respectively. Only about 3% or less of the radioactivity remained in the body as acid insoluble materials at 24–48 hr. The nitroguanidine did not seem to originate from the N-demethylation of N-methyl-N'-nitroguanidine since no $^{14}CO_2$ was detected in expired air of rats nor ^{14}C-labeled formaldehyde in vitro with rat liver homogenate after treatment with methyl-labeled N-methyl-N'-nitroguanidine. It is suggested that the nitroguanidine is formed as a result of the nucleophilic attack of amino groups on the guanidine carbon (525).

Unlike the nitrosamides, the dialkylnitrosamines require enzyme activity for their decomposition, and they persist in the body unchanged for much longer periods (6, 504, 526). N-Nitrosodimethylamine is rapidly and fairly evenly distributed in the body after parenteral injection (527) and is metabolized completely in about 6 hr when given to rats at a dose of 30 mg/kg body weight. After intraperitoneal injection of ^{14}C-N-nitrosodimethylamine (30 mg/kg), acid-soluble radioactivity was maximal at 20 min with concentrations ranging from 16μg/100 mg in the liver to 10 μg/100 mg in muscle. Tissue-bond radioactivity reached a maximum at 8 hr after injection and showed greater variation between organs. Administration of ^{14}C-N-nitrosodimethylamine to animals is followed rapidly by the appearance of $^{14}CO_2$ in the expired air (*526*). In rats receiving 30 mg N-nitrosodimethylamine/kg body weight (slightly below the median lethal dose) about 65% of the injected radioactivity is expired during the first 12 hr. The rate of metabolism of this nitrosamine may vary considerably from animal to animal (*528*). N-Nitrosodiethylamine (200 mg/kg body weight) was metabolized at a rate of about 4% of the dose per hour in the rat. N-Nitrosomorpholine was fairly evenly distributed in the rat after intraperitoneal injection (*529*) and was eliminated more slowly from the body. Exhalation of $^{14}CO_2$ by rats given the radioactively labeled compounds at doses slightly below the median lethal level was (as a percentage of that injected) about 60% for N-nitrosodimethylamine, 45% for N-nitrosodiethylamine, and only 3% with N-nitrosomorpholine. The corresponding urinary excretions were about 4, 14, and 80%, respectively (*530*). There are surprisingly few studies of the urinary excretion of nitrosamines and their metabolites. Druckrey *et al.* (*195*) reported briefly on the metabolism of N-nitrosodibutylamine involving terminal hydroxylation and on the highly selective carcinogenic action of N-nitrosobutyl-4-hydroxybutylamine on rat bladder. Recently the metabolism of this compound was studied in the rat, and several metabolites were identified in the urine, including N-nitrosobutyl-3-carboxypropylamine, N-nitrosbutyl-3-carboxy-2-hydroxypropylamine, and the glucuronide of N-nitrosobutyl-4-hydroxybutylamine. None of the unchanged compound was found (*531*). The recent report of Hashimoto *et al.* (*235*) that N-nitrosobutyl-3-carboxypropylamine induced bladder tumors in rats is of interest in this connection. Blattman *et al.* (*532, 533, 534*) studied the urinary metabolites formed in rats following oral administration of a homologous series of dialkylnitrosamines from N-nitrosodiethylamine to N-nitrosodi-n-pentylamine. In agreement with the Japanese workers they found that the main metabolites containing the nitroso group were formed by ω-oxidation of the alkyl groups to give the corresponding alcohols and carboxylic acids. To a smaller extent ω$_{-1}$-oxidation anl alkyl chain shortening also occurred.

The metabolism rate of N-nitrosodimethylamine as well as its toxicity and carcinogenicity may be influenced by diet and other factors. Prior treatment of rats with a protein-deficient diet greatly reduced the toxicity of the nitrosamine with an almost twofold increase in the LD_{50} (*477, 535, 536*). Following the earlier observation that dietary protein deficiency reduced the metabolism rate of carbon tetrachloride with concomitant reduction in its toxicity (*537*), Swann and McLean (*381, 478*) demonstrated that the metabolism rate of N-nitrosodimethylamine was approximately halved in the protein-deficient rats. The incidence of kidney tumors in those animals surviving the larger single dose was 100%, in contrast to the 20% incidence obtained with rats on a normal diet surviving the maximally tolerated dose of N-nitrosodimethylamine (382). Similar effects on the induction of kidney tumors in rats by N-nitrosodimethylamine were obtained by prior exposure of the animals to a diet consisting only of sucrose (87). The protective action of amino-acetonitrile against the acute toxicity of N-nitrosodimethylamine (474) is associated with a marked reduction in the metabolism rate of the nitrosamine and in the methylation of nucleic acids ($475, 476$). This compound was also reported to reduce the carcinogenic action of N-nitrosodimethylamine on rat liver (375). The reduced toxicity of N-nitrosodimethylamine in rats and mice pretreated with tetraethylthiuramdisulfide (disulfiram, Antabuse) (538) is also associated with reduced alkylation of cellular components by this nitrosamine. However, no protective effects were observed against the toxic actions of N-nitrosodiethyl-, dipropyl-, dibutyl- or methylpropylamine. Treatment with disulfiram had no effect on carcinogenesis by N-nitrosodimethylamine (539) and thus resembled the action of chloramphenicol which reduced the toxicity of N-nitrosodiethylamine but did not affect its carcinogenic action (540). Pretreatment of mice with unlabeled N-nitrosodimethylamine in their drinking water followed by injection of the ^{14}C nitrosamine reduced methylation in the liver by a factor of about two with increases of varying extent in methylation in the lung and kidney (541). This effect was reversible after discontinuing the pretreatment with N-nitrosodimethylamine and was associated with a considerable inhibition of the enzyme responsible for N-demethylation of the nitrosamine in the liver microsomes, which was also reversible (542). Ethanol protects against the disaggregation of mouse liver polysomes by N-nitrosodimethylamine (543). All these factors which reduce the toxic and carcinogenic actions of N-nitrosodimethylamine seem to depend on reducing the ability of the liver to metabolize the compound or to increase formation of nontoxic or noncarcinogenic metabolites. In contrast, Somogyi *et al.* (544) recently reported protection against N-nitrosodimethylamine toxicity by pregnenolone-16α-carbonitrile, which does not affect the metabolism rate and must, therefore, act by some other mechanism. Although there are several reports of metabolism of the dimethyl- and other nitrosamines by microsomal systems ($6, 507$), the enzymes involved appear, under the conditions used, to have relatively low activity. It proved relatively simple to incubate the ^{14}C-labeled nitrosamine with tissue slices *in vitro* and to measure the production of $^{14}CO_2$ or methylation of the tissue nucleic acid. Using this method, Montesano and Magee (545) showed that N-nitrosodimethylamine is metabolized by human liver slices at a rate slightly slower but comparable with that of rat liver slices and concluded that this nitrosamine would probably be carcinogenic in man. The same procedure was used to compare the production of $^{14}CO_2$ from ^{14}C-N-nitrosodimethyl- and ^{14}C-N-nitrosodiethylamine by rat and hamster tissues *in vitro*. $^{14}CO_2$ production from hamster lung slices occurred at about the same rate as from hamster liver slices while production from lung with ^{14}C-N-nitrosodimethylamine was only a fraction of that with liver slices. Since liver tumors are induced by both nitrosamines in the hamster but lung tumors only with the diethyl compound, these results suggested that the organ-specific action might be explained, at least in part, by the varying capacities of the different tissues to metabolize the carcinogens (*546, 547*). The metabolism of *N*-nitrosodimethylamine by microsomal preparations *in vitro* was measured by the amount of formaldehyde produced. Using this method the highest levels of activity were found in the liver with lower levels in the kidney and other tissues (*548*).

The reported effects of known inducers of liver *N*-demethylase enzymes, such as phenobarbital or 3-methylcholanthrene, on demethylation of nitrosamines by liver microsomal preparations *in vitro* were atypical. Kato *et al.* (*549*) found that *N*-demethylation of *N*-nitrosodimethylamine and of *N*-nitrosomethylaniline by rat liver microsomes *in vitro* occurred at a greater rate than that of *N,N*-dimethyl-4-phenylazoaniline (4-dimethylaminoazobenzene) and that preparations from males were about 50% more active than those from females. Phenobarbital had no effect on the activity of female microsomes and slightly decreased the activity of male preparations. 3-Methylcholanthrene decreased the activity in both sexes. Venkatesan *et al.* (*550*) also observed reduction rather than stimulation of demethylation of *N*-nitrosodimethylamine by liver microsomes from rats pretreated with phenobarbital or 3-methylcholanthrene and other polycyclic hydrocarbons. Lung microsomes from untreated or pretreated animals were inactive. Pretreatment with 3-methylcholanthrene reduced the acute toxicity of the nitrosamine. The same authors (*551, 552*) studied the effects of 3-methylcholanthrene pretreatment and of various dietary factors on demethylation of *N*-nitrosodimethylamine in greater detail and concluded that the level of the enzyme in liver is under the control of multiple regulatory factors. Earlier work by the same group showed that feeding *N*-nitrosodimethylamine together with 3-methylcholanthrene to rats for about 25 weeks did not change the incidence of liver tumors but did induce lung tumors which were not induced by the nitrosamine alone (*111*).

The effects of inducers on metabolism of *N*-nitrosodiethylamine *in vitro* were studied by Magour and Nievel (*553*) who found increased acetaldehyde production with liver microsomal fractions from rats pretreated with phenobarbitone, 3-methylcholanthrene, butylated hydroxytoluene, or DDT. Simultaneous treatment with phenobarbitone lowered the toxicity of repeated doses of *N*-nitrosodiethylamine. Simultaneous phenobarbitone administration reduced the incidence of liver tumors induced in NMRI mice by *N*-nitrosodiethylamine given daily in their drinking water. This nitrosamine induces predominantly tumors of the stomach in this strain, and their incidence was reduced by phenobarbtone (*162*).

Reactions with Cellular Components by Nitroso Compounds *in Vitro* and *in Vivo*. As expected from their differing chemical stabilities, the nitrosamides can react directly with nucleic acids, proteins, and other compounds *in vitro*, but the dialkyl- and other nitrosamines cannot. Reactions with nucleic acids were the most extensively studied and were discussed in detail by Lawley (*554*) and by Singer and Fraenkel-Conrat (*555*). Aspects of the alkylation of nucleic acids *in vivo* were discussed in the reviews cited above (*6, 503–508*).

Alkylation of Nucleic Acids by Methylnitroso Compounds. Several nitrosamides, including N-methyl-N-nitrosourethane, N'-nitro-N-nitrosoguanidine, and N-methyl-N-nitroso-p-toluenesulfonamide, alkylate nucleic acids *in vitro* under physiological conditions of pH and temperature (*515, 556, 557, 558*). Craddock (*559*) found no evidence of deamination of DNA after treatment *in vitro* with N-methyl-N'-nitro-N-nitrosoguanidine. The rate and extent of methylation of DNA by the latter compound was increased by the presence of thiols, as was that by N-methyl–N-nitrososourethane, but that by N-methyl–N–nitroso–p-toluenesulfonamide was considerably reduced (*556, 557, 558*). Lawley (*560*) reviewed his recent studies on the action of various nitrosamides on nucleic acids *in vitro* and after treatment of microorganisms and cells in culture. N-Methyl-N'-nitro-N-nitrosoguanidine and other nitrosamides may undergo activation by alkaline-catalyzed hydrolysis to yield the diazohydroxide ($CH_3–N{=}N–OH$) which is presumed to react or to ionize to give $CH_3N_2^+$ which may react or further dissociate yielding the CH_3^+ ion. Other possibilities are reaction with a thiol group on an electron-deficient C atom or reaction with thiol at a nitroso group (*515*).

Direct effects of N-methyl-N-nitrosourea and of N-methyl-N-nitrosourethane on DNA *in vitro* were demonstrated by physicochemical means, including decrease in sedimentation coefficient both before denaturation and in the presence of formamide. N-Nitrosodimethylamine caused similar changes in the DNA, leading the authors to postulate a role for the nitroso function since they assumed that the nitrosamine required metabolic activation before it could act as an alkylating agent (*561*).

The main site of alkylation in the nucleic acids by the alkyl nitroso compounds is the $N(7)$-position of guanine, as with other alkylating agents. As with the latter agents, other sites are attacked, and these are being studied in several laboratories (*560*). A notable advance was made by Loveless (*576*) who showed that alkylation on the $O(6)$-position of guanine occurred when salmon sperm DNA was treated *in vitro* with N-methyl- or N-ethyl-N-nitrosourea. Although this reaction was reported previously by Friedman *et al.* (*562, 563*), it had been overlooked by later workers who hydrolyzed the nucleic acids in $1M$ hydrochloric acid. Loveless found that, in addition to the two nitrosamides, ethyl methanesulfonate also caused alkylation on the $O(6)$-position of guanine, but he could not detect any reaction at this position with methyl methanesulfonate. The possible importance of $O(6)$-alkylation for biological activity was suggested because the nitrosamides (*564*) and ethyl methanesulfonate are mutagenic in bacteriophage, but methyl methanesulfonate is not (*565*). The demonstration that hydrolysis of nucleic acids in $0.1M$ hydrochloric acid at 37°C did not cause degradation of O^6-methylguanine (*566*), and the use of enzymic hydrolysis methods have led to the finding of this methylated base in a number of nucleic acids methylated by N-nitroso compounds *in vivo* as well as *in vitro*. A small extent of methylation at $O(6)$ of guanine in DNA by methyl methanesulfonate *in vitro* was recently detected (*567*) but considerably less than that found with the nitrosamides. Thus, it appears that the behavior difference of methyl methanesulfonate is quantitative rather than qualitative. Although $N(7)$ of guanine is the main site of alkylation of nucleic acids *in vivo* as well as *in vitro*, it is clear that a number of other sites are alkylated to various smaller extents (560). Problems have arisen in identifying bases alkylated *in vivo* because of the small quantities involved. Even with the use of labeled nitroso compounds of high specific radioactivity progress has been slow, and the various methylated bases are only now being firmly identified. As well as 7-methylguanine, 1- and 3-methyladenine and 3-methylcytosine were identified in DNA and RNA prepared from livers of rats treated with ^{14}C-N-nitrosodimethylamine and hydrolyzed by $1M$ hydrochloric acid at 100°C for 1 hr (568). This procedure would of course have destroyed any O^6-methylguanine present. Subsequent work (569, 570) has shown that O^6-methylguanine is present in ribosomal RNA of DNA of livers from rats treated with N-nitrosodimethylamine, but none was detected after treatment of the animals with methyl methanesulfonate. Similarly O^6-methylguanine was found in the brain nucleic acids of rats treated with N-methyl-N-nitrosourea but not with methyl methanesulfonate (571). These findings may, of course, reflect the sensitivity of the methods used rather than an absolute lack of O^6-methylguanine in the brain nucleic acids of the rats treated with methyl methanesulfonate.

Recent comparative studies of methylation of nucleic acids *in vitro* and *in vivo* by various N-nitroso compounds and by dimethyl sulfate and methyl methanesulfonate (567, 572, 573, 574) were summarized by Lawley (560). The following methylation products have been identified—1-methyladenine, 3-methyladenine, 7-methyladenine, 3-methylcytosine, 3-methylguanine, 7-methylguanine (which was the major product with both types of reagent in both nucleic acids), and O^6-methylguanine (which was only formed in very small amounts or was undetectable after treatment with methyl methanesulfonate). 3-Methylthymine was not detected in DNA with either type of reagent, and Craddock (575) failed to find this methylated base in DNA prepared from livers of rats treated with N-nitrosodimethylamine. Lawley (560) concluded that the N-nitroso compounds differed significantly in their mechanism of action from the simpler methylating agents such as methyl methanesulfonate. The nitroso compounds react through intermediates derived from N-nitroso-monomethylamine and can be classified as S_N1 reagents in part while dimethyl sulfate and methyl methanesulfonate behave as typical S_N2 reagents. These differences are reflected in the pattern of minor products of methylation of nucleic acids which they produce. As mentioned above, the nitroso compounds have considerably greater capacity to methylate the $O(6)$ atom of guanine residues, but they show less tendency to react at the $N(1)$ atom of adenine or at the $N(3)$ of cytosine. Both types of reagent react to a small extent at the $N(3)$ of guanine and the $N(7)$ of adenine, the nitroso compounds rather more than the simpler methylating agents. It is not possible to correlate these differences in nucleic acid methylation with differences in the biological behavior of the compounds. Although methyl methanesulfonate is inactive as a mutagen in the bacteriophage studied by Loveless (576), it is mutagenic in other systems. As a carcinogen also, methyl methanesulfonate has been considered less active than the nitroso methylating agents, but its neuro-oncogenic action (577), particularly by the transplacental route (578), leaves little doubt of its carcinogenic potency. Lawley has pointed out that methylation on the O^6 atom of guanine could account for mutagenesis since this would be expected to cause mispairing of bases and thus induce transition mutations.

Based on the assumption that alkylation by the nitroso compounds *in vivo* would be similar to that occurring *in vitro*, it was widely thought that diazomethane must be an intermediate formed *in vivo*. Recent work by Lijinsky *et al.* (579), however, has made this postulate less likely to be correct. These authors prepared nucleic acids from the livers of rats treated with fully deuterated *N*-nitrosodimethylamine and isolated 7-methylguanine by conventional extraction procedures. Examination of the 7-methylguanine in the mass spectrometer clearly showed that the methyl group transferred from the carcinogen was $-CD_3$ and not $-CD_2H$. These important findings indicate that diazomethane is unlikely to be an intermediate and that the methyl group is transferred intact from the nitrosamine to the nucleic acid *in vivo*. Similar findings were reported in experiments with *N*-methyl-*N*-nitrosourea, *N*-nitrosodiethylamine and *N*-methyl-*N*-nitrosocyclohexylamine *in vivo* in which the alkyl group was transferred intact (276, 580, 581, 582), and in work on mutagenesis in *E. coli* by Lingens *et al.* using fully deuterated *N*-methyl-*N'*-nitro-*N*-nitrosoguanidine (583, 584, 585).

It is clearly well established that several carcinogenic nitroso compounds methylate nucleic acids and other cellular components after administration to experimental animals, but the significance of these reactions is not apparent. The marked preponderance of methylation on the 7-position of guanine in the liver and kidney of rats treated with *N*-nitrosodimethylamine suggested that this interaction might be important in carcinogenesis. Ways in which methylation at this site could induce mutations were also suggested (586). Comparative studies of the extent of formation of 7-methylguanine of DNA and RNA in various organs of rats treated with *N*-nitrosodimethylamine, *N*-methylnitrosourea, methyl methanesulfonate, and dimethyl sulfate were reported by Swann and Magee (587). Clear correlation between the organs with maximum methylation (liver, kidney, and lung) and the tumor formation sites was found with *N*-nitrosodimethylamine and a fairly uniform level of methylation in the organs studied after treatment with *N*-methyl-*N*-nitrosourea was consistent with the wide range of organs susceptible to carcinogenesis by the latter compound. In particular, the extent of guanine conversion to 7-methylguanine was closely similar in the kidneys with that of the two nitroso compounds, both of which induce tumors in this organ. With dimethyl sulfate the level of methylation in several organs was considerably lower than with the nitroso compounds, and, in view of the very brief existence of this compound after injection into the animals, it was concluded that it failed to reach effective concentrations in the organs even after toxic doses. With methyl methanesulfonate, however, the conversion to 7-methylguanine in the kidney nucleic acids was of the same order as that found with the nitroso compounds although the methylation of DNA was greater than with RNA, in contrast to the findings with the latter compounds. Recently, higher methylation on the 7-position of guanine in DNA than in RNA was also found in the brains of rats treated with methyl methanesulfonate (571). Since no kidney tumors were observed in the rats surviving the same dose of methyl methanesulfonate, doubt was thrown on the significance of N(7)-alkylation for carcinogenesis. Kleihues *et al.* (588) found no difference between the extent of interaction of N-methyl-N-nitrosourea with neuronal and glial cells, as determined by the formation *in vivo* of 7-methylguanine in nuclear DNA, and the failure to induce neuronal tumors by this compound was attributed to the incapacity of these cells to divide. Further doubt was cast by Schoental (589) who failed to find correlation between the presence of 7-methylguanine in nucleic acids and the localization of tumors induced by N-methyl-N-nitrosourethane. The failure to induce tumors of the liver, where nucleic acid methylation was maximal, was emphasized. Intraportal injection of N-methyl- or N-ethyl-N-nitrosourea produced tumors at a number of sites but only one liver tumor. Similar treatment with the deuterium-labeled nitrosamides was followed by no detectable alkylation of the DNA. 7-Methylguanine was present, however, in the RNA of rats receiving N-methyl-N-nitrosourea, and mass spectroscopic analysis confirmed the transfer of the intact methyl group (276). The failure to detect alkylation of DNA may have been the result of the lower sensitivity of mass spectrometry than methods using radioactively labeled nitroso compounds of high specific activity. However, a single treatment with N-nitrosodimethyl or diethylamine or N-methyl-N'-nitro-N-nitrosoguanidine after partial hepatectomy induced liver tumors in rats whereas usually no liver tumors are observed in intact rats. Methyl methanesulfonate failed to induce liver tumors even when given after partial hepatectomy (371). O^6-Methylguanine is formed in liver DNA of partially hepatectomized rats treated with N-nitrosodimethylamine, but none was detected in animals treated with methyl methanesulfonate (590). Mice treated with carcinogenic doses of ^{14}C-N-methyl-N-nitrosourea showed similar levels of 7-methylguanine and O^6-methylguanine in a range of organs, but there were tissue-dependent differences in the distribution of 3-methyladenine which occurred in disproportionately high relative amounts in bone marrow, thymus, and spleen which are the organs thought to play an important part in the genesis of thymic lymphomas (591). Krüger *et al.* (592) studied the alkylating action and tumor inhibition of ^{14}C-N-nitrosodimethylamine and ^{14}C-N-methyl-N-nitrosourea in transplanted tumors of rats and mice. After intravenous injection of N-nitrosodimethylamine no 7-methylguanine was found in the tumors, but it was present after injection of N-methyl-N-nitrosourea. The nitrosamide exerted a chemotherapeutic action on transplanted reticulum cell sarcoma in the mouse, but N-nitrosodimethylamine had no such action. The authors suggest the intermediate formation of N-methyl-N-nitrosocarbamic acid as a common stage in the formation of a methyl carbonium ion from both carcinogens.

Failure to detect methylation of liver nucleic acids in trout treated with N-nitrosodimethylamine led to the conclusion that this reaction was not related to the carcinogenic action of the compound (593). However, N-nitrosodimethylamine diffuses very rapidly out of the bodies of fish into the surrounding water which probably accounts for its very low toxicity in these animals. Methylation of nucleic acids of fish liver slices incubated with ^{14}C-N-nitrosodimethylamine was demonstrated (594). Similar methylation was also observed in nucleic acids of monkey liver and kidney slices by ^{14}C-N-nitrosodimethylamine (547).

In the work so far discussed, nucleic acid methylation of total unfractionated tissue nucleic acids was studied. Recent studies have been extended to subcellular fractions and to different molecular species of RNA. Greater methylation of mitochondrial than nuclear DNA occurred in the livers of rats or hamsters treated with N-methyl-N-nitrosourea (595) or N-nitrosodimethylamine (596). Muramatsu et al. (597) studied the labeling patterns of mouse nuclear and cytoplasmic RNA at various times after injection of ^{3}H-N-nitrosodimethylamine and ^{14}C-orotate. Sedimentation analysis showed that most RNA species—including cytoplasmic ribosomal 28S, 18S, and 4S RNA, nuclear ribosomal and low molecular weight RNA (4 to 7S), and possibly rapidly labeled nRNA—were all labeled by N-nitrosodimethylamine. The average specific radioactivity of nuclear RNA was almost the same as that of cytoplasmic RNA. The methylated RNA was unstable in vivo—a fraction of the ribosomal RNA having a half-life of about one and a half days and the remainder about three to four days while the normal rRNA had a half-life of about five days. The variance of these findings from those of McElhone et al. (598), which are discussed later, may be explained by the much larger dose of N-nitrosodimethylamine used by the Japanese workers.

Liver RNA from mice treated 12 hr previously with ^{14}C-N-nitrosodimethylamine has been characterized by column chromatography and density gradient centrifugation. The methylated RNA fractions were different from the naturally occurring methylated RNA species which were only lightly labeled. The highest incorporation of the label from ^{14}C-N-nitrosodimethylamine was found in the high molecular weight nRNA fractions. Methylation occurred predominantly on the N(7)-position of guanine. Thus, methylation of messenger RNA may lead to disaggregation of liver polysomes which may play an important part in the heaptotoxic action of the nitrosamine (599).

Earlier work had indicated that maximum levels of RNA methylation were reached about 4–5 hr after a single dose of ^{14}C-N-nitrosodimethylamine (30 mg/kg) to rats and that the amount of labeled 7-methylganine in RNA began to decline between 12 and 24 hr after injection (600). Subsequent studies on the stability of ribosomal RNA methylated in vivo by lower doses of N-nitrosodimethylamine (2 mg/kg body weight) led to the conclusion that it was intrinsically stable in vivo with a similar biological half-life to normal rRNA (598). In contrast, rat liver and kidney DNA methylated in vivo by N-nitrosodimethylamine becomes unstable with loss of 7-methylguanine. This loss probably occurs mainly by excision of the methylated base or breakdown of the DNA because there is evidence for the excretion in the urine of 7-methylguanine derived from DNA following injection of the nitrosamine (601).

Comparison of the disappearance rates of 7-methylguanine from DNA during two days following varying doses of *N*-nitrosodimethylamine to rats with those found on incubation under simulated physiological conditions *in vitro* revealed a higher rate *in vivo* with bigger doses (26 mg/kg body weight) which may have been related to cell damage in the liver. With lower doses of *N*-nitrosodimethylamine (1 or 2 mg/kg body weight), however, there was insufficient difference to indicate the presence of a specific enzyme for excision of the abnormal base (*602*). The excretion of increased amounts of 7-methylguanine by rats treated with *N*-nitrosodimethylamine has been confirmed, but no such increase was found with rats treated with relatively high doses of other carcinogens, including *N*-nitrosodiethylamine, *N*-nitrosomorpholine, *trans*-4-dimethylaminostilbene, and 7,12-dimethylbenz(*a*)anthracene, which immediately decrease 7-methylguanine excretion (*603*). A survey of the urinary excretion of 7-methylguanine and other minor purines by human subjects with and without diagnosed cancer of various organs or liver cirrhosis revealed no significant differences between the healthy and diseased groups (*604*). The fate of 7-^{14}C-methylguanine after injection into rats was studied. No evidence of incorporation into DNA or RNA was found even in organs of rapid cell turnover such as the small intestine or into the rapidly growing tissues of the fetus. The major part (about 95%) of the dose was excreted unchanged in the urine with only a small amount of *N*-demethylation as indicated by the expiration of $^{14}CO_2$ (*605*). Long-term administration of 7-methylguanine to rats failed to reveal carcinogenic activity (*606*).

Alkylation of Nucleic Acids by Higher Alkyl, Aryl-Alkyl, and Cyclic Nitroso Compounds. As indicated above, most work on metabolism of carcinogenic nitroso compounds has been with methyl derivatives. Recently, however, investigation was extended to higher alkyl, aryl alkyl, and cyclic nitroso compounds. Administration of *N*-1-^{14}C-ethyl-*N*-nitrosourea to rats did not cause ethylation of nucleic acids, but methylation was confirmed after injection of ^{14}C–*N*–methyl-*N*-nitrosourea by the same workers (*607*). Subsequently ethylation of DNA and RNA with formation of 7-ethylguanine was demonstrated in the liver and other organs of rats treated with ^{14}C-*N*-nitrosodiethylamine or *N*-^{14}C-ethyl-*N*-nitrosourea. Although alkylation of the nucleic acids was clearly demonstrated, the extent of the reaction was considerably less, and the proportion of the alkylation occurring on the N(7)-position of guanine was lower than with the methylating compounds (*522*). The smaller extent of ethylation may have accounted for the earlier failure to detect it. Ethylation of the nucleic acids of the fetus was observed after injection of *N*-1-^{14}C-ethyl-*N*-nitrosourea into mother rats on the 18th day of pregnancy. The conversion of guanine to 7-ethylguanine in the fetus was about one-half that in the livers of the mother rats (*608*, *609*). As mentioned earlier, *N*-ethyl-*N*-nitrosourea is a very potent inducer of tumors of the nervous system by the transplancental route. The cancer chemotherapeutic agent 1-(2-chloroethyl)-3-cyclohexyl-1-nitrosourea (CCNU) has recently been shown to interact with nucleic acids and proteins *in vivo* and *in vitro* (*610*).

The metabolism of *N*-nitroso–1-(^{14}C)-di-*n*-propylamine and *N*-nitroso–1-

(^{14}C)-di-n-butylamine was studied in the rat by Krüger who showed that their administration led to the formation of 7-(^{14}C)-n-propyl- and 7-(^{14}C)-n-butyl-guanine respectively in small amounts in liver RNA. In both cases 7-(^{14}C-methyl)guanine was also formed, but when the rats were given 2-(^{14}C)-N-nitrosodi-n-propylamine, it was not detected—only 7-(^{14}C)-n–propylguanine was found (611, 612). In vivo administration to rats of 1-(^{14}C)-N-nitroso-propyl-2-hydroxyproylamine, (^{3}H)-N-nitrosopropyl-2-oxopropylamine, and N-nitrosopropyl(^{3}H)methylamine (but not 2-(^{14}C)-N-nitrosopropyl-2-hydroxy-propylamine) resulted in the formation of 7-methylguanine in nucleic acids of liver (613, 614). These results suggest that β-oxidation of these ali-phatic nitrosamines occurs in vivo with metabolic splitting between the α- and β-carbon atoms and the formation of a methylating intermediate. This inter-pretation is consistent with the earlier observation that N-nitroso-n-butyl-methylamine produces 7-methylguanine in the nucleic acids of the liver after administration to rats (615).

Alkylation of rat liver RNA by cyclic nitrosamines was reported after experiments in which tritiated N-nitrosopyrrolidine, N-nitrosopiperidine, or N-nitrosomorpholine were given to rats. In each case, 7-methylguanine ap-peared to be present in acid hydrolysates of the nucleic acids, and no other alkylated component was detected (616). In subsequent work, Lijinsky and Ross, also using tritium- or deuterium-labeled compounds, reported that, except for N-nitrosocyclohexylmethylamine, no alkylation could be detected with some cyclic nitrosamines while apparent alkylation occurred in organs where tumors were not induced or by cyclic nitrosamines which were not carcinogenic. It was concluded that alkylation of rat liver nucleic acids was not related to carcinogenesis by nitrosamines (581, 617). More recently the metabolism of 2,5- and 3,4-^{14}C-N-nitrosopyrrolidine was investigated in rats. With both agents radioactivity was incorporated into liver RNA, and analysis of 1M acid hydrolysates revealed radioactive components distinct from the major purine or pyrimidine bases. Although these components were not identified, they were shown not to be 7-methyl–, 7-ethyl-, or 7-(3-carboxy-propyl)guanine (612). Somewhat similar results were obtained after treat-ment of rats with 2-^{14}C-N-nitrosomorpholine. Incorporation of radioactivity was found in DNA and RNA, and the presence of 7-methylguanine in 1M acid hydrolysates of the nucleic acids was excluded. Six distinct radioactive com-ponents other than the major bases were observed, one of which appeared to be 7-(2-hydroxyethyl)guanine. The presence of 7-(2-carboxymethyl)guanine was excluded (530).

Effects on Template Functions of Synthetic Polynucleotides. The effects of various alkylating agents and nitroso compounds on the template activities of synthetic polynucleotides in vitro were studied to clarify the effects of these agents on nucleic acid function in vivo. The presence of 7-methylguanine appears to have no effect on the coding properties of such polynucleotides although it reduces their template activity (618, 619). Methyl substitution in poly C templates by methyl methansulfonate, however, caused anomalous incorporation of UTP and reduced incorporation of GTP by RNA polymerase (*620, 621*). Similar effects were observed after reaction of poly C with N-methyl-N′-nitro-N-nitrosoguanidine (*622*) and N-methyl or N-ethyl-N-nitrosourea (*623*). However, as originally suggested by Loveless (*576*), Gerchman and Ludlum (*624*) demonstrated that there is an aberrant base pairing with a polymer containing O^6-methylguanine.

The importance of alkylation in the O(6)-position of guanine was further substantiated by Goth and Rajewsky (*625*). They found that the initial degree of alkylation in the O(6)-position of guanine in the DNA of a given tissue is apparently not correlated to the tissue-specific carcinogenicity of N-ethyl-N-nitrosourea, which induced brain, but not liver, tumors in rats. However, O^6-ethylguanine is characterized by a high degree of persistence in brain DNA; its elimination rate from brain DNA being much lower than from liver DNA and also distinctly reduced in comparison with the elimination rates from brain DNA of 3-ethylguanine and 3-ethyladenine. This might be a determining factor in the neoplastic transformation by N-ethyl-N-nitrosourea in the nervous system, and it might suggest that the excision of the alkylated base might be caused by an enzyme and not by hydrolytic removal from DNA.

Recently, the ability of the enzyme endonucleose II (EC3.1.4.30) of *Escherichia coli* to release O^6-methylguanine and 3-methyladenine, but not 7-methylguanine, from DNA alkylated *in vitro* by N-methyl-N-nitrosourea, was reported (*626*). The significance of these *in vitro* studies for the interpretation of the reactions of the carcinogenic nitroso componds *in vivo* remains to be established.

Alkylation of Proteins. Relatively little work has been done on the reactions of the nitroso carcinogens with proteins. N-Methyl-N′-nitro-N-nitrosoguanidine reacts with lysine residues in proteins *in vitro* with the formation of a nitroguanido derivative which yields nitrohomoarginine after enzymic hydrolysis (*627, 628, 629*). The concentration of the nitrosamide which is lethal to various cell types and rapidly inactivates transforming DNA would not be expected to form nitroguanido groups in any significant proportion of protein molecules. It was concluded that damage to protein cannot be the primary biological effect of this compound (*627*). Nitroamidination of the SH group of cysteine was also observed (*519*). Comparison of the reactions of ^{14}C-methyl- and ^{14}C-guanidine labeled N-methyl-N′-nitro–N–nitrosoguanidine with various proteins and polynucleotides showed that the methyl group became bound preferentially to the polynucleotides, particularly DNA while the guanido group was preferentially bound to protein with little reaction with polynucleotides. A possible role of protein guanidation in mutagenesis by alteration in the properties of DNA polymerase was suggested (*628*). Reaction of cytochrome C with N-methyl-N′-nitro-N-nitrosoguanidine induced modifications in its properties including increase in its negative charge and in its oxidation–reduction potential, as well as reduction in ts rate of enzymic reduction by NADH with rat liver mitochondria in comparison with native cytochrome C (*630*). Some years ago N-nitrosodimethylamine was shown to methylate imidazole groups of histidine in proteins of rat liver slices after incubation *in vitro* (*631, 632*) and reacted with SH groups of cysteine of rat liver proteins *in vivo*. More recently a detailed study of the methylation of nuclear proteins of rat liver by N-nitrosodimethylamine was reported. Administration of ^{14}C-labeled N-nitrosodimethylamine to rats produced labeled S-methylcysteine, 1-methylhistidine, 3-methylhistidine, and ϵ-N-methyllysine in the liver histones. The extent of alkylation of liver histones was about four times greater than those of kidney and was maximal at about 5 hr, subsequently declining between 5 and 24 hr. N-Nitrosodiethylamine also alkylated liver histones *in vivo* (*633*).

The effects of pretreatment with various agents on the labeling of liver proteins of rats treated with ^{3}H-N-nitrosodimethylamine were reported. Protein labeling was slightly inhibited when the animals were pretreated with 3-methylcholanthrene or phenobarbitone and more severely inhibited after treatment with dimethylformamide, diethylformamide, or aminoacetonitrile. The labeling was also inhibited by toxic doses of ethionine or carbon tetrachloride. Since several of these agents are known to have effects on hepatic protein biosynthesis, the above findings are difficult to interpret in terms of inhibition of protein methylation as opposed to total incorporation of label (*634*).

Apart from the metabolic pathways leading to the formation of alkylating intermediates, very little is known of the metabolism of the nitrosamines. Early work by Heath and Dutton (*635*) using N-nitrosodimethylamine labeled with ^{15}N revealed incorporation of the isotope into cellular components and into urinary urea. These findings indicate that metabolic pathways exist which are different from the formation of a methyl carbonium ion *via* N-nitrosomonomethylamine and methyldiazohydroxide, which has been postulated by most authors. Neunhoeffer *et al.* (*636*) reported the conversion of carcinogenic nitrosamines into the corresponding amidoximes by incubation with acetone powder preparations from rat liver or kidney homogenates. The amidoximes were hydrolyzed to give the corresponding primary amine and hydroxamic acid in a further enzymic reaction. The occurrence of these reactions *in vivo* might explain the findings of Dutton and Heath. Reduction of N-nitrosomorpholine to the corresponding hydrazine derivative after anaerobic incubation with rat liver microsomes *in vitro* was observed by Süss (*637*) who suggested that such reductive reactions occurring *in vivo* might have significance in carcinogenesis.

Formation of N-Nitroso Compounds in the Body

The synthesis of N-nitroso compounds from secondary amines and nitrosating agents has been well known since 1865 when it was found that dimethylamine hydrochloride treated with sodium nitrite in an aqueous solution at an acid pH formed a high yield of N-nitrosodimethylamine (*9*). It was suggested (*638, 639, 640, 641, 642*) that this reaction could occur in the acid conditions of the mammalian stomach from ingested nitrites and amines, and there is now substantial evidence that nitrosamines can be formed in this way.

Nitrates and, to a lesser extent, nitrites are widely distributed in nature.

The major human intake of nitrates in foodstuffs comes from vegetables or water supplies or from nitrates used as additives in the meat-curing processes. Spinach, beets, lettuce, radishes, eggplant, celery, and turnips are vegetables with the highest concentrations of nitrates (*643, 644*). Nitrates have relatively low toxicity while nitrites are considerably more toxic, inducing methemoglobinemia.

The reduction of nitrates to nitrites occurs in the upper gastrointestinal tract in adults suffering from achlorhydria or infants with a low gastric acidity. These conditions allow the upper part of the gastrointestinal tract to be invaded by the nitroreductase-containing bacteria which normally inhabit the lower bowel and are responsible for converting nitrates to nitrites (*644*). This conversion occurs also during storage of some vegetables, mainly spinach, as well as in damp forage materials with high nitrate content (*643, 645*). However, cured meat or fish products are the major sources of nitrites in the human diet. In many countries(*e.g.*, Statutory Instrument 1962, No. 1532, HMSO, London; US Code of Federal Regulations, Title 21, Sec. 12-1064 and Sec. 121, 1230; Canadian Food and Drug Act and Regulations, Table XI) the permissible concentrations of sodium nitrate and nitrite in a limited number of meat and fish products for preservation and color fixation are 500 and 200 ppm, respectively. The average human daily intake of nitrite has been estimated by Sander (*639*) at 1.5 mg sodium nitrite. The daily intake of nitrates could be much higher than this and is affected by the concentration in the drinking water, which can vary considerably.

Nitrosatable substances in the environment include secondary and tertiary amines, quaternary ammonium compounds, ureas, carbamates and guanidines. Secondary amines occur ubiquitously in nature and have been identified in vegetables, wine, spirits, beer, tea, fish, and other items (*646*). Various flavoring agents are prepared from secondary amines (*642, 647, 648, 649, 650*). Some drugs, such as piperazine, are secondary amines. Tobacco and tobacco smoke contain several secondary amines including pyrrolidine, dimethylamine, and piperidine (*651*). The occurrence and use of ureas, carbamates, and guanidines were reviewed recently by Mirvish (*652*) and Sander (*648, 649, 650*). The presence of various aliphatic and heterocyclic amines of endogenous and exogenous origin, including dimethylamine, piperidine and pyrrolidine, were identified in human blood and urine (*653, 654*). The mean basal excretion in the urine over 24 hr amounted to 15.3 mg for dimethylamine and 5.7 mg for piperidine (*653, 655*).

The synthesis of *N*-nitroso compounds from nitrite and secondary and tertiary amines or amides has been demonstrated *in vitro* with animal and human gastric juice and *in vivo* in animals.

The kinetics of dimethylamine nitrosation was examined by Mirvish (*656*) in buffered aqueous solution using tritium-labeled amine. The reaction rate was proportional to the nonionized dimethylamine concentration and to that of nitrogen trioxide and to the square of HNO_2 concentration, the highest yield of *N*-nitrosodimethylamine being at pH 3.4.

Various other aliphatic or aromatic amines (dipropylamine, dipentylamine, N-methylbenzylamine, piperidine, morpholine, mononitrosopiperazine, piperazine, N-methylaniline, diphenylamine) were nitrosated *in vitro* in aqueous solution at an optimum pH between 1 and 3. The yield of nitrosamines, as measured by ultraviolet absorption or by the amount of nitrite after photochemical decomposition of the nitrosamines, depended on the basicity of the amines, increasing from the strongest to the weakest base (*657, 658*). The nitrosation rate of the different amines depended on the proportion of the reactive nonionized amine present which is related to the basicity of the amine. Nitrosation *in vitro* in an aqueous solution of the amino acids L-proline, L-hydroxyproline, and sarcosine occurs at the optimum pH 2.25–2.5, and the reaction rate is proportional to the concentration of the amino acid and the square of nitrite concentration as with the secondary amines (*657*). Nonenzymatic nitrosation occurs under neutral and basic conditions in the presence of appropriate catalysts. Aqueous buffer solutions of diethylamine, sodium nitrite, and formaldehyde led to significant yields of N-nitrosodiethylamine over a pH range 6.4 to 11.0 (*659*).

The nitrosation of N-alkylureas and N-alkylurethanes proceeds very rapidly. The rate of methylurea nitrosation to give N-methyl-N-nitrosourea is proportional to the concentration of the amide and the nitrous acidium ion which in turn is proportional to the concentration of hydrogen ion and nitrous acid and, unlike the amines, is not pH dependent. The nitrosation of ethylurea, N-methylurethane and N-ethylurethane proceeds more slowly than with methylurea and follows the same reaction rate (*660, 661*). Nitrosation of DL-citrulline gives N-δ-nitroso-DL-citrulline, and methylguanidine produces N-methyl-N-nitrosourea, nitrosocyanamide, and probably N-methyl-N-nitrosoguanidine (*660*). Under strong acidic conditions the guanidino–amino acids, arginine, and N-α-acetylarginine were nitrosated, and the butanol extracts showed ultraviolet absorption maxima indicating the formation of N-nitrosoureas (*660*).

Other naturally occurring guanidine derivatives, creatine and creatinine, react with nitrite under acid conditions to produce N-nitrososarcosine and creatinine-5-oxime or 1-methylhydantoin-5-oxime, respectively (*662*). Lijinsky *et al.* (*663, 664*) examined the nitrosation in aqueous solutions (pH 2.1–4.4) of various drugs (aminopyrine, oxytetracycline, disulfiram, nikethamide, tolazamide, 3-hexahydroazepinyl-nitropropiophenone, chlorpromazine, dextropropoxyphene, chlorpheniramine, methadone, methapyrilene, quinacrine, lucanthone, and cyclizine) and showed the formation of carcinogenic nitrosamines such as N-nitrosodimethyl- and diethylamine, nitrosohexamethyleneimine, dinitrosopiperazine, and N-nitrosopiperidine. The yield of nitrosamines from the various compounds varied largely, ranging from 40% for aminopyrine to 0.03% for dextropropoxyphene at 37°C. The nitrosation of the antitubercular drug, ethambutol, was reported by Montesano *et al.* (*665*). The nitrosation of a variety of tertiary amines was studied by Lijinsky *et al.* (*666*). The formation of carcinogenic nitroso compounds from nitrite and some pesticides, herbicides, or fungicides has been described (*667, 668, 669*).

Many N-nitroso compounds whose formations are reported above are toxic and carcinogenic (*see* Table II), but for some the toxic and carcinogenic effects are not known (*N*-δ-nitrosocitrulline) or have been shown to be negative (*N*-nitrosodiphenylamine). Nitrosation of various aliphatic and aromatic secondary amines were also demonstrated *in vitro* using gastric juices and *in vivo* in the mammalian and human stomach.

Sen *et al.* (*670*) demonstrated the *in vitro* formation of *N*-nitrosodiethylamine when diethylamine and sodium nitrite were incubated with gastric juice from rats, rabbits, cats, dogs, and man. Human and rabbit gastric juices (pH 1.3–2) produced more nitrosamine than juice from the rat (pH 4.4–4.6). The nitrosation reaction was also demonstrated *in vivo* in cats and rabbits after feeding diethylamine hydrochloride (450–1000 mg) and sodium nitrite (300–1000 mg). The identity of the nitrosamine formed was established by thin-layer and gas chromatography. Similar results were obtained by Sander (*639*) who observed nitrosation *in vitro* of various secondary amines including dimethyl- and diethylamine using human gastric juice. The formation of the carcinogenic *N*-nitrosopiperidine from nitrate and/or nitrite and piperidine was described by Alam *et al.* (*671, 672*), *in vitro* with rat gastric contents and also *in vivo* in the rat stomach and small intestine. The yields of *N*-nitrosopiperidine *in vivo* were higher in the stomach than in the small intestine.

In vivo synthesis of the corresponding nitrosamines following administration to rats of dimethylamine (*640*), *N*-methylaniline, and *N*-methylbenzylamine (*658*) with nitrite were demonstrated. As observed *in vitro*, the nitrosamine yield was much greater with weakly basic than with strongly basic secondary amines. Similar results were obtained by Greenblatt *et al.* (*673*) who described the formation of *N*-nitrosophenmetrazine in rabbit and rat stomachs after administration of the drug phenmetrazine and nitrite. Negative results were obtained with the corresponding tertiary amine, phendimetrazine, or when nitrates were used instead of nitrite.

High doses of amines and nitrites were used in these *in vivo* experiments because of the difficulty in detecting small amounts of nitrosamines in intact animals because of their rapid absorption and metabolism. These difficulties were overcome by using biochemical and toxicological effects caused by the nitrosamine itself as indirect indices of *in vivo* formation of nitrosamines. Magee (*674*) administered ^{14}C-dimethylamine and sodium nitrite orally to rats and found methylation of liver nucleic acids following nitrosation of dimethylamine in the stomach. Epstein reported similar findings (*675*) after observing methylation of mouse liver DNA after combined oral administration of ^{14}C-dimethylamine and sodium nitrite, but not with ^{14}C-dimethylamine alone. Combined oral administration of sodium nitrite and dimethylamine or methylbenzylamine to mice induced mortality, liver necrosis, and inhibition of liver protein and RNA synthesis (*676, 677*).

Centrilobular liver necrosis, typical of the effect of *N*-nitrosodimethylamine itself, and increased levels of serum glutamic pyruvic transaminase and carcinogenic effect were also observed in rats treated orally with the analgesic aminopyrine and sodium nitrite (*678, 679*). Methylation of nucleic acids of the stomach, liver, and small intestine of rats given ^{14}C-N-methylurea and sodium nitrite simultaneously was demonstrated by Montesano and Magee (*674*). Since no evidence of nucleic acid methylation was obtained with ^{14}C-N-methylurea alone, these data indicate that the unstable and potent carcinogen N-methyl-N-nitrosourea was formed in the stomach and absorbed into the circulation of the rat.

In addition to demonstrating the formation of N-nitroso compounds *in vitro* and *in vivo*, simultaneous feeding of nitrite and nitrosatable amines resulted in the induction of tumors similar to those produced by the corresponding N-nitroso compounds. In the rat, tumors developed following chronic feeding of nitrite and several amines or amides, namely morpholine, heptamethyleneimine, N-methylbenzylamine, N-methylaniline, 2-imidazolidone, methylcyclohexylamine, methylurea, dimethylurea, and ethylurea (*376, 648, 649, 650, 679, 680, 681, 682, 683*).

Administration of mixtures of sodium nitrite (0.05%–0.1%) and various secondary amines (pyrrolidine, piperidine, piperazine, morpholine, heptamethyleneimine) to rats for 75 weeks at a concentration of 0.025–0.2% in the diet did not produce a carcinogenic effect (*684*). In these conditions, nitrosamine formation was insufficient. In mice, an increased incidence and number of lung tumors was observed after oral treatment with sodium nitrite and various amines or amides (piperazine, morpholine, N-methylaniline, methylurea, and ethylurea) (*222, 685*). Various authors (*451, 452, 686*) reported the induction of neurogenic tumors in the offspring of mothers treated intragastrically with ethylurea and sodium nitrite. The lack of carcinogenicity observed with diethylamine, piperidine, phenylurea, and N-methylthiourea in rats (*638, 648, 683*) or with dimethylamine, proline, hydroxyproline, and arginine in mice or rats (*222, 243, 687*) has been attributed to the low rate of their nitrosation or to the noncarcinogenicity of the corresponding N-nitroso compounds.

The intestine has been suggested as a site for formation of nitrosamines by bacterial action. Sander (*688*) demonstrated that nitrosamines can be formed by four strains of nitrate reducing bacteria (*E. coli, E. dispor, Proteus vulgaris*, and *Serratia marcescens*) from aromatic and aliphatic amines and nitrate at neutral pH. Under these pH conditions spontaneous reaction between the amines and sodium nitrite could occur only very slowly. Subsequently, bacterial reduction of nitrate to nitrite in the human stomach was reported by Sander and Seif (*689*), and N-nitrosodiphenylamine was identified in the stomach contents of 31 human subjects who had received sodium nitrate and diphenylamine intragastrically. In accordance with these findings, Klubes and Jondorf (*690*) and Klubes *et al.* (*691*) reported the formation of N-nitrosodimethylamine on incubation of ^{14}C-dimethylamine and sodium nitrite with rat cecal contents. Of 10 strains of *Escherichia coli* isolated from the human intestinal tract, 5 were able to form nitrosamines when incubated aerobically at neutral pH with sodium nitrate and the secondary amines diphenylamine, dimethylamine, diethylamine, piperidine, pyrrolidine, and N-methylaniline. A number of strains of enterococci, clostridia, bacterioides, and bifidobacteria with no nitrate-reductase activity formed nitrosamines when nitrite replaced the nitrate (*692*). The same authors (*693, 694*) suggest that the infected bladder may be a more important site than the intestine for the nitrosamine formation by bacteria, and they found that rats with experimentally induced bladder infections of *E. coli* excreted *N*-nitrosopiperidine after they were treated orally with the amine and sodium nitrate. *N*-Nitrosodimethylamine was identified in the urine of two different individuals infected with *Proteus mirabilis* (*695*) and also reported in pooled human cervical and vaginal discharge matter (*696*).

Nitrosation of several amines or amides may occur *in vivo* either by simple chemical reaction or as a result of the metabolic activity of microorganisms, and the nitrosation rate is affected by many factors such as amine basicity, substrate concentration, and pH. Thiocyanate increases the rate of nitrosamine formation (*697, 698*) whereas ascorbic acid may inhibit it (*699, 700*).

These experimental data indicate that the formation of carcinogenic *N*-nitroso compounds in the human stomach is a realistic possibility which may represent a hazard to human beings. More information is needed concerning the naturally occurring amines and their human intake, the pH change in the stomach during digestion, the absorption rate of the reactants, the influence of other substances which may accelerate or inhibit the nitrosation reaction, and the role of bacteria.

Occurrence of N-Nitroso Compounds in the Environment

Although studies on the toxicity and carcinogenicity of nitrosamines were started after indications of human toxicity resulting from the industrial use of *N*-nitrosodimethylamine (*1, 8*), only in recent years has there been an increasing interest in the occurrence of these compounds in situations other than the industrial environment. The outbreak of serious, sometimes fatal, liver disease in sheep fed with a diet containing fish meal preserved with nitrite (*701*) and the identification of *N*-nitrosodimethyamine as the toxic principle in this meal (*702*) stimulated research on the occurrence of such compounds in food for human and animal consumption.

There is now no doubt that these compounds do occur in trace amounts in various environmental situations. The occurrence of nitrosamines was reported in various meat products, fish, milk, cheese, flour, mushrooms, alcoholic drinks, tobacco and tobacco smoke (*see* Table IV). The findings are sometimes contradictory because of the lack of sufficiently sensitive and specific analytical methods. Various methods have been developed, including polarography, thin-layer chromatography, gas–liquid chromatography, and mass spectrometry. Recently a better standardization of the methodology, using gas–liquid chromatography and mass spectrometry, has yielded more reliable identification of the nitrosamines (*703, 704, 705*).

Various authors (*706, 707, 708, 709*) reported the presence of various nitrosamines (*e.g.*, *N*-nitrosodimethyl and diethylamine, *N*-nitrosopyrrolidine, and *N*-nitrosopiperidine) in different meat products in concentrations ranging

Table IV. Nonindustrial Sources

Sources	Detection Methods[a]
Meat Products	
Smoked sausages, bacon, ham	TLC
Cured meat (Kasserel)	TLC
Salami, dry sausages	TLC, GC, MS
Fried bacon	GC, MS
Luncheon meat, salami, pork chopped Danish	GC, MS
Pressed ham, hamburger	TLC
Uncooked and fried bacon	TLC, GC, MS
Mettwurst sausages	TLC, GC, MS
Fish	
Smoked herring, haddock, mackerel, kipper	TLC
Chinese marine salted fish	GC, MS
Raw smoked and smoked nitrite–nitrate treated salmon, shad, sable	GC, MS
Fresh, salted, fried cod; fresh, fried hake	GC, MS
Dried mackerel pike, salted salmon roe	TLC
Other Foods	
Fruit (*Solanum incanum*)	TLC, IR, GC, NMR
Cheese, milk	TLC, GC
Cheese	GC, MS
Flour, wheat	TLC, GC
Mushrooms	TLC
	TLC
Spinach	TLC
Alcoholic Spirits	
Kachasu (Zambia)	PL, TLC
British whiskey	PL, TLC, MS
Spirits (Western Kenya, Southern Uganda)	PL
	GC
	MS
Miscellaneous	
Tobacco smoke condensate	TLC
	TLC, GC
	TLC
	GC, MS
Tobacco leaf	TLC, GC
Surveyor III	MS
Soya bean oil	TLC, GC, MS

[a] TLC—thin-layer chromatography; GC—gas chromatography; MS—mass spectrometry; IR—infrared spectroscopy; NMR—nuclear magnetic resonance spectroscopy; PL—polarography.

[b] DMN—*N*-nitrosodimethylamine (dimethylnitrosamine); DEN—*N*-nitrosodiethylamine (diethylnitrosamine); NPYR—*N*-nitrosopyrrolidine; NPIP—*N*-nitrosopiperidine; N-4-MAB—*N*-nitroso-4-methylaminobenzaldehyde; MEN—*N*-nitrosoethylme-

of Human Exposure to Nitrosamines

Nitrosamines[b]	Concentration[c]	References
unidentified	0.6–6.5	*710*
DEN	40	*711*
DMN	10–80	*706*
DMN, DEN, NPYR, NPIP	1–40	*709*
DMN, DEN	1–4	*709*
DMN	15–25	*712*
DMN, NPYR	2–30	*707*
NPYR, NPIP	13–105	*708*
unidentified	0.5–40	*710*
DMN	0.05–0.3 ppm	*713*
DEN	1.2–21 ppm	
DMN	0–26	*735*
DMN	1–9	*709*
DMN, DEN	trace	*712*
DMN	ND	*736*
DEN	ND	*737, 738*
DMN	1–4	*709*
DEN	0–10	*737–743*
N–4–MAB	ND	*744*
unidentified	0.4–30	*710*
DEN	neg.	*745*
DMN	1–3 ppm	*726*
DMN, DEN	neg.	*728*
DMN, DEN, MEN, DPN EBN, DBN, NPIP	1–21 ppm	*729*
DMN	0.1–0.9 ppm	
DMN	neg.	
MBN, 2 unidentified	ND	*746, 747*
DMN, DEN, NPIP	ND	*748*
DEN, NPIP	0.2 ppm/1200 cigarettes	*740*
DMN, DEN, MEN, MBN, DPN, NPYR, NPIP, DBN, NNN	0–180 ng/ cigarette	*720, 721, 722*
NPIP	ND	*749*
DMN	ND	*750*
DMN, DEN	ND	*751*

thylamine (methylethylnitrosamine); DPN—*N*-nitrosodipropylamine (dipropylnitrosamine); EBN—*N*-nitrosobutylethylamine (ethylbutylnitrosamine); MBN—*N*-nitrosobutylmethylamine (methylbutylnitrosamine); DBN—*N*-nitrosodibutylamine (dibutylnitrosamine); NNN—*N*-nitrosonornicotine.

[c] The concentrations are expressed as ppb (parts per billion) unless otherwise specified; ND—not determined; Neg.—negative.

from 1 to 80 ppb. In these studies the presence of nitrosamines was confirmed by mass spectrometry whereas in other studies (710, 711, 712) the nitrosamines were determined by thin-layer chromatography and colorimetry, which give less reliable results. In fresh, salted, smoked, or fried fish the concentration of the nitrosamines observed varied from 1 to 26 ppb (Table IV). Samples of Cantonese salted fish obtained from markets in Hong Kong contained N-nitrosodimethylamine (713), and its formation was related to the contamination of the food with nitrate-reducing staphylococci. This bacterium isolated from the salted fish increased the nitrosamine content in salted fish broth (714). Nitrosamine formation in sewage by microorganisms was suggested by Ayanaba et al. (715).

The formation of nitrosamines in food products by nitrosation of secondary, tertiary, quaternary, and other biogenic amines was recently emphasized (716, 717). Recently, N-nitrosodimethylamine (0.12–0.45 ppm) was detected in fish meal which had been implicated in liver disease in mink (718).

The possible occurrence of nitrosamines in cigarette smoke was suggested by Druckrey and Preussmann (719) since tobacco contains several secondary amines, including dimethylamine, nornicotine, anabasine, piperidine, pyrrolidine, and nitrosating agents (486). Various nitrosamines were found in cigarette condensates, reaching a concentration of 180 ng per cigarette made from tobacco grown in a high nitrogen soil (720, 721, 722). The levels of nitrosamines seem dependent on the level of total volatile bases in the tobacco and on the tobacco nitrate content. There is always the possibility of nitrosamine artifacts in the condensate formation.

The presence of nitrosamines in wheat flour (Table IV) was detected only in some instances. Recently, various authors (723, 724) were unable to detect various nitrosamines in spite of the application of large amounts of nitrogen fertilizers and of various amines.

The geographical variation of esophageal cancer strongly suggests a relation to etiological factors in the environment. A high incidence of this cancer occurs in Southern, Central, and East Africa (725), and it was suggested that a nitrosamine might be responsible since a variety of these carcinogens induce tumors of the esophagus in experimental animals. The presence of nitrosamine-like substances was reported in spirits distilled locally from sugar and maize husks from a high incidence area of Zambia (726, 727). However, the methods used for detecting the nitrosamines were too unspecific (728), and subsequent analysis by gas–liquid chromatography and mass spectrometry of spirit samples from areas of high and low frequency in East Africa did not show the presence of nitrosamines (729). N-Nitrosodimethylamine was isolated from alcoholic extracts of a fruit Solanum incanum, which is used in South Africa to sour milk. The high incidence rate of rumenal cancer observed in a valley of Kenya was associated with abnormal forest grazing of the cattle, and the presence of nitrosamines in the plants has been suggested (730).

A high level of cancer of the stomach and esophagus in humans was linked with the formation in vivo of nitrosamines caused by the high intake of nitrates (731, 732, 733).

The majority of these studies on the presence of nitrosamines was done in samples of food for human consumption. However, recently nitrosamines were detected in the atmosphere of factories producing secondary amines. Concentrations ranging from 0.001 to 0.43 ppb of *N*-nitrosodimethylamine were found in the air of a factory producing dimethylamine, and the nitrosamine concentration was correlated with the atmospheric concentrations of nitrogen dioxide and dimethylamine (*734*).

Possible Carcinogenic Hazard to Man

The possible hazard from nitrosamines and the related alkylhydrazines in industry was reviewed by Magee (*752*). Cases of human toxicity caused by exposure to *N*-nitrosodimethylamine (*8*) and 1,1-dimethylhydrazine (*753*, *754*) were reported. Although there is no direct proof that nitrosamines are carcinogenic for man, *N*-nitrosodimethylamine appears to have induced toxic liver changes very similar to those observed in experimental animals (*8*). Recently *N*-nitrosodimethylamine was reported in pooled human cervical and vaginal discharge matter of southern African women (*696*). That a wide range of species is susceptible to the carcinogenic action of nitrosamines (*755*) suggests that man is probably not resistant. Human liver metabolized *N*-nitrosodimethylamine *in vitro* in a way very similar to the rat liver (*545*). The risk for man from nitrosamine formation in the body was recently emphasized (*704*). It is clear that chemists and others who are exposed to nitrosamines in their work should handle these materials with extreme caution. Good knowledge of the carcinogenic potential of nitrosamines for man can be obtained only by epidemiological studies.

Conclusions

Many *N*-nitroso compounds are powerfully carcinogenic in experimental animals, and, although there is no firm proof, it is highly probable that they are also carcinogenic in man. All personnel in the laboratory or elsewhere who handle these compounds should be aware of their great carcinogenic potential and should treat them with correspondingly great care.

The carcinogenic nitroso compounds are effective in a wide range of species, including birds, reptiles, fish, and mammals. Variation in the chemical structure of the compounds results in cancer induction in different organs. Tumors have been induced by one or more nitroso carcinogens in most organs of the rat, which has been more extensively studied than other species, and there may be considerable organ specificity. Most of the evidence suggests that decomposition or metabolism of the parent nitroso compound is necessary before carcinogenesis or other biological activities can occur. Alkylation of nucleic acids and proteins occurs after exposure of animals or cellular preparations *in vitro* to the compounds. *N*-Nitroso compounds were used extensively in the experimental investigation of mechanisms of chemical carcinogenesis.

It is now well established that carcinogenic nitrosamines may be present in minute amounts in certain foods for human consumption, particularly where nitrites are used as food additives. Carcinogenic nitrosamines may also be formed from secondary or tertiary amines and nitrites in the body, particularly in the acid conditions of the stomach after simultaneous ingestion. Secondary and tertiary amines occur in some foods, and a number of drugs and other environmental chemicals have secondary or tertiary amino structures. Humans also are exposed to secondary amines and nitrosating agents in various industries. The significance of these types of exposure to nitrosamines in causing human cancer is not yet known.

Cycasin

The carcinogenic activity of cycasin, the glucoside of methylazoxymethanol (Figure 1), was discovered by Laqueur *et al.* (*756*) who observed the induction of benign and malignant tumors, mainly of the liver and kidney, in rats fed cycad nut meal as part of their diet. This study was initiated because

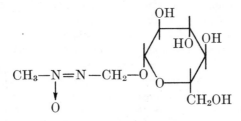

Figure 1.   Structure of cycasin

it was suggested that consumption of cycad material might be responsible for the greatly increased incidence of the neurological disorder amyotrophic lateral sclerosis in the human population on Guam (*757, 758, 759*). There is no doubt that cycad plants do contain neurotoxic components, for example α-amino-β-methylaminopropionic acid (*760*) and also that cycasin, when administered in the neonatal period or transplacentally, can cause malformation of the nervous system in rodents, particularly in the cerebellum (*761, 762, 763*). However, this section is concerned primarily with the carcinogenic, mutagenic, and some relevant toxic properties of cycasin and other glycosides of methylazoxymethanol. These topics were discussed in a number of detailed reviews (*764, 765, 766, 767*). In addition the proceedings of the Third Conference on the Toxicity of Cycads (1964) (*768*) and of the Sixth International Cycad Conference (1972) (*769*) have been published, and a bibliography of cycad research appeared in 1972 (*770*). For accounts of other classes of naturally occurring carcinogens, see the two following chapters.

The cycads belong to an ancient botanical family which predominated over other vegetation during most of the Mesozoic period. They now occur only in tropical and subtropical regions, and they have the capacity to survive adverse climatic conditions when other plants are destroyed. This resistance has led to more extensive consumption by humans when other vegetable foods are unavailable. The cycad may represent an intermediate evolutionary stage between ferns and flowering plants. Cycads belong to the family *Cycadaceae* of the Gymnospermae (771) of which there are nine genera: *Bowenia, Cerato-zamia, Cycas, Dioon, Encephalartos, Microcycas, Macrozamia, Stangeria,* and *Zamia* (764). Cycads have been used for various medicinal purposes and also as human food. Their toxic properties have been long recognized and are reduced by soaking the plant material in water before consumption (759, 764, 765). A fairly recent example of such food use by a human population occurred in the Miyako islands, south of Japan, about 170 miles west of Okinawa. Continuous typhoons destroyed virtually all the agricultural prod-ucts normally used for food, and the population subsisted largely on cycads during the ensuing famine. A statistical survey of the mortality from cancer in the islands from 1961 to 1966 revealed no significant difference in the incidence of liver tumors from that in the mainland, and the incidence of stomach cancer was lower. There was, however, a higher incidence of liver cirrhosis, but the natives had been eating cycads for many years before the famine and were apparently well aware of the methods for removing the toxic factor by soaking (772). There is thus no direct evidence for the carcinogenic activity of cycads in man.

Chemistry of the Glucosides of Methylazoxymethanol. Earlier work on the chemistry of the toxic components of cycads was reviewed by Whiting (764). Nishida and Yamada (773) produced formaldehyde from *Cycas revoluta* by the action of the enzyme emulsin which is present in the seeds, and cycasin was isolated from the same plant and its chemical structure proposed (774). A similar crystalline material was isolated from *Macrozamia spiralis* seeds by Cooper in 1941 (775) and called macrozamin. The carbo-hydrate component of macrozamin is primeverose (775) and its aglycone is methylazoxymethanol (777). It was subsequently found in seeds of some *Cycadaceae* and *Macrozamia* (778), but only glucose and no primeverose was detected in *Cycas circinalis*, indicating the absence of macrozamin (779). The structure of cycasin (Figure 1) was confirmed by Korsch and Riggs (780) from evidence derived from proton magnetic resonance spectra. Similar conclusions on the structure of cycasin were made by Nishida *et al.* (774) who also determined the amounts of the glycoside in cycad seeds (781).

Cycas circinalis nuts were chemically separated into nine fractions, three of which were acutely toxic to rats. Pure crystalline cycasin was prepared from these toxic fractions, and evidence was obtained that one fraction con-tained the free aglycone which appeared to be reasonably stable (782). Meth-ylazoxymethanol was prepared from cycasin by hydrolysis with an enzyme prepared from cycad nuts or with a commercial almond emulsin. The product was extracted with ether and purified by repeated fractional distillation *in vacuo*. The purity was determined by ultraviolet absorption and formalde-hyde analysis. The ester, methylazoxymethanol acetate, was prepared from both crude and purified methylazoxymethanol by reaction with acetic an-hydride in pyridine followed by extraction with chloroform and purification by repeated vacuum distillation. Methylazoxymethanol benzoate and 3,5-dinitrobenzoate were also prepared (783, 784). Methylazoxymethanol acetate was synthesized by azomethane oxidation to azoxymethane followed by bromination by the Wohl–Ziegler reaction and subsequent conversion of the bromoazoxymethane to the acetate by reaction with silver acetate (785). A procedure for the preparation of the acetate labeled with ^{14}C or ^3H was described in which labeled 1,2-dimethylhydrazine is prepared from radioactive methyl iodide followed by oxidation to azomethane (786). The ester is hydrolyzed by an enzyme present in serum (787). Deacetylation is probably the initial step, mediated by a serum esterase sensitive to physostigmine inhibition (788).

Cycasin produced anisole in 40–50% yield when dissolved in molten phenol and treated with a drop of concentrated sulfuric acid (789). Methylazoxymethanol, however, methylated DNA, RNA, phenol, or p-chlorobenzoic acid in aqueous solution under physiological conditions at pH 7 and 37°C (790). The latter findings were consistent with the suggestion of Miller (791) that cycasin and its aglycone might act biologically in a similar manner to N-nitrosodimethylamine. This received further support from in vivo studies discussed later.

Procedures for quantitatively measuring cycasin in cycad material were based on determination of the formaldehyde content by the chromotropic acid method (782). This was because one mole of formaldehyde is produced when one mole of azoxyglycoside is hydrolyzed with acid (777) or on separation of the cycasin by paper chromatography and determination of the sugar component colorimetrically (781). Using a modification of the latter procedure, Palekar and Dastur (792) determined the cycasin content of Cycas circinalis in various materials obtained from Guam. Interestingly, dried cycad chips, prepared by the Guamanians for human consumption, contained no detectable cycasin while extracts of freshly removed kernels and of powder from dried nuts contained clearly measurable amounts of 0.5 to 1% cycasin by weight. The same authors quote cycasin levels in cycad materials reported by other workers to be in the range 0.15–5% and suggest that the variation is caused not only by differences in species of cycad but also by factors affecting the enzymes (emulsins) that decompose cycasin. Prolonged storage of cycasin under inadequate refrigeration or boiling for 80 min or more resulted in increased amounts of the glycoside, apparently because of inactivation of the endogenous β-glucosidase (793). More recently a rapid and sensitive method for the quantitative determination of cycasin by gas–liquid chromatography after trimethylsilylation was described (794). The average content of cycasin from 10 separate analyses of one lot of cycad flour by this method was about 0.4% (794).

Toxicity of Cycasin and Methylazoxymethanol. Earlier work on cycad toxicity was reviewed by Whiting (764). All the evidence supports the conclusion first put forward by Nishida and his colleagues (795), that cycasin itself is not toxic but that it is cleaved, probably by microbial enzymes of the intestinal tract, to yield the aglycone methylazoxymethanol, which is responsible for the toxic action. The Japanese workers showed that toxic effects of cycasin appeared about 24 hr after oral administration, but intravenous injection of the glycoside was ineffective. These findings were confirmed and extended by Kobayishi and Matsumoto (*783, 784*) who showed that cycasin had no apparent toxicity after intraperitoneal administration to rats and that it was almost quantitatively excreted unchanged in the urine. On the other hand, methylazoxymethanol, prepared by enzymic hydrolysis of cycasin, was toxic when injected intraperitoneally and induced hepatic changes morphologically similar to those resulting from oral cycasin (*789*). The importance of the intestinal microorganisms for the activation of cycasin was confirmed by its lack of toxicity in germ-free rats (*796*), which is further discussed later. A detailed account of the acute changes caused by oral administration of cycasin was provided by Laqueur *et al.* (*756*). In their demonstration of tumor induction in rats chronically ingesting cycad meal, these workers noted pathological changes in the liver within 24 hr of the start of the experiment. These changes consisted of loss of glycogen and cytoplasmic basophilia from isolated liver cells around the central veins which were followed, at 48 hr, by cytoplasmic eosinophilia and focal cellular necrosis. The alterations progressed to involve all the liver lobules uniformly, and there was usually hemorrhage into the necrotic areas, and the lesions resembled those induced by *N*-nitrosodimethylamine. This resemblance was subsequently confirmed at the ultrastructural level by Ganote and Rosenthal (*797*) who reported closely similar hepatic changes induced by methylazoxymethanol and by *N*-nitrosodimethylamine in contrast to those caused by two other hepatotoxins, carbon tetrachloride and hydrazine. The hepatic parenchymal cells (Megalocytosis) increased in size during continued feeding of methylazoxymethanol acetate (*798*).

Carcinogenicity of Cycasin and Methylazoxymethanol. In the first demonstration of the carcinogenicity of cycad material, Laqueur *et al.* (*756*) fed untreated flour prepared from cycad nuts, indigenous to Guam, to rats and obtained benign and malignant tumors mainly in the liver and kidneys, with one in the lung and two in the intestine. The tumors of the liver were decribed as hepatomas and reticuloendothelial neoplasms which occurred simultaneously but independently of one another. All the hepatomas were hepatocellular and many showed a striking vascular component often associated with hemorrhage into the tumor. There was massive fatal intraabdominal hemorrhage in several animals following rupture of the capsule of the liver lying over the tumor. Secondary tumor deposits in the lungs resembled the primary tumors in the liver and were also associated with massive hemorrhage into the tumor and into the surrounding pulmonary tissue. The authors emphasized the strong resemblance between these changes and those produced in the rat by *N*-nitrosodimethylamine.

The kidney tumors were of two types described as adenomas and undifferentiated tumors; again the resemblance to the renal tumors induced in rats by *N*-nitrosodimethylamine was striking. The epithelial lesions included solid and papillary intracystic adenomas, and occasionally clear-cell tumors were seen, resembling those that occur in man. The undifferentiated proliferative tumors were thought to originate from cells between tubules and capillaries in the inner cortex and grew infiltratively between pre-existing renal structures, again resembling the N-nitrosodimethylamine-induced mesenchymal tumors of rat kidney ($97, 393$). The one primary lung tumor was an alveolar cell adenoma with foci of squamous metaplasia, and the tumors of the large intestine were primary mucinous adenocarcinomas. The authors drew attention to the resemblance between the chemical structures of methylazoxymethanol and N-nitrosodimethylamine and suggested that metabolism of the two carcinogens might lead to the formation of an active metabolite common to both. Similar liver and kidney tumors were found in rats given diets containing 0.5–2% dry cycad husk which is eaten as candy by natives of Guam ($799, 800$) or the related plant $Encephalartos\ hildebrandtiae$ ($801, 802$). In contrast, cycad flour processed by the Guamanians for human consumtion (772) was not carcinogenic in rats (803). Most subsequent experimental work was done with the purified carcinogenic components of the crude materials.

Sprague–Dawley rats proved sensitive to administration of cycasin in the drinking water ($10\ \text{mg/kg}$ body weight/day) for 10 days, followed by withdrawal of the carcinogen. Hepatic tumors, described as hepatoma and hepatic sarcoma, were induced in more than 80% of the animals, with a few kidney tumors (804). The pathology of the renal tumors in the rat was studied in detail by Gusek and his co-workers, using light and electron microscopy as well as histochemical methods. In their earlier studies, special attention was given to the "interstitial tumor" described by Laqueur. It was concluded that this tumor is a nephroblastoma, corresponding to the Wilms tumor in man and that it may be derived from relatively primitive, pre-existing interstitial cells ($805, 806, 807$). Subsequently the epithelial tumors were investigated with the conclusion that they correspond morphologically with the renal adenomas found in human subjects and that they arise from islets of tubular proliferation or from cysts (808).

Like N-nitrosodimethylamine, cycasin is capable of inducing tumors in the rat after a single dose (809). Following subcutaneous injection in newborn Fischer rats or single administration to weanling Osborne–Mendel rats, tumors morphologically similar to those induced by cycasin in adult animals appeared (in descending order of frequency) in the kidneys, intestine, liver, lung, and brain. The tumor induction period was not shortened in the neonatally treated animals (809). The development of carcinogenesis following subcutaneous injection of cycasin was surprising in view of the probable necessity for enzymic release of the aglycone by a β-glucosidase and is discussed later. Tumors induced by crude cycad meal, cycasin, or its aglycone were transplanted, including several renal tumors of both types and some liver and colonic tumors (810). Successful transplantation of the nephroblastomas, but not of the renal sarcomas, depended on the sex of the recipient animals. Attempts to convert transplanted kidney tumors into the ascites form failed. A detailed account of the intestinal tumors induced in the rat by crude cycad material, cycasin and methylazoxymethanol, was given by Laqueur (811). The glycoside produced tumors only in the large intestine, while the aglycone, after intraperitoneal injection, induced tumors also in the small intestine (*811*). Tumors of the mammary gland were induced in rats by cycasin (*812*), and the target organs for cycasin carcinogenesis are considerably influenced by the dosage regimen in rats and mice (*813*).

Several other species in addition to the rat were sensitive to cycasin carcinogenesis. Hepatic and renal tumors were induced in mice by topical application of aqueous extracts of cycad nuts to artificial skin ulcers (*814*). The rationale of this experiment was to imitate the conditions of use of such extracts by human beings in some parts of the world to promote the healing of skin ulceration. Newborn C57Bl/6 mice showed early development of reticulum cell tumors and a high incidence of hepatomas following injection of a single dose of cycasin, but adult mice were less susceptible to the carcinogen (*815*). Newborn mice of the dd strain that received single subcutaneous injections of 0.5 mg cycasin/g body weight within 24 hr of birth developed a high incidence of lung tumors and liver tumors in more than half of the survivors. In the same experiment mice receiving 1.0 mg cycasin/g body weight showed neurological disorders with severe ataxia, but the tumor incidence in the less severely affected animals that survived was similar in the lung but smaller in the liver. The mice with the nervous system disorders showed changes in the cerebellum that are discussed later (*816*). Syrian golden hamsters that survived the acute toxic effects of a single subcutaneous injection of cycasin within 24 hr after birth (0.2–0.6 mg/kg body weight) showed neurological disorders, and the more severely affected died relatively quickly. The less affected animals developed bile duct or hepatocllular carcinomas. Single intragastric doses of cycasin given to adult (two month old) hamsters produced bile duct carcinomas only in the liver and very few kidney tumors (*817*). Guinea pigs fed crude cycad meal at a level of 10% in the diet developed acute hemorrhagic centrilobular necrosis of the liver, similar to that seen in the rat, and continued feeding at the 5% dietary level induced hepatic parenchymal tumors (*818*). Aquarium fish exposed to *Cycas circinalis* also showed hepatic neoplasms (*819*) but prolonged feeding of 0.5 or 1% cycad kernel or husk to chickens did not produce tumors although toxicity was observed at higher dose levels (*820*). The carcinogenicity of cycasin in different species was discussed by Hirono (*821*). He compared the incidence and localization of tumors in rats and mice receiving a single dose of cycasin with the findings in hamsters, rabbits, and guinea pigs given similar treatment. Tumors of the kidney and small intestine were frequent in rats but uncommon in mice or the other species. Hepatocellular carcinomas were as readily induced in new born hamsters as bile duct carcinomas, but the former type of tumor was not found after treatment of adult animals. No tumors were observed in rabbits or guinea pigs that survived single intragastric doses of cycasin (*821*).

As already mentioned, cycasin did not cause toxic manifestations in germ-free rats, and it also failed to increase the incidence of tumors in such animals when fed at a level of 200 mg/100 g of basal diet for 20 days and observed for a period of two years. Conventional rats fed the same cycasin-containing germ-free diet showed marked reduction in weight gain and severe liver necrosis. Methylazoxymethanol acetate or the free aglycone proved to be effectively carcinogenic at low dose levels in germ-free rats inducing tumors of the large intestine, kidney, and liver, as in conventional animals (822). Excretion of unchanged cycasin in the germ-free rats was virtually complete, mainly in the urine while only 18–35% of the administered glycoside was recovered in conventional rats. This confirmed that intestinal microbial flora containing β-glucosidase are required to decompose cycasin in the body (823). This conclusion was substantiated by experiments in which germ-free rats were monocontaminated with several strains of bacteria before being given cycasin. The toxicity of the cycasin and the amounts excreted unchanged were found to correlate closely with the level of the glucosidase in the organisms (824).

The induction of kidney tumors in neonatal rats following subcutaneous injection of cycasin (809) was apparently inconsistent with a requirement for bacterial enzymes, but it was subsequently shown that a β-D-glucosidase, which is capable of hydrolyzing cycasin, is present in the subcutaneous tissue of newborn rats (825, 826). An alternative suggestion was put forward that the tumors might have resulted from cycling of cycasin from the urine of the newborn rats to their mothers followed by excretion of methylazoxymethanol and undegraded cycasin in the maternal milk (827). Toxic material is known to be excreted in the milk of animals fed crude cycad (828). The situation has been considerably clarified by a detailed study of the tissue distribution and activity with increasing age after birth of β-glucosidase in the rat, carried out by Matsumoto and his colleagues (829). These authors found that the enzyme activity of the small intestine increased gradually to a maximum at about the 15th postnatal day and decreased rapidly to a minimum shortly after weaning at 21 days. There was comparatively little activity in other tissues, including the skin, and there was no evidence of enzyme induction by administration of cycasin. The incidence of tumors induced appeared to correlate well with the level of β-glucosidase activity at the time of injection, and the authors conclude that their data tend to support the hypothesis that the incidence of tumor induction is related to the β-glucosidase activity of the small intestine (829).

Tumors have been induced transplacentally by feeding crude cycad meal to pregnant rats during the first, second, and third weeks of gestation. Animals exposed during the first week developed neoplasms of the jejunum, but there was no correlation between site of tumor induction, frequently the brain, and time of exposure to the carcinogen during the second two weeks. The main sites of transplacental carcinogenesis by cycad material were thus different from those reported in immature or adult rats but the time necessary for tumor production was essentially the same (830). The transformation in vitro by methylazoxymethanol acetate of rat embryo cells infected with Rauscher leukemia virus was recently reported (831).

Teratogenicity and Mutagenicity of Cycasin and Methylazoxymethanol. The transplacental induction of tumors suggested that cycasin and/or its aglycone were able to cross the placenta. This was shown by Spatz and Laqueur (*832*) who demonstrated the presence of both materials in rat or hamster fetuses after oral or intravenous administration. Both compounds were also excreted in the milk during lactation (*832*). Methyl-azoxymethanol injected intravenously into golden hamsters on the eighth day of pregnancy caused growth retardation of the progeny and a variety of malformations, including hydrocephalus, microcephalus, cranioschisis, exencephaly, spina bifida, rachischisis, anophthalmia, microophthalmia, and oligo-dactyl (*833*). Microencephaly was induced transplacentally in the rat by intraperitoneal injection of the mother animals on the 14th or 15th day of pregnancy. The condition was found uniformly in all litter mates, and the effect was independent of the rat strain—Fishcer or Osborne–Mendel. Gliomas were found in about 10% of the microencephalic rats permitted to live beyond one year (*834*). The changes induced in the cerebellum in mice and hamsters were subjected to detailed study (*761, 762, 763*), and the repair of the damage to the extrenal granular layer was described (*835*). Mental defects were found in rats exposed to methylazoxymethanol *in utero* (*836*).

Methylazoxymethanol is an effective mutagen, increasing the frequency of reversion to histidine independence of several histidine-requiring mutants of *Salmonella typhimurium*. Most of the mutants were revertible with a variety of alkylating agents while the one frame-shift mutant tested was not reverted by alkylating agents or methylazoxymethanol. Cycasin was not mutagenic in this system, presumably because the *Salmonella* lacked the necessary deglucosylating enzyme (*837*). Methylazoxymethanol and its acetate were mutagenic in *Drosophilia*, inducing sex-linked recessive lethal mutations, but cycasin was inactive. Homogenates of *Drosophila* contained substantial esterase activity but very little or no detectable β-glucosidase (*838*). When tested by the host-mediated assay in mice, however, cycasin and the aglycone were both mutagenic. In this procedure histidine auxotrophs of *Salmonella typhimurium* were injected intraperitoneally and the test compounds given orally. Reversions from histidine dependence were detected and scored in the organisms recovered from the peritoneal cavity after 2-hr incubation. In these experiments the cycasin was presumably activated by the organisms of the intestinal tract of the mice (*839*). Cycasin also induced chromosome aberrations in root tip cells of *Allium cepa* (*840, 841*).

Cycads are used as food by larvae of the Lepidopteran *Seirarctia echo* which is surprising in view of the powerful toxicity of these plants for other animal species. An interesting explanation of this phenomenon was provided by Teas (*842*) who showed that this organism is able to synthesize cycasin when fed a diet containing added methylazoxymethanol. Homogenates of whole caterpillars showed strong β-glucosidase activity, and studies of the distribution revealed the highest enzyme activity in the gut with very little in other organs. It was concluded that the azoxyglycosides were hydrolyzed in the gut and resynthesized into the relatively nontoxic cycasin which is accumulated in those parts of the insect with low or absent β-glucosidase activity (*842*).

Biochemical Actions of Cycasin and Methylazoxymethanol.
Feeding crude cycad material or cycasin (0.2% in the diet) resulted in loss
of RNA and phospholipid from rat liver cells, first observed 24 hr after starting the treatment, and the effect was dose dependent. These changes correlated
closely with the loss of cytoplasmic basophilia observed with the light microscope and the loss of ribosomes from the endoplasmic reticulum seen with
the electron microscope. There was no effect on hepatic DNA concentration
while the cholesterol and neutral glycerides increased (843). Oral administration of cycasin (500 mg/kg body weight) to rats inhibited protein synthesis
in liver but not in kidney, spleen, or ilium. The inhibition was not evident
until about 5 hr after cycasin administration, but once established, it persisted
for the next 20 hr. (844). Both cycasin and methylazoxymethanol acetate
disaggregated polysomes of rat liver. The acetate was more effective than
the glycoside, and cycasin inhibited strongly the induction of hepatic tryptophan pyrrolase by cortisone (845). Zedeck et al. (846) reported that single
nonlethal doses of methylazoxymethanol acetate inhibited thymidine incorporation into liver, small intestine, and kidney of rats. The effect was most
marked in the liver which was the only organ to show inhibition of RNA
and protein synthesis. In the mouse there was only a slight inhibitory effect
on DNA synthesis in the liver with earlier inhibition of RNA and protein
synthesis and no detectable effects on the kidney or small intestine. The
corresponding morphological changes reported by these authors were described in the section on toxicity. Detailed studies of the effects of methylazoxymethanol acetate on hepatic RNA synthesis (847) revealed inhibition
of UTP incorporation into RNA of hepatic nuclei isolated from rats treated
with the ester. This suggests an effect on either DNA template or RNA
polymerase activity. Orotic acid incorporation into nucleolar RNA was unaffected 30 min after treatment when ultrastructural changes were already
present, but cytidine incorporation was significantly decreased suggesting an
early selective inhibition of cytidylate uptake into nucleolar RNA (847).
The same group (848) showed that the inhibition of UTP incorporation into
nuclear RNA was probably not caused by failure of the precursor to penetrate
the nucleus because RNA synthetic activity of "aggregate" enzyme (a preparation containing chromatin and RNA polymerase) was also significantly
inhibited 3 hr after treatment of the animals with methylazoxymethanol
acetate. The template capacity of hepatic DNA chromatin preparations from
the carcinogen-treated animals only differed very slightly, or not at all, from
the control preparations with RNA polymerase from *E. coli* or from rat liver
(848). The possibility that decreased RNA synthesis following treatment
with methylazoxymethanol acetate might be caused by interaction with proteins, perhaps RNA polymerase, was suggested by a report that the aglycone
reacted with L-histidine *in vitro* to produce *N*-1 and *N*-3-methylhistidines
(849). Grab et al. (848) obtained evidence from circular dichroism analysis
of the "aggregate" enzyme preparation indicating a change in conformation
of the protein component and concluded that the induction of such changes in
hepatic nuclear proteins may result in decreased RNA synthesis (848). Evi-

dence of methylation of liver nucleic acids *in vivo* in rats treated with cycasin or methylazoxymethanol was obtained by Shank and Magee (*844*), and brain nucleic acids were shown to be methylated in fetal rats after treatment with methylazoxymethanol (*850*). Like other methylating agents, methylazoxy-methanol acetate induced single strand breaks in rat liver DNA *in vivo* and its potency in this respect was comparable with that of *N*-nitrosodimethyl-amine. The repair of DNA damage induced by these two liver carcinogens appeared to be slower than that with other methylating agents (*N*-methyl-*N*-nitrosourea and methyl methanesulfonate) that are not carcinogenic for rat liver (*851*). It may be concluded that, as with their toxic, carcinogenic, and mutagenic properties, cycasin and other methylazoxymethanol derivatives closely resemble the nitrosamines in their biochemical actions.

Acknowledgments

P. N. Magee would like to acknowledge a generous grant from the Cancer Research Campaign of Great Britain. The authors wish to thank Margaret Blamire, Amanda Pickett, and Susan Huckle for their secretarial assistance in the preparation of this manuscript.

Literature Cited

1. Barnes, J. M., Magee, P. N., *Br. J. Ind. Med.* (1954) **11**, 167.
2. Magee, P. N., Barnes, J. M., *Br. J. Cancer* (1956) **10**, 114.
3. Schoental, R., *Nature* (1960) **188**, 420.
4. Druckrey, H., Preussmann, R., Schmähl, D., Müller, M., *Naturwissenschaften* (1961) **48**, 165.
5. Magee, P. N., Schoental, R., *Br. Med. Bull.* (1964) **20**, 102.
6. Magee, P. N., Barnes, J. M., *Adv. Cancer Res.* (1967) **10**, 163.
7. Druckrey, H., Preussmann, R., Ivankovic, S., Schmähl, D., *Z. Krebsforsch.* (1967) **69**, 103.
8. Freund, H. A., *Ann. Int. Med.* (1937) **10**, 1144.
9. Fridman, A. L., Mukhametshin, F. M., Novikov, S. S., *Russian Chem. Rev.* (1971) **40**, 34.
10. Feuer, H., "The Chemistry of the Nitro and Nitroso Groups, Part 2, Wiley Interscience, New York, 1970.
11. Cadogan, J. L., *Accounts Chem. Res.* (1971) **4**, 187.
12. Eiter, K., Hebenbrock, K., Kabbe, M., *Liebig's Ann. Chem.* (1972) **765**, 55.
13. Geuther, A., *Liebig's Ann. Chem.* (1863) **128**, 151.
14. Renouf, E., *Chem. Ber.* (1880) **13**, 2170.
15. Ladenburg, A., *Chem. Ber.* (1879) **12**, 948.
16. Graymore, J., *J. Chem. Soc.* (1938) 1311.
17. Jones, J., Urbanski, T., *J. Chem. Soc.* (1949) 1768.
18. Löffler, K., *Chem. Ber.* (1910) **43**, 2035.
19. Forlander, D., Wallis, Th., *Liebig's Ann. Chem.* (1906) **345**, 277.
20. Jones, E., Kenner, J., *J. Chem. Soc.* (1933) 363.
21. Klement, U., Schmidpeter, A., *Angew. Chem.* (1968) **80**, 444.
22. Eisenbrand, G., Preussmann, R., *Arzeim. Forsch.* (1970) **20**, 1513.
23. Baliga, B. T., *J. Org. Chem.* (1970) **35**, 2031.
24. Fischer, E., *Chem. Ber.* (1879) **8**, 1587.
25. Wieland, H., Fressel, H., *Liebig's Ann. Chem.* (1912) **392**, 133.
26. Paal, C., Yao, W. N., *Chem. Ber.* (1930) **63**, 65.
27. Bailey, J., Snyder, D., *J. Am. Chem. Soc.* (1915) **37**, 935.

28. Rohde, W., *Liebig's Ann. Chem.* (1869) **151**, 366.
29. Poirier, H., Benington, F., *Am. Chem. Soc.* (1951) **73**, 3192.
30. Hanna, C., Schueler, F., *J. Am. Chem. Soc.* (1952) **74**, 3693.
31. Jaffé, B. F., Sabinian, E. I., *Zhur Obshch. Khim.* (1963) **33**, 2188.
32. Iversen, P. E., *Chem. Ber.* (1972) **105**, 358.
33. Overberger, C., Anselme, J., Lombardino, J., "Organic Compounds with Nitrogen-Nitrogen Bonds," New York, 1966.
34. Smith, P., "The Chemistry of Open-Chain Organic Nitrogen Compounds, Vol. II," New York, 1966.
35. Emmons, W., *J. Am. Chem. Soc.* (1954) **76**, 3468.
36. Cowell, G. W., Ledwith, A., *Quart. Rev.* (1970) **24**, 119.
37. Zollinger, H., "Azo and Diazo Chemistry," Interscience, New York, 1961.
38. Curtis, T., *Chem. Ber.* (1883) **16**, 2030.
39. Fields, R., Haszeldine, R. N., *J. Chem. Soc.* (1964) 1881.
40. Shepard, R. A., Sciaraffa, P. L., *J. Org. Chem.* (1966) **31**, 964.
41. Huisgen, R., *Angew. Chem.* (1955) **67**, 439.
42. Franchimont, A. P. N., *Rec. Trav. Chim.* (1890) **9**, 146.
43. Werner, E. A., *J. Chem. Soc.* (1919) 1093.
44. Horak, V., Prechazka, M., *Czech.* (1959) 98007.
45. De Boer, T. J., Backer, H. J., *Org. Synth.* (1956) **36**, 16.
46. Reimlinger, H. K., *Chem. Ber.* (1961) **94**, 2547.
47. Applequist, D. E., McGreer, D. E., *J. Am. Chem. Soc.* (1960) **82**, 1965.
48. Kirmse, W., Wächtershäuser, G., *Ann. Chem.* (1967) **707**, 44.
49. Moss, R. A., *J. Org. Chem.* (1966) **31**, 1082.
50. Kirmse, W., Schütte, H., *Chem. Ber.* (1968) **101**, 1674.
51. Friedman, L., Bayless, J. H., *J. Am. Chem. Soc.* (1969) **91**, 1790.
52. Newman, M. S., Beard, C. D., *J. Am. Chem. Soc.* (1969) **91**, 5677.
53. *Ibid.* (1970) **92**, 4309.
54. Newman, M. S., Patrick, T. B., *J. Am. Chem. Soc.* (1969) **91**, 6461.
55. *Ibid.* (1970) **92**, 4312.
56. Newman, M. S., Okorodudu, A. O. M., *J. Org. Chem.* (1969) **34**, 1220.
57. White, E. H., *J. Am. Chem. Soc.* (1955) **77**, 6011.
58. Overberger, C. G., Lombardino, J. G., Hiskey, R. G., *J. Am. Chem Soc.* (1958) **80**, 3009.
59. Carpino, L. A., *J. Am. Chem. Soc.* (1957) **79**, 4427.
60. Baumgardner, C. L., Martin, K. J., Freeman, J. P., *J. Am. Chem. Soc.* (1963) **85**, 97.
61. Baumgardner, C. L., Freeman, J. P., *J. Am. Chem. Soc.* (1964) **86**, 2233.
62. Carter, P., Stevens, T. S., *J. Chem. Soc.* (1961) 1743.
63. Hünig, S., *Helv. Chim. Acta* (1971) **54**, 1721.
64. Hünig, S., Geldern, L., Lücke, E., *Angew. Chem.* (1963) **75**, 476.
65. Hünig, S., Büttner, G., Cramer, J., Geldern, L., Hausen, H., Lücke, E., *Chem. Ber.* (1969) **102**, 2093.
66. Hünig, S., Hausen, H., *Chem. Ber.* (1969) **102**, 2109.
67. Eicher, T., Hünig, S., Nikolaus, P., *Angew. Chem.* (1967) **79**, 682.
68. Eicher, T., Hünig, S., Hausen, H., *Angew. Chem.* (1969) **102**, 2889.
69. Eicher, T., Hünig, S., Hausen, H., Nikolaus, P., *Angew. Chem.* (1969) **102**, 3159.
70. Eicher, T., Hünig, S., Nikolaus, P., *Angew. Chem.* (1969) **102**, 3176.
71. Büttner, G., Hünig, S., *Chem. Ber.* (1971) **104**, 1088.
72. *Ibid.*, 1104.
73. Büttner, G., Cramer, J., Geldern, L., Hünig, S., *Chem. Ber.* (1971) **104**, 1118.
74. D'Agostino, J. T., Jaffé, H. H., *J. Org. Chem.* (1971) **36**, 992.
75. Fraser, R. R., Wigfield, Y. Y., *Tetrahedron Lett.* (1971) 2515.
76. Apsimon, J. W., Cooney, J. D., *Can. J. Chem.* (1971) **49**, 2377.
77. Mannschreck, A., Münsch, H., *Angew. Chem.* (1967) **79**, 1004.

78. Kessler, H., *Angew. Chem.* (1970) **82,** 237.
79. Karabatos, G. J., Taller, R. A., *J. Am. Chem. Soc.* (1964) **86,** 4373.
80. Chow, K. L., *Angew. Chem.* (1967) **79,** 51.
81. D'Agostino, J. T., Jaffé, H. H., *J. Am. Chem. Soc.* (1969) **91,** 3383.
82. Pensabene, J. W., Fiddler, W., Dooley, C. J., Doerr, R. C., Wassermann, A. E., *J. Agr. Food Chem.* (1972) **20,** 274.
83. Apsimon, J. W., Cooney, J. D., *Arch. Mass Spectral Data* (1972) **3,** 536.
84. Apsimon, J. W., Cooney, J. D., *Can. J. Chem.* (1971) **49,** 1367.
85. Billets, S., Jaffé, H. H., Kaplan, F., *J. Am. Chem. Soc.* (1970) **92,** 6964.
86. Axenrod, R., Milne, G. W. A., *Chem. Commun.* (1968) 67.
87. Hard, G. C., Butler, W. H., *Cancer Res.* (1970) **30,** 2796.
88. Hard, G. C., Butler, W. H., *J. Pathol.* (1970) **102,** 201.
89. Bannasch, P., "The Cytoplasm of Hepatocytes During Carcinogenesis," Springer-Verlag, Heidelberg and New York, 105, 1968.
90. Schoental, R., Magee, P. N., *Br. J. Cancer* (1962) **16,** 92.
91. Leaver, D. D., Swann, P. F., Magee, P. N., *Br. J. Cancer* (1969) **23,** 177.
92. Malling, H. V., *Muta. Res.* (1971) **13,** 425.
93. Legator, M. S., Malling, H. V., "Chemical Mutagens: Principles and Methods for their Detection," A. Hollaender, Ed., **2,** 569, Plenum, New York and London, 1971.
94. Pielsticker, K., Mohr, U., Klemm, J., *Naturwissenschaften* (1967) **54,** 340.
95. Ehrentraut, W., Juhls, H., Kupfer, G., Kupfer, M., Zintzsch, J., Rommel, P., Wähmer, R., Schnurrbusch, U., Möckel, P., *Arch. Geschwulstforsch.* (1969) **33,** 31.
96. Magee, P. N., Barnes, J. M., *Acta Unio Int. Contra Cancrum* (1959) **15,** 187.
97. Magee, P. N., Barnes, J. M., *J. Pathol. Bacteriol.* (1962) **84,** 19.
98. Schmähl, D., Preussmann, R., *Naturwissenschaften* (1959) **46,** 175.
99. Zak, F. G., Holzner, J. H., Singer, E. J., Popper, H., *Cancer Res.* (1960) **20,** 96.
100. Argus, M. F., Arcos, J. C., Hoch-Ligeti, C., *J. Natl. Cancer Inst.* (1965) **35,** 949.
101. Riopelle, J.-L., Jasmin, G., *Rev. Can. Biol.* (1963) **22,** 365.
102. *Ibid.* (1964) **23,** 129.
103. Riopelle, J.-L., Jasmin, G., *J. Natl. Cancer Inst.* (1969) **42,** 643.
104. Terracini, B., Magee, P. N., *Nature* (1964) **202,** 502.
105. Terracini, B., Magee, P. N., Barnes, J. M., *Br. J. Cancer* (1967) **21,** 559.
106. Terracini, B., Palestro, G., Ruà, S., Trevisio, A., *Tumori* (1969) **55,** 357.
107. Thomas, C., *Z. Krebsforsch.* (1965) **67,** 1.
108. Ito, N., Johno, I., Marugami, M., Konishi, Y., Hiasa, Y., *Gann* (1966) **57,** 595.
109. Schmidt, J. D., Murphy, G. P., *Invest. Urol.* (1966) **4,** 57.
110. Hadjiolov, D., *Z. Krebsforsch.* (1968) **71,** 59.
111. Hoch-Ligeti, C., Argus, M. F., Arcos, J. C., *J. Natl. Cancer Inst.* (1968) **40,** 535.
112. Takayama, S., Imaizumi, T., *Int. J. Cancer* (1969) **4,** 373.
113. Takayama, S., Oota, K., *Gann* (1963) **54,** 465.
114. *Ibid.* (1965) **56,** 189.
115. Toth, B., Magee, P. N., Shubik, P., *Cancer Res.* (1964) **24,** 1712.
116. Toth, B., Shubik, P., *Cancer Res.* (1967) **27,** 43.
117. Terracini, B., Palestro, G., Ramella Gigliardi, M., Montesano, R., *Br. J. Cancer* (1966) **20,** 871.
118. Clapp, N. K., Craig, A. W., Toya, R. E., *J. Natl. Cancer Inst.* (1968) **41,** 1213.
119. Clapp, N. K., Tyndall, R. L., Otten, J. A., *Cancer Res.* (1971) **31,** 196.
120. Clapp, N. K., Toya, R. E., *J. Natl. Cancer Inst.* (1970) **45,** 495.
121. Vesselinovitch, S. D., *Cancer Res.* (1969) **29,** 1024.
122. Frei, J. V., *Cancer Res.* (1970) **30,** 11.
123. Mirvish, S. S., Kaufman, L., *Int. J. Cancer* (1970) **6,** 69.

124. Otsuka, H., Kuwahara, A., *Gann* (1971) **62,** 147.
125. Shabad, L. M., Savluchinskaya, L. A., *Bull. Exp. Biol. Med.* (1971) **71,** 76.
126. Armuth, V., Berenblum, I., *Cancer Res.* (1972) **32,** 2259.
127. Kuwahara, A., Otsuka, H., Nagamatsu, A., *Gann* (1972) **63,** 499.
128. Den Engelse, L., Hollander, C. F., Misdorp, W., *Eur. J. Cancer* (1974) **10,** 129.
129. Tomatis, L., Magee, P. N., Shubik, P., *J. Natl. Cancer Inst.* (1964) **33,** 341.
130. Tomatis, L., Cefis, F., *Tumori* (1967) **53,** 447.
131. Herrold, K. M., *J. Natl. Cancer Inst.* (1967) **39,** 1099.
132. Kowalewski, K., Todd, E. F., *Proc. Soc. Exp. Biol. Med.* (1971) **136,** 482.
133. Stenback, F., Ferrero, A., Montesano, R., Shubik, P., *Z. Krebsforsch.* (1973) **79,** 31.
134. LePage, R. N., Christie, G. S., *Br. J. Cancer* (1969) **23,** 125.
135. Fujii, K., Sato, H., *Gann* (1970) **61,** 425.
136. LePage, R. N., Christie, G. S., *Pathol.* (1969) **1,** 49.
137. Ashley, L. M., Halver, J. E., *J. Natl. Cancer Inst.* (1968) **41,** 531.
138. Ingram, A. J., *Br. J. Cancer* (1972) **26,** 206.
139. Khudolei, V. V., *Vop. Onkol.* (1971) **17,** 67.
140. Sato, S., Matsushima, T., Tanaka, N., Sugimura, T., Takashima, F., *J. Natl. Cancer Inst.* (1973) **50,** 765.
141. Koppang, N., *Acta Pathol. Microbiol. Scand. Suppl.* (1970) **215,** 30.
142. Mohr, U., Haas, H., Hilfrich, J., *Br. J. Cancer* (1974) **29,** 359.
143. Schmähl, D., Preussmann, R., Hamperl, H., *Naturwissenschaften* (1960) **47,** 89.
144. Schmähl, D., Thomas, C., König, K., *Z. Krebsforsch.* (1963) **65,** 529.
145. Argus, M. F., Hoch-Ligeti, C., *J. Natl. Cancer Inst.* (1961) **27,** 695.
146. Dontenwill, W., Mohr, U., *Z. Krebsforsch.* (1962) **65,** 166.
147. Druckrey, H., Schildbach, A., Schmähl, D., Preussmann, R., Ivankovic, S., *Arzneim. Forsch.* (1963) **13,** 841.
148. Druckrey, H., Steinhoff, D., Preussmann, R., Ivankovic, S., *Z. Krebsforsch.* (1964) **66,** 1.
149. Hoch-Ligeti, C., Lobl, L. T., Arvin, J. M., *Br. J. Cancer* (1964) **18,** 271.
150. Rajewsky, M. F., Dauber, W., Frankenberg, H., *Science* (1966) **152,** 83.
151. Reuber, M. D., Lee, C. W., *J. Natl. Cancer Inst.* (1968) **41,** 1133.
152. Svoboda, D., Higginson, J., *Cancer Res.* (1968) **28,** 1703.
153. Mohr, U., Hilfrich, J., *J. Natl. Cancer Inst.* (1972) **49,** 1729.
154. Yamamoto, R. S., Kroes, R., Weisburger, J. H., *Proc. Soc. Exp. Biol. Med.* (1972) **140,** 890.
155. Schmähl, D., Thomas, C., König, K., *Naturwissenschaften* (1963) **50,** 407.
156. Schmähl, D., Thomas, C., *Z. Krebsforsch.* (1965) **66,** 533.
157. Hoffmann, F., Graffi, A., *Acta Biol. Med. Ger.* (1964) **12,** 623.
158. Hoffmann, F., Graffi, A., *Arch. Geschwulstforsch.* (1964) **23,** 274.
159. Clapp, N. K., Craig, A. W., *J. Natl. Cancer Inst.* (1967) **39,** 903.
160. Clapp, N. K., Craig, A. W., Toya, R. E., *Int. J. Cancer* (1970) **5,** 119.
161. Gargus, J. L., Reese, W. H., Jr., Rutter, H. A., *Toxicol. Appl. Pharmacol.* (1969) **15,** 92.
162. Kunz, W., Schaude, G., Thomas, C., *Z. Krebsforsch.* (1969) **72,** 291.
163. Hilfrich, J., Althoff, J., Mohr, U., *Z. Krebsforsch.* (1971) **75,** 240.
164. Turusov, V., Tomatis, L., Guibert, D., Duperray, B., Pacheco, H., "Transplacental Carcinogenesis," *IARC Sci. Publ.* (1973) No. **4,** 84.
165. Dontenwill, W., Mohr, U., *Z. Krebsforsch.* (1961) **64,** 305.
166. Dontenwill, W., Mohr, U., Zagel, M., *Z. Krebsforsch.* (1962) **64,** 499.
167. Herrold, K. M., Dunham, L. J., *Cancer Res.* (1963) **23,** 773.
168. Herrold, K. M., *Br. J. Cancer* (1964) **18,** 763.
169. Herrold, K. M., *Cancer Res.* (1964) **17,** 114.
170. Herrold, K. M., *Arch. Pathol.* (1964) **78,** 189.

171. Mohr, U., Wieser, O., Pielsticker, K., *Naturwissenschaften* (1966) **53**, 229.
172. Montesano, R., Saffiotti, U., *Cancer Res.* (1968) **28**, 2197.
173. Montesano, R., Saffiotti, U., *J. Natl. Cancer Inst.* (1970) **44**, 413.
174. Mohr, U., Pielsticker, K., Wieser, O., Kinzel, V., *Eur. J. Cancer* (1967) **3**, 139.
175. Baker, J. R., Mason, M. M., Herganian, G., Weisburger, E. K., Weisburger, J. H., *Proc. Soc. Exp. Biol. Med.* (1974) **146**, 291.
176. Mohr, U., Althoff, J., Page, N., *J. Natl. Cancer Inst.* (1972) **49**, 595.
177. Druckrey, H., Steinhoff, D., *Naturwissenschaften* (1962) **49**, 497.
178. Argus, M. F., Hoch-Ligeti, C., *J. Natl. Cancer Inst.* (1963) **30**, 533.
179. Thomas, C., Schmähl, D., *Z. Krebsforsch.* (1963) **65**, 531.
180. Lombard, C., *Bull. Cancer* (1965) **52**, 389.
181. Arcos, J. C., Argus, M. F., Mathison, J. B., *Experientia* (1969) **25**, 296.
182. Dale, M. M., Easty, G. C., Tchao, R., Desai, H., Andjargholi, M., *Br. J. Cancer* (1973) **27**, 445.
183. Rapp, H. J., Carleton, J. H., Crisler, C., Nadel, E. M., *J. Natl. Cancer Inst.* (1965) **34**, 453.
184. Schmähl, D., Thomas, C., *Naturwissenschaften* (1965) **52**, 165.
185. Schmähl, D., Thomas, C., Scheld, G., *Naturwissenschaften* (1964) **51**, 466.
186. Schmähl, D., Osswald, H., Mohr, U., *Naturwissenschaften* (1967) **54**, 341.
187. Schmähl, D., Osswald, H., Goerttler, K., *Z. Krebsforsch.* (1969) **72**, 102.
188. Halver, J. A., *Res. Rep. U.S. Fish Wild Serv.* (1963) **160**, 22.
189. Stanton, M. F., *J. Natl. Cancer Inst.* (1965) **34**, 117.
190. Schmähl, D., Osswald, H., Karsten, C., *Naturwissenschaften* (1966) **53**, 437.
191. Kelly, M. G., O'Gara, R. W., Adamson, R. H., Gadekar, K., Botkin, C. C., Reese, W. H., Kerber, W. T., *J. Natl. Cancer Inst.* (1966) **36**, 323.
192. O'Gara, R. W., Adamson, R. H., Dalgaro, D. W., *Proc. Am. Ass. Cancer Res.* (1970) **11**, 60.
193. Druckrey, H., Preussmann, R., Schmähl, D., Müller, M., *Naturwissenschaften* (1961) **48**, 134.
194. *Ibid.* (1962) **49**, 19.
195. Druckrey, H., Preussmann, R., Ivankovic, S., Schmidt, C. H., Mennel, H. D., Stahl, K. W., *Z. Krebsforsch.* (1964) **66**, 280.
196. Kunze, E., Schauer, A., *Z. Krebsforsch.* (1971) **75**, 146.
197. Kunze, E., Schauer, A., Spielmann, J., *Z. Krebsforsch.* (1971) **76**, 236.
198. Okajima, E., Hiramatsu, T., Motomiya, Y., Iriya, K., Ijuin, M., Ito, N., *Gann* (1971) **62**, 163.
199. Bertram, J. S., Craig, A. W., *Br. J. Cancer* (1970) **24**, 352.
200. Wood, M., Flaks, A., Clayson, D. B., *Eur. J. Cancer* (1970) **6**, 433.
201. Mohr, U., Althoff, J., Schmähl, D., Krüger, F. W., *Z. Krebsforsch.* (1970) **74**, 112.
202. Althoff, J., Krüger, F. W., Mohr, U., Schmähl, D., *Proc. Soc. Exp. Biol. Med.* (1971) **136**, 168.
203. Althoff, J., Pour, P., Cardesa, A., Mohr, U., *Z. Krebsforsch.* (1973) **79**, 85.
204. Ivankovic, S., Bücheler, T., *Z. Krebsforsch.* (1968) **71**, 183.
205. Krüger, F. W., Pour, P., Althoff, J., *Naturwissenschaften* (1974) **61**, 328.
206. Druckrey, H., Preussmann, R., *Naturwissenschaften* (1962) **49**, 111.
207. Boyland, E., Carter, R. L., Gorrod, J. W., Roe, F. J. C., *Eur. J. Cancer* (1968) **4**, 233.
208. Druckrey, H., Ivankovic, S., Mennel, H. D., Preussmann, R., *Z. Krebsforsch.* (1964) **66**, 138.
209. Lesch, R., Meinhardt, K., Oehlert, W., *Z. Krebsforsch.* (1967) **70**, 267.
210. Pour, P., Krüger, F. W., Cardesa, A., Althoff, J., Mohr, U., *J. Natl. Cancer Inst.* (1974) **52**, 457.
211. Heath, D. F., Magee, P. N., *Br. J. Ind. Med.* (1962) **19**, 276.
212. Druckrey, H., Landschütz, C., Preussmann, R., *Z. Krebsforsch.* (1968) **71**, 135.

213. Druckrey, H., Landschütz, C., Z. Krebsforsch. (1971) **75,** 221.
214. Brune, H., Henning, S., Z. Krebsforsch. (1967) **69,** 307.
215. Dontenwill, W., Food Cosmet. Toxicol. (1968) **6,** 571.
216. Pour, P., Krüger, F. W., Althoff, J., Cardesa, A., Mohr, U., J. Natl. Cancer Inst. (1974) **52,** 1245.
217. Althoff, J., Hilfrich, J., Krüger, F. W., Bertram, B., Z. Krebsforsch. (1974) **81,** 23.
218. Goodall, C. M., Lijinsky, W., Tomatis, L., Wenyon, C. E. M., Toxicol. Appl. Pharmacol. (1970) **17,** 426.
219. Druckrey, H., Preussmann, R., Schmähl, D., Blum, G., Naturwissenschaften (1961) **48,** 722.
220. Boyland, E., Roe, F. J. C., Gorrod, J. W., Mitchley, B. C. V., Br. J. Cancer (1964) **18,** 265.
221. Napalkov, N., Pozharisski, K. M., J. Natl. Cancer Inst. (1969) **42,** 927.
222. Greenblatt, M., Mirvish, S., So, B. T., J. Natl. Cancer Inst. (1971) **46,** 1029.
223. Druckrey, H., Preussmann, R., Blum, G., Ivankovic, S., Afkham, J., Naturwissenschaften (1963) **50,** 100.
224. Sander, J., Schweinsberg, F., Z. Krebsforsch. (1973) **79,** 157.
225. Ivankovic, S., Arzeim. Forsch. (1964) **66,** 541.
226. Litvinov, N. N., Govorchenko, V. I., Kurylev, V. N., Bull. Exp. Biol. Med. (1971) **8,** 84.
227. Hadidian, Z., Fredickson, T. N., Weisburger, E. K., Weisburger, J. H., Glass, R. M., Mantel, N., J. Natl. Cancer Inst. (1968) **41,** 985.
228. Schmähl, D., Thomas, C., Scheld, G., Naturwissenschaften (1963) **50,** 717.
229. Ito, N., Hiasa, Y., Tamai, A., Okajima, E., Kitamura, H., Gann (1969) **60,** 401.
230. Ito, N., Hiasa, Y., Toyoshima, K., Okajima, E., Kamamoto, Y., Makiura, S., Yokota, Y., Sukihara, S., Matayoshi, K., "Topics in Chemical Carcinogenesis," W. Nakahara et al., Eds., 175, University of Tokyo, 1972.
231. Ishikawa, M., Okajima, E., Imoto, T., Hiramatsu, T., Ito, N., Konishi, Y., Hiasa, Y., J. Urol. (1969) **60,** 99.
232. Akagi, G., Akagi, A., Kimura, M., Otsuka, H., Gann (1973) **64,** 331.
233. Hashimoto, Y., Suzuki, K., Okada, M., Gann (1974) **65,** 69.
234. Bertram, J. S., Craig, A. W., Eur. J. Cancer (1972) **8,** 587.
235. Hashimoto, Y., Suzuki, E., Okada, M., Gann (1972) **63,** 637.
236. Okada, M., Hashimoto, Y., Gann (1974) **65,** 13.
237. Druckrey, H., Preussmann, R., Blum, G., Ivankovic, S., Naturwissenschaften (1963) **50,** 99.
238. Güttner, J., Schmidt, A., Jungstand, W., Z. Krebsforsch. (1971) **75,** 296.
239. Lijinsky, W., Lee, K. Y., Tomatis, L., Butler, W. H., Naturwissenschaften (1967) **54,** 518.
240. Lijinsky, W., Ferrero, A., Montesano, R., Wenyon, C. E. M., Z. Krebsforsch. (1970) **74,** 185.
241. Garcia, H., Lijinsky, W., Z. Krebsforsch. (1972) **77,** 257.
242. Greenblatt, M., Lijinsky, W., J. Natl. Cancer Inst. (1972) **48,** 1687.
243. Ibid., 1389.
244. Ito, N., Kamamoto, Y., Makiura, S., Sugihara, A., Marugami, M., Gann (1971) **62,** 435.
245. Takayama, S., Naturwissenschaften (1969) **56,** 142.
246. Althoff, J., Wilson, R., Cardesa, A., Pour, P., Z. Krebsforsch. (1974) **81,** 251.
247. O'Gara, R. W., Adamson, R. H., Dalgaro, D. W., Proc. Am. Ass. Cancer Res. (1970) **11,** 60.
248. Wiessler, M., Schmähl, D., Z. Krebsforsch. (1973) **79,** 118.
249. Garcia, H., Keefer, L., Lijinsky, W., Wenyon, C. E. M., Z. Krebsforsch. (1970) **74,** 179.
250. Schmähl, D., Thomas, C., Z. Krebsforsch. (1965) **67,** 11.
251. Bannasch, P., Müller, H. A., Arzeim. Forsch. (1964) **14,** 803.

252. Bannasch, P., Schacht, U., *Virchows. Arch. A. B.* (1968) **1**, 95.
253. Bannasch, P., Reiss, W., *Z. Krebsforsch.* (1971) **76**, 193.
254. Müller, H. A., *Z. Krebsforsch.* (1964) **66**, 303.
255. Wiessler, M., Schmähl, D., *Z. Krebsforsch.* (1973) **79**, 114.
256. Goodall, C. M., Lijinsky, W., Tomatis, L., *Cancer Res.* (1968) **28**, 1217.
257. Schmähl, D., *Naturwissenschaften* (1968) **55**, 653.
258. Althoff, J., Pour, P., Cardesa, A., Mohr, U., *Z. Krebsforsch.* (1972) **78**, 78.
259. Lijinsky, W., Tomatis, L., Wenyon, C.E.M., *Proc. Soc. Exp. Biol. Med.* (1969) **130**, 945.
260. Goodall, C. M., Lijinsky, W., Keefer, L., D'Ath, E. F., *Int. J. Cancer* (1973) **11**, 369.
261. Carter, R. L., *Br. J. Cancer* (1969) **23**, 408.
262. Yamamoto, R. S., Richardson, H. L., Weisburger, E. K., Weisburger, J. H., Benjamin, T., Bahner, C. T., *J. Natl. Cancer Inst.* (1973) **51**, 1313.
263. Druckrey, H., Steinhoff, D., Preussmann, R., Ivankovic, S., *Naturwissenschaften* (1963) **50**, 735.
264. Druckrey, H., Ivankovic, S., Preussmann, R., *Naturwissenschaften* (1964) **51**, 144.
265. Druckrey, H., Ivankovic, S., Preussmann, R., *Z. Krebsforsch.* (1965) **66**, 389.
266. Graffi, A., Hoffmann, F., Schutt, M., *Nature* (1967) **214**, 611.
267. Jänisch, W., Schreiber, D., Stengel, R., Steffen, U., *Exp. Pathol.* (1967) **1**, 243.
268. Schreiber, D., Jänisch, W., *Exp. Pathol.* (1967) **1**, 331.
269. Thomas, C., Sierra, I. L., Kersting, G., *Naturwissenschaften* (1967) **54**, 228.
270. *Ibid.* (1968) **55**, 183.
271. Stroobandt, J., Brucher, J. M., *Neurochirurgie* (1968) **14**, 515.
272. Schiffer, D., Fabiani, A., Grossi-Paoletti, E., Paoletti, P., *J. Neurol. Sci.* (1970) **11**, 559.
273. Terracini, B., Testa, M. C., *Br. J. Cancer* (1970) **24**, 588.
274. Weiss, J. F., Grossi-Paoletti, E., Paoletti, P., Schiffer, D., Fabiani, A., *Cancer Res.* (1970) **30**, 2107.
275. Hicks, R. M., Wakefield, J. St. J., *Chem. Biol. Interactions* (1972) **5**, 139.
276. Lijinsky, W., Garcia, H., Keefer, L., Loo, J., Ross, A. E., *Cancer Res.* (1972) **32**, 893.
277. Swenberg, J. A., Koestner, A., Wechsler, W., *Lab. Invest.* (1972) **26**, 74.
278. Druckrey, H., Ivankovic, S., Gimmy, J., *Z. Krebsforsch.* (1973) **79**, 282.
279. Murthy, A. S. K., Vawter, G. F., Bhaktaviziam, A., *Arch. Pathol.* (1973) **96**, 53.
280. Fort, L., Taper, H. S., Brucher, J. M., *Z. Krebsforsch.* (1974) **81**, 51.
281. Graffi, A., Hoffmann, F., *Acta Biol. Med. Ger.* (1966) **16**, K1.
282. *Ibid.*, **17**, K33.
283. Terracini, B., Stramignoni, A., *Eur. J. Cancer* (1967) **3**, 435.
284. Kelly, M. G., O'Gara, R. W., Yancey, S. T., Botkin, C., *J. Natl. Cancer Inst.* (1968) **41**, 619.
285. Joshi, V. V., Frei, J., *J. Natl. Cancer Inst.* (1970) **44**, 379.
286. *Ibid.*, **45**, 335.
287. Eckert, H., Seidler, E., *Arch. Geschwulstforsch.* (1971) **38**, 7.
288. Denlinger, R. H., Koestner, A., Wechsler, W., *Int. J. Cancer* (1974) **13**, 559.
289. Herrold, K. M., *J. Pathol. Bacteriol.* (1966) **92**, 35.
290. Herrold, K. M., *O.S.O.M.O.P.* (1968) **25**, 262.
291. Herrold, K. M., *Pathol. Vet.* (1969) **6**, 403.
292. Herrold, K. M., *Int. J. Cancer* (1970) **6**, 217.
293. Druckrey, H., Ivankovic, S., Bücheler, J., Preussmann, R., Thomas, C., *Z. Krebsforsch.* (1968) **71**, 167.
294. Osske, G., Schreiber, D., Schneider, J., Jänisch, W., *Eur. J. Cancer* (1969) **5**, 525.

295. Schreiber, D., Jänisch, W., Warzok, R., Tausch, H., *Z. Ges. Exp. Med.* (1969) **150,** 76.
296. Stavrou, D., *Z. Krebsforsch.* (1969) **73,** 98.
297. Kleihues, P., Zülch, K. J., Matsumoto, S., Radke, U., *Z. Neurol.* (1970) **198,** 65.
298. Warzok, R., Schneider, J., Schreiber, D., Jänisch, W., *Experientia* (1970) **26,** 303.
299. Stavrou, D., Haglid, K. G., *Naturwissenschaften* (1972) **59,** 317.
300. Druckrey, H., Schagen, B., Ivankovic, S., *Z. Krebsforsch.* (1970) **74,** 141.
301. Hadjiolov, D., *Z. Krebsforsch.* (1972) **77,** 98.
302. Frei, J. V., *Chem. Biol. Interactions* (1971) **3,** 117.
303. Lombard, L. S., Vesselinovitch, S. D., *Proc. Soc. Am. Ass. Cancer Res.* (1971) **12,** 55.
304. Rice, J. M., Davidson, J. K., *Cancer Res.* (1971) **31,** 2008.
305. Vesselinovitch, S. D., Lombard, L. S., Mihailovich, N., Itze, L., Rice, J. M., *Proc. Am. Ass. Cancer Res.* (1971) **12,** 56.
306. Searle, C. E., Jones, E. L., *Nature* (1972) **240,** 559.
307. Vesselinovitch, S. D., Itze, L., Mihailovich, N., Rao, K. V. N., Manojlovski, B., *Cancer Res.* (1973) **33,** 339.
308. Schoental, R., Bensted, J. P. M., *Br. J. Cancer* (1968) **22,** 316.
309. Druckrey, H., Preussmann, R., Afkham, J., Blum, G., *Naturwissenschaften* (1962) **49,** 451.
310. Schoental, R., *Acta Unio Int. Cancer* (1963) **19,** 680.
311. Caulet, T., Pluot, M., *Z. Krebsforsch.* (1970) **74,** 227.
312. Herrold, K. M., *J. Natl. Cancer Inst.* (1966) **37,** 389.
313. Schoental, R., *Nature* (1965) **208,** 300.
314. Schoental, R., Bensted, J. P. M., *Cancer Res.* (1971) **31,** 573.
315. Hiraki, S., *Gann* (1971) **62,** 135.
316. Ivankovic, S., Druckrey, H., Preussmann, R., *Z. Krebsforsch.* (1965) **66,** 541.
317. Druckrey, H., Preussmann, R., Ivankovic, S., So, B. T., Schmidt, C. H., Bücheler, J., *Z. Krebsforsch.* (1966) **68,** 87.
318. Odashima, S., *Gann* (1970) **61,** 245.
319. Yokoro, K., Imamura, N., Takizawa, S., Nishihara, H., Nishihara, E., *Gann* (1970) **61,** 287.
320. Takizawa, S., Nishihara, H., *Gann* (1971) **62,** 495.
321. Takizawa, S., Yamasaki, T., *Gann* (1971) **62,** 485.
322. Hosokawa, M., Gotohda, E., Kobayashi, H., *Gann* (1971) **62,** 557.
323. Matsuyama, M., Suzuki, H., *Experientia* (1971) **27,** 1459.
324. Preussmann, R., Druckrey, H., Bücheler, J., *Z. Krebsforsch.* (1968) **71,** 63.
325. Sugimura, T., Nagao, M., Okada, Y., *Nature* (1966) **210,** 962.
326. Sugimura, T., Fujimura, S., *Nature* (1967) **216,** 943.
327. Craddock, V. M., *Experientia* (1968) **24,** 1148.
328. Schoental, R., Bensted, J. P. M., *Br. J. Cancer* (1969) **23,** 757.
329. Bralow, S. P., Gruenstein, M., Meranze, D. R., *Oncology* (1973) **27,** 168.
330. Bralow, S. P., Gruenstein, M., Meranze, D. R., Bonakdarpour, A., Shimkin, M. B., *Cancer Res.* (1970) **30,** 1215.
331. Sugimura, T., Fujimura, S., Baba, T., *Cancer Res.* (1970) **30,** 455.
332. Fujimura, S., Kogure, K., Sugimura, T., Takayama, S., *Cancer Res.* (1970) **30,** 842.
333. Narisawa, T., Sato, T., Hayakawa, M., Sakuma, A., Nakano, H., *Gann* (1971) **62,** 231.
334. So, B. T., Magadia, N. E., Wynder, E. L., *J. Natl. Cancer Inst.* (1973) **50,** 927.
335. Takayama, S., Kuwabara, N., Azama, Y., Sugimura, T., *J. Nat. Cancer Inst.* (1971) **46,** 973.
336. Sugimura, T., Fujimura, S., Kogure, K., Baba, T., Saito, T., Nagao, M., Hosoi, H., Shimosato, Y., Yokoshima, T., *Gann Monogr.* (1969) **8,** 157.

337. Fujimura, S., Kogure, K., Oboshi, S., Sugimura, T., *Cancer Res.* (1970) **30,** 1444.
338. Shimosato, Y., Tanaka, N., Kogure, K., Fujimura, S., Kawachi, T., Sugimura, T., *J. Natl. Cancer Inst.* (1971) **47,** 1053.
339. Sugimura, T., Tanaka, N., Kawachi, T., Kogure, K., Shimosato, Y., *Gann* (1971) **62,** 67.
340. Nakamura, T., Matsuyama, M., Kishimoto, H., *J. Natl. Cancer Inst.* (1974) **52,** 519.
341. Kawachi, T., Kogure, K., Tanaka, N., Tokunaga, A., Fujimura, S., Sugimura, T., *Z. Krebsforsch.* (1974) **81,** 29.
342. Kurihara, M., Shirakabe, H., Murakami, T., Yasui, A., Izumi, T., Sumida, M., Igarashi, A., *Gann* (1974) **65,** 163.
343. Druckrey, H., Landschütz, C., *Z. Krebsforsch.* (1971) **76,** 45.
344. Druckrey, H., Ivankovic, S., Preussmann, R., *Z. Krebsforsch.* (1970) **75,** 23.
345. Ungerer, O., Eisenbrand, G., Preussmann, R., *Z. Krebsforsch.* (1974) **81,** 217.
346. Druckrey, H., Preussmann, R., Matzkies, F., Ivankovic, S., *Naturwissenschaften* (1967) **54,** 285.
347. Druckrey, H., "Carcinoma of the Colon and Antecedent Epithelium," W. J. Burdette, Ed., 267, C. C. Thomas, Springfield, 1970.
348. Schauer, A., Völlnagel, T., Wildanger, F., *Z. Ges. Exp. Med.* (1969) **150,** 87.
349. Springer, P., Springer, J., Oehlert, W., *Z. Krebsforsch.* (1970) **74,** 236.
350. Wittig, Von G., Wildner, G. P., Ziebarth, D., *Arch. Geschwulstforsch.* (1971) **37,** 105.
351. Kelly, M. G., O'Gara, R. W., Yancey, S. T., Gadekar, K., Botkin, C., Oliverio, V. T., *J. Natl. Cancer Inst.* (1969) **42,** 337.
352. Weibecke, B., Lohrs, U., Gimmy, J., Eder, M., *Z. Ges. Exp. Med.* (1969) **149,** 277.
353. Pegg, A. E., Hawks, A., *Biochem. J.* (1971) **122,** 121.
354. Toth, B., Wilson, R. B., *Am. J. Pathol.* (1971) **64,** 585.
355. Thurnherr, N., Deschner, E., Liplin, M., *Proc. Am. Ass. Cancer Res.* (1972) **13,** 120.
356. Osswald, H., Krüger, F. W., *Arzeim. Forsch.* (1969) **19,** 1891.
357. Toth, B., *Cancer Res.* (1972) **32,** 804.
358. *Ibid.,* 2818.
359. Roe, F. J. C., Grant, G. A., Millican, D. M., *Nature* (1967) **216,** 375.
360. Toth, B., *J. Natl. Cancer Inst.* (1973) **50,** 181.
361. Druckrey, H., Preussmann, R., Matzkies, F., Ivankovic, S., *Naturwissenschaften* (1966) **53,** 557.
362. Druckrey, H., Preussmann, R., Ivankovic, S., Schmidt, C. H., So, B. T., Thomas, C., *Z. Krebsforsch.* (1965) **67,** 31.
363. Arison, R. N., Feudale, E. L., *Nature* (1967) **214,** 1254.
364. Mauer, S. M., Lee, C. S., Najarian, J. S., Brown, D. M., *Cancer Res.* (1974) **34,** 58.
365. Berman, L. D., Hayes, J. A., Sibay, T. M., *J. Natl. Cancer Inst.* (1973) **51,** 1287.
366. Schoental, R., *Nature* (1969) **221,** 765.
367. Druckrey, H., Ivankovic, S., Preussmann, R., *Naturwissenschaften* (1967) **54,** 171.
368. Preussmann, R., Ivankovic, S., Landschütz, C., Gimmy, J., Flohr, E., Griesbach, U., *Z. Krebsforsch.* (1974) **81,** 285.
369. Ivankovic, S., Wohlenberg, H., Mennel, H. D., Preussmann, R., *Z. Krebsforsch.* (1972) **77,** 217.
370. Druckrey, H., "Potential Carcinogenic Hazards from Drugs—Evaluation of Risks," R. Truhaut, Ed., **7,** 60, UICC Monograph Series, 1967.
371. Craddock, V. M., *Nature* (1973) **245,** 386.
372. Pound, A. W., Lawson, T. A., Horn, L., *Br. J. Cancer* (1973) **27,** 451.

373. Craddock, V. M., *J. Natl. Cancer Inst.* (1971) **47,** 889.
374. Schmähl, D., Thomas, C., *Allg. Pathol.* (1963) **104,** 578.
375. Hadjiolov, D., *Z. Krebsforsch.* (1971) **76,** 91.
376. Newberne, P. M., Shank, R. C., *Food Cosmet. Toxicol.* (1973) **11,** 819.
377. Takayama, S., *J. Natl. Cancer Inst.* (1968) **40,** 629.
378. Takayama, S., *Z. Krebsforsch.* (1968) **71,** 246.
379. Haas, H., Mohr, U., Krüger, F. W., *J. Natl. Cancer Inst.* (1973) **51,** 1295.
380. Jasmin, G., Riopelle, J.-L., *Rev. Can. Biol.* (1964) **23,** 129.
381. Swann, P. F., McLean, A. E. M., *Biochem. J.* (1968) **107,** 14.
382. McLean, A. E. M., Magee, P. N., *Br. J. Exp. Pathol.* (1970) **51,** 587.
383. Thomas, C., Schmähl, D., *Z. Krebsforsch.* (1964) **66,** 125.
384. Murphy, G. P., Mirand, E. A., Johnston, G. S., Schmidt, J. D., Scott, W. W., *Invest. Urol.* (1966) **4,** 39.
385. Ito, N., Hiasa, Y., Kamamoto, Y., Makiura, S., Sugihara, A., Marugami, M., Okajima, E., *Gann* (1971) **62,** 435.
386. Jasmin, G., Riopelle, J.-L., *Arch. Pathol.* (1968) **85,** 298.
387. Hard, G. C., Butler, W. H., *Cancer Res.* (1971) **31,** 366.
388. *Ibid.,* 1496.
389. Taper, H. S., *Pathol. Eur.* (1967) **2,** 394.
390. Yang, Y. H., *Urol. Int.* (1966) **21,** 229.
391. Ito, N., Hiasa, Y., Tamai, A., Yoshida, K., *Gann* (1969) **60,** 319.
392. Ireton, H. J. C., McGiven, A. R., Davies, D. J., *J. Pathol.* (1972) **108,** 181.
393. Hard, G. C., Butler, W. H., *Cancer Res.* (1970) **30,** 2806.
394. *Ibid.* (1971) **31,** 337.
395. Jasmin, G., Riopelle, J.-L., *Int. J. Cancer* (1969) **4,** 299.
396. Takayama, S., Imaizumi, T., *Gann* (1969) **60,** 353.
397. Toyoshima, K., Ito, N., Hiasa, Y., Kamamoto, Y., Makiura, S., *J. Natl. Cancer Inst.* (1971) **47,** 979.
398. Flaks, A., Flaks, B., *Cancer Res.* (1973) **33,** 3285.
399. Ito, N., Makiura, S., Yokota, Y., Kamamoto, Y., Hiasa, Y., Sugihara, S., *Gann* (1971) **62,** 359.
400. Pour, P., Cardesa, A., Althoff, J., Mohr, U., *Cancer Res.* (1974) **34,** 16.
401. Montesano, R., *Tumori* (1970) **56,** 335.
402. Gibel, W., *Arch. Geschwulstforsch.* (1968) **31,** 5.
403. Ito, N., Kamamoto, Y., Hiasa, Y., Makiura, S., Marugami, M., Yokota, Y., Sugihara, S., Hirao, K., *Gann* (1971) **62,** 445.
404. Druckrey, H., Preussmann, R., Schmähl, D., *Acta Unio Int. Contra Cancrum* (1963) **19,** 510.
405. Druckrey, H., Landschütz, C., Preussmann, R., Ivankovic, S., *Z. Krebsforsch.* (1971) **75,** 229.
406. Toledo, J. D., *Beitr. Pathol. Anat. Allg. Pathol.* (1965) **131,** 63.
407. Bücheler, J., Thomas, C., *Beitr. Path. Bd.* (1971) **142,** 194.
408. Saito, T., Inokuchi, K., Takayama, S., Sugimura, T., *J. Natl. Cancer Inst.* (1970) **44,** 769.
409. Bosch, D. A., Gerrits, P. O., Ebels, E. J., *Z. Krebsforsch.* (1972) **77,** 308.
410. Denlinger, R. H., Swenberg, J. A., Koestner, A., Wechsler, W., *J. Natl. Cancer Inst.* (1973) **50,** 87.
411. Druckrey, H., Landschütz, C., Ivankovic, S., *Z. Krebsforsch.* (1970) **73,** 371.
412. Koestner, A., Swenberg, J. A., Wechsler, W., *Am. J. Pathol.* (1971) **63,** 37.
413. Kleihues, P., Matsumoto, S., Wechsler, S., Zülch, K. J., *Verh. Deut. Ges. Pathol.* (1968) **52,** 371.
414. Wechsler, W., Kleihues, P., Matsumoto, S., Zülch, K. J., Ivankovic, S., Preussmann, R., Druckrey, H., *Ann. N.Y. Acad. Sci.* (1969) **159,** 360.
415. Zülch, K. J., Mennel, H. D., *Zb. Neurochir.* (1971) **32,** 225.
416. Wechsler, W., Ramadan, M. A.-E., *Naturwissenschaften* (1971) **58,** 577.
417. Wechsler, W., Pfeiffer, S. E., Swenberg, J. A., Koestner, A., *Naturwissenschaften* (1972) **59,** 370.

418. Thust, R., Warzok, R., Batka, H., *Arch. Geschwulstforsch.* (1972) **40**, 300.
419. Pfeiffer, S. W., Wechsler, W., *Proc. Nat. Acad. Sci.* (1972) **69**, 2885.
420. Thomas, C., Kersting, G., *Naturwissenschaften* (1964) **51**, 144.
421. Kodama, T., Hosokawa, M., Gotohda, E., Sendo, F., Kobayashi, H., *Gann* (1972) **63**, 261.
422. Tomatis, L., "Modern Trends in Oncology, Part I," R. W. Raven, Ed., 99, *Research Progress*, Butterworths, London, 1973.
423. Napalkov, N. P., Alexandrov, V. A., *Z. Krebsforsch.* (1968) **71**, 32.
424. Napalkov, N. P., "Transplacental Carcinogenesis," *IARC Sci. Publ.* (1973) No. **4**, 1.
425. Druckrey, H., "Transplacental Carcinogenesis," *IARC Sci. Publ.* (1973) No. **4**, 45.
426. Alexandrov, V. A., *Nature* (1968) **218**, 280.
427. Magee, P. N., "Transplacental Carcinogenesis," *IARC Sci. Publ.* (1973) No. **4**, 143.
428. Alexandrov, V. A., *Nature* (1969) **222**, 1064.
429. Ivankovic, S., Druckrey, H., *Z. Krebsforsch.* (1968) **71**, 320.
430. Jänisch, W., Schreiber, D., Warzok, R., Schneider, J., *Arch. Geschwulstforsch.* (1972) **39**, 99.
431. Druckrey, H., Preussmann, R., Ivankovic, S., *Ann. N.Y. Acad. Sci.* (1969) **163**, 676.
432. Swenberg, J. A., Koestner, A., Wechsler, W., Denlinger, R. H., *Cancer Res.* (1972) **32**, 2656.
433. Grossi-Paoletti, E., *Arch. J. Pathol. Tumori* (1970) **13**, 3.
434. Zülch, K. J., *J. Génét. Hum.* (1969) **17**, 511.
435. Diwan, B. A., Meier, H., *Cancer Res.* (1974) **34**, 764.
436. Tomatis, L., Hilfrich, J., Turusov, V., *Int. J. Cancer* (1975) **15**, 385.
437. Smetanin, E. E., *Vop. Onkol.* (1971) **17**, 75.
438. Pielsticker, K., Wieser, O., Mohr, U., Wrba, H., *Z. Krebsforsch.* (1967) **69**, 345.
439. Thomas, C., Bollmann, R., *Z. Krebsforsch.* (1968) **71**, 129.
440. Mohr, U., Althoff, J., *Z. Krebsforsch.* (1965) **67**, 152.
441. Likhachev, A. Ya., *Vop. Onkol.* (1971) **17**, 45.
442. Mohr, U., Althoff, J., *Naturwissenschaften* (1964) **51**, 515.
443. Mohr, U., Althoff, J., Authaler, A., *Cancer Res.* (1966) **26**, 2349.
444. Alexandrov, V. A., *Vop. Onkol.* (1969) **15**, 55.
445. Druckrey, H., Ivankovic, S., Preussmann, R., *Nature* (1966) **210**, 1378.
446. Grossi-Paoletti, E., Paoletti, P., Schiffer, D., Fabiani, A., *Z. Neurol. Sci.* (1970) **11**, 573.
447. Graw, J., Zeller, W. J., Ivankovic, S., *Z. Krebsforsch.* (1974) **81**, 169.
448. Rice, J. M., *Ann. N.Y. Acad. Sci.* (1969) **163**, 813.
449. Diwan, B. A., Meier, H., Huebner, R. J., *J. Natl. Cancer Inst.* (1973) **51**, 1965.
450. Kupfer, M., Kupfer, G., Zintsch, I., Juhls, H., Ehrentraut, W., *Arch. Geschwulstforsch.* (1969) **34**, 25.
451. Ivankovic, S., Preussmann, R., *Naturwissenschaften* (1970) **9**, 460.
452. Osske, G., Warzok, R., Schneider, J., *Arch. Geschwulstforsch.* (1972) **40**, 244.
453. Ivankovic, S., Zeller, W. J., *Arch. Geschwulstforsch.* (1972) **40**, 99.
454. Tanaka, T., "Transplacental Carcinogenesis," *IARC Sci. Publ.* (1973) No. **4**, 100.
455. Druckrey, H., Ivankovic, S., Preussmann, R., Landschütz, C., Stekar, J., Brunner, V., Schagen, B., *Experientia* (1968) **24**, 561.
456. Ivankovic, S., *Arzeim. Forsch.* (1972) **22**, 905.
457. Huberman, E., Salzberg, S., Sachs, L., *Proc. Nat. Acad. Sci. U.S.* (1968) **59**, 77.
458. Takayama, S., Inui, N., *Gann* (1968) **59**, 437.

459. Sanders, F. K., Burford, B. O., *Nature* (1967) **213**, 1171.
460. DiPaolo, J. A., Nelson, R. L., Donovan, P. J., *Nature* (1972) **235**, 278.
461. Montesano, R., Saint Vincent, L., Tomatis, L., *Br. J. Cancer* (1973) **28**, 215.
462. Williams, G. M., Elliott, J. M., Weisburger, J. H., *Cancer Res.* (1973) **33**, 606.
463. Frei, J. V., Oliver, J., *Exp. Cell Res.* (1972) **70**, 49.
464. Takii, M., Takaki, R., Okada, N., *Jap. J. Exp. Med.* (1971) **41**, 563.
465. Inui, N., Takayama, S., Sugimura, T., *J. Natl. Cancer Inst.* (1972) **48**, 1409.
466. Di Mayorca, G., Greenblatt, M., Trauthen, T., Soller, A., Giordano, R., *Proc. Nat. Acad. Sci. U.S.* (1973) **70**, 46.
467. Borland, R., Hard, G. C., *Eur. J. Cancer* (1974) **10**, 177.
468. Freeman, A. E., Price, P. J., Igel, H. J., Young, J. C., Maryak, J. M., Huebner, R. J., *J. Natl. Cancer Inst.* (1970) **44**, 65.
469. Gross, L., *Proc. Soc. Exp. Biol. Med.* (1951) **76**, 27.
470. Goodall, C. M., *N.Z. Med. J.* (1968) **67**, 32.
471. Lee, K. Y., Goodall, C. M., *Biochem. J.* (1968) **106**, 767.
472. Jänisch, W. A., Warzok, E., Schreiber, D., *Bull. Eksp. Biol. Med.* (1969) **67**, 64.
473. Ivankovic, S., *Arzeim. Forsch.* (1969) **19**, 1040.
474. Fiume, L., *Sperimentale* (1963) **112**, 365.
475. Fiume, L., Campadelli-Fiume, G., Magee, P. N., Holsman, J., *Biochem. J.* (1970) **120**, 601.
476. Hadjiolov, D., Mundt, D., *J. Natl. Cancer Inst.* (1974) **52**, 753.
477. McLean, A. E. M., Verschuuren, H. G., *Brit. J. Exp. Pathol.* (1969) **50**, 22.
478. Swann, P. F., McLean, A. E. M., *Biochem. J.* (1971) **124**, 283.
479. Pound, A. W., Horn, L., Lawson, T. A., *Pathology* (1973) **5**, 233.
480. Lacassagne, A., Buu-Hoi, N. P., Giao, N. B., Hurst, L., Ferrando, R., *Int. J. Cancer* (1967) **2**, 425.
481. Osswold, H., Schmähl, D., *Naturwissenschaften* (1966) **53**, 255.
482. Kawachi, T., Hirata, Y., Sugimura, T., *Gann* (1968) **59**, 523.
483. Weisburger, E. K., Ward, J. M., Brown, C. A., *Toxicol. Appl. Pharmacol.* (1974) **28**, 477.
484. Cardesa, A., Pour, P., Rustia, M., Althoff, J., Mohr, U., *Z. Krebsforsch.* (1973) **79**, 98.
485. Dontenwill, W., *Arzeim. Forsch.* (1964) **14**, 774.
486. Wynder, E. L., Hoffmann, D., "Tobacco and Tobacco Smoke: Studies in Experimental Carcinogenesis," 173, Academic, New York, London, 1967.
487. Montesano, R., Saffiotti, U., Shubik, P., "Inhalation Carcinogenesis," M. G. Hanna, P. Nettesheim. J. R. Gilbert, Eds., 353, AEC Symposium, 1970.
488. Feron, V. J., Emmelot, P., Vossenaar, T., *Eur. J. Cancer* (1972) **8**, 445.
489. Montesano, R., Ferrero, A., Saffiotti, U., *J. Natl. Cancer Inst.* (1974) **53**, 1395.
490. Schmidt-Ruppin, K. H., Papadopulu, G., *Z. Krebsforsch.* (1972) **77**, 150.
491. Schreiber, H., Nettesheim, P., Lijinsky, W., Richter, C. B., Walburg, H. E., *J. Natl. Cancer Inst.* (1972) **49**, 1107.
492. Kordac, V., Schön, E., Braun, A., *Neoplasma* (1969) **16**, 485.
493. Weisburger, J. H., Hadidian, Z., Fredrickson, T. N., Weisburger, E. K., "Bladder Cancer, A Symposium," K. F. Lampe, Ed., 45, Aescular Publ. Co., Birmingham, Alabama, 1967.
494. Flaks, A., Hamilton, J. M., Clayson, D. B., Burch, P. R. J., *Br. J. Cancer* (1973) **28**, 227.
495. Ivankovic, S., Zeller, W. J., Schmähl, D., *Naturwissenschaften* (1972) **59**, 369.
496. Zeller, W. J., Ivankovic, S., *Naturwissenschaften* (1972) **59**, 82.
497. Carlton, W. W., Price, P. S., *Food Cosmet. Toxicol.* (1973) **11**, 827.
498. Rogers, A. E., Sanchez, O., Feinsod, F. M., Newberne, P. M., *Cancer Res.* (1974) **34**, 96.

499. Montesano, R., Mohr, U., Magee, P. N., Hilfrich, J., Haas, H., *Br. J. Cancer* (1974) **29**, 50.
500. Druckrey, H., *Ärztliche Praxis* (1972) **24**, 2537, 2593, 2621.
501. Druckrey, H., *Xenobiotica* (1973) **3**, 271.
502. Lijinsky, W., *N.Z. Med. J.* (1968) **67**, 100.
503. Magee, P. N., *N.Z. Med. J.* (1968) **67**, 59.
504. Magee, P. N., *Ann. N.Y. Acad. Sci.* (1969) **163**, 717.
505. Magee, P. N., *Cancer Res.* (1971) **31**, 599.
506. Magee, P. N., "Topics in Chemical Carcinogenesis," W. Nakahara *et al.*, Eds., 259, University of Tokyo, 1972.
507. Magee, P. N., Swann, P. F., *Br. Med. Bull.* (1969) **25**, 240.
508. Wunderlich, V., *Arch. Geschwulstforsch.* (1971) **38**, 310.
509. Nagata, C., Imamura, A., *Gann* (1970) **61**, 169.
510. Miller, J. A., *Cancer Res.* (1970) **30**, 559.
511. Miller, E. C., Miller, J. A., "Chemical Mutagens: Principles for their Detection," A. Hollaender, Ed., Vol. I, 83, Plenum, New York and London, 1971.
512. Nakahara, W., Takayama, S., Sugimura, T., Odashima, S., "Topics in Chemical Carcinogenesis," W. Nakahara *et al.*, Eds., 1, University of Tokyo, 1972.
513. Daiber, D., Preussmann, R., *Z. Anal. Chem.* (1964) **206**, 344.
514. Ballweg, H., Schmähl, D., *Naturwissenschaften* (1967) **54**, 116.
515. Lawley, P. D., *Nature* (1968) **218**, 580.
516. McCalla, D. R., Reuvers, A., Kitai, R., *Can. J. Biochem.* (1968) **46**, 807.
517. Haga, J. J., Russell, B. R., Chapel, J. F., *Cancer Res.* (1972) **32**, 2085.
518. Schoental, R., Rive, D. J., *Biochem. J.* (1965) **97**, 466.
519. Schulz, U., McCalla, D. R., *Can. J. Chem.* (1969) **47**, 2021.
520. Wheeler, G. P., Bowdon, B. J., *Biochem. Pharmacol.* (1972) **21**, 265.
521. Swann, P. F., *Biochem. J.* (1968) **110**, 49.
522. Swann, P. F., Magee, P. N., *Biochem. J.* (1971) **125**, 841.
523. Kleihues, P., Patzschke, K., *Z. Krebsforsch.* (1971) **75**, 193.
524. Kawachi, T., Kogure, K., Kamijo, Y., Sugimura, T., *Biochim. Biophys. Acta* (1970) **222**, 409.
525. Tanaka, A., Sano, T., *Experientia* (1971) **27**, 1007.
526. Heath, D. F., *Biochem. J.* (1962) **85**, 72.
527. Knecht, M., *Z. Krebsforsch.* (1967) **69**, 293.
528. Heath, D. F., *Biochem. Pharmacol.* (1967) **16**, 1517.
529. Stewart, B. W., Magee, P. N., *Biochem. J.* (1972) **126**, 21P.
530. Magee, P. N., Hawks, A., Stewart, B. W., Swann, P. F., *Proc. Congr. on Pharmacol., 5th* (1973) **2**, 140.
531. Okada, M., Suzuki, E., *Gann* (1972) **63**, 391.
532. Blattmann, L., Preussmann, R., *Z. Krebsforsch.* (1973) **79**, 3.
533. *Ibid.* (1974) **81**, 75.
534. Blattmann, L., Joswig, N., Preussmann, R., *Z. Krebsforsch.* (1974) **81**, 71.
535. McLean, A. E. M., Witschi, H. P., *Biochem. J.* (1966) **100**, 11P.
536. McLean, A. E. M., McLean, E. K., *Br. Med. Bull.* (1969) **25**, 278.
537. McLean, A. E. M., McLean, E. K., *Biochem. J.* (1966) **100**, 564.
538. Schmähl, D., Krüger, F. W., Ivankovic, S., Preissler, P., *Arzeim. Forsch.* (1971) **21**, 1560.
539. Schmähl, D., Krüger, F. W., "Topics in Chemical Carcinogenesis," W. Nakahara *et al.*, Eds., 199, University of Tokyo, 1972.
540. Alonso, A., Herranz, G., *Naturwissenschaften* (1970) **57**, 249.
541. Den Engelse, L., Bentvelzen, P. A. J., Emmelot, P., *Chem. Biol. Interact.* (1970) **1**, 395.
542. Den Engelse, L., Emmelot, P., *Chem. Biol. Interact.* (1971/2) **4**, 321.
543. Plapp, F. V., Updike, R. D., Chiga, M., *FEBS Lett.* (1971) **18**, 121.

544. Somogyi, A., Conney, A. H., Kuntzman, R., Solymoss, B., *Nature New Biol.* (1972) **237,** 61.
545. Montesano, R., Magee, P. N., *Nature* (1970) **228,** 173.
546. Montesano, R., Magee, P. N., *Proc. Amer. Ass. Cancer Res.* (1971) **12,** 14.
547. Montesano, R., Magee, P. N., "Chemical Carcinogenesis Essays," *IARC Sci. Publ.* (1974) No. **10,** 39.
548. Knecht, M., *Naturwissenschaften* (1966) **53,** 85.
549. Kato, R., Shoji, H., Takanaka, A., *Gann* (1967) **58,** 467.
550. Venkatesan, N., Arcos, J. C., Argus, M. F., *Life Sci.* (1968) **7,** 1111.
551. Venkatesan, N., Argus, M. F., Arcos, J. C., *Cancer Res.* (1970) **30,** 2556.
552. Venkatesan, N., Arcos, J. C., Argus, M. F., *Cancer Res.* (1970) **30,** 2563.
553. Magour, S., Nievel, J. C., *Biochem. J.* (1971) **123,** 8p.
554. Lawley, P. D., *Progr. Nucleic Acid Res. Mol. Biol.* (1966) **5,** 89.
555. Singer, B., Fraenkel–Conrat, H., *Progr. Nucleic Acid Res. Mol. Biol.* (1969) **9,** 1.
556. Schoental, R., *Biochem. J.* (1967) **102,** 5c.
557. Craddock, V. M., *Biochem. J.* (1968) **106,** 921.
558. McCalla, D. R., *Biochim. Biophys. Acta* (1968) **155,** 114.
559. Craddock, V. M., *Biochem. J.* (1969) **111,** 615.
560. Lawley, P. D., "Topics in Chemical Carcinogenesis," W. Nakahara *et al.,* Eds., 237, University of Tokyo, 1972.
561. Rosenkranz, H. S., Rosenkranz, S., Schmidt, R. M., *Biochim. Biophys. Acta* (1969) **195,** 262.
562. Friedman, O. M., Mahapatra, G. N., Stevenson, R., *Biochim. Biophys. Acta* (1963) **68,** 144.
563. Friedman, O. M., Mahapatra, G. N., Dash, B., Stevenson, R., *Biochim. Biophys. Acta* (1965) **103,** 286.
564. Loveless, A., Hampton, C. L., *Mutat. Res.* (1969) **7,** 1.
565. Loveless, A., *Nature* (1969) **223,** 206.
566. Lawley, P. D., Thatcher, C. J., *Biochem. J.* (1970) **116,** 693.
567. Lawley, P. D., Shah, S. A., *Chem. Biol. Interact.* (1972) **5,** 286.
568. Lawley, P. D., Brookes, P., Magee, P. N., Craddock, V. M., Swann, P. F., *Biochim. Biophys. Acta* (1968) **157,** 646.
569. O'Connor, P. J., Capps, M. J., Craig, A. W., Lawley, P. D., Shah, S. A., *Biochem. J.* (1972) **129,** 519.
570. O'Connor, P. J., Capps, M. J., Craig, A. W., *Br. J. Cancer* (1973) **27,** 153.
571. Kleihues, P., Magee, P. N., *J. Neurochem.* (1973) **20,** 595.
572. Lawley, P. D., Orr, D. J., Shah, S. A., *Chem. Biol. Interact.* (1971) **4,** 431.
573. Lawley, P. D., Shooter, K. V., House, W. L., Shah, S. A., *Biochem. J.* (1971) **122,** 22P.
574. Lawley, P. D., Shah, S. A., *Biochem. J.* (1972) **128,** 117.
575. Craddock, V. M., *Chem. Biol. Interact.* (1972) **4,** 149.
576. Loveless, A., *Proc. Roy. Soc.* (1959) **150,** 497.
577. Swann, P. F., Magee, P. N., *Nature* (1969) **223,** 947.
578. Kleihues, P., Mende, C. H. R., Reucher, W., *Eur. J. Cancer* (1972) **8,** 641.
579. Lijinsky, W., Loo, J., Ross, A. E., *Nature* (1968) **218,** 1174.
580. Ross, A. E., Keefer, L., Lijinsky, W., *J. Natl. Cancer Inst.* (1971) **47,** 789.
581. Lijinsky, W., Keefer, L., Loo, J., Ross, A. E., *Cancer Res.* (1973) **33,** 1634.
582. Lawley, P. D., Shah, S. A., *Chem. Biol. Interact.* (1973) **7,** 115.
583. Haerlin, R., Sussmuth, R., Lingens, F., *FEBS Lett.* (1970) **9,** 175.
584. Lingens, F., Haerlin, R., Sussmuth, R., *FEBS Lett.* (1971) **13,** 241.
585. Sussmuth, R., Haerlin, R., Lingens, F., *Biochim. Biophys. Acta* (1972) **269,** 276.
586. Brookes, P., Lawley, P. D., *Br. Med. Bull.* (1964) **20,** 91.
587. Swann, P. F., Magee, P. N., *Biochem. J.* (1968) **110,** 39.
588. Kleihues, P., Magee, P. N., Austoker, J., Cox, D., Mathias, A. P., *FEBS Lett.* (1973) **32,** 105.

589. Schoental, R., *Biochem. J.* (1969) **114**, 55P.
590. Craddock, V. M., *Biochim. Biophys. Acta* (1973) **312**, 202.
591. Frei, J. V., *Int. J. Cancer* (1971) **7**, 436.
592. Krüger, F. W., Osswald, H., Walker, G., Schelten, E., Z. *Krebsforsch.* (1970) **74**, 434.
593. Krüger, F. W., Walker, G., Wiessler, M., *Experientia* (1970) **26**, 520.
594. Montesano, R., Ingram, A. J., Magee, P. N., *Experientia* (1973) **29**, 599.
595. Wunderlich, V., Schütt, M., Böttger, M., Graffi, A., *Biochem. J.* (1970) **118**, 99.
596. Wunderlich, V., Tetzlaff, I., Graffi, A., *Chem. Biol. Interact.* (1971/2) **4**, 81.
597. Muramatsu, M., Azama, Y., Nemoto, N., Takayama, S., *Cancer Res.* (1972) **32**, 702.
598. McElhone, M. J., O'Connor, P. J., Craig, A. W., *Biochem. J.* (1971) **125**, 821.
599. Hennig, W., Kunz, W., Petersen, K., Schnieders, B., Krüger, F. W., Z. *Krebsforsch.* (1971) **76**, 167.
600. Craddock, V. M., Magee, P. N., *Biochem. J.* (1963) **89**, 32.
601. *Ibid.* (1967) **104**, 435.
602. Craddock, V. M., *Biochem. J.* (1969) **111**, 497.
603. Weyland, P., Gross, H. J., Dannenberg, H., Z. *Krebsforsch.* (1972) **77**, 141.
604. Mirvish, S. S., Medalie, J., Linsell, C. A., Yousuf, E., Reyad, S., *Cancer* (1971) **27**, 736.
605. Craddock, V. M., Mattocks, A. R., Magee, P. N., *Biochem. J.* (1968) **109**, 75.
606. Krüger, F. W., Schmähl, D., Z. *Krebsforsch.* (1971) **75**, 253.
607. Krüger, F. W., Ballweg, H., Maier-Borst, W., *Experientia* (1968) **24**, 592.
608. Goth, R., Rajewsky, M. F., Z. *Naturforsch.* (1971) **26b**, 1076.
609. Goth, R., Rajewsky, M. F., *Cancer Res.* (1972) **32**, 1501.
610. Cheng, C. J., Fujimura, S., Grunberger, D., Weinstein, I. B., *Cancer Res.* (1972) **32**, 22.
611. Krüger, F. W., Z. *Krebsforsch.* (1971) **76**, 145.
612. Krüger, F. W., "Topics in Chemical Carcinogenesis," W. Nakahara *et al.*, Eds., 213, University of Tokyo, 1972.
613. Krüger, F. W., Z. *Krebsforsch.* (1973) **79**, 90.
614. Krüger, F. W., Bertram, B., Z. *Krebsforsch.* (1973) **80**, 189.
615. Magee, P. N., Lee, K. Y., *Biochem. J.* (1964) **91**, 35.
616. Lee, K. Y., Lijinsky, W., *J. Natl. Cancer Inst.* (1966) **37**, 401.
617. Lijinsky, W., Ross, A. E., *J. Natl. Cancer Inst.* (1969) **42**, 1095.
618. Wilheim, R. C., Ludlum, D. B., *Science* (1966) **153**, 1403.
619. Ludlum, D. B., *J. Biol. Chem.* (1970) **245**, 477.
620. Ludlum, D. B., Wilhelm, R. C., *J. Biol. Chem.* (1968) **243**, 2750.
621. Ludlum, D. B., *Biochim. Biophys. Acta* (1970) **213**, 142.
622. Singer, B., Fraenkel-Conrat, H., *Biochem.* (1970) **9**, 3694.
623. Ludlum, D. B., Magee, P. N., *Biochem. J.* (1972) **128**, 729.
624. Gerchman, L. L., Ludlum, D. B., *Biochim. Biophys. Acta* (1973) **308**, 310.
625. Goth, R., Rajewsky, M. F., *Proc. Natl. Acad. Sci. U.S.* (1974) **71**, 639.
626. Kirtikar, D. M., Goldthwait, D. A., *Proc. Nat. Acad. Sci. U.S.* (1974) **71**, 2022.
627. McCalla, D. R., Reuvers, A., *Can. J. Biochem.* (1968) **46**, 1411.
628. Sugimura, T., Fujimura, S., Nagao, M., Uokoshima, T., Hasegawa, M., *Biochim. Biophys. Acta* (1968) **170**, 427.
629. Nagao, M., Yokoshima, T., Hosoi, H., Sugimura, T., *Biochim. Biophys. Acta* (1969) **192**, 191.
630. Nagao, M., Hosoi, H., Sugimura, T., *Biochim. Biophys. Acta* (1971) **237**, 369.
631. Magee, P. N., Hultin, T., *Biochem. J.* (1962) **83**, 106.
632. Craddock, V. M., *Biochem. J.* (1965) **94**, 323.
633. Turberville, C., Craddock, V. M., *Biochem. J.* (1971) **124**, 725.

634. Mirvish, S. S., Sidransky, H., *Biochem. Pharmacol.* (1971) **20**, 3493.
635. Heath, D. F., Dutton, A., *Biochem. J.* (1958) **70**, 619.
636. Neunhoeffer, O., Wilhelm, G., Lehmann, G., *Z. Naturforsch.* (1970) **25b**, 302.
637. Suss, A., *Z. Naturforsch.* (1965) **20b**, 714.
638. Druckrey, H., Steinhoff, D., Beuthner, H., Schneider, H., Klärner, P., *Arzeim. Forsch.* (1963) **13**, 320.
639. Sander, J., *Arch. Hyg. Bakteriol.* (1967) **151**, 22.
640. Magee, P. N., "Alkylierend wirkende Verbindungen, Wissenschaftliche Forschungsstelle im Verband der Cigarettenindustrie," 79, Hamburg, 1968.
641. *Lancet* (1968) **i**, 1071.
642. Lijinsky, W., Epstein, S. S., *Nature* (1970) **225**, 21.
643. Lee, D. H. K., *Environ. Res.* (1970) **3**, 484.
644. Phillips, W. E. J., *Food Cosmet. Toxicol.* (1971) **9**, 219.
645. Wolff, I. A., Wassermann, A. E., *Science* (1972) **177**, 15.
646. Neurath, G. B., Schreiber, O., "*N*-Nitroso Compounds in the Environment," *IARC Sci. Publ.* (1974) No. **9**, 211.
647. Wick, E. L., Underriner, E., Paneras, E., *J. Food Science* (1967) **32**, 365.
648. Sander, J., *Arzeim. Forsch.* (1971) **21**, 1572.
649. *Ibid.*, 1707.
650. *Ibid.*, 2034.
651. Neurath, G., *Experientia* (1967) **23**, 400.
652. Mirvish, S. S., "Topics in Chemical Carcinogenesis," W. Nakahara *et al.*, Eds., 279, University of Tokyo Press, 1972.
653. Asatoor, A. M., Simenhoff, M. L., *Biochim. Biophys. Acta* (1965) **111**, 384.
654. Perry, T. L., Shaw, K. N. F., Walker, D., Redlich, D., *Pediatrics* (1962) **30**, 576.
655. Blau, K., *Biochem. J.* (1961) **80**, 193.
656. Mirvish, S. S., *J. Nat. Cancer Inst.* (1970) **44**, 633.
657. Mirvish, S. S., "*N*-Nitroso Compounds: Analysis and Formation," *IARC Sci. Publ.* (1972) No. **3**, 104.
658. Sander, J., Schweinsberg, F., Menz, H. P., *Hoppe-Seyler's Z. Physiol. Chem.* (1968) **349**, 1691.
659. Keefer, L. K., Roller, P. P., *Science* (1973) **181**, 1245.
660. Mirvish, S. S., *J. Nat. Cancer Inst.* (1971) **46**, 1183.
661. Sander, J., Bürkle, G., Flohe, L., Aeiken, S., *Arzeim. Forsch.* (1971) **21**, 411.
662. Archer, M. C., Clark, S. D., Thilly, J. E., Tannenbaum, S. R., *Science* (1971) **174**, 1341.
663. Lijinsky, W., Conrad, E., Van de Bogart, R., *Nature* (1972) **239**, 165.
664. Lijinsky, W., *Cancer Res.* (1974) **34**, 255.
665. Montesano, R., Bartsch, H., Brésil, H., *J. Nat. Cancer Inst.* (1974) **52**, 907.
666. Lijinsky, W., Keefer, L., Conrad, E., Van de Bogart, R., *J. Nat. Cancer Inst.* (1972) **49**, 1239.
667. Elespuru, R. K., Lijinsky, W., *Food Cosmet. Toxicol* (1973) **11**, 807.
668. Sen, N. P., Donaldson, B. D., Charbonneau, C., "*N*-Nitroso Compounds in the Environment," *IARC Sci. Publ.* (1974) No. **9**, 75.
669. Eisenbrand, G., Ungerer, O., Preussmann, R., "*N*-Nitroso Compounds in the Environment," *IARC Sci. Publ.* (1974) No. **9**, 71.
670. Sen, N. P., Smith, D. C., Schwinghamer, L., *Food Cosmet. Toxicol.* (1969) **7**, 301.
671. Alam, B. S., Saporoschetz, I. B., Epstein, S. S., *Nature* (1971) **232**, 116.
672. *Ibid.*, 199.
673. Greenblatt, M., Kommineni, V., Conrad, E., Wallcave, L., Lijinsky, W., *Nature New Biol.* (1972) **236**, 25.
674. Montesano, R., Magee, P. N., *Int. J. Cancer* (1971) **7**, 249.
675. Epstein, S. S., "*N*-Nitroso Compounds: Analysis and Formation," *IARC Sci. Publ.* (1972) No. **3**, 109.

676. Asahina, S., Friedman, M. A., Arnold, E., Millar, G. N., Mishkin, M., Bishop, Y., Epstein, S. S., *Cancer Res.* (1971) **31,** 1201.
677. Friedman, M. A., Millar, G., Sengupta, M., Epstein, S. S., *Experientia* (1972) **28,** 21.
678. Lijinsky, W., Greenblatt, M., *Nature New Biol.* (1972) **236,** 177.
679. Lijinsky, W., Taylor, H. W., Snyder, C., Nettesheim, P., *Nature* (1973) **244,** 176.
680. Sander, J., Bürkle, G., *Z. Krebsforsch.* (1969) **73,** 54.
681. *Ibid.* (1971) **75,** 301.
682. Sander, J., *Arzeim. Forsch.* (1970) **20,** 418.
683. Sander, J., *Z. Krebsforsch.* (1971) **76,** 93.
684. Garcia, H., Lijinsky, W., *Z. Krebsforsch.* (1973) **79,** 141.
685. Mirvish, S. S., Greenblatt, M., Choudari Kommineni, V. R., *J. Natl. Cancer Inst.* (1972) **48,** 1311.
686. Rustia, M., Shubik, P., *J. Nat. Cancer Inst.* (1974) **52,** 605.
687. Greenblatt, M., Kommineni, V. R., Lijinsky, W., *J. Natl. Cancer Inst.* (1973) **50,** 799.
688. Sander, J., *Hoppe Seyler's Z. Physiol. Chem.* (1968) **349,** 429.
689. Sander, J., Seif, F., *Arzeim. Forsch.* (1969) **19,** 1091.
690. Klubes, P., Jandorf, W. R., *Chem. Pathol. Pharmacol.* (1971) **2,** 24.
691. Klubes, P., Cerna, I., Rabinowitz, A. D., Jondorf, W. R., *Food Cosmet. Toxicol.* (1972) **10,** 757.
692. Hawksworth, G. M., Hill, M. J., *Br. J. Cancer* (1971) **25,** 520.
693. Hill, M. J., Hawksworth, G., "*N*-Nitroso Compounds: Analysis and Formation," *IARC Sci. Publ.* (1972) No. **3,** 116.
694. Hawksworth, G., Hill, M. J., *Brit. J. Cancer* (1974) **29,** 353.
695. Brooks, J. B., Cherry, W. B., Thacker, L., Alley, C. C., *J. Inf. Dis.* (1972) **126,** 143.
696. Harington, J. S., Nunn, J. R., Irwig, L., *Nature* (1973) **241,** 49.
697. Boyland, E., Nice, E., Williams, K., *Food Cosmet. Toxicol.* (1971) **9,** 639.
698. Boyland, E., Walker, S. A., "*N*-Nitroso Compounds in the Environment," *IARC Sci. Publ.* (1974) No. **9,** 132.
699. Mirvish, S. S., Wallcave, L., Eagen, M., Shubik, P., *Science* (1972) **177,** 65.
700. Kamm, J. J., Dashman, T., Conney, A. H., Burns, J. J., *Proc. Nat. Acad. Sci. U.S.* (1973) **70,** 747.
701. Sakshaug, J., Sögnen, E., Hansen, M. A., Koppang, N., *Nature* (1965) **206,** 1261.
702. Ender, F., Havre, G., Helgebostad, A., Koppang, N., Madsen, R., Čeh, L., *Naturwissenschaften* (1964) **51,** 637.
703. Preussmann, R., Eisenbrand, G., "Topics in Chemical Carcinogenesis," W. Nakahara *et al.*, Eds., 323, University of Tokyo, 1972.
704. Bogovski, P., Preussmann, R., Walker, E. A., Eds., *IARC Sci. Publ.* (1972) No. **3.**
705. *IARC Sci. Publ.* (1974) No. **9.**
706. Sen, N. P., *Food Cosmet. Toxicol.* (1972) **10,** 219.
707. Sen, N. P., Donaldson, B., Iyengar, J. R., Panalaks, T., *Nature* (1973) **241,** 473.
708. Sen, N. P., Miles, W. F., Donaldson, B., Panalaks, T., Iyengar, J. R., *Nature* (1973) **245,** 104.
709. Crosby, N., Foreman, J. K., Palframan, J. F., Sawyer, R., *Nature* (1972) **238,** 342.
710. Ender, F., Čeh, L., "Alkylierend wirkende Verbindungen, Wissenschaftliche Forschungsstelle im Verband der Cigarettenindustrie," 83, Hamburg, 1968.
711. Freimuth, U., Gläser, E., *Nahrung* (1970) **14,** 357.
712. Ishidate, M., Tanimura, A., Ito, Y., Sakay, A., Sakuta, H., Kawamura, T., Sakai, K., Miyazana, F., "Topics in Chemical Carcinogenesis," W. Nakahara *et al.*, Eds., 313, University of Tokyo, 1972.

713. Fong, Y. Y., Chan, W. C., *Food Cosmet. Toxicol.* (1973) **11**, 841.
714. Fong, Y. Y., Chan, W. C., *Nature* (1973) **243**, 421.
715. Ayanaba, A., Verstraete, W., Alexander, M., *J. Natl. Cancer Inst.* (1973) **50**, 811.
716. Ender, F., Čeh, L., *Z. Lebensmittel. Untersuch. Forsch.* (1971) **145**, 133.
717. Fiddler, W., Pensabene, J. W., Doerr, R. C., Wassermann, A. E., *Nature* (1972) **236**, 307.
718. Sen, N. P., Schwinghamer, L. A., Donaldson, B. A., Miles, W. F., *Agr. Food Chem.* (1972) **20**, 1280.
719. Druckrey, H., Preussmann, R., *Naturwissenschaften* (1962) **49**, 498.
720. Rhoades, J. W., Johnson, D. E., *Nature* (1972) **236**, 307.
721. McCormick, A., Nicholson, M. J., Baylis, M. A., Underwood, J. G., *Nature* (1973) **244**, 237.
722. Hoffman, D., Rathkamp, G., Liu, Y. Y., "*N*-Nitroso Compounds in the Environment," *IARC Sci. Publ.* (1974) No. **9**, 159.
723. Sander, J., Aeikens, B., Schweinsberg, F., Eisenbrand, G., *Z. Krebsforsch.* (1973) **80**, 11.
724. Heyns, K., Röper, H., "*N*-Nitroso Compounds in the Environment," *IARC Sci. Publ.* (1974) No. **9**, 166.
725. Cook, P., *Brit. J. Cancer* (1971) **25**, 853.
726. McGlashan, N. D., Walters, C. L., McLean, A. E. M., *Lancet* (1968) **ii**, 1017.
727. McGlashan, N. D., *Gut* (1969) **10**, 643.
728. McGlashan, N. D., Patterson, R. L. S., Williams, A. A., *Lancet* (1970) **ii**, 1138.
729. Collis, C. H., Cook, P., Foreman, J. K., Palframan, J. F., *Gut* (1971) **12**, 1015.
730. Plowright, W., Linsell, C. A., Peers, F. G., *Br. J. Cancer* (1971) **25**, 72.
731. Zaldivar, R., *Z. Krebsforsch.* (1970) **75**, 1.
732. Hill, M. J., Hawksworth, G. M., Tattersall, G., *Br. J. Cancer* (1973) **28**, 562.
733. Hawksworth, G. M., Hill, M. J., Gordillo, G., Cuello, C., "*N*-Nitroso Compounds in the Environment," *IARC Sci. Publ.* (1974) No. **9**, 229.
734. Bretschneider, K., Matz, J., *Arch. Geschwulstforsch.* (1973) **42**, 36.
735. Fazio, T., Damico, J. N., Howard, J. W., White, R. H., Watts, J. O., *J. Agr. Food Chem.* (1971) **19**, 250.
736. Du Plessis, L. S., Nunn, J. R., Roach, W. A., *Nature* (1969) **222**, 1198.
737. Hedler, L., Marquardt, P., *Food Cosmet. Toxicol.* (1968) **6**, 341.
738. Petrowitz, H. J., *Arzeim. Forsch.* (1968) **18**, 1486.
739. Marquardt, P., Hedler, L., *Arzeim. Forsch.* (1966) **16**, 778.
740. Kröller, E., *Deut. Lebensm. Rundsch.* (1967) **63**, 303.
741. Thewlis, B. H., *Food Cosmet. Toxicol.* (1967) **5**, 333.
742. *Ibid.* (1968) **6**, 822.
743. Mohler, K., Mayrhofer, O. L., *Z. Lebensm. Unters. Forsch.* (1968) **135**, 313.
744. Hermann, H., *Hoppe Seyler's Z. Physiol. Chem.* (1961) **326**, 13.
745. Keybets, M. J. H., Groot, E. H., Keller, G. H. M., *Food Cosmet. Toxicol.* (1970) **8**, 167.
746. Neurath, G., Pirmann, B., Wichern, H., *Beitr. Tabakforsch.* (1964) **2**, 311.
747. Neurath, G., Pirmann, B., Luttich, W., Wichern, H., *Beitr. Tabakforsch.* (1965) **3**, 251.
748. Serfontein, W. J., Hurter, P., *Cancer Res.* (1966) **26**, 575.
749. Serfontein, W. J., Smit, J. H., *Nature* (1967) **214**, 169.
750. Simoneit, B. R., Burlingame, A. L., *Nature* (1971) **234**, 210.
751. Hedler, L., Kaunitz, H., Marquardt, P., Fales, H., Johnson, R. E., "*N*-Nitroso Compounds: Analysis and Formation," P. Bogovski, R. Preussmann, E. A. Walker, Eds., *IARC Scientific Publication, 1972*, No. **3**, 71.
752. Magee, P. N., *Ann. Occup. Hyg.* (1972) **15**, 19.
753. Shook, B. S., Cowart, H. O., *Ind. Med. Surg.* (1957) **26**, 333.

754. Petersen, P., Bredahl, E., Lauritsen, O., Laursen, T., *Brit. J. Ind. Med.* (1970) **27**, 141.
755. Schmähl, D., Osswald, H., *Experientia* (1967) **23**, 497.
756. Laqueur, G. L., Mickelsen, O., Whiting, M. G., Kurland, L. T., *J. Nat. Cancer Inst.* (1963) **31**, 919.
757. Kurland, L. T., *Neurology* (1954) **4**, 355.
758. *Ibid.*, 438.
759. Whiting, M. G., *Fed. Proc.* (1964) **23**, 1343.
760. Vega, A., Bell, E. A., *Phytochemistry* (1967) **6**, 759.
761. Hirono, I., Shibuya, C., *Nature, London* (1967) **216**, 1311.
762. Hirono, I., Shibuya, C., Hayashi, K., *Proc. Soc. Exp. Biol. Med.* (1969) **131**, 593.
763. Spatz, M., Laqueur, G. L., *Proc. Soc. Exp. Biol. Med.* (1968) **129**, 705.
764. Whiting, M. G., *Econ. Bot.* (1963) **17**, 271.
765. Whiting, M. G., Spatz, M., Matsumoto, H., *Econ. Bot.* (1966) **20**, 98.
766. Laqueur, G. L., Spatz, M., *Cancer Res.* (1968) **28**, 2262.
767. Spatz, M., *Ann. N.Y. Acad. Sci.* (1969) **163**, 848.
768. *Third Conference on the Toxicity of Cycads. Fed. Proc.* (1964) **23**, 1337.
769. *Sixth International Cycad Conference. Fed. Proc.* (1972) **31**, 1458.
770. Yang, M. G., Kobayashi, A., Mickelsen, O., *Fed. Proc.* (1972) **31**, 1543.
771. Birdsey, M. R., *Fed. Proc.* (1972) **31**, 1467.
772. Hirono, I., Kachi, H., Kato, T., *Acta Pathol. Jap.* (1970) **20**, 327.
773. Nishida, K., Yamada, A., *J. Agr. Chem. Soc. Japan* (1935) **11**, 357.
774. Nishida, K., Kobayashi, A., Nagahama, T., *Bull. Agr. Chem. Soc. Jap.* (1955) **19**, 77; *Chem. Abs.* (1956) **50**, 13756g.
775. Cooper, J. M., *J. Proc. Roy. Soc. N.S.W.* (1941) **74**, 450.
776. Lythgoe, B., Riggs, N. V., *J. Chem. Soc.* (1949) 2716.
777. Langley, B. W., Lythgoe, B., Riggs, N. V., *J. Chem. Soc.* (1951) 2309.
778. Riggs, N. V., *Aust. J. Chem.* (1954) **7**, 123.
779. Riggs, N. V., *Chem. Ind.* (1956) 926.
780. Korsch, B. H., Riggs, N. V., *Tetrahedron Lett.* (1964) **10**, 523.
781. Nishida, Y., Kobayashi, A., Nagahama, T., *Bull. Agr. Chem. Soc. Jap.* (1956) **20**, 74; *Chem. Abs.* (1956) **50**, 15761e.
782. Matsumoto, H., Strong, F. M., *Arch. Biochem.* (1963) **101**, 299.
783. Kobayashi, A., Matsumoto, H., *Fed. Proc.* (1964) **23**, 1354.
784. Kobayashi, A., Matsumoto, H., *Arch. Biochem.* (1965) **110**, 373.
785. Matsumoto, H., Nagahama, T., Larson, H. O., *Biochem. J.* (1965) **95**, 13c.
786. Horisberger, M., Matsumoto, H., *J. Label. Compounds* (1968) **4**, 164.
787. Ball, C. R., Van Den Berg, H. W., *Proc. Amer. Ass. Cancer Res.* (1972) **13**, 9.
788. Poynter, R. W., Ball, C. R., Goodban, J., Thackrah, T., *Chem. Biol. Interactions* (1972) **4**, 139.
789. Riggs, N. V., *Nature, Lond.* (1965) **207**, 632.
790. Matsumoto, H., Higa, H. H., *Biochem. J.* (1966) **98**, 20c.
791. Miller, J. A., *Fed. Proc.* (1964) **23**, 1361.
792. Palekar, R. S., Dastur, D. K., *Nature, Lond.* (1965) **206**, 1363.
793. Dastur, D. K., Palekar, R. S., *Nature, Lond.* (1966) **210**, 841.
794. Wells, W. W., Yang, M. G., Bolzer, W., Mickelsen, O., *Anal. Biochem.* (1968) **25**, 325.
795. Nishida, K., Kobayashi, A., Nagahama, T., Kojima, K., Yamane, M., *Seikagaku* (1956) **28**, 218; *Chem. Abs.* (1959) **53**, 8451c.
796. Laqueur, G. L., *Fed. Proc.* (1964) **23**, 1386.
797. Ganote, C. E., Rosenthal, A. S., *Lab. Invest.* (1968) **19**, 382.
798. Zedeck, M. S., Sternberg, S. S., McGowan, J., *Proc. Amer. Ass. Cancer Res.* (1973) **14**, 7.
799. Yang, M. G., Sanger, V. L., Mickelsen, O., Laqueur, G. L., *Proc. Soc. Exp. Biol. Med.* (1968) **127**, 1171.

800. Hoch-Ligeti, C., Stutzman, E., Arvin, J. M., *J. Nat. Cancer Inst.* (1968) **41,** 605.
801. Mugera, G. M., Nderito, P., *Brit. J. Cancer* (1968) **22,** 563.
802. Mugera, G..M., *Brit. J. Cancer* (1969) **23,** 755.
803. Yang, M. G., Mickelsen, O., Campbell, M. E., Laqueur, G. L., Keresztesy, J. C., *J. Nutr.* (1966) **90,** 153.
804. Fukunishi, R., Terashi, S., Watanabe, K., Kawaji, K., *Gann* (1972) **63,** 575.
805. Gusek, W., Buss, H., Krüger, C. H., *Verh. Deut. Ges. Pathol.* (1966) **50,** 337.
806. Gusek, W., Buss, H., Laqueur, G. L., *Beitr. Pathol. Anat.* (1967) **135,** 53.
807. Gusek, W., *Verh. Deut. Ges. Pathol.* (1968) **52,** 410.
808. Gusek, W., Mestwerdt, W., *Beitr. Pathol. Anat.* (1969) **139,** 199.
809. Hirono, I., Laqueur, G. L., Spatz, M., *J. Nat. Cancer Inst.* (1968a) **40,** 1003.
810. *Ibid.* (1968b) **40,** 1011.
811. Laqueur, G. L., *Virchows Arch. Pathol. Anat.* (1965) **340,** 151.
812. Kawaji, K., Fukunishi, R., Terashi, S., Higashi, J., Watanabe, K., *Gann* (1968) **59,** 361.
813. Fukunishi, R., Watanabe, K., Terashi, S., Kawaji, K., *Gann* (1971) **62,** 353.
814. O'Gara, R. W., Brown, J. M., Whiting, M. G., *Fed. Proc.* (1964) **23,** 1383.
815. Hirono, I., Shibuya, C., Fushimi, K., *Cancer Res.* (1969) **29,** 1658.
816. Hirono, I., Shibuya, C., *Gann* (1970) **61,** 403.
817. Hirono, I., Hayashi, K., Mori, H., Miwa, T., *Cancer Res.* (1971) **31,** 283.
818. Spatz, M., *Fed. Proc.* (1964) **23,** 1384.
819. Stanton, M. F., *Fed. Proc.* (1966) **25,** 661.
820. Sanger, V. L., Yang, M. G., Mickelsen, O., *J. Nat. Cancer Inst.* (1969) **43,** 391.
821. Hirono, I., *Fed. Proc.* (1972) **31,** 1493.
822. Laqueur, G. L., McDaniel, E. G., Matsumoto, H., *J. Nat. Cancer Inst.* (1967) **39,** 355.
823. Spatz, M., McDaniel, E. G., Laqueur, G. L., *Proc. Soc. Exp. Biol. Med.* (1966) **121,** 417.
824. Spatz, M., Smith, D. W. E., McDaniel, E. G., Laqueur, G. L., *Proc. Soc. Exp. Biol. Med.* (1967) **124,** 691.
825. Spatz, M., *Proc. Soc. Exp. Biol. Med.* (1968) **128,** 1005.
826. Spatz, M., Laqueur, G. L., Hirono, I., *Fed. Proc.* (1968) **27,** 722.
827. Yang, M. G., Mickelsen, O., Sanger, V. L., *Proc. Soc. Exp. Biol. Med.* (1969) **131,** 135.
828. Mickelsen, O., Yang, M. G., *Fed. Proc.* (1966) **25,** 104.
829. Matsumoto, H., Nagata, Y., Nishimura, E. T., Bristol, R., Haber, M., *J. Nat. Cancer Inst.* (1972) **49,** 423.
830. Spatz, M., Laqueur, G. L., *J. Nat. Cancer Inst.* (1967) **38,** 233.
831. Freeman, A. E., Weisburger, E. K., Weisburger, J. H., Wolford, R. G., Maryak, J. M., Huebner, R. J., *J. Nat. Cancer Inst.* (1973) **51,** 799.
832. Spatz, M., Laqueur, G. L., *Proc. Soc. Exp. Biol. Med.* (1968) **127,** 281.
833. Spatz, M., Dougherty, W. J., Smith, D. W. E., *Proc. Soc. Exp. Biol. Med.* (1967) **124,** 476.
834. Hirano, A., Dembitzer, H. M., Jones, M. G., *Neuropathol. Exp. Neurol.* (1972) **31,** 113.
835. Shimada, M., Langman, *J. Teratology* (1970) **3,** 119.
836. Haddad, R. K., Rabe, A., Laqueur, G. L., Spatz, M., Valsamis, M., *Science* (1969) **163,** 88.
837. Smith, D. W. E., *Science* (1966) **152,** 1273.
838. Teas, H. J., Dyson, J. G., *Proc. Soc. Exp. Biol. Med.* (1967) **125,** 988.
839. Gabridge, M. G., Denunzio, A., Legator, M. S., *Science* (1969) **163,** 689.
840. Teas, H. J., Sax, H. J., Sax, K., *Science* (1965) **149,** 541.
841. Porter, E. D., Teas, H. J., *Radiat. Bot.* (1971) **11,** 21.
842. Teas, H. J., *Biochem. Biophys. Res. Commun.* (1967) **26,** 686.

843. Williams, J. N., Laqueur, G. L., *Proc. Soc. Exp. Biol. Med.* (1965) **118**, 1.
844. Shank, R. C., Magee, P. N., *Biochem. J.* (1967) **105**, 521.
845. Shank, R. C., *Biochim. Biophys. Acta* (1968) **166**, 578.
846. Zedeck, M. S., Sternberg, S. S., Poynter, R. W., McGowan, J., *Cancer Res.* (1970) **30**, 801.
847. Zedeck, M. S., Sternberg, S. S., McGowan, J., Poynter, R. W., *Fed. Proc.* (1972) **31**, 1485.
848. Grab, D. J., Zedeck, M. S., Swislocki, N. I., Sonenberg, M., *Chem. Biol. Interactions* (1973) **6**, 259.
849. Morita, N., Hayashi, T., Yunoki, K., "Abstracts of Papers," 10th International Cancer Congress, Houston, 1970, 5.
850. Nagata, Y., Matsumoto, H., *Proc. Soc. Exp. Biol. Med.* (1969) **132**, 383.
851. Damjanov, I., Cox, R., Sarma, D. S. R., Farber, E., *Cancer Res.* (1973) **33**, 2122.

12

Carcinogens in Plants and Microorganisms

R. Schoental, Royal Veterinary College, Department of Pathology, Royal College Street, London, NW1 OTU, England

CANCER HAS AFFLICTED animals and man, probably since the inception of life on earth. It used to be attributed to the "wrath of gods," the "evil eye," witchcraft, etc. With the discovery that it is possible to induce cancer in animals by the application of tar or of pure chemicals, cancer shed much of its mystery and became the subject of scientific investigations. In the last 60 years tumors have been induced in experimental animals by various physical, chemical, and viral agents. Genetic and immunological factors play a part in the induction of experimental tumors by affecting the susceptibility of a particular animal. It was learned that man can also be affected by similar carcinogenic agents through industrial and/or accidental exposure.

Great anxiety is often expressed about the hazards to health, especially in relation to cancer, from the use of synthetic chemicals—such as insecticides, fungicides, weed killers, and food additives, which modern industry has introduced into our environment. Such anxieties are well justified, and it is good to know that appropriate authorities keep a watch on adequate screening of new chemicals before these are sold to the general public.

However, the synthetics have been introduced only within the last century. Cancer in earlier times must have been caused by carcinogenic agents in the "natural" environment. These include viruses, ultraviolet and ionizing radiation, heat and cold, asbestos, certain metals, radioactive minerals, estrogens, and certain secondary metabolites of plants and microorganisms. These agents continue to be a hazard to animals and man.

In any particular case of cancer considered as "spontaneous" in man or animals, it is likely that more than one contributing factor is involved. Some of the factors cannot be controlled, but elimination of even a single agent would be of practical value and could reduce the incidence of cancer. The residual combination of carcinogenic agents would be less effectual and the appearance of the tumor accordingly delayed, hopefully beyond the life span of the individual. Identification of sources of carcinogens is of primary importance, especially as some of these might be readily eliminated without undue cost or hardship.

As regards "natural" carcinogens, much could still be learned from epidemiological studies of malignant and certain other diseases which prevail in some developing countries. These include various types of liver disease and primary liver cancer, naso-pharyngeal, esophageal and stomach tumors, skin cancer, tumors of the sex organs, Burkitt lymphoma, Kaposi sarcoma, etc. (*1*). Most of these types of tumors can be reproduced in experimental animals with the already known carcinogens, but no doubt many more carcinogenic substances will come to light among natural products in the coming years.

Since about 196,000 species of flowering plants and also large numbers of fungi and microorganisms are known, the problem of systematic testing of all these materials for carcinogens is daunting. Some clues are needed in order to select those that would warrant priority for investigation. Carcinogenic agents can usually induce also some subacute "illness," especially when their dosage is excessive or when they act on the very young. Many of the known natural carcinogens have been discovered as a result of their effects on livestock. Accurate observations and astute deductions of veterinarians and farmers often led to correct identification of the causative factors. The clues derived from field poisoning or from unthriftiness among livestock caused by fodder are not yet exhausted and deserve detailed evaluation. Valuable information can be found in the selected books and articles which deal with the toxic and medicinal plants and fungi of various countries (*2–31*).

In this review of natural carcinogens, the term "tumor" is used for neoplastic conditions, whether benign or malignant, as distinction between these is not always possible. Genetic, viral, and immunological factors have not been considered in discussing specific carcinogens, although they are obviously very important. Particular problems are, however, stressed which appear important for the prevention of cancer and which require further studies.

Pyrrolizidine Alkaloids

Pyrrolizidine alkaloids (PA) occur in many plant species of unrelated botanical families and genera, the list of which is continuously increasing. The content of the alkaloids in different plants varies greatly, from traces up to about 5% of dried weight. It can vary even in the same species depending on the season and the climatic and soil conditions. The concentration varies also in different parts of the plant; it is usually higher in the roots, seeds, and flowers than in the leaves or stems. The chemistry, synthesis, and biogenesis of the alkaloids have been reviewed (*32, 33, 34, 35*) as well as their toxicity, pharmacology, their teratogenic, mutagenic, carcinogenic, and certain other effects (*35, 36, 37, 38, 39*) up to about 1970.

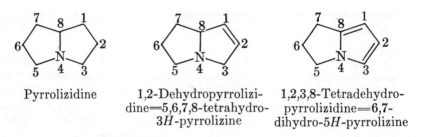

| Pyrrolizidine | 1,2-Dehydropyrrolizi-
dine=5,6,7,8-tetrahydro-
3H-pyrrolizine | 1,2,3,8-Tetradehydro-
pyrrolizidine=6,7-
dihydro-5H-pyrrolizine |

Figure 1. Structures of pyrrolizidine and some of its dehydrogenation products

The interest in the pyrrolizidine (*Senecio*) alkaloids started as a result of livestock losses from liver or lung lesions when the animals were grazing on *Senecio, Crotalaria, Heliotropium,* and *Amsinckia* plants (*35, 36*). This interest has greatly increased since the discovery of carcinogenic potentials of some members of this group of alkaloids (*37*) and the possibility that they may be involved in human liver diseases, including kwashiorkor (*40, 41*), veno-occlusive disease (*42*), and primary liver cancer (*37, 43*) which often occur in communities using the respective plants in folklore medicines (*8, 9, 26, 28, 31, 44*) (*see* also p. 669).

More than 100 pyrrolizidine alkaloids and their *N*-oxides have already been isolated from plants (and insects) and their structures established. They include simple derivatives of pyrrolizidine, of 1,2-dehydropyrrolizidine, and of 1,2,3,8-tetradehydropyrrolizidine (Figure 1) which are not all hepatotoxic.

Only a few alkaloids have as yet been examined for biological action. The available evidence indicates that the alkaloids which can cause liver

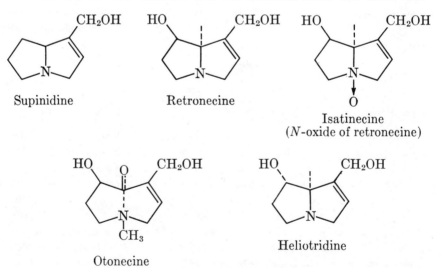

Figure 2. Structures of various necines present in toxic pyrrolizidine alkaloids

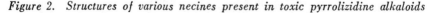

damage are esters of the basic amino alcohols, the necines (Figure 2) which include supinidine (1-hydroxymethyl-8α-1,2-dehydropyrrolizidine or 1-hydroxymethyl-5,6,7,8α-tetrahydro-3H-pyrrolizine), its 7-α- and 7-β-hydroxy derivatives, retronecine (the 7-β-HO) and heliotridine (7-α-HO), their N-oxides, and otonecine, the N-methyl derivative. The esterifying acids, necic acids, represent a variety of C_4–C_6-chain acids, which are mostly branched-chain, unsaturated, epoxidized, or hydroxylated mono- or dicarboxylic acids. Some of these alkaloids, their biological action (*35, 38*, Schoental unpublished), trivial and systematic names (*45*) are shown in Tables I, II, and III. The systematic names proposed for the pyrrolizidine alkaloids (*45*) are rather cumbersome. In order to avoid confusion, trivial names have been used in this text, as these appear in the original papers dealing with the biological studies of the alkaloids.

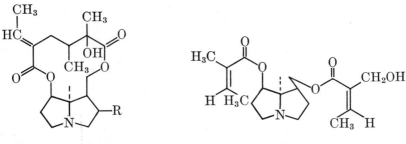

R = H;   Platyphylline
R = OH;   Rosmarinine

Sarracine

Figure 3.   Structures of diester saturated alkaloids which are not hepatotoxic

Ester alkaloids which have no 1,2-double bond in the pyrrolizidine moiety, such as platyphylline, rosmarinine and sarracine (Figure 3) are not hepatotoxic.

Many animal species, including birds, rodents, ruminants, monkeys, and man, are susceptible to the toxic action of hepatotoxic alkaloids (*36*). The toxic doses vary greatly depending on the structural features of the alkaloids (*35, 38*) and on the susceptibility of the recipient. The degree of susceptibility depends not only on the species, the strain, and sex of the animal, but also on the age, the type of diet, and the enzymatic "fitness" at the time of exposure to the alkaloids (*36*).

The acute toxicities of the various macrocyclic diester alkaloids of retronecine (Table I) differ by a factor of two to three from that of the most toxic compound, retrorsine (LD$_{50}$ 35mg/kg body weight). Lasiocarpine, the open diester of heliotridine is two to three times, and the diesters of otonecine five to six times less toxic than retrorsine (Figures 4, 5, 6). Particularly great differences in toxicities are encountered among the open

Table I.   Cyclic Diester Alkaloids Effective in Inducing

Alkaloid	Necine Base[f]
Retrorsine[a]	R
Isatinine[a]	I
Senecionine	R
Seneciphylline[b]	R
Riddelliine[b]	R
Jacobine	R
Sceleratine[c]	R
Chlorodeoxysceleratine[c]	R
Senkirkine[c]	O
Hydroxysenkirkine[c]	O
Emiline[d]	O
Dicrotaline[e]	R
Fulvine	R

Chronic Disease in Rats with One or a Few Doses

	Trivial Name of Acid
Necic Acid	

$$\underset{HOOC\underset{\|}{-}C-CH_2-CH-C(OH)-COOH}{\overset{HC-CH_3\quad CH_3\ CH_2OH}{}}$$

retronecic

$$\underset{HOOC-C-CH_2-CH-C(OH)-COOH}{\overset{H_3C-CH\qquad CH_3\ CH_2OH}{}}$$

isatinecic

$$\underset{HOOC-C-CH_2-CH-C(OH)-COOH}{\overset{H_3C-CH\qquad CH_3\ CH_3}{}}$$

senecic

$$\underset{HOOC-C-CH_2-C\underline{\quad}C(OH)-COOH}{\overset{H_3C-CH\qquad CH_2\ CH_3}{}}$$

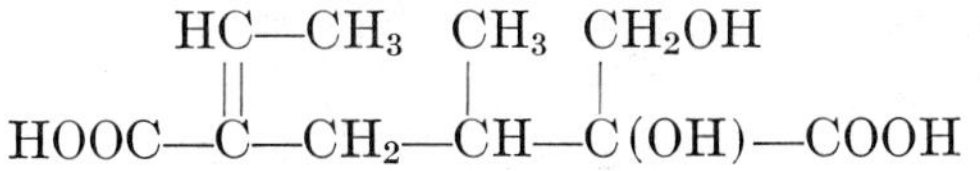

seneciphyllic

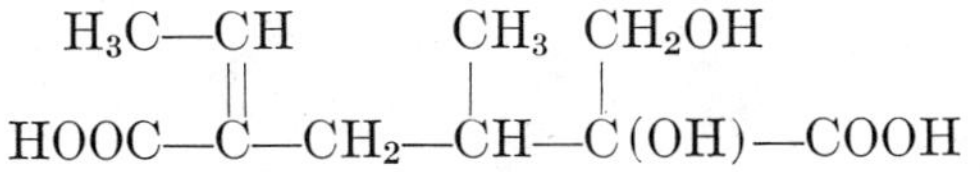

$$\underset{HOOC-C-CH_2-C\underline{\quad}C(OH)-COOH}{\overset{HC-CH_3\quad CH_2\ CH_2OH}{}}$$

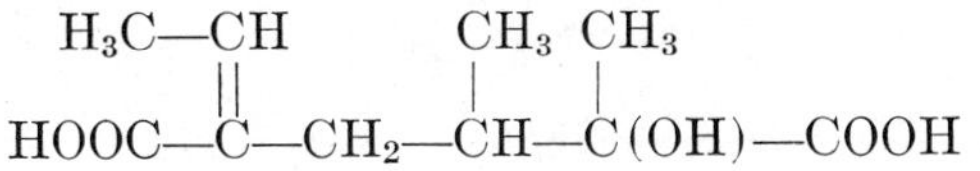

riddelliic

$$\underset{HOOC-C-CH_2-CH-C(OH)-COOH}{\overset{H_3C-CH\diagdown O\qquad CH_3\ CH_3}{}}$$

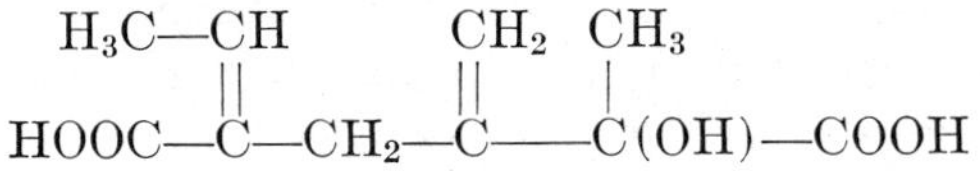

jacobinecic

$$\underset{HOOC-C(OH)-CH-CH-C(OH)-COOH}{\overset{CH_3\qquad CH_3\ CH_3\ CH_2OH}{}}$$

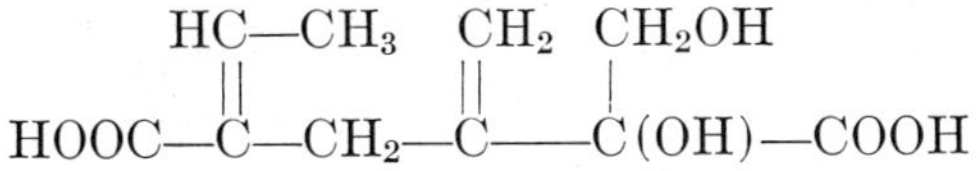

sceleranecic

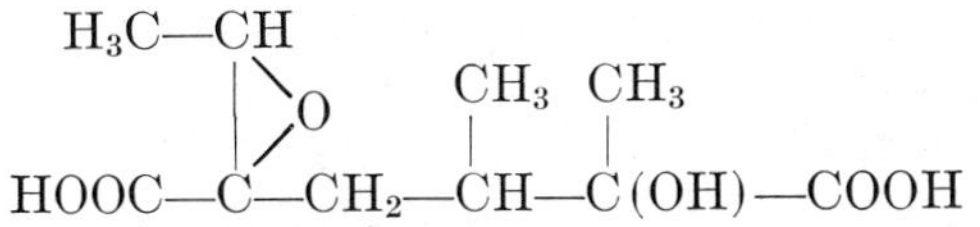

$$\underset{HOOC-C(OH)-CH-CH-C(OH)-COOH}{\overset{CH_3\qquad CH_3\ CH_3\ CH_2Cl}{}}$$

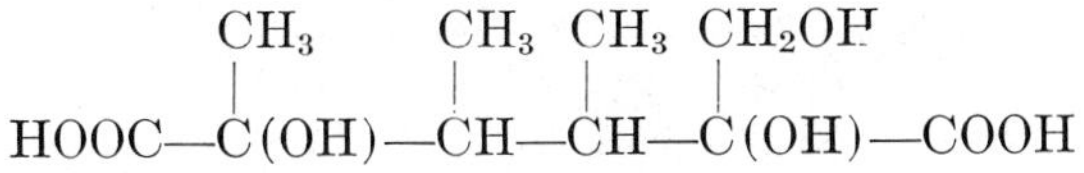

sceleratinic

$$\underset{HOOC-C-CH_2-CH-C(OH)-COOH}{\overset{H_3C-CH\qquad CH_3\ CH_3}{}}$$

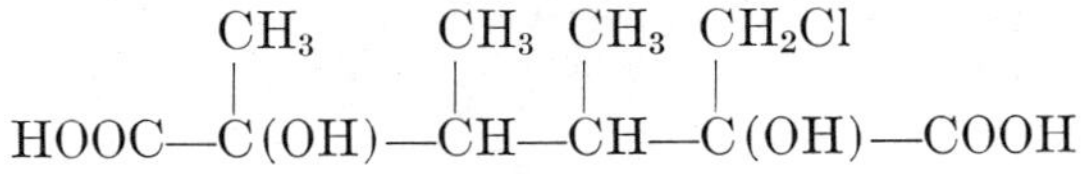

senecic

$$\underset{HOOC-CH-CH_2-CH-C(OH)-COOH}{\overset{H_3C-CH\qquad CH_3\ CH_2OH}{}}$$

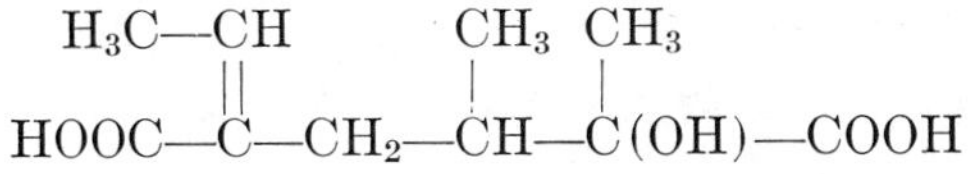

isatinecic

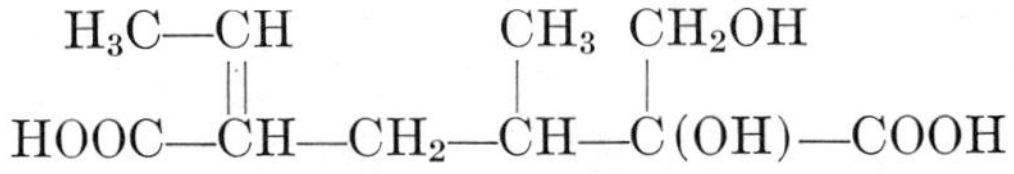

$$\underset{HOOC-C(CH_3)-C\underline{\quad}C(OH)-COOH}{\overset{CH_2CH_3\quad CH_2\ CH_3}{}}$$

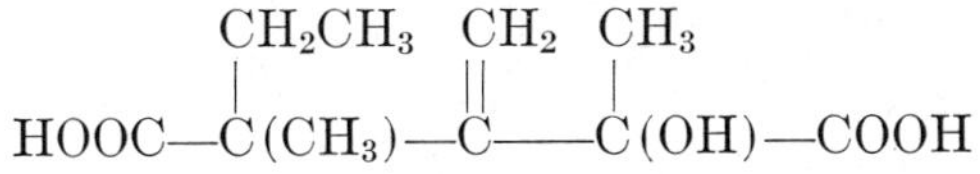

emilinic

$$\underset{HOOC-CH_2-C(OH)-CH_2-COOH}{\overset{CH_3}{}}$$

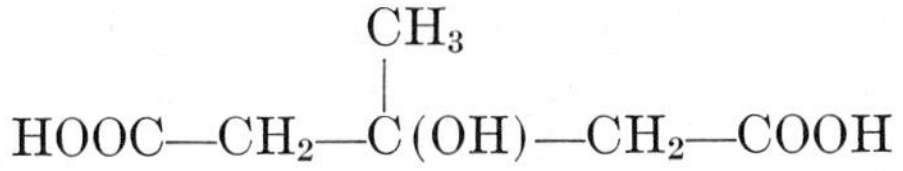

dicrotalic

$$\underset{HOOC-CH-C(OH)-CH-COOH}{\overset{CH_3\ CH_3\qquad CH_3}{}}$$

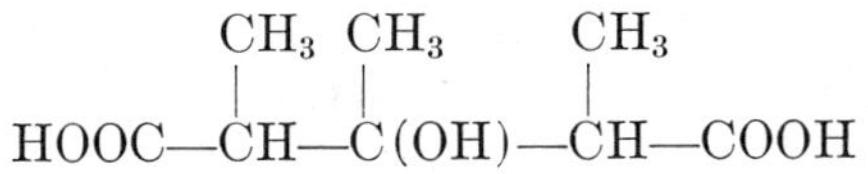

fulvinic

Table I.

Alkaloid   *Necine Base*

Monocrotaline[b]   R

[a] Gift of F. L. Warren.
[b] Gift of R. Adams.
[c] Gift of D. H. G. Crout.

monoesters of supinidine, heliotridine, and retronecine, some of which are
shown in Table II (*35*).

The quoted LD_{50} values refer arbitrarily to death that occurs within three
to seven days after the dose. The pathological lesions found in the animals
which die within the first week after the dose are mainly hemorrhagic
necrosis of the liver, edema of the pancreas, and/or congestion and edema
of the lungs. Among the animals that survive one week, some will die later
after various time intervals from more chronic lesions. A second peak of
high mortality usually occurs one to two months after dosing with the
alkaloid.

The differences in the toxicities of the various alkaloids depend in part
on their water solubility and on the distribution coefficient between the lipid
and aqueous tissue compartments. These characteristics are related to the
number of free hydroxyls and basicity of the PA and affect their rate of
excretion from the body (*35*). Accessibility to the ester groupings and to
the double bond in the necines affects the hydrolysis, metabolism, and
relative rates of formation and degradation of various metabolites.

The metabolic "fitness" of an individual is partly genetically determined
by the enzymatic endowment, but can be influenced by age, hormonal,

**Table II. Monoester Pyrrolizidine Alkaloids: Trivial Names
and Toxicities in Relation to Their Basic
and Acidic Moieties (*35*)[a]**

Acid	Number of HO and MeO Groups	Base		
		Supinidine	*Heliotridine*	*Retronecine*
Helio-tric	1 + 1	heleurine 140	heliotrine 300	
Viridi-floric	2	cynaustine 260	echinatine 350	lycopsamine + inter-medine >1000
Trache-lanthic	2	supinine 450	rinderine 550	
Lasio-carpic	2 + 1		europine >1000	indicine >1000

The Pyrrolizidine Alkaloids

[a] Approx. LD_{50} in mg/kg body weight.

Continued

| | *Trivial Name* |
| *Necic Acid* | *of Acid* |

$$CH_3 \quad CH_3 \qquad CH_3$$
$$HOOC—CH—C(OH)—C(OH)—COOH$$ monocrotalic

[d] Gift of S. Kohlmünzer.
[e] Gift of J. S. C. Marais.
[f] R = retronecine; I = isatinecine (retronecine-N-oxide); O = otonecine.

Table III.   Trivial and Systematic Names of Some Pyrrolizidine Alkaloids (45)

Alkaloids	*Systematic Name*
Supinidine	1-hydroxymethyl-5,6,7,8α-tetrahydro-3H-pyrrolizine
Heliotridine	7α-hydroxy-1-hydroxymethyl-5,6,7,8α-tetrahydro-3H-pyrrolizine
Retronecine	7β-hydroxy-1-hydroxymethyl-5,6,7,8α-tetrahydro-3H-pyrrolizine
7-Angelylheliotridine	(1-hydroxymethyl-5,6,7,8α-tetrahydro-3H-pyrrolizin-7α-yl) angelate
Supinine	(5,6,7,8α-tetrahydro-3H-pyrrolizin-1-yl) methyl-2,3-dihydroxy-2-isopropylbutyrate
Heliotrine	(5,6,7,8α-tetrahydro-7α-hydroxy-3H-pyrrolizin-1-yl) methyl-2-hydroxy-2-isopropyl-3-methoxybutyrate
Lasiocarpine	(7α-angelyloxy-5,6,7,8α-tetrahydro-3H-pyrrolizin-1-yl) methyl-2,3-dihydroxy-2-(1′-methoxyethyl)-3-methylbutyrate
Dicrotaline	13β-hydroxy-13α-methylcrotal-1-enine
Fulvine	13β-hydroxy-12α,13α,14α-trimethylcrotal-1-enine
Monocrotaline	12β,13β-dihydroxy-12α,13α,14α-trimethylcrotal-1-enine
Jacobine	12β-hydroxy-12α,13β-dimethylsenec-1-enine-15S-spiro-2′-(3′R-methyloxiran)
Senecionine	*trans*-15-ethylidene-12β-hydroxy-12α,13β-dimethylsenec-1-enine
Seneciphylline	*trans*-15-ethylidene-12β-hydroxy-12α-methyl-13-methylenesenec-1-enine
Retrorsine	*trans*-15-ethylidene-12β-hydroxy-12α-hydroxymethyl-13β-methylsenec-1-enine
Sceleratine	12ξ,15ξ-dihydroxy-12ξ-hydroxymethyl-13ξ,14ξ,15ξ-trimethylsenec-1-enine
Senkirkine	*trans*-15-ethylidene-12β-hydroxy-4,12α,13β-trimethyl-8-oxo-4,8-secosenec-1-enine
Hydroxysenkirkine	*trans*-15-ethylidene-12β-hydroxy-12α-hydroxymethyl-4,13β-dimethyl-8-oxo-4,8-secosenec-1-enine

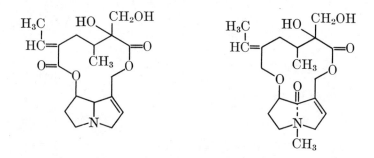

*Figure 4. Structure of the hepatocarcinogenic retrorsine (left)
and hydroxysenkirkine (right)*

dietary, and other factors. These factors also play a role in the carcinogenic
response of an organism.

Carcinogenic Action of Pyrrolizidine Alkaloids. Pyrrolizidine
alkaloids were the first among the extrinsic "natural" products which have
been found to induce tumors of the liver and occasionally of the lung, etc.,
in white rats on repeated intermittent administration (*46, 47*), with a few
doses (*48, 49*), or even with a single dose (*50*). The pyrrolizidine alkaloids
have a strikingly insidious action. Many months may elapse after dosing before the chronic effects and tumors fully "ripen" and become apparent. This
feature has not been recognized by some of the workers in this field, who
found no tumors when they killed the animals at predetermined times, pre-
maturely, or when the animals died from liver atrophy caused by excessive
treatment (*35*). The controversy about the carcinogenic potentialities of
pyrrolizidine alkaloids is resolved now. By appropriate treatment of rats with
various plant materials or with pure alkaloids, tumors of the liver and of certain other organs have been induced by several groups of workers (*51–56a*).

The experiments of Harris and Chen (*52*) illustrate the difficulties of
finding appropriate dosage schedules which would allow the animals to
survive for long periods and yet be sufficient for tumor induction. These

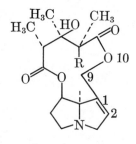

*Figure 5. Structures of the car-
cinogenic monocrotaline and fulvine*

R = OH;   Monocrotaline
R = H;   Fulvine

workers used more than 600 rats and several feeding schedules of *Senecio longilobus* L, a plant that contains several cyclic diester alkaloids, including retrorsine (Figure 4) (*32, 33*). When a diet containing 0.5% of this plant material was given intermittently every other week, malignant liver tumors developed in 14 males and 3 females among 47 rats which survived for more than 217 days. On other feeding schedules tumors developed only occasionally (*52*).

Monocrotaline (Figure 5), the alkaloid of *Crotalaria spectabilis* and of several other *Crotalaria* species, induced malignant liver tumors in the rat (*56*) when given intragastrically once weekly (25 mg/kg body weight for four weeks, then 7 mg/kg body weight for 38 weeks). Among rats maintained on normal diet, 10 out of 42 developed liver cell carcinomas while on a diet marginal in lipotropes (low in choline and in vitamin B_{12}) such tumors developed in 14 out of 35 rats that survived several months after cessation of the treatment (*56*). Although low-lipotrope diet protects rats against the acute toxic effects of monocrotaline, it does not protect them from tumors.

When monocrotaline was given to rats in conjunction with aflatoxin B_1, it appeared to act synergistically. Among rats exposed to both carcinogens simultaneously, mortality and the liver tumor incidence was higher than among rats receiving only one of the carcinogens (*56*).

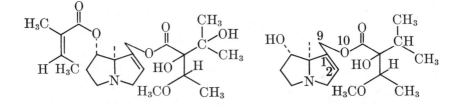

Figure 6.   Structures of the open-ester carcinogenic lasiocarpine (left) and heliotrine (right)

Among plants of the Boraginaceae, such as *Heliotropium, Cynoglossum, Amsinckia, Echium*, etc., the alkaloids are mostly mono- and di-open esters of supinidine, heliotridine, or retronecine and of their *N*-oxides. Angelic acid usually esterfies the 7-hydroxyl; substituted C_4-chain acids esterify the 1-hydroxymethyl group (Table II) (*35*).

The diester lasiocarpine (Figure 6) is an effective carcinogen. Though hepatomas were found only occasionally in animals given single doses of $LD_{30\text{-}60}$ (Schoental, unpublished) prolonged intermittent treatment resulted in a variety of malignant tumors (*54*). No tumors were found in the rats within about one year, during the time that the animals were treated with lasiocarpine by approximately weekly intraperitoneal injections (7.8 mg/kg body weight) (*57*). After the treatment was stopped however, 16 out of 18 survivors developed malignant tumors of the liver, skin, lungs, and certain other organs, some with metastases within the following 4–20 weeks (*54*).

Monoesters of retronecine, such as indicine (from *Heliotropium indicum* L),
intermedine, and lycopsamine (from *Amsinckia intermedia* Fisch and Mey)
are only slightly toxic for the liver, but can occasionally induce tumors in
other organs such as the islet cells of the pancreas, the bladder, kidneys,
CNS, etc. (*51, 55, 58*). Heliotrine (Figure 6), the monoester of heliotridine,
can induce hepatomas in the liver and tumors of the pancreatic islet cells
especially when the rats are pretreated with nicotinamide (*58a*).

It is now evident that pyrrolizidine alkaloids are more versatile carcinogens that was previously believed. They can induce tumors in organs other
than the liver and the lung, namely of the skin, gastrointestinal tract (*54*),
brain and spinal cord (*55*), the pancreas, (notably of the islet cells) (*18, 58a*),
kidneys (*58*), etc. The extrahepatic tumors are more likely to develop if
the particular alkaloid (or rather its activated metabolite) is less effectively
sequestered by the liver and can survive in the blood stream to reach other
organs.

Not all the pyrrolizidine alkaloids are carcinogenic (*37*). An allylic
carbonyl group and accessibility to the 1,2-double bond of the pyrrolizidine
moiety appear essential for this action. These features are present in the
macrocyclic diester alkaloids in which the necines, retronecine, isatinecine,
and otonecine (Figure 2) are esterified with substituted adipic and glutaric
acids. Such alkaloids are found in many *Senecio* and *Crotalaria* plants.

Some of these alkaloids (listed in Table I) were tested in long term
experiments in which they were given to weanling or suckling white rats.
All induced similar chronic liver and/or lung lesions with one or a few
appropriate doses (*40, 48, 50, 58a–61*, Schoental, unpublished). Tumors
usually developed among animals which survived longer than one year
from the time of treatment. In view of the similarity of the chronic lesions
and their evolution after a single dose, all the macrocyclic alkaloids with
the 1,2-double bond in the pyrrolizidine moiety might induce tumors in
white rats when the treatment is appropriate.

Very large doses of all the pyrrolizidine alkaloids cause convulsions
and immediate death of many animal species. The non-hepatotoxic alkaloids
which are esters of the saturated necines (Figure 3) have pronounced
pharmacological activity (anticholinergic action) (*36, 62, 63*) and have
been used medicinally as substitutes for atropine (*64*).

Of the alkaloids found in Crotalaria plants, dicrotaline (Table I) is
present in *C. dura,* which has been considered in South Africa to be the
cause of "jagsiekte" in horses, a condition characterized by emphysema and
adenomatosis of the lungs (*65*). In Australia, a similar chronic, often fatal,
condition known as the "Kimberley disease" occurs in horses (*66*) which
graze on *C. cryspata,* containing the alkaloids monocrotaline, cryspatine,
and its diastereoisomer, fulvine. Fulvine (Figure 5) may cause "veno-occlusive" liver disease in children in Jamaica, where the plant *C. fulva* L is used in
"bush teas" (*42, 67*). In North Queensland, Australia, certain varieties of
C. trifoliastrum Willd and *C. aridicola* Domin (which contain nonesterified
alkaloids, mainly derivatives of 1-methoxymethyl-1,2-dehydro-8α-pyrrolizidine,

some having 1,2-epoxy rings (Figure 7)) have been suspected to cause chronic lesions of the esophagus and of the stomach in horses (*68*).

A plant used as a remedy in Ayurvedic medicine in India, *C. medicaginea* Lamk., is considered identical with certain forms of *C. trifoliastrum* (*68*). The use of this plant may have some relation to tumors of the palate and of the esophagus among the Gujarati and elsewhere in India. 1-Methoxymethyl-1,2-dehydro-8α-pyrrolizidine and its 7-hydroxy-derivative (Figure 7) were found in the Indian plant (*69*). The epoxy-pyrrolizidines that are present in *C. trifoliastrum* have been synthesized (*68*). Their biological action, if any, has not yet been reported.

The effects in experimental animals of the cyclic diester alkaloids, such as fulvine from *C. fulva* L. and monocrotaline from *C. spectabilis*, *C. retusa*, and certain other *Crotalaria* species, are similar. Hypertension, arteritis, corpulmonale, changes in the vascular endothelium (not unlike those seen in veno-occlusive liver disease (*70*)), congestion of the liver, centrilobular liver, hemorrhagic necrosis, lung edema or pleural effusions, thickening of the alveolar wall, etc., have been seen in various animal species, including primates (*36, 39, 71, 72*). The lesions can progress to more chronic ones. Tumors of the lung and of the liver in the rat have already been mentioned (*48, 56*).

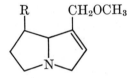

R = H, α-OH, β-OH
or β-OCOCH₃

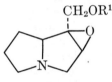

R¹ = H or CH₃

Australian Journal of Chemistry

Figure 7.   Nonesterified alkaloids from Crotalaria trifoliastrum *Willd. and* C. aridicola *Domin.* (36)

Karyotypic studies of lymphocyte chromosomes in the peripheral blood of children in the acute and recovering phase of veno-occlusive disease in Jamaica and in rats given fulvine showed abnormalities (*73*) similar to those described in rat liver hepatocytes. These chromosomal aberrations may correspond to the mutagenic action of fulvine in *Drosophila* (*74*). Given to pregnant rats fulvine is fetotoxic and teratogenic (*75*). Various pyrrolizidine alkaloids or their metabolites can induce mutations and chromosomal aberration in *Drosophila*, microorganisms, and plants (*36*).

A variety of animal species are evidently susceptible to various chronic effects, but so far tumors have been induced with PA only in rats and chickens (*37*). Vervet monkeys, *Cercopithecus aethiops,* given retrorsine orally (20 mg/kg body weight once weekly for 30 weeks, then once every 14 days) developed various chronic lesions, including some resembling veno-occlusive disease, but died within 20–72 weeks of treatment, mostly in hepatic coma (76). Such lesions might lead to tumors, if the monkeys were to survive longer on less intense treatment.

Metabolism of Pyrrolizidine Alkaloids. The PA, like many other foreign substances, undergo metabolic changes in the animal body by more than one pathway. The metabolites so far identified are similar to the pyrrolizidine compounds encountered in plants or insects (35). The known metabolites represent products of N-oxidation and dehydrogenation of the pyrrolizidine moiety, of O-demethylation of methoxy groups when these are present in the acidic moiety, and products of hydrolysis of the ester linkages (35, 77, 78, 79, 80). In the metabolic studies, open ester alkaloids have been mainly used. In Figure 8 several pathways (A–E) are indicated (of which only N-oxidation is reversible) as well as the probable stepwise formation of known and certain putative metabolites (the latter in square brackets).

The part of the administered dose that is excreted in the urine as the unchanged parent alkaloid depends mainly on its basic properties and water solubility. Lasiocarpine is excreted in trace quantities, heliotrine in about 30% of the administered dose; heliotridine trachelanthate, about 35%; heliotridine, 40%; and heliotridine-N-oxide, 62% (35).

It is evident that products of metabolic oxidation and hydrolysis of PA, if not bound immediately at the site of formation, would be readily excreted as soon as they reach the circulating blood. The levels of such metabolites found in the urine of animals given, e.g., heliotrine, represented about 35% of the administered dose in addition to the 30% excreted as unchanged alkaloid (35). The remaining one third of the dose, corresponding in the case of heliotrine to about 100 mg/kg remains unaccounted for. Part of it is likely to remain bound in the liver and in other tissues, but the actual amount and the nature of the bound metabolite(s) still remains to be established. Some metabolites in the liver give a magenta color on treatment with the Ehrlich pyrrol reagent, 4-dimethylaminobenzaldehyde (77). The term "metabolic pyrrols" has been used for the unidentified tissue-bound metabolites, which are considered to be related to dehydro-alkaloids. These represent a small fraction of the administered alkaloid. The urinary compounds which give colored derivatives with the Ehrlich reagent have been estimated to represent 0.2–12.4% of the dose, depending on the alkaloid used (77). By chemical oxidation of the pyrrolizidine alkaloids, dehydro-products are obtained, which indeed give color tests with the Ehrlich reagent, but their respective absorption spectra differ from those given by the metabolic products (77).

The chemically prepared dehydro-ester alkaloids are unstable compounds in aqueous solutions and rapidly hydrolyze to the respective necic acids, the 1,2,3,8-tetradehydronecines and other unidentified products (77, 79). They are irritants and cause necrotizing lesions at the site of application; when injected intravenously into rats they induce lung edema or chronic lung lesions (81). Tumors have not been induced in rats within two years after a single dose of dehydroretrorsine injected into mesenteric vein (J. M. Barnes, personal communication) nor after twice weekly subcutaneous injections of dehydromonocrotaline for more than a year (82).

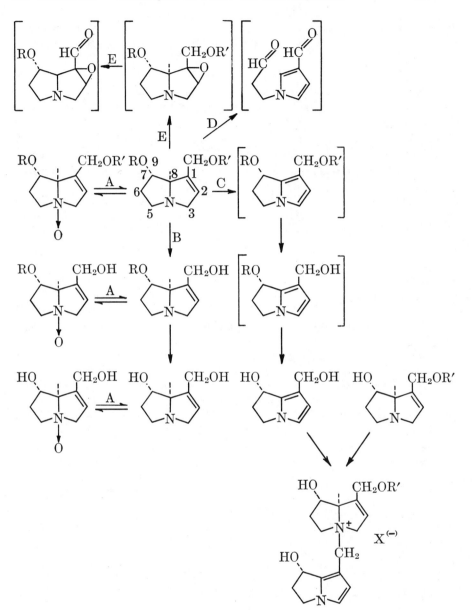

Figure 8. Metabolism of open ester alkaloids by known and putative pathways.
The compounds in square brackets are suggested as possibilities; so far, no experimental
evidence exists for their formation in the animal body. A. N-oxidation (reversible). B.
Stepwise hydrolysis of ester groups. C. Dehydrogenation. D. Oxidative fission of bond
C₇–C₈, possibly preceded by B or C and dehydrogenation of the 1-hydroxymethyl group.
E. Epoxidation of the 1,2-double bond and dehydrogenation of the 1-hydroxymethyl group.
R = H, or angelyl group; R′ = lasiocarpyl, heliotryl, trachelanthyl, etc. group.

Dehydroretronecine, the non-esterified metabolite of monocrotaline, induced rhabdomyosarcomas in rats given biweekly subcutaneous injections of 20 mg/kg body weight for four months, then 10 mg/kg for additional eight months. In these animals tumors of internal organs were not present, although rats treated in a similar way with monocrotaline, 5 mg/kg, developed tumors of the liver, the lung, and acute myelogenous leukemia, besides rhabdomyosarcomas (*56a*).

A urinary rat metabolite of lasiocarpine or heliotrine, which gives the Ehrlich reaction, has been isolated and identified as dehydroheliotridine, 7α-hydroxy-1-hydroxymethyl-6,7-dihydro-5*H*-pyrrolizine (*78*); the same compound is formed *in vitro* by the action of rat liver microsomal preparations on the alkaloids (*79*). Dehydroheliotridine has been reported to possess antimitotic activity and to cause atrophic changes in hair follicles, in the mucosa of the gastrointestinal tract, bone marrow, testes, thymus, spleen, etc., and mild melagocytosis in the liver when given to rats by intraperitoneal injection (*79*). Cytotoxic effects have been observed when KB cells were treated with dehydroheliotridine in tissue culture (*78*), but its long term effects in animals have not yet been reported. A quaternary compound *N*-[6,7-dihydro-7α-hydroxy-1-(5*H*-pyrrolizino)]methylheliotrine chloride (Figure 8) from dehydroheliotridine and the parent alkaloid has been isolated from *Heliotropium europeum* and has also been found as product of *in vitro* metabolism of heliotrine by rat liver microsomal preparations (*79*). Similar alkylation by dehydroheliotridine (and possibly also by dehydroretronecine) of the ring nitrogen in nicotinamide may be responsible for the depletion of NAD coenzymes, and for some of the acute and subacute effects caused by the pyrrolizidine alkaloids (*83 83a*).

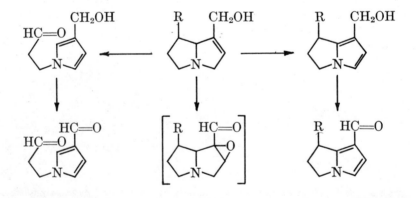

Australian Journal of Chemistry

Figure 9. Some of the products isolated from chemical oxidations of necines with manganese dioxide in chloroform (84). 1-Formyl-1,2-epoxy-derivatives (in square brackets) have been included as a hypothetical possibility, in analogy with some of the putative metabolites suggested in Figure 8.

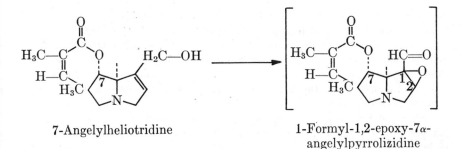

7-Angelylheliotridine   1-Formyl-1,2-epoxy-7α-
                                               angelylpyrrolizidine

Figure 10.   7-Angelylheliotridine (left) and its hypothetical metabolite 1-formyl-
1-2-epoxy-7α-angelylpyrrolizidine (right)

Chemical oxidation of certain pyrrolizidine alkaloids and of their necines gives complicated mixtures of products (*84*) which include, in the case of oxidations with manganese dioxide in chloroform; derivatives of 1-hydroxy-methyl-1,2-dehydropyrrolizidines, 1-formyl-1,2,3,8-tetradehydropyrrolizidines, *N*-2′-formylethyl, 3-hydroxymethylpyrrol, 3-formyl-1-(2′formylethyl) pyrrol, etc. (Figure 9). 7α-Angeloxy- and 7α-hydroxy-1-formyl-1,2,3,8-tetradehydro-pyrrolizidines give magenta colors with the Ehrlich reagent (*85*). It is not unlikely that in the course of metabolic oxidation of the pyrrolizidine alkaloids some of such formyl derivatives may be formed and that ring fission at the C_7–C_8 bond might also occur in the course of metabolic degradation as tentatively indicated in Figure 8.

Clearly, pyrrolizidine alkaloids are metabolized by several unrelated pathways; metabolic intermediates which are precursors of the specific metabolite, which is responsible for tumor induction, would obviously be carcinogenic. The alkaloids and their N-oxides are reversibly interconvertible depending on the redox potential of tissues. Regardless of the route of administration of PA, N-oxides are excreted in the urine (*35*). The N-oxide of fulvine induced chronic lesions of the liver and lung in rats, indistinguish-able from those caused by a similar single dose of fulvine (*86*). Isatidine, the N-oxide of retrorsine, induced chronic liver lesions and tumors whether given orally, intraperitoneally, or by skin application (*47*).

7-Angelylheliotridine is not an allylic ester and, although it does not produce acute liver necrosis, it can induce megalocytosis in the liver (*35*). It is not yet known whether under appropriate conditions it could induce tumors. Necrotizing action is not a prerequisite for tumor induction. An epoxy-formyl metabolite might be the active form (Figure 10).

The nonesterified necine, retronecine, is not hepatotoxic but it appeared to be responsible for a rat's spinal cord tumor (*55*). High doses of PA kill the animal because of their effects on the CNS. The conditions under which PA can induce tumors of the CNS require further studies.

As already indicated, the 1,2-double bond in the pyrrolizidine moiety appears essential for the carcinogenic action. This is likely to undergo metabolic epoxidation (*58, 61*). Chemically prepared α- and β-epoxides of monocrotaline (*87*) had no cytotoxic effects when tested on KB cells in tissue culture (*78*). Their long-term effects in rats have not yet been reported.

The crystal structures of jacobine (*88*), fulvine, and heliotrine (*89*) indicate that the dihedral angle between the bonds C_1–C_2 and C_9–O_{10} (which would affect the accessibility to $\Delta^{1,2}$) is 114° for jacobine, 64.° for fulvine, and 12° for heliotrine; this agrees with the order of the biological efficacies of these alkaloids (*89, 89a*).

The metabolism of pyrrolizidine alkaloids (including the suggested but not yet experimentally demonstrated epoxidation) is catalyzed by enzymes mainly located in the endoplasmic reticulum, such as the cytochrome P-450 enzyme, "microsomal mixed function oxidases," epoxide hydrase, etc. The enzymes can be affected by various substances, inducers, and inhibitors. When more is known of how to influence preferentially any one of the various reactions involved in the metabolic formation and degradation of the specific carcinogenic entity, it might be possible to prevent tumor initiation by pyrrolizidine alkaloids (and by other carcinogens) without the need for their complete eradication from the environment. It would appear particularly important to induce and/or stimulate the action of epoxide hydrase, the enzyme that transforms epoxides into more water-soluble and usually inactive diols (*90*) as a possibly tumor preventive measure.

Mechanism of Action. The mechanism of action of "natural" and synthetic carcinogens, is not known. How is it that compounds with such a variety of chemical structures can induce similar tumors and that the tumors sometimes develop even after a single dose and emerge only a long time after its administration? Evidently, certain of the events that take place during the encounter of the carcinogen with cell constituents determine subsequent neoplasia. Although the morphological and biochemical effects that take place in the tissues of animals given carcinogens have been extensively studied, the fateful event specific for neoplastic transformation has yet to be identified.

MORPHOLOGICAL CHANGES. Cytotoxic effects that lead to cell necrosis are not specific and are probably not essential for carcinogenic action. Segregation of the nucleolar material into granular and fibrillar components (cap formation), seen by electron microscopy in rat hepatocytes less than 30 min after dosing with aflatoxin, lasiocarpine, etc. (*91*), is reversible, and the appearance of the cell nucleolus is restored to normal within 48 hr. Cytoplasmic changes, including the release of ribosomes, proliferation of the smooth endoplasmic reticulum, loss of glycogen, etc., are also reversible. Similar changes have been seen after treatment of rats with compounds which do not induce liver tumors.

The most common effects of carcinogens are inhibition of cell division (*92*) and the development of enlarged cells. Greatly enlarged cells are found in the skin within a week after local application of carcinogenic polycyclic hydrocarbons (*93*), in the gastric mucosa (another tissue that is undergoing constant wear and tear) within a few days after *N*-methyl-*N*-nitrosourethane (*94*), but usually only within three to four weeks in the liver after ingestion of hepatocarcinogens. Particularly conspicuous are the enlarged cells which appear in young rat livers after pyrrolizidine alkaloids (*35, 59, 60*). The parenchymal cells vary greatly in their size, in the size of their nuclei, in the size and number of their nucleoli, etc. The cells that grow large are evidently able to synthesize nucleic acids, proteins, and other constituents essential for survival and growth (*95*). Why are these cells unable to divide? Mitotic figures are rarely found in enlarged cells and if present these show numerous chromosomes, suggestive of higher ploidy. The chromosomes are often clumped or fragmented and "pulverized." Whether some of the enlarged cells could overcome the inhibition of division, and on dividing start new cell lines with different, possibly neoplastic characteristics, is at present a matter for conjecture. Electron microscopy of the enlarged cells present in rat liver about one month after a single dose of retrorsine showed, in addition to an enlarged nucleus and one or more nucleoli, an increase in annuli in the nuclear membrane, proliferation of the rough-surfaced endoplasmic reticulum, enlargement of the Golgi complexes, increased number of perichromatin granules, and the presence of centrioles. The numbers of lysosomes, fat droplets, and microbodies appeared rather low (*95*).

These features are usually related to signs of increased metabolic activity. Indeed, the enlarged hepatocytes can incorporate effectively ^{14}C-adenine into their nucleic acids (*95*). Factors that regulate the normal distribution of the cellular organelles and that determine cell division appear missing in the enlarged cells, but their nature is still unknown.

BIOCHEMICAL CHANGES. The role of thiols in relation to cell division and to the mechanism of carcinogenesis has received much attention (*96*). Alkylation of nucleic acids by carcinogens, including the PA (*35, 78, 97*), has been widely believed to be the primary reaction responsible for tumorigenesis. Selenium, an essential microelement recently found to be a cofactor of glutathione peroxidase, may however also be involved in the carcinogenic process, as well as proteins and lipids. It may also be significant that many natural carcinogens possess reactive carbonyl groups as part of allylic ester groups, of α, β-unsaturated aldehydes and lactones, etc. The respective ethylenic double bonds may become epoxidized in the course of their metabolism.

The resulting putative metabolites of several types of carcinogens (*98*) have these electrophilic groups in similar positions. This would appear to be significant and may indicate involvement of these groups binding to cellular elements. The striking nuclear abnormalities and chromosomal aberrations seen in the tissues in which tumors will eventually appear justify the assumption that interaction of carcinogens with nuclear elements, probably with chromatin, may be involved.

Chromatin, the material that makes up the chromosomes, is composed of DNA, some RNA, basic and acidic proteins, and lipids (*99*). It is replicated during the S phase of the mitotic cycle, possibly after appropriate unwinding, dissociation, rearrangement, etc. Consideration should be given to the situation arising if the carcinogenic entity should crosslink, for example nucleic acid with protein, and prevent their usual dissociation.

The putative metabolic intermediates of carcinogenic PA with electrophilic epoxy and carbonyl functions could be expected to react with nucleophilic sulfhydryl, selenohydryl, and amino groups, etc. The epoxide ring could be opened by thiols to form covalent bonds with a peptide; a carbonyl group could also react with thiols or form Schiff base-type links with amino groups of nucleic acid bases, etc. The carcinogenic residue might thus form a "bridge" between nucleic acid and other constituents of chromatin. The particular site at which such a bridge is formed may be crucial for the carcinogenic process. During the mitotic cycle, this particular site of chromatin may become exposed only for a short time, and the relevant constituents may remain in juxtaposition just long enough for a concerted interaction with appropriate molecules to take place. For this to happen, the carcinogenic entity, *in statu nascendi*, must be present at the right time, at the right site, and with the appropriate orientation of the reactive groups.

Considering the many possibilities that exist for the reactive carcinogenic metabolite to react with soluble cell constituents, such as glutathione or even water, and to become inactivated before reaching the nucleus, it is clear that its concentration must be critical for the "fateful" interaction to ensue. On the molecular level, the latter would be a very rare event.

Carcinogens acting on young, growing tissues, in which mitotic divisions of cells are frequent, have a greater chance of hitting the relevant site. Moreover, an epoxide ring is likely to persist longer when the level of epoxyhydrase (the enzyme that catalyzes its opening, addition of water, and formation of noncarcinogenic diols) is low; the level of this enzyme increases with the age and maturation of the animal (*90*). The very young and actively regenerating tissues are often particularly susceptible to the action of carcinogens (*100*); they evidently possess the enzyme systems, etc., necessary for the formation of the relevant activated metabolites.

Besides the active groups, the molecular structure of the carcinogenic entity is critical. In order to form a bridge it must "fit" into the available space; its geometry, size and shape, and charge distribution would all affect the ease of its intercalation. If the fit is just right, the residue of the carcinogen could persist, or "stick", at the site where it crosslinks constituents of chromatin, and prevent its normal functioning. "The primary change may involve a segment of the genome that controls its own replication and the division of the cell (*101*)." A cell that succeeds in dividing may have some of its chromosomes carrying characteristics of the carcinogenic residue, imprinted into the relevant part of the chromatin. Recent karyotypic analyses indeed suggest that chromosomal patterns in some tumors are not random, but appear to depend on the carcinogenic agent with which the tumor has been induced (*102, 103*).

In a similar way by the formation of carbonyl-oxidation products from alkyl or alkoxy groups, alkylnitrosamines, and alkylazoxy carcinogens have been suggested to form bridges cross-linking constituents of chromatin (*104*). Recent experimental results appear to support this idea (*105*). The carcinogenic entity must probably be able to "hit, fit, and stick," in order to induce tumors.

Methylenedioxy-, Polymethoxy-allyl-, and propenylbenzenes and Certain Other Compounds

Ring-substituted allyl- and propenylbenzenes (Table IV) are constituents of essential oils derived from various plant species (*106*). Some have been used for flavoring foods and beverages, for medicinal purposes, etc., because of their carminative and certain other biological properties. Elemicine (3,4,5-trimethoxy-1-allylbenzene), isoelemicine (3,4,5-trimethoxy-1-propenyl-

Table IV. Derivatives of Allyl- and Propenylbenzene, Their Names, and Carcinogenic Activity

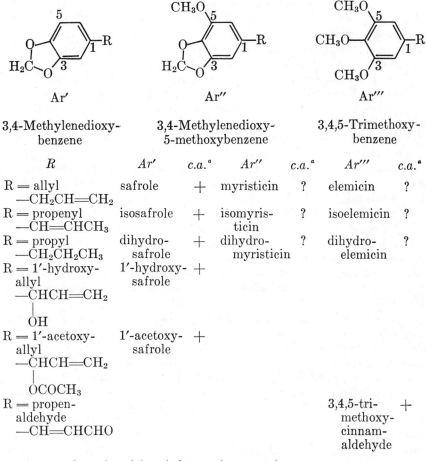

	Ar'		Ar''		Ar'''	
	3,4-Methylenedioxy-benzene		3,4-Methylenedioxy-5-methoxybenzene		3,4,5-Trimethoxy-benzene	
R	Ar'	c.a.[a]	Ar''	c.a.[a]	Ar'''	c.a.[a]
R = allyl —CH_2CH=CH_2	safrole	+	myristicin	?	elemicin	?
R = propenyl —CH=$CHCH_3$	isosafrole	+	isomyristicin	?	isoelemicin	?
R = propyl —$CH_2CH_2CH_3$	dihydro-safrole	+	dihydro-myristicin	?	dihydro-elemicin	?
R = 1'-hydroxy-allyl —CHCH=CH_2 | OH	1'-hydroxy-safrole	+				
R = 1'-acetoxy-allyl —CHCH=CH_2 | $OCOCH_3$	1'-acetoxy-safrole	+				
R = propen-aldehyde —CH=CHCHO					3,4,5-tri-methoxy-cinnam-aldehyde	+

[a] c.a., carcinogenic activity; +, known; ?, not tested.

benzene), and myristicine (3,4-methylenedioxy-5-methoxy-1-allylbenzene) have hallucinogenic properties (*107, 108*).

Safrole (3,4-methylenedioxy-1-allylbenzene), isosafrole (3,4,-methylene-dioxy-1-propenylbenzene), and dihydrosafrole (3,4-methylenedioxy-1-propyl-benzene) are weak carcinogens (*109, 110, 111*). When given for prolonged periods in diet (at about 0.5–1.0%) liver tumors were induced in mice and in rats. Infant mice given four doses of safrole by subcutaneous injections developed liver and lung tumors (*112*). A commercial sample of dihydrosafrole, such as is used for flavoring, induced tumors of the esophagus (*111*) when given to rats for long periods in the diet (1% and 0.25%).

In the course of its metabolism (Figure 11), safrole is oxidized to 1'-hydroxysafrole, which is excreted conjugated as glucuronide in the urine of rats, mice, hamsters, and guinea pigs (*113*). Urinary 1'-hydroxysafrole accounted for 1–3% of the administered dose in the rat, hamster, and guinea pig and for about 30% in the mouse (*113*). 1'-Hydroxysafrole is considered to be the proximate carcinogenic metabolite of safrole (*114*). When given for long periods in the diet (about 0.5%), it induced liver tumors in rats and mice, also a few tumors of the stomach in rats, and sarcomas in the interscapular region in mice. When 1'-hydroxysafrole was repeatedly injected subcutaneously, a small incidence of sarcomas developed locally. 1'-Acetoxysafrole was more effective in inducing tumors of the stomach when fed and sarcomas at the site of subcutaneous injections. No skin tumors have been induced in mice given repeated applications of safrole or of 1'-hydroxy-, 1'-acetoxy-, or 1'-methoxysafrole; nor by corresponding 2',3'-dihydrosafrole derivatives, when tested in conjunction with the co-carcinogen phorbol-12,13-didecanoate (*114*).

However, the metabolic fate of the major part of the administered dose of safrole is still not accounted for, and it is possible that in addition to 1'-hydroxysafrole and its derivatives, (a putative ester of 1'-hydroxy-safrole has been suggested as the ultimate carcinogenic form of safrole (*114*)), some other carcinogenic metabolites may be formed in the animal body. In particular, it would be of interest to know whether, in the rat, safrole might undergo stepwise changes by additional metabolic pathways similar to those found in the case of *p*-methoxyallylbenzene, which led to the formation of epoxides and of the respective cinnamoyl derivatives as in Figure 12 (*115*).

In a recent detailed study of the metabolism in the rat of *p*-methoxy-allylbenzene (estragole) and of *p*-methoxypropenylbenzene (anethole), 60–90% of the administered dose of estragole and almost 100% of anethole have been accounted for in the form of various metabolic intermediates (*115*). About half of the administered dose gave *p*-O-demethylated products. In the remainder, the side chain underwent several oxidative reactions (Figure 12)—epoxidation of the double bond, alpha and/or omega oxidation, and chain shortening. The propenyl compound appears to undergo oxidation more readily than the allylic estragole. Because of migration of the double bond from the 2',3'- to 1',2'-position, both estragole and anethole yield a number of common metabolites as propenyl derivatives. Some of the more

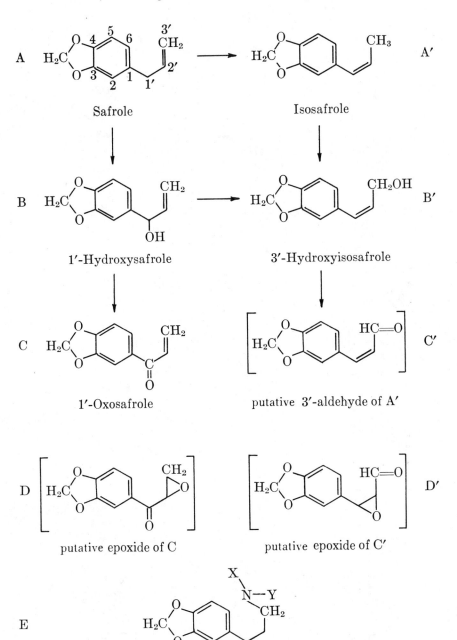

Figure 11. Metabolism of safrole (A) and isosafrole (A'). B, B', C, and E are known metabolites; C', D, and D' are suggested as possible metabolites.

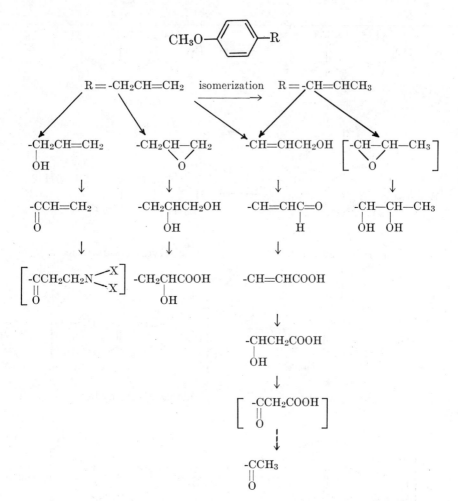

Xenobiotica

Figure 12. Metabolic pathways of p-methoxyallylbenzene (estragole) and p-methoxypropenylbenzene (anethole), in which the p-methoxy group is retained (115)

reactive metabolites have been detected only in the bile (*e.g.*, the epoxide of estragole) or were found only in traces in the urine (*e.g.*, the epoxide of anethole).

The problem arises—does the metabolism of the related ring polysubstituted methoxy-, methylenedioxyallyl-, and propenylbenzenes follow pathways similar to those shown in Figure 12? In the case of safrole, the operation of the first pathway leads to 1'-hydroxysafrole (Figure 11) (*113*). The formation of 1'-keto safrole could be inferred from the isolation of 1'-keto-3'-dimethylamino-2',3'-dihydrosafrole and the corresponding *N*-piperidyl- and *N*-pyrrolidinyl-derivatives from rat and guinea pig urine (*116*). Tertiary aminopropiophenone derivatives are urinary metabolites also in the case of myristicin (*117*) and elemicin (*118*). The migration of the allylic double bond in the side chain from position 2′,3′ to 1′,2′ under acidic conditions takes place not only in the case of the hydrocarbons, but also in the case of 1′-hydroxysafrole, from which the 3′-hydroxyisosafrole is readily formed (*113*).

The significance of cinnamic metabolites in relation to the carcinogenic action of safrole and of its congeners deserves attention because 3,4,5-trimethoxycinnamaldehyde (TMCA; Table IV) is carcinogenic (*119*). 3,4,5-Trimethoxycinnamaldehyde (3,4,5-trimethoxybenzenepropenaldehyde) (Figure 13) induced, among other tumors, two nasal squamous carcinomas in a small scale experiment in which two doses—100 and 150 mg/kg body weight—were given to young rats by subcutaneous and intraperitoneal injections respectively (*119*). Unsubstituted cinnamaldehyde did not induce tumors (Schoental and Gibbard, unpublished data). TMCA was tested for carcinogenic action in connection with an investigation into possible etiological factors of nasal and nasopharyngeal tumors in man (*120*). The high incidence of nasopharyngeal cancer reported among the Southern Chinese, the Highland Kenyans, etc., might possibly be related to exposure to wood smoke (*121*) while the high frequency of nasal ethmoid tumors among woodworkers in England (*122*) and elsewhere (*123*) may be related to the deposition of fine dust in the nasal ethmoids during machining of

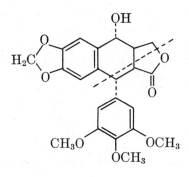

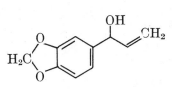

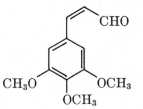

Figure 13. Structures of 1′-hydroxysafrole (left), podophyllotoxin (top), and 3,4,5-trimethoxycinnamaldehyde (right)

hard woods. Constituents of wood lignins (124) such as sinapaldehyde and related compounds (124, 125) present in wood and in its smoke (125) came under suspicion. TMCA, the p-O-methyl derivative of sinapaldehyde, appeared worthy of testing, as p-methoxy groups increase the carcinogenic efficacy of carcinogens (126).

The search for carcinogens in woods is a new field, the exploration of which has hardly begun. A number of known constituents are already under suspicion and deserve priority testing for carcinogenic activity. These include the lignin constituents, methoxy-substituted cinnamaldehydes, and cinnamalcohols (124), (the latter would obviously yield the respective aldehydes in the course of metabolic oxidations by alcohol dehydrogenases), as well as the methylenedioxy and polymethoxylignans (127). Of the latter, podophyllotoxin (Figure 13) is present (about 0.1%) in the dry needles of red cedar (*Juniperus virginiana* L.) and in certain other plants and *Juniperus* species. It is the active constituent of "podophyllin" from *Podophyllum peltatum* (127, 128), which is a mitotic poison and a cytotoxic and antitumor agent (129, 130), able to induce striking hyperplastic lesions and occasionally tumors when applied to the mouse uterine cervix or given in the diet (131, 132).

Podophyllotoxin may be responsible for some of the carcinogenic effects of red cedar wood bedding, recently demonstrated in Australia, where the high incidence of "spontaneous" tumors in C3H-A^vyfB mice imported from the U.S. dropped considerably when other wood shavings (from Douglas Fir, *Pseudotsuga* spp.) were used as bedding instead of red cedar wood chips (133) (*see* also p. 662). The structure of podophyllotoxin (Figure 13) indicates that in the course of its metabolic or microbial degradation it might yield methylenedioxyphenyl- and 3,4,5-trimethoxyphenyl-derivatives (134).

Unidentified esters of 3,4,5-trimethoxycinnamic acid have been found in the root of *Polygala senega*, which is used medicinally as a stimulant, expectorant, etc. (135). Methylation of phenolic hydroxy groups changes greatly the biological properties of substances. Their acute toxicity is usually reduced while other activities, including carcinogenic action, may become prominent. Methylenedioxy- (equivalent to two methoxy groups) and polymethoxy-substituents are present (among other natural products) in certain flavonoids and isoflavonoids (136). The heartwood of *Cordyla*

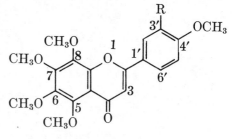

Figure 14.   Structures of tangeretin and nobiletin

R = H; tangeretin

R = OCH₃; nobiletin

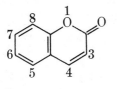

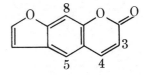

5,7-Dimethoxycoumarin
= limettin

5-Methoxypsoralen = bergapten
8-Methoxypsoralen = methoxalen
= xanthotoxin

Figure 15. Structures of coumarin (left) and psoralens (right)

africana (*Leguminosae*) is particularly rich in such isoflavonoids, which impart resistance to fungal attack (137).

Polymethoxyflavonoids, such as tangeretin (5,6,7,8,4′-pentamethoxy-flavone) and nobiletin (5,6,7,8,3′,4′-hexamethoxyflavone) (Figure 14), which are present in certain citrus oils, effectively induce microsomal hydroxylating enzymes in the liver (138). Safrole acts similarly (139). The related flavonoid 3,5,6,3′, 4′-pentamethyl ether of quercetin inhibits the development of skin tumors by local application of benzo[a]pyrene (140). On the other hand, lime oil has a co-carcinogenic action (141). Freshly pressed lime oil contains a high concentration of "solids" (about 10%), which include polymethoxyflavonoids, 5,7-dimethoxycoumarin (limettin), and 5-methoxypsoralen (bergapten) (Figure 15) (142). The latter may be a cause of dermatitis in lime pickers.

Rats fed coumarin for long periods developed bile duct adenomas and carcinomas (143). Substitution of particular positions in coumarins (5, 7, and 8) with methoxy or other groups greatly affects the biological activity (142, 144). Certain of the methoxy-substituted furo- and pyranocoumarins have narcotic, piscicidal, and antimicrobial action while some affect blood clotting. The inhibition of certain enzymes (such as peroxidase and indole-acetic acid oxidase) is probably caused by the interaction of the 3,4-double bond of the respective coumarins with thiols and amino groups (142, 144). The furocoumarins or psoralens (Figure 15) are present in many plants traditionally used as medicines; they are highly fluorescent and can cause photosensitization. Albino mice irradiated after treatment with 8-methoxy-psoralen (a compound used for vitiligo and in suntan preparations) developed tumors on their ears (145).

Polymethoxy compounds usually undergo metabolic and microbial degradation less readily than the respective polyphenols (146). Some poly-methoxy compounds are psychotropic and some have hallucinogenic action, e.g., mescaline (Figure 16) and some other *Anhalonium lewinii* Henning and *Rauwolfia* alkaloids (Figure 17) (147, 148), and some of the constituents of nutmeg (*Myristica fragrans*), e.g., myristicin and its congeners (Table IV) (107, 108, 149). Appropriate long term testing of the various poly-methoxy compounds for carcinogenic action appears desirable (150, 150a).

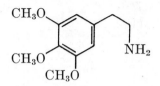

Figure 16.   Structure of mescaline

Tannins are a group of poorly defined polyphenolic plant constituents used for tanning hides. The interest in tannins as potential carcinogens started as a result of observations made during World War II, when patients treated for burns with tannic acid dressings developed liver lesions (*151*). Experimentally, certain tannins can induce tumors of the liver and local sarcomas when given to rats by subcutaneous injections (*151*).

Recently, catechin tannins have been suggested by Morton (*152*) to be involved in the high incidence of esophageal cancer reported among certain communities in Transkei, Kenya, Curaçao, in the Honan Province of North China (*153*), in Kazakhstan (*154*), and in some parts of the Caspian

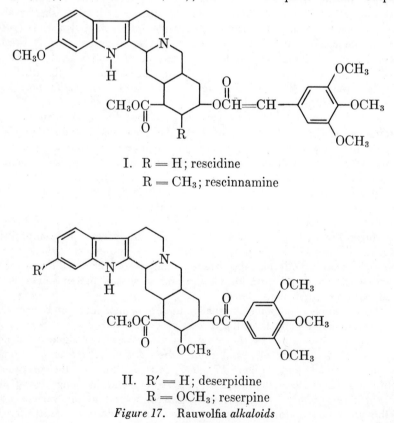

I. R = H; rescidine
R = CH₃; rescinnamine

II. R′ = H; deserpidine
R = OCH₃; reserpine

Figure 17.   Rauwolfia *alkaloids*

Littoral (*155*). This type of tumor is found not only in man but also in livestock, *e.g.*, among cattle in Scotland (*156*), in Masai cattle in Kenya (*157*), and in sheep in the Cape Province of South Africa (but only when the sheep were drenched with nicotine sulfate and copper sulfate and were grazing on a plateau at 4000-ft altitude (*158*). Its occurrence in circumscribed geographical areas suggests the involvement of "natural" products with some specific characteristics. Multifactorial etiology appears likely; certain plant materials may act in conjunction with other factors, *e.g.*, fungal metabolites such as the highly irritant 12,13-epoxytrichothecenes (Figure 18) (*159*). These are secondary metabolites of certain strains of *Fusaria* and related fungi which sometimes contaminate cereals and other plant

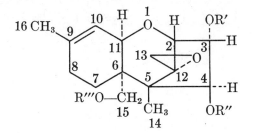

I.   R′ = R″ = R‴ = H; 3α,4β,15-trihydroxy-12,13-epoxy-Δ^9-trichothecene

II. R′ = H, R″ = R‴ = Ac; 3α-hydroxy-4β,15-diacetoxy-12,13,epoxy-Δ^9-
     Δ^9-trichothecene

III. R′ = R″ = R‴ = Ac; or other acids 3α,4β,15-triacetoxy-12,13-epoxy-
     Δ^9-trichothecene

Figure 18

materials. Barley, contaminated by *Fusarium sporotrichiella* because of wet harvesting conditions, has caused the occasional "epidemics" of beer "gushing" (the overflow of beer on opening the shaken container because of excessive formation of gas bubbles) (*160*). Traditionally esophageal cancer in man has been connected with alcoholic beverages—the basis for such a relationship may be the occasional use of Fusaria-contaminated cereals for alcoholic fermentations—but the etiology of these tumors in man is also likely to be multifactorial (*161*). T-2 toxin (4β,15-diacetoxy-8α-(3-methyl-butyryloxy)-12,13-epoxy-trichothec-9-en-3-ol) has been found to be carcinogenic for the brain and the digestive tract of rats (*381*).

Experimentally, esophageal tumors have been induced by dihydrosafrole (*111*) and by various nitroso compounds (*162*). The role of nitroso compounds, whether present as such in foodstuffs or formed in the stomach from nitrite and secondary or tertiary amines, is difficult to assess and impossible to exclude. The finding that heavy metal salts (copper sulfate or cobalt chloride) enhance the local carcinogenic action of ethylnitrosourea (*163*) may be relevant to the esophageal tumors found only among sheep that have been subjected to drenching with copper sulfate (*158*).

An α,β-unsaturated lactone moiety is frequently encountered in nature. A number of simple α,β-unsaturated lactones (Figure 19) induce subcutane-

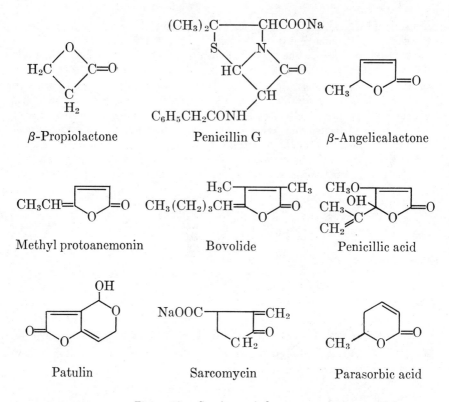

β-Propiolactone   Penicillin G   β-Angelicalactone

Methyl protoanemonin   Bovolide   Penicillic acid

Patulin   Sarcomycin   Parasorbic acid

Figure 19.   Carcinogenic lactones

ous sarcomas in rats (some also in mice) at the site of twice weekly subcutaneous injections repeated over prolonged periods (32–78 weeks) (*164, 165*). Coumarin, which is also an α,β-unsaturated lactone, did not induce tumors under these conditions. Most of the active compounds of this type have substituents on the carbon vicinal to the oxygen of the lactone group, which may be necessary in order to hinder too-ready hydrolysis of the lactone ring.

Among compounds the carcinogenic potentialities of which require further evaluation is colchicine (Figure 20), the very toxic alkaloid of

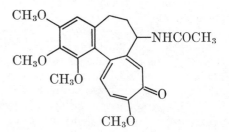

Figure 20.   Structure of colchicine

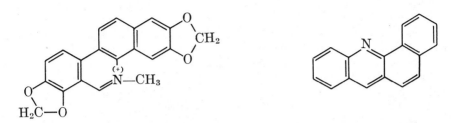

Figure 21.   Structures of sanguinarine (left) and benz[c]acridine (right)

Colchicum autumnale L., which has striking effects on cell division, by arresting mitosis in the metaphase (*166*). Colchicine applied repeatedly to the skin in conjunction with croton oil, gave a single skin tumor among eight mice that survived this treatment (*167*).

Sanguinarine (Figure 21) the benzphenanthridine alkaloid present in *Argemone mexicana* L and in many other poppy-fumaria species, may be involved in "epidemic dropsy" in India (allegedly because of adulteration of edible oils with argemone seed oil) and possibly even in causing tumors of the esophagus in India and elsewhere as a result of medicinal uses of the plant (*168*). Sanguinarine forms, among other metabolites, benz[*c*]-acridine (Figure 21), which has been detected in the milk of animals treated with sanguinarine during lactation (*169*). When sanguinarine or benz[*c*]-acridine were applied for prolonged periods to the skin of mice or implanted in paraffin pellets into the bladder of rats, a few tumors developed (*168*).

Cycasin and its Congeners. Cycasin (Figure 22), a glucoside of methylazoxymethanol, and its congeners (macrosamin, neocycasin), which have the same aglycone but different sugar moieties, are present in various plant species belonging to the botanical family, Cycadaceae (*170*). Their toxic and carcinogenic activity arises from the aglycone methylazoxymethanol (Figure 22), which is released by the action of the enzyme β-glucosidase, derived mainly from the intestinal microorganisms (*171*). The carcinogenic entity may be a metabolic oxidation product, methylazoxyformaldehyde (*104*). The biological action of cycasin, which closely resembles that of *N*-nitrosodimethylamine, is described in detail in Chapter 11.

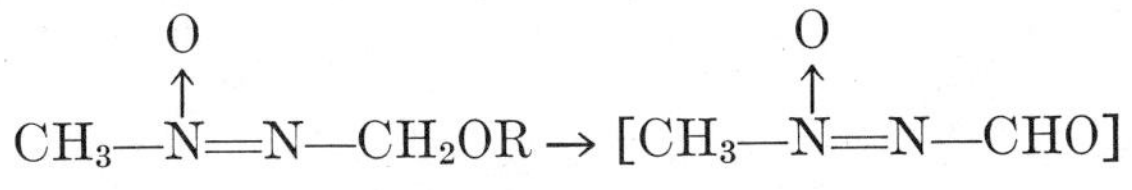

$$CH_3{-}\overset{\overset{O}{\uparrow}}{N}{=}N{-}CH_2OR \rightarrow [CH_3{-}\overset{\overset{O}{\uparrow}}{N}{=}N{-}CHO]$$

R = β-D-glucopyranosyl; cycasin
R = 6-(β-D-xylosido)-D-glucosyl (= primeverosyl); macrosamin
R = H; methylazoxymethanol

Figure 22.   Structures of cycasin, macrosamin, methylazoxymethanol, and a postulated active metabolite, methylazoxyformaldehyde

Phorbol Esters and Co-carcinogenesis. Among plant materials, croton oil from the seeds of *Croton tiglium* L, a strong irritant that has been used in human and veterinary medicine, has striking co-carcinogenic activity. It accelerates the development of skin tumors initiated by local application of a single dose of carcinogenic polycyclic aromatic hydrocarbons (*172*) or by injection of urethane (*173*). The active constituents of croton oil are diesters of a tetracyclic diterpene, phorbol (Figure 23). Fourteen diesters have been isolated from croton oil, all having a long chain acid at C_{12} and a short one at C_{13}. The most active biologically is 12-*O*-tetra-decanoylphorbol-13-acetate or phorbol myristate acetate (PMA) (Figure 23).

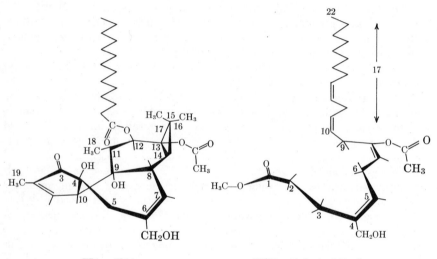

TPA = PMA   PUFA methyl ester derivative

Nature

Figure 23.   The structure of phorbol-12-O-tetradecanoyl-13-acetate (TPA) = phorbol-myristyl-acetate (PMA) and of 4-hydroxymethyl-8-acetoxy-4,7,10,13-docosatetraenoic acid methyl ester, (polyunsaturated fatty acid methyl ester = PUFA-methylester derivative) (177)

The free hydroxyl at C_{20}, the $4\beta,10\alpha$-configuration of the junction between the five and the seven-membered rings, and the double bond $\Delta^{6,7}$ are essential for the co-carcinogenic action (*174, 175*).

A number of related compounds have been isolated from various other species of *Euphorbiaceae*. Some have co-carcinogenic but others only irritant action (*175*). The mechanism of the tumor promoting activity may be related to an interaction of PMA with certain specific receptors on the membranes of sensitive cells (*176*). Attention has been directed to the similarity of the tridimensional structure of PMA to that of a derivative of 4,7,10,13-docosatetraenoic acid methyl ester (Figure 23). Polyunsaturated fatty acids in association with phospholipids are membrane constituents. They may also act as cellular regulators and be involved in cell growth (*177*).

The essential double bond of PMA, $\Delta^{6,7}$ and the corresponding $\Delta^{4,5}$ in the natural polyunsaturated fatty acid would be expected to become metabolically epoxidized and are probably involved in the binding to cellular elements. Epoxidation of the double bond $\Delta^{7,8}$ of the polyunsaturated fatty acid would simulate the cyclopropanoid 3-membered ring of $C_{13,14}$ of phorbol.

Co-carcinogenic action has been reported for certain citrus fruit oils. Their active principles have yet to be identified. The subject of co-carcinogenesis and the phorbol esters is reviewed in Chapter 2.

Other Miscellaneous Carcinogenic Plant Materials. Plants used as food or remedy have been receiving increasingly more attention, with the findings that some have carcinogenic potentialities. Extracts and purified fractions from bracken, *Pteridium aquilinum*, induce intestinal and bladder tumors (*see* Chapter 13).

Among plants collected by Morton (*178*) on the island of Curaçao, where the incidence of esophageal cancer is particularly high, were *Krameria ixina* L, *Acacia villosa* L, and *Melochia tomentosa* L. Fibrosarcomas developed in all the rats which were given crude extracts of these plants by subcutaneous injections over long periods (*179*). These plants are being used as tonics and remedies for various ills by many inhabitants, including the esophageal cancer patients. When the extracts from *Krameria ixina* were freed from tannin, tumors were not induced (*180*).

Among Japanese plants screened for carcinogenic action, *Petasites japonicus* (a kind of coltsfoot) induced tumors in the rats given the dried powdered flower stalk in diet (4% or 8%) for 430 days. The tumors included hemangioendothelial liver sarcomas, liver cell adenomas, and hepatocellular carcinomas (*181*).

Conclusions. The high dosage of safrole, 3,4-methylenedioxyallylbenzene (and its congeners), required for tumor induction indicates that the active carcinogenic entity formed in the course of its metabolism, may represent only a minute fraction of the administered dose and might be very difficult to identify. This is illustrated by the metabolism of the related *p*-methoxyallylbenzene and *p*-methoxypropenylbenzene, in which the identified metabolites accounted for almost 100% of the administered dose (*115*). These compounds are metabolized by several pathways to many metabolites, among which the reactive epoxy and aldehydic metabolites are present only in traces.

Preliminary data indicate that 3,4,5-trimethoxycinnamaldehyde is a potent carcinogen and may be involved in the carcinogenic action of certain woods and their products. Examples are given of compounds which would be of interest to test for carcinogenic action; these include "natural" methylenedioxy, polymethoxy, and certain other compounds which are used medicinally or otherwise and some of which have various biological activities. The use of infant animals for the testing, as well as for the metabolic studies, appears advisable and might facilitate the task.

"Natural" Estrogens

Since Lacassagne (*182*) first demonstrated that folliculin (estrone) can induce mammary tumors in male mice, estrogens have been found capable, in susceptible animals under appropriate conditions, of inducing tumors in several target organs—the breast, uterus, vagina, anterior pituitary, adrenal, thyroid, etc. (*183, 184, 185, 186, 187*). In hamsters (*Cricetus auratus*) estrogens induce kidney tumors in males and also in females when treated before puberty (*188*). The younger the animal, the more susceptible it is to the action of estrogens, as it frequently is to other carcinogens (*189, 190*).

In order to prevent pregnancy in mice and rats, high daily doses of oral contraceptives are required (0.3–5 mg/kg/day for mice, 1–5 mg/kg/day in rats, as compared with 0.02–0.08 mg/kg/day required by humans. When rodents are given contraceptive steroids (mice: 0.3–30 mg/kg, rats: 7–15 mg/kg) for one to three days during the second week of pregnancy, the fetuses removed at the end of gestation show teratogenic effects, growth retardation, skeletal, urogenital, brain, and various other abnormalities, but no tumors (*191*). When oral contraceptives are given to rodents by subcutaneous injections, their efficacy is about five times higher than when given orally (*191*).

Even a single large dose of estrogens can have carcinogenic and certain other deleterious effects. A single dose of the synthetic diethylstilbestrol (DES) (Figure 24) induces multiple cysts of the epididymis in male mice while in female mice tumors of the vagina and of the uterus (myoblastoma) have been found (*192*). Similar results have been reported when the oral contraceptive Enovid containing norethynodrel and mestranol was used (*193, 194*). Continuous administration of Enovid in diet induced uterine tumors in all the treated mice (*193*). Although these results have been obtained in small-scale experiments, their significance became apparent in the light of certain epidemiological findings in humans.

As a consequence of large doses of estrogens given medicinally to women for threatened abortion, masculization of the female offspring (*195, 196*) and the development of various malformations have been reported (*197, 198*). Moreover, seven cases of the very rare vaginal tumors which occurred among very young women, less than 22 years old, in one hosiptal, have resulted from treatment of the patients' mothers for threatened abortion with diethylstilbestrol (*199*). Other cases of similar iatrogenic origin also have been reported (*200, 201, 202*). In cases of vaginal tumors in young women whose mothers were not treated with estrogens during pregnancy (*203*), other sources of estrogenic substances (*vide infra*) including those that may be present in certain foodstuffs must be considered.

Oral contraceptives containing steroidal, estrogenic, and progestational substances taken over prolonged periods present a carcinogenic hazard which depends on the cumulative total dose and may take 20–30 years to become epidemiologically recognized. They are known to cause various unwanted side effects. Among the mild ones are nausea, photophobia, depression, headaches, weight gain, and hair loss; more serious effects include thromboembolism, liver injury, bile stasis, and cardiovascular disease. The reduction of fertility can be followed by superfertility when the oral contraceptives are stopped or by complete sterility (*204*). Thromboembolic disease is about ten-fold, and gallbladder disease two-fold higher among the women using oral contraceptives than among the non-users (*205*). Jaundice among breast-fed babies of mothers that used oral contraceptives several years before the child's conception has also been reported (*206*).

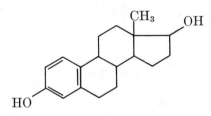

I. Estradiol

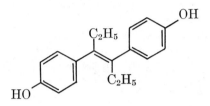
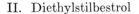

II. Diethylstilbestrol

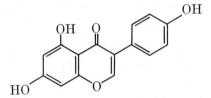

III. Genistein

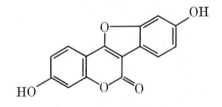
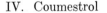

IV. Coumestrol

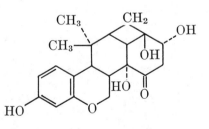

V. Mirestrol

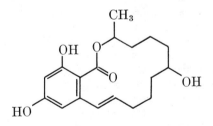

VI. Zearalenone (reduced)

Figure 24. Structures representing the types of compounds with estrogenic activity

The oral contraceptives came into wide use about 1960, and by 1971 about 13,000,000 women were taking them (*207*). At present the numbers are probably even higher. According to a Report by the Committee on Safety of Medicines (H. M. Stationery Office, London, 1972), benign hepatomas as well as pituitary, mammary, and certain other tumors have been found among mice and rats in carcinogenicity tests of oral contraceptives.

Since similar tumors were present in the controls, as in some of the test series the diet of these animals might have contained some additional estrogenic substances.

A recent report described a possible association between benign hepatomas (a type of tumor very rare in western countries) found in seven women aged 25–39 years with use of various oral contraceptives for up to 12 years (*208*). Additional cases are already coming to light (*209*), as well as cases of gonadal abnormalities in young men, who were exposed during gestation to estrogens given to their mothers on medical grounds (*209a*). Male mice exposed experimentally to DES during gestation developed various lesions of the reproductive tract (*209b*).

Other steroids with anabolic properties also can cause tumors. Hepatocellular hepatomas have been reported in anemic young patients (male and female) who were treated with androgenic-anabolic steroids (*210*). These steroids (despite the carcinogenic hazard) are used in very large doses by male and female young athletes (*211*).

The health hazard probably arises from the cumulative action of estrogenic agents present in various sources which include:

1. The endogenous hormones,

2. Estrogenic constituents derived from plants or from certain fungi which contaminate foodstuffs,

3. Estrogenic agents which are added to livestock fodder or implanted in the form of pellets under the skin and may pass into milk, meat, etc.,

4. Estrogenic additives to cosmetics,

5. Oral contraceptives,

6. Estrogens used medicinally, especially for threatened abortion, for suppression of lactation, menstrual disorders, the treatment of certain forms of cancer, etc.

The estrogenic contribution by agents mentioned under 1. and 2. varies and cannot be readily estimated or avoided. This "natural" estrogenic load could occasionally already be excessive (at the end of pregnancy estriol levels can increase 1000-fold (*212*)). It is therefore the more important to avoid adding to it from sources mentioned under 3.–6. unless absolutely indicated on medical grounds. The chemical structures of representative types of compounds known to possess estrogenic activity are shown in Figure 24. The physiological female sex hormones are steroidal compounds, *e.g.*, estradiols (I); estrone has been found also in plant materials, *e.g.*, date palm kernels (*213*). Genistein (5,7,4'-trihydroxyisoflavone; III) is present in soybean and other plants (*214*). Its high concentration (about 0.5%) in subterranean clover (*Trifolium subterraneum* L.) was responsible for sheep sterility in Australia (*215*), even though its estrogenic activity is only 10^{-5} of that shown by diethylstilbestrol (II) (*216*). Many plants used as food or as fodder contain substances that have estrogenic activity. Coumestrol (IV) isolated from alfalfa and from other forage crops is a coumarin derivative (*217*) and has about 35-fold higher estrogenic activity than genistein. Other *iso*-flavonoids (Figure 25), especially those with methoxy groups (*214, 218*), have even lower estrogenic activity than genistein, but

may be present in high enough concentrations to present health and repro-
duction hazards (*219*). The estrogenic mirestrol (V) isolated from *Pueraria
mirifica* (Leguminosae), has been used in Thailand as a rejuvenating medicine for old men and women, but was wisely considered too dangerous for
young people (*220*).

Synthetic estrogens, mainly diethylstilbestrol (DES), have been used as
additives to livestock diets, in order to accelerate growth and fattening and
to achieve a better food conversion. The Food and Drug Administration of
the U.S. has prohibited its addition to animal fodder or the implantation of
its pellets into the ears of livestock (*221*), but another estrogen ("Ralgro")
has been developed to replace diethylstilbestrol (*222*). This preparation has
similar estrogenic activity, but it has a different structure (Figure 24, VI).
It consists of two stereoisomers which are hydroxylic reduction products of
zearalenone, a secondary metabolic product of *Fusarium graminearum*

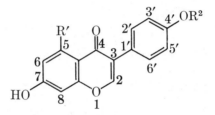

$R' = R^2 = H =$ daidzein (4',7-dihydroxyisoflavone)

$R' = H; R^2 = CH_3 =$ formononetin (7-hydroxy-4'-methoxyisoflavone)

$R' = OH; R^2 = H =$ genistein (5,7,4'-trihydroxyisoflavone)

$R' = OH; R^2 = CH_3 =$ biochanin A. (5,7-dihydroxy-4'-methoxyisoflavone)

$R' = OCH_3; R^2 = H =$ 5-*O*-methylgenistein (5-methoxy-7,4'-dihydroxyisoflavone).

Figure 25.   Estrogenic isoflavones in plants

(*Gibberella zeae*), and certain related fungi which often contaminate cereals
and other foodstuffs. The estrogenic activity of zearalenone was discovered
during investigation of the pathological condition vulvovaginitis in pigs,
which was traced to contamination of the diet with *Fusaria* (*222*).

Although the various estrogenic compounds differ in their chemical
structures, they show marked similarity in the positions of the hydroxyl
groups, which are essential for the estrogenic action. Indeed, of the two
stereoisomeric reduction products of zearalenone, which differ in the configuration of the hydroxyl at C_6, one is more active than the other.

The various plant and fungal estrogenic compounds have yet to be
tested for carcinogenic action. However, their effects on the target organs
are likely to be similar to those caused by diethylstilbestrol and by the
steroidal estrogens.

When estrogens are present in livestock fodder, small quantities are present not only in eggs, meat, etc., but also in milk and its products (223). Estrogens which are protein bound or in conjugated form are likely to be released in the gastrointestinal tract by enzymic action. Since milk is the main foodstuff of the very young who are extremely susceptible to the action of carcinogens, the hazard posed by the presence of estrogens, of whatever chemical structure, in cow's fodder may be far from negligible.

The normal liver is usually able to metabolize, conjugate, and inactivate estrogenic agents. In certain pathological conditions, however, it might be unable to cope with an excessive intake; the circulating estrogens could then affect the gonads and other organs.

Certain commercial animal rations, even those used for laboratory animals, can occasionally contain appreciable amounts of estrogen of unknown source (224). They may then interfere with the biological assay for estrogens or progesterone (224a).

An interesting observation has been recently reported from Australia. C3H A^{vy} mice, which have a high incidence of mammary and hepatic tumors in the laboratories of the National Cancer Institute (NIH) in the U.S., have developed fewer tumors when exported to Australia; the incidence declined strikingly in the subsequent generations of mice bred in Australia. However, when the mice were given the American diet, the incidence of the mammary tumors increased; it was restored to the American level when their Douglas fir bedding (*Pseudotsuga spp.*) was replaced by shavings of red cedar (*Juniperus virginiana*), which is used at NIH (225). The authors suspected that the red cedar shavings contain carcinogens. This would not be surprising in view of the carcinogenic activity of 3,4,5-trimethoxycinna-maldehyde, a derivative of the α,β-unsaturated aldehydes, which are normal constituents of wood lignins (226, 227). Other carcinogenic compounds may also be present in red cedar wood. However, the enhancing effect of the American diet on the induction of mammary cancer could be related to its content of estrogens (224). This remarkable instance of modification by environmental factors of the incidence of "spontaneous" tumors, which had been believed to be genetically determined, appears very important and warrants closer examination, especially in relation to breast cancer in women.

The activity of the steroidal, synthetic, and plant estrogens depends on the presence of hydroxyl groups at the extremities of their molecules (esterone has only about 1/10th of the activity of estradiol, to which it is metabolically reduced in the animal body). The hydroxyls are involved in the binding with specific receptor proteins, present in the cytosol of cells in the target organs. The resulting complexes are then carried into the nucleus, where they become tightly bound to acceptor proteins. This process has been detected *in vivo* and *in vitro*; it is susceptible to inhibition by thiol reagents (228).

The vaginal tumors in young women referred to earlier appeared after more than 12 years when estrogens acted transplacentally. The etiology of childhood and prenatal tumors (229, 230) remains unknown. It is possible that in such cases the causative agent(s) might have acted on the parental gonads at or preceding conception (*190*). However, the experimental induction prenatally of tumors in animals, which could serve as models for the etiology of the human neonatal cases, has yet to be demonstrated. As hormones affect the levels of drug metabolizing enzymes (*231*), they can also modify the action of environmental carcinogenic agents to which the parental gonads may be exposed.

Various "natural" estrogenic substances of plant or microbial origin have been reviewed here. Some are constituents of certain foodstuffs or herbal remedies and others may be present in food as a result of its contamination with secondary metabolites of certain microorganisms, e.g., *Fusaria*. Though these substances vary in their chemical structures, they have certain features in common which endow them with estrogenic and probably with other biological activities. These natural estrogens can add considerably to the estrogenic load of man and livestock and could present carcinogenic hazards. They need to be tested in long-term animal experiments. (Tumor induction by substances with estrogenic activity is reviewed in Chapter 3).

Aflatoxins and Other Secondary Metabolites of Microorganisms

It is remarkable that the carcinogenic hazards posed by metabolites of fungi and other microorganisms have been detected only within the last 15 years, although molds have contaminated foodstuffs probably as long as mankind has been on earth. It required the dramatic losses of more than 100,000 turkey poults in England during 1960 for investigations into the causes of this economic disaster to be initiated. Recognition soon followed that the fatal liver damage seen in these birds was caused by toxic and carcinogenic secondary metabolites of the fungus *Aspergillus flavus* Link ex Fries (named aflatoxins), which contaminated the moldy Brazilian ground nut (peanut) meal included in the turkey feeds (*232, 233*). This episode focused attention on secondary metabolites of various microorganisms which can contaminate inappropriately stored foodstuffs and may present potential health hazards to animals and man. Secondary metabolites of microorganisms have been studied mainly as possible sources of antibiotics and very few have been tested for carcinogenic action (*234*), yet in Japan moldy "yellowed rice" has been suspected since the end of the 19th century as a possible cause of human diseases (*234a*). The disastrous effects of "yellowed rice" imported to Japan after World War II led to the isolation of *Penicillium islandicum* Sopp. and to the recognition that metabolites of this fungus (luteoskyrin and cyclochlorotine (islanditoxin)) (Figure 26) are hepatotoxic and possibly hepatocarcinogenic (*235, 236*).

A disease known as alimentary toxic aleukia (ATA), which caused many fatalities in the Orenburg district of the USSR during World War II, has been traced to the consumption of bread made from "overwintered" grain which had remained in the fields unharvested throughout the winter and had become contaminated with toxic metabolites of *Fusarium poae* and

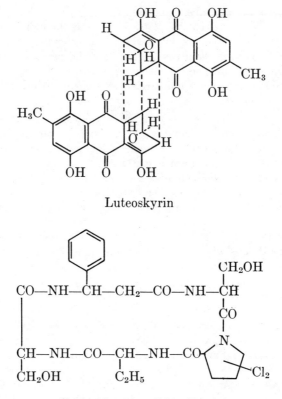

Luteoskyrin

Cyclochlorotine (islanditoxin)

Figure 26. The structures of hepatotoxic secondary metabolites of Penicillium islandicum. *Sopp.*

F. sporotrichioides (*237*). These metabolites may have some bearing on the gastric and esophageal tumors which occur in certain specific areas (*238*). Moldy feedstuffs have also been implicated in various livestock diseases (*239*). The problems related to mycotoxicoses are many; most remain to be solved (*239a*).

Aflatoxins. The finding that aflatoxins are not only effective hepatotoxins but also very potent hepatocarcinogens led to their extensive study, the results of which have been frequently reviewed (*240–245*). A comprehensive treatise on the aflatoxins and certain related compounds published in 1971 contains more than 900 references (*245*). These deal with the occurrence, chemistry, biosynthesis, metabolism, the toxic, mutagenic, carcinogenic, and other biological and biochemical effects of aflatoxins in plants, microorganisms, and various animal species and should be consulted for the earlier references.

The structures of a number of aflatoxins have been established (Table V; Figures 27, 28, 29) (*245–250*), and racemic aflatoxins B₂ (*251*) and

B_1, G_1, and M_1 (*252*) have been totally synthesized. Aflatoxin P has been prepared from natural aflatoxin B_1 by O-demethylation with lithium *t*-butyl-mercaptide in hexamethyl phosphoramide (Figure 27) (*253*). All these aflatoxins are simple derivatives of Af B_1 or of Af G_1 from which they derive in the course of metabolic hydrogenation, oxidation, O-demethylation, etc. Aflatoxin B_1 is biogenetically formed from acetate (*254, 255*), probably via oxidative coupling of a polyhydroxyanthraquinone with acetoacetic acid (*256*). Evidence has showed that biogenetically Af B_1 is a precursor of the other aflatoxins including Af G_1 (*257*).

Metabolites of aflatoxin from fungal cultures or from animal excreta have usually been given arbitrary names with the result that some of the metabolites have multiple designations. For example, the reduction product of Af B_1, aflatoxicol, has also been known as aflatoxin R_0 or aflatoxin F_1 (Figure 28) (*248*).

Systematic names of aflatoxins, such as are used in the Index Guide of the Chemical Abstracts (**71**, 1969), are cumbersome. When the structures of new metabolites become established, they could be related to Af B_1 or Af G_1 (Figure 27) by numbering the external ring positions consecutively starting from the oxygen of the terminal bifuranoid moiety of the parent compound as shown in Table V. Metabolites in which the rings of the parent structures are degraded would not be classified as aflatoxins. Accordingly, parasiticol (known also as aflatoxin B_3 (*258*)), a metabolite of *A. parasiticus* (*247*) which contains a hydroxyethyl group (Figure 28), in place of the

Table V.   Structural Relationships of Various Aflatoxins to Aflatoxin B_1 and Aflatoxin G_1 and Their Toxicities

Compound	Structure in Figure		Toxicity
Aflatoxin B_1	27	Af B_1	$++++$
Aflatoxin M_1	27	4-hydroxy-Af B_1	$++++$
Aflatoxicol (AfRo)	28	7-hydroxy-Af B_1	$++$
Aflatoxin Q	28	9-hydroxy-Af B_1	$++$
Aflatoxin P	27	10-O-demethyl-Af B_1	$++$
Aflatoxin B_2	29	2,3-dihydro-Af B_1	$\pm$
Aflatoxin M_2	29	2,3-dihydro-4-hydroxy-Af B_1	$\pm$
Aflatoxin B_{2a}	29	2-hydroxy-2,3-dihydro-Af B_1	$\pm$
Aflatoxin G_1	27	Af G_1	$+++$
Aflatoxin GM_1	27	4-hydroxy-Af G_1	$+++$
Aflatoxin G_2	29	2,3-dihydro-Af G_1	$\pm$
Aflatoxin G_{2a}	29	2-hydroxy-2,3-dihydro-Af G_1	$\pm$
Aflatoxin M_{2a}	29	2,4-dihydroxy-2,3-dihydro-aflatoxin B_1	?
Aflatoxin GM_{2a}	29	2,4-dihydroxy-2,3-dihydro-aflatoxin G_1	?
—	29	2,3-dihydroxy-2,3-dihydro-aflatoxin B_1	—
—	29	2,3-dichloro-2,3-dihydro-aflatoxin B_1	$++++$

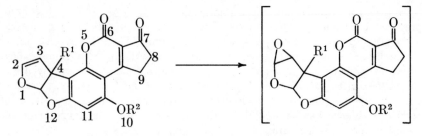

$R^1 = H, R^2 = CH_3$; aflatoxin $B_1 \rightarrow$ 2,3-epoxide of Af B_1

$R^1 = OH, R^2 = CH_3$; aflatoxin $M_1 \rightarrow$ 2,3-epoxide of Af M_1

$R^1 = R^2 = H$; aflatoxin $P_1 \rightarrow$ 2,3-epoxide of Af P_1

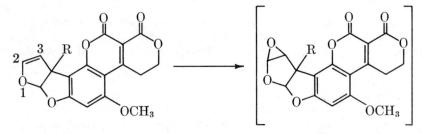

$R = H$; aflatoxin $G_1 \rightarrow$ 2,3-epoxide of Af G_1

$R = OH$; aflatoxin $GM_1 \rightarrow$ 2,3-epoxide of Af GM_1

Figure 27. The structures of aflatoxins and their putative metabolic epoxides

cyclopentenone ring of aflatoxin B_1 or of the terminal lactone ring of aflatoxin G_1, would no longer be considered an aflatoxin.

The intense fluorescence of aflatoxins allows their detection by thin
layer chromatography (TLC) in picogram quantities corresponding to levels
in foodstuffs as low as approximately 2 ppb. They have been detected in
various plant materials, including cereals, fruit, seeds and oils, and in
animal tissues, in milk and its products, etc. (245). High levels of aflatoxin
B_1 (more than 50 ppb) have been reported in pig tissues, even when the
animals did not appear affected (259). In certain samples of bacon and
lard levels as high as 1000–5000 ppb have been found (260). However,
because of the great differences in toxicities between some aflatoxins which
may have very similar fluorescence and TLC behavior, the duckling test
remains the most reliable for assessing the health hazards of foodstuffs
contaminated with aflatoxins.

Experimentally, certain strains of Aspergilli, when grown under optimal
conditions for the production of aflatoxins (at 28°–32°C, 20–33% moisture
content, about pH 5, aerobically) can produce on solid cereals or nuts up
to 100–900 mg/kg; in liquid media the yield of aflatoxins can be up to
200–300 mg/l. It is obvious that in the presence of appropriate strains of
Aspergilli, even wholesome foodstuffs can become toxic and carcinogenic

within a few days when stored under warm and humid conditions (*244, 245*).

No satisfactory method exists to detoxify food contaminated with aflatoxins, which would not interfere with the palatability and/or nutritive value. Practical preventive measures such as storage of foodstuffs in the cold, at lower than 15% moisture content, etc., would be desirable but difficult to achieve, especially in the tropics and subtropics. Dichlorvos (dimethyl-2,2-dichlorovinylphosphate) has been reported to prevent the formation of aflatoxins, even when the growth of the fungus is not affected (*261*).

A number of animal species among fish, birds, and mammals, including primates, have been found to be susceptible to the toxic effects of aflatoxin B_1. The LD_{50} values vary greatly, depending not only on the species and strains of the animals, but also on the age, sex, and diet. Newborn ducklings are among the most susceptible and are used as test animals. The rate of *in vitro* metabolic disappearance of aflatoxin added to microsomal preparations (reinforced with a NADPH generating system) from livers of several animal species correlates only to some extent with their vulnerability (*262*). However, the pattern of aflatoxin metabolism and the relative toxicities of the metabolites formed by a particular animal under particular conditions are also important (*262*).

In view of the small amounts of available individual adequately purified natural aflatoxins, carcinogenic data have been obtained mostly by using con-

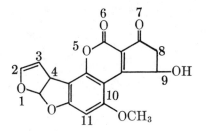

Aflatoxin Q = 9-hydroxy-aflatoxin B_1

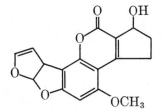

Aflatoxicol ≡ aflatoxin R_o
  ≡ aflatoxin F_1

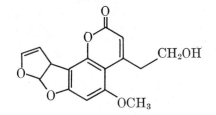

Parasiticol ≡ aflatoxin B_3

Figure 28.   The structures of some hydroxy derivatives of aflatoxins with a 2,3-double bond

taminated diets in which the levels of aflatoxins have been estimated, usually fluorimetrically, after extraction and chromatographic separation. Such data would not include derivatives which are not extractable into organic solvents, or which may undergo decomposition in the course of the extraction and purification processes. The quantitative aspect of biological results obtained in different laboratories, using variably purified preparations of "natural" aflatoxins, can therefore be considered only approximate (compare *263*) Table VI.

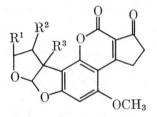

$R^1 = R^2 = R^3 = H$; 2,3-dihydroaflatoxin B_1 (Af B_2)

$R^1 = R^2 = H$; $R^3 = OH$; 2,3-dihydro-4-hydroxy-Af.B_1 (Af M_2)

$R^1 = OH$; $R^2 = R^3 = H$; 2-hydroxy-2,3-dihydro-Af.B_1 (Af B_{2a})

$R^1 = R^3 = OH$, $R^2 = H$; 2,4-dihydroxy-2,3-dihydro-Af.B_1 (Af M_{2a})

$R^1 = R^2 = OH$, $R^3 = H$; 2,3-dihydroxy-2,3-dihydro-Af B_1

$R^1 = R^2 = Cl$, $R^3 = H$; 2,3-dichloro-2,3-dihydro-Af B_1

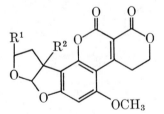

$R^1 = R^2 = H$; 2,3-dihydroaflatoxin G_1 (Af G_2)

$R^1 = OH$, $R^2 = H$; 2-hydroxy-2,3-dihydro-Af.G_1 (Af G_{2a})

$R^1 = R^2 = OH$; 2,4-dihydroxy-2,3-dihydro-AfG_1 (Af GM_{2a})

Figure 29.   The structures of aflatoxins with no 2,3-double bond

Liver tumors have been induced in several animal species, trout (*Salmo gairdnerii*), ducks, rats, guinea pigs, ferrets, sheep (*264*), Sockeye salmon, (*Oncorhynchus nerka*) (*265*), and monkeys (*266, 267*). Although the liver is the organ most frequently affected, tumors have been found occasionally also in other organs, in the rat kidneys (*268*) particularly after aflatoxin G_1 (*269*), in the glandular stomach (*270*), and in the colon (*271*). Sarcomas developed at the site of subcutaneous injections in both mice and rats (*234*). Mice are usually resistant to aflatoxin-induced liver tumors, but when treated early in life, C57BL $\times$ C_3H F_1 hybrid mice developed hepatic tumors (*272*). A high susceptibility of the very young and of the fetus to the carcinogenic action of aflatoxins has been shown also in rats (*273*).

The evidence of human susceptibility to the heaptotoxic or carcinogenic action of aflatoxins is fragmentary and inconclusive. Illness and liver damage have been reported to result from occasional ingestion of foodstuffs contaminated with high levels of aflatoxins (*274, 275, 276*). Correlations have been presented between the levels of aflatoxins found in diets consumed in certain areas of Thailand (*277*) or East Africa (*278, 279*) and the frequency of occurrence in these areas of primary liver cancer. However, liver tumors in these areas may arise from more than one etiological factor; other hepatocarcinogenic fungal metabolites (*e.g.*, sterigmatocystin (*316*), elaiomycin, p. 677) or plant constituents (*see* p. 628) may also be involved. In experimental animals, the pyrrolizidine alkaloids lasiocarpine or monocrotaline act synergistically with aflatoxins (*280, 281*), as did some other hepatotoxins (*282*).

The levels of proteins, fat, lipotropes, vitamin A, and certain other dietary constituents as well as of enzyme inducers, affect the response to aflatoxins (*283–288*). The factors that protect from acute toxicity, *e.g.*, low lipotropes (*286*), increase the carcinogenic response while the inverse is true for protein deficiency, which enhances the toxicity of aflatoxins (*283*). Phenobarbitone appears to protect rats from aflatoxin-induced tumors (*288*), possibly by inducing the enzyme epoxyhydrase.

Purified natural aflatoxins B_1, G_1, and M_1 are carcinogenic, and their relative efficacy in this respect parallels to some extent the order of their respective toxicities. Aflatoxin B_1 is the most active, not only among the aflatoxins, but among hepatocarcinogens in general; it is almost twice as active as Af G_1. The toxicity of Af M_1 (4-hydroxyaflatoxin B_1) almost equals that of Af B_1, as does its carcinogenic potency for the trout (*289*).

Synthetic racemic Af B_1 and Af M_1 are only about half as toxic as the highly purified natural materials, indicating that only one diastereoisomer has biological activity (*290*). The synthetic racemic Af M_1 induced within 100 weeks only one hepatocellular carcinoma among 29 rats given 40 doses (1 mg/kg *in toto*) while the natural Af B_1 in parallel experiments induced such tumors in nine out of nine treated rats given similar dosage (*291*).

There is some uncertainty about the carcinogenic action of Af B_2 (2,3-dihydroaflatoxin B_1). A preparation obtained by hydrogenation of Af B_1 and extensive purification induced liver tumors in four out of nine rats given 40 intraperitoneal doses (150 mg/rat *in toto*) but no sarcomas when given by repeated subcutaneous injections amounting to 12 mg/rat. Under similar conditions Af B_1 induced sarcomas in nine out of nine treated rats with a total dose of 0.4 mg/rat (*292*). Af B_2 may become partly dehydrogenated in the animal body (*292*). The fact that Af B_2 is toxic to the duckling at 1.76 mg/kg but not to the rat (even at 200 mg/kg (*292*)) indicates the need for its detailed metabolic study in the two species.

Hydroxy derivatives of aflatoxins other than Af M_1, which have the C_2–C_3 double bond (Figure 28) are less toxic than the parent compounds, but have not been available in sufficient quantities to be adequately tested for carcinogenic action. This applies also to parasiticol (Figure 28) and to the hydroxy derivatives of aflatoxins which have no C_2–C_3 double bond (Figure 29). Comparative studies of the carcinogenic response in various species would also become possible if sufficient quantities of the individual compounds were available. Certain synthetic compounds, with structures which resemble the coumarin part of aflatoxins but without the bifuranoid moiety, were not carcinogenic for the rat (292) or for the trout (293).

X-ray studies of the crystal structures of Af G_1 (294), B_1, and B_2 (295) showed that the molecules are almost planar, except for the terminal furanoid ring which forms a second plane inclined at an angle of about 110° to the main structure (295). The configuration of the natural aflatoxins has been established (246) (Figure 30).

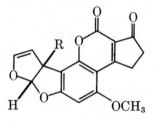

Figure 30. Configuration of the natural aflatoxins (B_1, R = H; M_1, R = OH)

Two features, a reactive C_2–C_3 double bond and an unsaturated lactone ring, appear essential for the induction of tumors by aflatoxins. The very reactive synthetic compound, Af B_1-2,3-dichloride (Figure 29), is, however, a potent carcinogen (306).

Metabolism of Aflatoxins. Aflatoxins, like other foreign substances, are metabolized in the body by more than one pathway and give rise to a number of products, of which only some are likely to be involved in the initiation of the carcinogenic process. The precursors of the active entities would obviously possess carcinogenic potentialities, as do the parent compounds. The ultimate carcinogenic entities are probably bound immediately after formation to cell constituents of the liver and of other organs or become metabolized further, degraded, and eliminated.

Aflatoxin M_1 (4-hydroxyaflatoxin B_1) is a milk and urinary metabolite of Af B_1 in many animal species including man (296). It represents only a small fraction of the administered dose (0.3–3%). Its toxicity and its carcinogenic efficacy resemble but do not exceed, those of Af B_1. Aflatoxin P_1, a phenolic O-demethylation product of Af B_1, represents a major urinary metabolite in the rhesus monkey and accounts for about 20% of the administered dose. It is excreted predominantly in the form of its water-soluble glucuronide and sulfate (249).

The finding that liver microsomal preparations reinforced with a NADPH generating system can metabolize aflatoxin B_1 *in vitro* (297) allowed the identification of several metabolites, many identical with those found in cultures of Aspergilli: Afs M_1, B_{2a}, P_1, F_1, G_{2a}, etc. (262). Their production can vary depending on the animal species from which the liver preparations are derived (*262*, *298*). Monkey liver microsomes produce Af Q (9-hydroxy Af B_1) in 16–52% yield, Af M_1 (1–3% yield) (*250*), and also Af P_1 (*298*). The rate and the pattern of metabolism *in vitro* only partly reflect the susceptibility of the animals to the toxic or carcinogenic effects of aflatoxin, possibly because *in vivo* the transport of aflatoxin into the liver cell and the conjugation and excretion of metabolites formed, can vary depending not only on the species and strain, but also on the nutritional, hormonal, and other specific conditions of the individual animal. Hence studies *in vitro* should proceed parallel with those *in vivo*.

It is of interest that the mouse, which resists the carcinogenic action of aflatoxins, forms little aflatoxin M_1 but produces at least three other, as yet unidentified, fluorescent metabolites which are not formed by the rat (*299*). The biochemical basis for this species differences in response to aflatoxin, especially in regard to liver RNA synthesis, is being investigated (*300*, *301*).

The course of metabolic reactions in the body is determined by integrated interaction of various factors including age, sex, hormonal status, diet, temperature, etc. The very young, although lacking certain enzyme systems, are more susceptible than adults to the carcinogenic action of aflatoxins and also to that of other carcinogens which require metabolic activation. Clearly they must be able to form the relevant carcinogenic entities from Af B_1 and G_1. It has been suggested that epoxides formed on the critical 2,3-double bond of the bifuranoid moiety might represent the active carcinogenic entity (*302*). This view is supported by recent experimental evidence. In tissue culture, Af B_1 usually does not affect rat kidney fibroblasts. However, in the presence of liver cells, a metabolite is formed from Af B_1 which is cytotoxic for the fibroblasts (*303*).

Liver microsomal preparations fortified with a NADPH-generating system activate added aflatoxin B_1 to a derivative which is lethal to microorganisms such as *Salmonella typhimurium* (TA–1530) (*304*). This derivative becomes covalently bound to added nucleic acids and on treatment with acid produces 2,3-dihydro-2,3-dihydroxyaflatoxin B_1 (*305*). The metabolite could not be isolated as such, and so far its identity with 2,3-epoxyaflatoxin B_1 could not be directly established, because its synthesis has not yet been accomplished. The reactive 2,3-dichloride of Af B_1 (Figure 29) proved to be a very effective initiator of skin carcinogenesis and lethal to 58% of mice within six weeks after skin application of 148μg/mouse (*306*).

The 2,3-double bond has exceptional characteristics. It is the shortest bond in the molecule, as x-ray crystallographic data have shown (*295*). More recently, theoretical molecular orbital calculations have indicated that the 2,3-double bond in the aflatoxins and in related bifuranoid fungal metabolites has the highest bond order (*307*) and accordingly would be the most active in addition reactions. Af B_1 and Af G_1 readily add water to the double bond under acid catalysis and form the respective 2-hydroxy-2,3-dihydro derivatives. This bond would be expected to undergo facile epoxidation (*302*). Chemically, two epoxides are possible, one facing the lactone ring, the other facing away from it. Metabolically, however, one epoxide only is likely to be formed, and this might be responsible for the biological action on which depend the mutagenic effects and possibly also the induction of tumors by Af B_1 (*304, 308*).

The mutagenic metabolite formed from Af B_1 in fortified liver microsomal preparations *in vitro* becomes inactivated when 2,3-dimercaptopropanol is added. This indicates its interaction with the vicinal sulfhydryl groups, behavior compatible with an epoxide structure (*308*).

It is now believed that there is a close relationship between the mutagenic and carcinogenic activity. A recent review of the naturally occurring mutagens lists some known "natural" carcinogens (*309*). However, the mutagenic activity is usually detected under conditions which allow metabolic activation of the parent compounds. Appropriate *in vitro* systems have been developed (*309*).

It has to be stressed, however, that various new metabolites of Af B_1 of unknown structures have been occasionally reported, some of which were toxic (*310*), but the chromatographic characteristics of the compounds were not compatible with an epoxide structure. The nature of the metabolites involved in the induction of tumors by aflatoxins still needs clarification.

From cultures of *A. flavus*, new derivatives have been isolated (Af M_{2a} and Af GM_{2a}) which appear to be the 2,4-dihydroxy-2,3-dihydroaflatoxins B_1 and G_1, respectively (Figure 29) (*311*). The substitution positions in these aflatoxin derivatives have been assigned by analogy with dothistromin, a metabolite of *Dothistroma pini* (*312*) isomeric with 2,4-dihydroxyversicolorin B (Figure 31) (*326*). The biological activities of these compounds have not yet been reported, but they are not likely to be carcinogenic.

The recognition that aflatoxins require metabolic activation for their biological effects is relatively new. Reinterpretation of some of the previous biochemical data will therefore be necessary, especially of those obtained *in vitro*.

Sterigmatocystin and Other Bifuranoid Compounds. Sterig-matocystin (St) (Figure 32), a secondary metabolite of *Aspergillus versicolor* (Vuillemin) Tiraboshi, like the aflatoxins, contains a bifuranoid moiety, which is attached to a xanthone instead of a coumarin moiety. Its

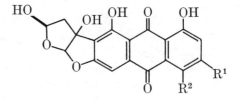

$R^1 = H, R^2 = OH$; dothistromin
$R^1 = OH, R^2 = H$; 2,4-dihydroxyversicolorin B

Figure 31.   The structures of dothistromin and of 2,4-dihydroxyversicolorin B

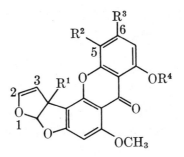

R^1 = R^2 = R^3 = R^4 = H; sterigmatocystin (St)
R^1 = R^2 = R^3 = H; R^4 = CH$_3$; *O*-methyl-St
R^1 = R^3 = R^4 = H; R^2 = OCH$_3$; 5-methoxy-St
R^1 = R^2 = R^4 = H; R^3 = OCH$_3$; 6-methoxy-St
R^1 = OH, R^2 = R^3 = H; R^4 = CH$_3$; aspertoxin
   = 4-hydroxy-*O*-methyl-St.

Figure 32. Sterigmatocystin and its congeners

structure was established before that of the aflatoxins (*313*). It is produced
by several Aspergillus species, by *Penicillium luteum,* and by some other
fungi that contaminate cereals, sometimes in considerable quantity (up to
0.1%) (*314*). Thus it can present health hazards even though its toxicity
and carcinogenic efficacy are much lower than those of aflatoxin B$_1$ or G$_1$
(*315, 316*). In rats sterigmatocystin induced sarcomas and liver tumors on
repeated subcutaneous injections (*315*), liver tumors by the oral route
(*316*), and skin tumors on repeated applications to the skin (*317*). It has
induced a hepatoma also in a vervet monkey (*318*). In the monkey more
than 50% of the administered dose of sterigmatocystin (14 mg/kg b.wt.)
was excreted in the form of a glucuronide conjugate (*319*).

O-Methylsterigmatocystin (*320*) and aspertoxin (4-hydroxy-*O*-methyl-
sterigmatocystin) (Figure 32) have been isolated from cultures of *A. flavus*
which produced aflatoxins (*321*). A total synthesis of *O*-methylsterigmato-
cystin has been reported (*322*). 5-Methoxysterigmatocystin (Figure 32)
has been isolated as a secondary metabolite of *A. versicolor* (*323*). Other
metabolites isolated from a variant strain of *A. versicolor* (versicolorin A
and B, and aversin) (Figure 33), also contain a difuranoid moiety, which is
attached to anthraquinone structures (*324, 325, 326*).

Data on carcinogenic activity, if any, of the various derivatives of
sterigmatocystin and related bifuranoid compounds have not yet been
reported. In a microsomal activation assay, *in vitro,* compounds having the
2,3-double bond at the end of the bifuranoid moiety were lethal to *E. coli*
(AB 2480), but 10–150 times less effective than Af B$_1$. Versicolorin B and
Af B$_2$ (in which the 2,3-double bond is saturated) were not active (*308*).

Griseofulvin. Griseofulvin (Figure 34), 7-chloro-4,6-dimethoxycou-
maran-3-one-2-spiro-1′-(2′-methoxy-6′-methylcyclohex-2′-en-4′-one), is a me-

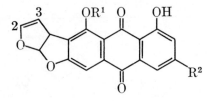

$R^1 = H$, $R^2 = OH$; versicolorin A
$R^1 = H$, $R^2 = OH$, $\Delta^{2,3}$ absent; versicolorin B
$R^1 = R^2 = H$; deoxyversicolorin A
$R^1 = CH_3$, $R^2 = H$, $\Delta^{2,3}$ absent; aversin

Figure 33. Versicolorin and its congeners

tabolite of *Penicillium griseofulvum* Dierck (*327*), a mutant of *P. patulum* and of certain other *Penicillium* species (*328*); its structure has been established by Grove *et al.* (*329*). Griseofulvin is an effective and specific antifungal agent used for the control of ringworm, *Tinea capitis*, in children (*330*) and also in veterinary medicine (*331*). The treatment may require prolonged administration (*332*). Given to mice in the diet (1%), griseofulvin inhibits their growth, causes hepatic porphyria and liver damage, and male mice develop liver tumors (*333, 334*). When given subcutaneously to infant Swiss white mice, griseofulvin induces hepatomas in the males with four doses not exceeding 3.0 mg, corresponding to about 200 mg/kg total (*335*). Griseofulvin arrests mitotic division of plants and animal cells, including those of transplanted Walker carcinoma and lymphosarcoma (*336*). It can act as a co-carcinogen in skin carcinogenesis by 3-methylcholanthrene (*337*).

Griseofulvin undergoes 4-, 6-, and 2′-*O*-demethylation by various fungi (*338*); the resulting metabolites are no more active. Two additional polar products, the 5′-hydroxy and the 6′-hydroxymethyl derivatives of griseofulvin are formed by the fungus *Cephalosporium curtipes* (*339*).

In mammals, including man, dog, rabbit, rat, and mouse, the main metabolite of griseofulvin is the 6-desmethylgriseofulvin (*340, 341, 34 343, 344*). The liver of the mouse and of the rat demethylates also   4-methoxy group, and conjugates the resulting phenol with glucuronic   d *in vivo* and *in vitro* (*342, 343, 344*). Using radioactive ^{14}C-griseof· .n,

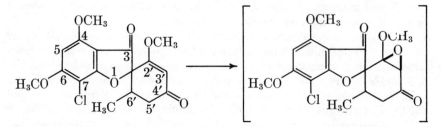

Figure 34. Griseofulvin and its putative metabolic epoxide

$$CH_2—S—C_2H_5$$
$$CH_2$$
$$CH—NH_2$$
$$COOH$$

$$CH_2—S—CH_3$$
$$CH_2$$
$$CH—NH_2$$
$$COOH$$

Figure 35. The structures of ethionine (left) and of methionine (right)

traces of 4-desmethylgriseofulvin and of several unidentified minor metabolites have also been detected in human urine (*345*). The rabbit can split the molecule of griseofulvin, and excretes 3-chloro-4,6-dimethoxysalicyclic acid in the urine (*346*). The carcinogenic action of griseofulvin is likely to be mediated by its putative epoxide (Figure 34).

Ethionine. Ethionine, L-*S*-ethylhomocysteine, the toxic analog of the amino acid methionine (Figure 35), is produced by *Escherichia coli* and by various other microorganisms (*347*). Its hepatotoxic and hepatocarcinogenic actions in the rat have been much studied and have been well reviewed by Farber (*348*). The optimal induction of liver tumors requires continuous feeding of synthetic DL-ethionine (0.25 % in diet) for about five months. Ethionine forms *S*-adenosylethionine and acts as a methionine antagonist. DL-Methionine at 0.6–0.8 % in the diet fed simultaneously with ethionine prevents the development of liver tumors. Though ethionine causes acute degenerative lesions in the pancreatic acini and prevents alloxan diabetes, no pancreatic tumors have been reported.

Daunomycin (Figure 36), a secondary metabolite of *Streptomyces peucetius*, has been used for the treatment of leukemia and as an antitumor agent. It is nephrotoxic and can induce in rats tumors of the kidneys and

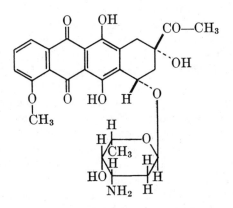

Figure 36.   The structure of daunomycin

of the sex organs with a single intravenous dose, 5–10 mg/kg body weight (*349*).

Actinomycins, the polypeptide secondary metabolites of Actinomycetales, can also induce tumors. Actinomycin D (Figure 37) already synthesized (*350*), inhibits nucleic acid synthesis and has been used clinically as antitumor agent. When given to rats by intraperitoneal injections, doses as low as 0.8 mg/rat induced mesotheliomas (*351*). Actinomycins A, L, and S induced sarcomas in mice by repeated subcutaneous injections (quoted in *240*).

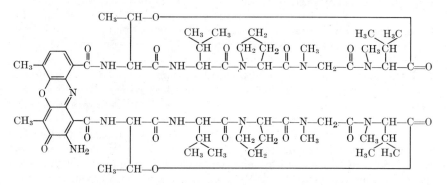

Figure 37.   The structure of actinomycin D (synthetic)

Streptozotocin. This 2-desoxy-D-glucose derivative of *N*-methyl-*N*-nitrosourea (Figure 38), is a secondary metabolite of *Streptomyces achromogenes* var. 128. It was isolated in the laboratories of the Upjohn Co. where its structure was established (*352*). It has antibiotic (*253, 254*), diabetogenic (*355, 356*), mutagenic (*357, 358*), antitumor (*359, 360, 361*), and carcinogenic (*362–367*) activity. A single dose of streptozotocin (50–65 mg/kg) induces in the rat tumors of the kidneys (*362, 366*), the liver (*364*), and the pancreatic islet cells (*367*). Liver tumors also have been reported in Chinese hamsters (*Cricetus griseus*) given streptozotocin (100 mg/kg) in a single intraperitoneal dose or in four divided doses (*365*). The action of streptozotocin probably arises from the release of *N*-methyl-*N*-nitrosourea in the liver. Hence, it can affect organs such as the liver and pancreas in which the latter compound does not usually induce tumors. Streptozotocin differs from *N*-methyl-*N*-nitrosourea in its action on microorganisms (*368*). Both compounds lower the concentration of NAD in mouse pancreatic islets, but the damage to the cells is more severe with streptozotocin (*369*).

Streptozotocin damages preferentially the pancreatic islet β-cells (*370*) and is diabetogenic for several animal species—the rat, mouse, hamster, guinea pig, and monkey (*356*). It has been recommended for the treatment of tumors (*359*), particularly those of the pancreatic islet cells (insulinomas) (*360*) and of metastatic carcinoid tumors (*365*).

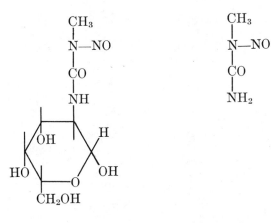

Figure 38. Structures of streptozotocin (left) and N-methyl-N-nitrosourea (right)

Streptozotocin depresses the levels of pyridine nucleotides (NAD and NADH) in the mouse liver and pancreas but this can be prevented by pretreatment with nicotinamide (*371, 372, 373*). Nicotinamide (but not nicotinic acid) modifies the diabetogenic action of streptozotocin without lessening its antitumor activity (*371*). The diabetogenic action of streptozotocin appears to be related to the decrease of pyridine nucleotides in the pancreatic β-cells. Studies of isolated mouse pancreatic islets, treated with streptozotocin *in vitro,* demonstrated reduced uptake of precursors and decreased synthesis of NAD (*373*). Pretreatment of rats with nicotinamide 10 min before giving streptozotocin inhibits the induction of kidney tumors and greatly increases the incidence of pancreatic islet cell tumors, from 4 up to 64% (*367*). Although nicotinamide protects the pancreatic islet β-cells from the acute cytotoxic and necrogenic affects of streptozotocin and prevents diabetes (*370, 374, 375*) it does not prevent the induction of islet cell tumors, but rather increases their yield (*367*).

Elaiomycin. Elaiomycin, 4-methoxy-3-(1-octenyl-*N-O-N*-azoxy)-2-butanol (Figure 39), is a metabolite of a soil organism, *Streptomyces hepaticus,* which has been isolated and its structure determined in the laboratories of Parke, Davis and Co. (*374, 375, 376*). Elaiomycin has been isolated also

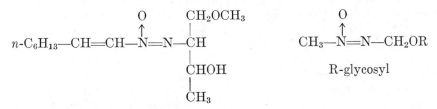

Figure 39. Structures of elaiomycin (left) and cycasin (right)

Table VI.   Carcinogenic Activity of Certain

Compound	Structure in Figure	Parent Microorganisms
Aflatoxin B_1	27	*A. flavus* and *A. parasiticus*
Aflatoxin G_1	27	*A. flavus* and *A. parasiticus*
Aflatoxin M_1	27	*A. flavus* and *A. parasiticus*
Sterigmatocystin	32	*A. versicolor*
Griseofulvin	34	*P. griseofulvum*
Luteoskyrin	26	*P. islandicum*
Streptozotocin	38	*Streptomyces achromogens*
Elaiomycin	39	*Streptomyces hepaticus*
Actinomycin D	37	*Streptomyces*
Actinomycin A	—	*Streptomyces*
Actinomycin S	—	*Streptomyces*
Actinomyces L	—	*Streptomyces*
Ethionine	35	*E. coli, Ps. aeruginosa*, and others
Patulin	19	*P. patulum* and other *penicilli* and *aspergilli*

ᵃ The total "effective" dose for tumor induction is: $++++$, less than 10 mg/kg body weight; $+++$, between 10–100 mg/kg body weight; $++$, between 100–1000

from a Japanese species of *Streptomyces*, No. 1252 (*377*). Although tuber-culostatic *in vitro*, elaiomycin proved devoid of therapeutic action when tested *in vivo* and caused liver damage in mice and guinea pigs (*374, 375*). In young rats, doses of elaiomycin exceeding 40 mg/kg caused death within a few days from acute lesions of the liver, lung, kidney, and stomach. Among rats which survived longer than 1.5 years after single or divided smaller doses, tumors developed in various organs, including the liver, kidneys, stomach, thymus, and brain (*378, 379, 380*). Elaiomycin thus resembles cycasin (Figure 39) not only chemically but also in its carcinogenic action.

Conclusions. "Natural" carcinogens occur in the environment of animals and man as constituents of plants or as metabolites of microor-ganisms. They may be inadvertently ingested in food or in medicines or otherwise enter the body. Some may not be detectable by smell or taste and may have no immediately recognizable ill effects on health, although they initiate an irreversible process which may lead to chronic disease or cancer. In the course of a lifetime, man and beast are likely to be exposed to more than one carcinogenic hazard which may act additively or synergistically. It is essential to reduce exposures to any known carcinogens that could be avoided; even a single exposure may, in some cases, tip the balance.

The presence of carcinogens in the natural environment has been recognized only in the last quarter of a century. It is likely that many more will be discovered in the future among natural products which hitherto have not been suspected of carcinogenic potentialities. "Natural" carcinogens already known can induce tumors in many organs of animals which are similar to cancers encountered in man. The type of tumor induced depends on the carcinogen, its route of entry, the dosage and duration of exposure,

Secondary Metabolites of Microorganisms

Carcinogenic Activity[a]	Tumors Induced	
	Species	Tissues
++++	many species incl. monkey	liver, kidney, s.c. sarcoma, etc.
++++	rat, duck	liver, kidney
+++	trout, rat	liver
++	rat, monkey	liver, skin, s.c. sarcoma
++	mouse	liver
++	mouse	liver
+++	rat	kidney, liver, etc.
+++	rat	kidney, liver, etc.
++++	rat	i.p. mesothelioma
+++++	mouse	s.c. sarcoma
+++++	mouse	s.c. sarcoma
+++	mouse	s.c. sarcoma
+	rat	liver
+++	rat	s.c. sarcoma

mg/kg body weight; +, higher than 1000 mg/kg body weight.

and also on the age, sex, and metabolic "fitness" of the individual. The earlier in the biological existence the exposure to carcinogens occurs, the greater is the hazard.

Although the natural carcinogens have chemical structures of many different types, they possess certain features in common—a reactive carbonyl group and an ethylenic double bond in close proximity, which in the course of metabolic oxidation in the body (*e.g.*, epoxidation) are transformed into polyfunctional intermediates. These may then interact in a concerted manner with several reactive groups of chromatin which become exposed momentarily in the course of the mitotic cycle. The carcinogenic residues, by forming a stable "bridge" between constituents of chromatin, may bring about permanent changes in some chromosomes which eventually lead to neoplasia.

Acknowledgment

I thank N. Brewster for excellent and devoted secretarial help.

Literature Cited

1. Clifford, P., Linsell, C. A., "Cancer in Africa," *East Afr. Med. J.* (1968).
2. Abd Al-Rahman, Ismail, "Folk Medicine in Modern Egypt," 1934.
3. Arbelaez, E. P., "Plantas Utiles de Colombia," *Imprenta Nacional.* (1936).
4. Biegeleisen, H., "Lecznictwo ludu polskiego," *Polska Akad. Umiejetnosci* (1929).
5. Brooker, S. G., Cooper, R. C., "New Zealand Medicinal Plants," University Press, 1961.
6. Chopra, R. N., "Indian Flora and Its Toxic and Medicinal Preparation," 1940.

7. "Culpeper's Complete Herbal," C. F. Lloyd, Ed., Herbert Joseph Ltd., London, 1947.
8. Dalziel, J. M., "The Useful Plants of West Tropical Africa," Crown Agents, London, 1937.
9. Dragendorff, G., "Die Heilpflanzen der verschiedenen Völker und Zeiten," Stuttgart, 1898.
10. Dymock, W., "Pharmacographia Indica," 1899, reprinted by Hamdard, Jonsa Institute Health and Tibbi (Med.) Research, Pakistan, 1972.
11. "Dioscorides Greek Herbal," R. T. Gunter, Ed., Oxford University, London, 1934.
12. Forsyth, A. A., "British Poisonous Plants," H.M. Stationery Office, London, 1954.
13. Forgacs, J., Carll, W. T., Adv. Vet. Sci. (1962) 7, 273.
14. Gan, Woei-Song, "Manual of Medicinal Plants in Taiwan," National Research Institute of Chinese Medicine, 1960.
15. Gerarde, J., "The Herball or Generall Histori of Plants," London, 1597.
16. Gimlette, J. D., Burkill, I. H., "The Medical Book of Malayan Medicine," The Gardens Bull., Straits Settlements (1930) 6, No. 11-15.
17. Hooper, D., "Useful Plants and Drugs of Iran and Iraq," Chicago, 1937.
18. Kingsbury, J. M., "The Poisonous Plants of the United States and Canada," Prentice-Hall, Inc., Englewood Cliffs, 1964.
19. Kirtikar, K. R., Basu, B. D., An, I. C. S., "Indian Medicinal Plants," 2nd ed., Allahabad, 1936.
20. Lemordant, D., "Les Plantes Ethiopiennes," Addis Ababa, 1960.
21. Long, H. C., "Plants Poisonous to Live Stock," Cambridge Agr. Monogr. 1924.
22. Martinez, M., "Las plantas medicinales de Mexico," 3rd ed., Ediciones Boras, Mexico, D.F., 1944 and 1959.
23. Murillo, A., "Plantes medicinales du Chile," Paris, 1889.
24. Read, B. E., "Chinese Medicinal Plants," Peking Nat. Hist. Bull. (1936).
25. Verdcourt, B., Trump, E. C., "Common poisonous plants of East Africa," Collins, London, 1969.
26. Watt, M. J., Breyer-Brandwijk, M. G., "The Medicinal and Poisonous Plants of Southern and Eastern Africa," Livingstone, Edinburgh, 1962.
27. Weck, W., "Heilkunde und Volkstum auf Bali," F. Enke Verlag, Stuttgart, 1937.
28. de Wildeman, E., Bull. Séances, Inst. Roy. Colonial Belge (1946) 17, 317.
29. Everist, S. L., "Poisonous Plants of Australia," in press.
30. Morton, J. F., Cancer Res. (1968) 28, 2268.
31. Rose, E. F., South African Med. J. (1972) 46, 1039.
32. Warren, F. L., Prog. Chem. Org. Nat. Prod. (1955) 12, 198.
33. Ibid. (1966) 24, 330.
34. Warren, F. L., "The Alkaloids," R. H. F. Manske, Ed., 12, p. 245, Academic, New York, 1970.
35. Bull, L. B., Culvenor, C. C. J., Dick, A. T., "The Pyrrolizidine Alkaloids. Their Chemistry, Pathogenicity and other Biological Properties," North Holland, Amsterdam, 1968.
36. McLean, E. K., Pharmacol. Rev. (1970) 22, 429.
37. Schoental, R., Cancer Res. (1968) 28, 2237.
38. Schoental, R., Israel J. Med. Sci. (1968) 4, 1133.
39. Kay, J. M., Heath, D., "Crotalaria Spectabilis. The Pulmonary Hypertension Plant," in "Lectures in Living Chemistry," C. Thomas, Springfield, Ill., 1970.
40. Schoental, R., Voeding (1955) 16, 268.
41. Schoental, R., J. Trop. Pediatr. (1957) 2, 208.
42. Bras, G., Jelliffe, D. B., Stewart, K. L., Arch. Pathol. (1954) 57, 285.
43. Berman, C., "Primary Carcinoma of the Liver," Adv. Cancer Res. (1958) 5, 55.

44. Schoental, R., "Potential carcinogenic hazards from drugs," *U.I.C.C. Monogr. Ser.* (1967) **7**, 152.
45. Culvenor, C. C. J., Crout, D. H. G., Klyne, W., Mose, W. P., Renwick, J. D., Scopes, P. M., *J. Chem. Soc. (C)* (1971) 3653.
46. Cook, J. W., Duffy, E., Schoental, R., *Br. J. Cancer* (1950) **4**, 405.
47. Schoental, R., Head, M. A., Peacock, P. R., *Br. J. Cancer* (1954) **8**, 458.
48. Schoental, R., Head, M. A., *Br. J. Cancer* (1955) **9**, 229.
49. *Ibid.* (1957) **11**, 535.
50. Schoental, R., Bensted, J. P. M., *Br. J. Cancer* (1963) **17**, 242.
51. Schoental, R., Fowler, M. E., Coady, A., *Cancer Res.* (1970) **30**, 2127.
52. Harris, P. N., Chen, K. K., *Cancer Res.* (1970) **30**, 2881.
53. Williams, A. O., Schoental, R., *Trop. Geogr. Med.* (1970) **22**, 201.
54. Svoboda, D. J., Reddy, J. K., *Cancer Res.* (1972) **32**, 908.
55. Schoental, R., Cavanagh, J. B., *J. Natl. Cancer Inst.* (1972) **49**, 665.
56. Newberne, P. M., Rogers, A. E., *Plant Foods for Man* (1973) **1**, 23.
56a. Allen, J. R., Hsu, I. C., Carstens, L. A., *Cancer Res.* (1975) **35**, 997.
57. Reddy, J. K., Svoboda, D. J., *Arch. Pathol.* (1972) **93**, 55.
58. Schoental, R., Hard, G. C., Gibbard, S., *J. Natl. Cancer Inst.* (1971) **47**, 1037.
58a. Schoental, R., *Cancer Res.* (1975) **35**, 2020.
59. Schoental, R., Magee, P. N., *J. Pathol. Bacteriol.* (1957) **74**, 305.
60. *Ibid.* (1959) **78**, 471.
61. Schoental, R., *Oncology* (1970) **5**, 203.
62. McKenzie, J. S., *Aust. J. Exp. Biol. Med. Sci.* (1958) **36**, 11.
63. Pomeroy, A. R., Raper, C., *Br. J. Pharmacol.* (1971) **41**, 683.
64. Khylstov, V. G., *Klin. Med. (Moskow)* (1966) **44**, 85.
65. Theiler, A., 7th and 8th Report, Dir. Vet. Res., p. 58, S. Africa, 1920.
66. Gardiner, M. R., Royce, R., Bokor, A., *J. Pathol. Bacteriol.* (1965) **98**, 43.
67. Bras, G., McLean, E., *Ann. N.Y. Acad. Sci.* (1963) **111**, 392.
68. Culvenor, C. C. J., O'Donovan, G. M., Smith, L. W., *Aust. J. Chem.* (1967) **20**, 757.
69. Sawhney, R. S., Atal, C. K., *J. Indian Chem. Soc.* (1970) **47**, 741.
70. Brooks, S. E. H., Miller, C. G., McKenzie, K., Audretsch, J. J., Bras, G., *Arch. Pathol.* (1970) **89**, 507.
71. Allen, J. R., Carstens, L. A., Norback, D. H., Loh, P. M., *Cancer Res.* (1970) **30**, 1857.
72. Chesney, C. F., Allen, J. R., *Cardiovasc. Res.* (1973) **7**, 508.
73. Martin, P. A., Thorburn, M. J., Hutchinson, S., Bras, G., Miller, C. G., *Br. J. Exp. Path.* (1972) **53**, 374.
74. Cook, L. M., Holt, A. C. E., *J. Genetics* (1966) **59**, 273.
75. Persaud, T. V. N., Hoyte, D. A. N., *Exp. Pathol.* (1974) **9**, 59.
76. Van der Watt, J. J., Purchase, I. F. H., Tustin, R. C., *J. Pathol.* (1972) **107**, 279.
77. Mattocks, A. R., *Nature* (1968) **217**, 723.
78. Culvenor, C. C. J., Downing, D. T., Edgar, J. A., Jago, M. V., *Ann. New York Acad. Sci.* (1969) **163**, 837.
79. Jago, M. V., Edgar, J. A., Smith, L. W., Culvenor, C. C. J., *Molec. Pharmacol.* (1970) **6**, 402.
80. Mattocks, A. R., White, I. N. H., *Chem.-Biol. Interact.* (1971) **3**, 383.
81. Butler, W. H., Mattocks, A. R., Barnes, J. M., *J. Pathol.* (1970) **100**, 169.
82. Hooson, J., Grasso, P., Mattocks, A. R., *J. Pathol.* (1973) **110**, 8.
83. Schoental, R., *Biochem. Soc. Trans.* (1975) **3**, 292.
83a. Schoental, R., *FEBS Lett.* (1976) **61**, 111.
84. Culvenor, C. C. J., Edgar, J. A., Smith, L. W., Tweeddale, H. J., *Aust. J. Chem.* (1970) **23**, 1853.
85. *Ibid.*, 1869.

86. Barnes, J. M., Magee, P. N., Schoental, R., *J. Pathol. Bacteriol.* (1964) **88**, 521.
87. Culvenor, C. C. J., O'Donovan, G. M., Sawhney, R. S., Smith, L. W., *Aust. J. Chem.* (1970) **23**, 347.
88. Fridrichsons, J., Mathieson, A. McL., Sutor, D. J., *Acta Crystallogr.* (1963) **16**, 1075.
89. Sussman, J. L., Wodak, S. J., *Acta Crystallogr. B.* (1973) **29**, 2918.
89a. Wodak, S. J., *Acta Crystallogr. Sect. B.* (1975) **31**, 569.
90. Oesch, F., *Xenobiotica* (1972) **3**, 305.
91. Svoboda, D., Racela, A., Higginson, J., *Biochem. Pharmacol.* (1967) **16**, 651.
92. Oehlert, W., *Cell Tissue Kinet.* (1973) **6**, 325.
93. Pullinger, B. D., *J. Pathol. Bacteriol.* (1940) **50**, 463.
94. Toledo, J. D., *Beitr. Pathol. Anat.* (1965) **131**, 63.
95. Afzelius, B. A., Schoental, R., *J. Ultrastruct. Res.* (1967) **20**, 328.
96. Harington, J. S., *Adv. Cancer Res.* (1967) **10**, 247.
97. White, I. N. H., Mattocks, A. R., *Biochem. J.* (1972) **128**, 291.
98. Schoental, R., "Abstracts, XI Intern. Cancer Congress, Florence," (1974) **2**, 55.
99. Huberman, J. A., *Ann. Rev. Biochem.* (1973) **42**, 355.
100. Schoental, R., *Ann. Rev. Pharmacol.* (1974) **14**, 185.
101. Baserga, R., *Cell Cycle Cancer* (1971) **1**, 57.
102. Mittelman, F., Mark, J., Levan, G., Levan, A., *Science* (1972) **176**, 1340.
103. Rowley, J. D., *J. Natl. Cancer Inst.* (1974) **52**, 315.
104. Schoental, R., *Br. J. Cancer* (1973) **28**, 436.
105. Fahmy, O. G., Fahmy, M. J., *Cancer Res.* (1975) **35**, 3780.
106. Guenter, E., "Essential Oils," van Nostrand, New York, 1952.
107. Shulgin, A. T., *Nature* (1966) **210**, 380.
108. Farnworth, N. R., *Science* (1968) **162**, 1086.
109. Homburger, F., Boger, E., *Cancer Res.* (1968) **28**, 2372.
110. Long, E. L., Nelson, A. A., Fitzhugh, O. G., Hansen, W. H., *Arch. Pathol.* (1963) **75**, 595.
111. Long, E. L., Jenner, P. M., *Fed. Proc.* (1963) **22**, 275.
112. Epstein, S. S., Fujii, K., Andrea, J., Mantel, N., *Toxicol. Appl. Pharmacol.* (1970) **16**, 321.
113. Borchert, P., Wislocki, P. G., Miller, J. A., Miller, E. C., *Cancer Res.* (1973) **33**, 575.
114. Borchert, P., Miller, J. A., Miller, E. C., Shires, T. K., *Cancer Res.* (1973) **33**, 590.
115. Solheim, E., Scheline, R. R., *Xenobiotica* (1973) **3**, 493.
116. Oswald, E. O., Fishbein, L., Corbett, B. J., Walker, M. P., *Biochem. Biophys. Acta* (1971) **230**, 237.
117. *Ibid.* (1971) **244**, 322.
118. Oswald, E. O., Fishbein, L., Corbett, B. J., Walker, M. P., *J. Chromatogr.* (1972) **73**, 43.
119. Schoental, R., Gibbard, S., *Br. J. Cancer* (1972) **26**, 504.
120. Schoental, R., *Cancer Res.* (1970) **30**, 252.
121. Shanmugaratnam, K., *Int. Rev. Exp. Pathol.* (1971) **10**, 361.
122. Acheson, E. D., Cowdell, R. H., Hadfield, E., Macbeth, R. G., *Br. Med. J.* (1968) **2**, 587.
123. Adenis, L., Vankemmel, B., Egret, G., Demaille, A., *Arch. Mal. Prof.* (1973) **34**, 644.
124. Pearl, I. A., "The Chemistry of Lignin," Marcel Dekker, Inc., New York, 1967.
125. Gibbard, S., Schoental, R., *J. Chromatogr.* (1969) **44**, 396.
126. Schoental, R., *Nature* (1958) **182**, 719.
127. Hearon, W. M., MacGregor, W. S., *Chem. Rev.* (1955) **55**, 957.

128. Hartwell, J. L., Johnson, J. M., Fitzgerald, D. B., Belkin, M., *J. Am. Chem. Soc.* (1953) **75**, 235.
129. Kelly, M. G., Hartwell, J. L., *J. Natl. Cancer Inst.* (1954) **14**, 967.
130. Stähelin, H., *Planta Med.* (1972) **21**, 336.
131. Kaminetzky, H. A., McGrew, E. A., *Arch. Pathol.* (1962) **73**, 481.
132. O'Gara, R. W., *Cancer Res.* (1968) **28**, 2272.
133. Sabine, J. R., Horton, B. J., Wicks, M. B., *J. Natl. Cancer Inst.* (1973) **50**, 1237.
134. Petcher, T. J., Weber, H. P., Kuhn, M., von Wartburg, A., *J. Chem. Soc., Perkin Trans. 2* (1973) 288.
135. Corner, J. J., Harborne, J. B., Humphries, S. G., Ollis, W. D., *Phytochemistry* (1962) **1**, 73.
136. Dean, F. M., "Naturally occurring oxygen ring compounds," p. 176, Butterworth, London, 1963.
137. Campbell, R. V. M., Tannock, J., *J. Chem. Soc., Perkin Trans. 1* (1973) 2222.
138. Wattenberg, L. W., Page, M. A., Leong, J. L., *Cancer Res.* (1968) **28**, 934.
139. Parke, D. V., Rahman, H., *Biochem. J.* (1970) **119**, 53P.
140. Wattenberg, L. W., Leong, J. L., *Cancer Res.* (1970) **30**, 1922.
141. Roe, F. J. C., Field, W. E. H., *Food Cosmet. Toxicol.* (1965) **3**, 311.
142. Stanley, W. L., Jurd, L., *J. Agr. Food Chem.* (1971) **19**, 1106.
143. Griepentrog, T., *Toxicology* (1973) **1**, 93.
144. Scheel, L. D., "The Biological Action of the Coumarins," in *Microb. Toxins* (1972) **8**, 47.
145. Hakim, R. E., Griffin, A. C., Knox, J. M., *Arch. Dermatol.* (1960) **82**, 572.
146. Griffiths, L. A., Smith, G. E., *Biochem. J.* (1972) **130**, 141.
147. Reti, L., *Alkaloids* (1954) **4**, 7.
148. Schlittler, E., "The Alkaloids," R. H. F. Manske, Ed., **8**, p. 287, Academic, New York, 1965.
149. Kalbhen, D. A., *Angew. Chem. Int. Ed.* (1971) **10**, 370.
150. Schoental, R., *Lancet* (1974) **ii**, 1571.
150a. *Ibid* (1975) **i**, 858.
151. Korpassy, B., *Progr. Tumor Res.* (1961) **2**, 245.
152. Morton, J. F., *Econ. Bot.* (1970) **24**, 217.
153. Li Kuang-Heng, Kao Jen Ch'uan, Wu Ying K'ai *Chin. Med. J.* (1962) **81**, 489.
154. Doll, R., *Br. J. Cancer* (1969) **23**, 1.
155. Kmet, J., Mahboubi, E., *Science* (1972) **175**, 846.
156. Pirie, H. M., *Res. Vet. Sci.* (1973) **15**, 135.
157. Plowright, W., Linsell, C. A., Peers, F. G., *Br. J. Cancer* (1971) **25**, 72.
158. Schütte, K. H., *J. Natl. Cancer Inst.* (1968) **41**, 821.
159. Bamburg, J. R., Strong, F. M., *Microb. Toxins* (1971) **7**, 207.
160. Gjertsen, P., Trolle, B., Andersen, K., *Eur. Brewing Conv. Proc. Congr.* (1965) 428.
161. Burrell, R. J. W., *J. Natl. Cancer Inst.* (1962) **28**, 495.
162. Magee, P. N., Barnes, J. M., *Adv. Cancer Res.* (1967) **10**, 163.
163. Ivankovic, S., Zeller, W. J., Schmähl, D., *Naturwissenschaften* (1972) **59**, 369.
164. Dickens, F., "Potential Carcinogenic Hazards from Drugs," R. Truhaut, Ed., *UICC Monogr. Ser.* (1967) **7**, 144.
165. Ciegler, A., Detroy, R. W., Lillehoj, E. B., *Microb. Toxins* (1971) **6**, 409.
166. Ludford, R. J., *J. R. Microsc. Soc.* (1953) **73**, 1.
167. Roe, F. J. C., Salaman, M. H., *Br. J. Cancer* (1955) **9**, 177.
168. Hakim, S. A. E., *Indian J. Cancer* (1968) **5**, 183.
169. Hakim, S. A. E., Mijovic, V., Walker, J., *Nature* (1961) **189**, 201.
170. Whiting, M. G., *Econ. Bot.* (1963) **17**, 269.
171. Laqueur, G. L., Spatz, M., *Cancer Res.* (1968) **28**, 2262.
172. Berenblum, I., *Br. Med. Bull.* (1947) **4**, 343.

173. Salaman, M. H., Roe, F. J. C., *Br. Med. Bull.* (1964) **20,** 139.
174. Hecker, E., *Cancer Res.* (1968) **28,** 2338.
175. Furstenberger, G., Hecker, E., *Planta. Med.* (1972) **22,** 241.
176. van Duuren, B. L., Sivak, A., *Cancer Res.* (1968) **28,** 2349.
177. Rohrschneider, L. R., Boutwell, R. K., *Nature New Biol.* (1973) **243,** 212.
178. Morton, J. F., *Morris Arbor. Bull.* (1974) **25,** 24.
179. O'Gara, R. W., Lee, C., Morton, J. F., *J. Natl. Cancer Inst.* (1971) **46,** 1131.
180. O'Gara, R. W., Lee, C. W., Morton, J. F., Kapadia, G. J., Dunham, L. J., *J. Natl. Cancer Inst.* (1974) **52,** 445.
181. Hirono, I., Shimizu, M., Fushimi, K., Mori, H., Kato, K., *Gann* (1973) **64,** 527.
182. Lacassagne, A., *C. R. Acad. Sci. (Paris)* (1932) **195,** 630.
183. Gardner, E. U., *Adv. Cancer Res.* (1953) **1,** 173.
184. Mackenzie, I., *Br. J. Cancer* (1955) **9,** 284.
185. Kirschbaum, A., *Cancer Res.* (1957) **17,** 432.
186. Fürth, J., *Harvey Lect..* (1969) **63,** 47.
187. Mühlbock, O., *J. Natl. Cancer Inst.* (1972) **48,** 1213.
188. Kirkman, H., *J. Natl. Cancer Inst., Monogr.* No. **1,** 1.
189. Della Porta, G., Terracini, B., *Progr. Exp. Tumor Res.* (1969) **11,** 334.
190. Schoental, R., *Ann. Rev. Pharmacol.* (1974) **14,** 185.
191. Andrea, F. P., Christensen, H. D., Williams, T. L., Thompson, M. G., Wall, M. E., *Teratology* (1973) **7,** Abstract A.11.
192. Dunn, T. B., Green, A. W., *J. Natl. Cancer Inst.* (1963) **31,** 425.
193. Dunn, T. B., *J. Natl. Cancer Inst.* (1969) **43,** 671.
194. Dunn, T. B., *New England J. Med.* (1971) **285,** 1147.
195. Bongiovanni, A. M., Di George, A. M., Grumbach, M. M., *J. Clin. Endocrin.* (1959) **19,** 1004.
196. Wilkins, L. P., *J. Am. Med. Assoc.* (1960) **172,** 1028.
197. Karnofsky, D. A., *Ann. Rev. Pharmacol.* (1965) **5,** 447.
198. Nora, J. J., Nora, A. H., *Arch. Environ. Health* (1975) **30,** 17.
199. Herbst, A. L., Kurman, R. J., Scully, R. E., Poskanzer, D. C., *N. Engl. J. Med.* (1972) **287,** 1259.
200. Folkman, J., *New England J. Med.* (1971) **285,** 404.
201. Herbst, A. L., Ulfeder, H., Poskanzer, D. C., *N. Engl. J. Med.* (1971) **284,** 878.
202. Tsukada, Y., Hewett, W. J., Barlow, J. J., Pickren, J. W., *Cancer* (1972) **29,** 1208.
203. Greenwald, P., Barlow, J. J., Nasca, P. C. Burnett, W. S., *N. Engl. J. Med.* (1971) **285,** 390.
204. Kalman, S. M., *Ann. Rev. Pharmacol.* (1969) **9,** 363.
205. Report from the Boston Collaborative Drug Surveillance Program, *Lancet* (1973) **i,** 1399.
206. Wong, Y. K., Woods, B. S. B., *Br. Med. J.* (1971) **IV,** 403.
207. Doll, R., *Br. Med. Bull.* (1971) **27,** 25.
208. Baum, J. K., Bookstein, J. J., Holtz, F., Klein, E. W., *Lancet* (1973) **ii,** 926.
209. Contostavlos, D. L., *Lancet* (1973) **ii,** 1200.
209a. Hoefnagel, D., *Lancet* (1976) **i,** 152.
209b. McLachlan, J. A., Newbold, R. R., Bullock, B., *Science* (1975) **190,** 991.
210. Johnson, F. L., Feagler, J. R., Lerner, K. G., Majerus, P. W., Siegel, M., Hartmann, J. R., Thomas, E. D., *Lancet* (1972) **ii,** 1273.
211. Wade, N., *Science* (1972) **176,** 1399.
212. Kellie, A. E., *Ann. Rev. Pharmacol.* (1971) **11,** 97.
213. Butenandt, A., Jacobi, H., *Hoppe-Seyler's Z. Physiol. Chem.* (1933) **218,** 104.
214. Liener, J. E., "Miscellaneous Toxic Factors," in "Toxic Constituents of Plant Foodstuffs," J. E. Liener, Ed., p. 409, Academic, 1969.
215. Bradbury, R. B., White, D. E., *Vitam. Horm.* (1954) **12,** 207.

216. Bickoff, E. M., Livingston, A. L., Hendrickson, A. P., Booth, A. N., *J. Agr. Food Chem.* (1962) **10,** 410.
217. Bickoff, E. M., Booth, A. N., Lyman, R. L., Livingston, A. L., Thompson, C. R., de Eds, F., *Science* (1957) **126,** 969.
218. Chopin, J., Bouillant, M. L., Lebreton, P., *Bull. Soc. Chim. France* (1964) 1038.
219. Leavitt, W. W., Meismer, D. M., *Nature* (1968) **218,** 181.
220. Cain, I. C., *Nature* (1960) **188,** 774.
221. *Nature* (1973) **243,** 6.
222. Mirocha, C. J., Christensen, C. M., Nelson, G. H., "F2-(Zearalenone) Estrogenic Mycotoxin from Fusarium," in *Microb. Toxins* (1971) **7,** 107.
223. Lunaas, T., *Nature* (1963) **198,** 288.
224. Drane, H., Patterson, D. S. P., Roberts, B. A., Saba N., *Food Cosmet. Toxicol.* (1975) **13,** 491.
224a. Zarrow, M. X., Lazo-Wasem, E. A., Shoger, R. L., *Science* (1953) **118,** 650.
225. Sabine, J. R., Horton, B. J., Wicks, N. M., *J. Natl. Cancer Inst.* (1973) **50,** 1237.
226. Schoental, R., *Cancer Res.* (1974) **34,** 2419.
227. Schoental, R., *Laboratory Animals* (1973) **7,** 47.
228. Jensen, E. V., De Sombre, E. R., "Estrogens and Progestins," in *Biochem. Action Horm.* (1972) **2,** 215.
229. Wells, H. G., *Arch. Pathol.* (1940) **30,** 535.
230. Miller, R. W., "Prenatal Origin of Cancer in Man: Epidemiological Evidence," in "Transplacental Carcinogenesis," L. Tomatis, U. Mohr, W. Davis, Eds., No. **4,** 175, Publ. I.A.R.C., 1973.
231. Gillette, J. R., *Ann. New York Acad. Sci.* (1971) **179,** 43.
232. Sargeant, K., Sheridan, A., O'Kelly, J., Carnaghan, R. B. A., *Nature* (1961) **192,** 1096.
233. Lancaster, M. C., Jenkins, F. P., Philp, J. M., *Nature* (1961) **192,** 1095.
234. Dickens, F., in "Carcinogenesis: A Broad Critique," p. 447, Williams & Wilkins, Baltimore, 1967.
234a. Uraguchi, K., Tatsuno, T., Sakai, F., Tsukioka, M., Sakai, Y., Yonemitsu, O., Ito, H., Miyake, M., Saito, M., Enomoto, M., Shikata, T., Ishiko, T., *Jap. J. Exp. Med.* (1961) **31,** 19.
235. Enamoto, M., Saito, M., *Ann. Rev. Microbiol.* (1972) **26,** 279.
236. Uraguchi, K., Saito, M., Noguchi, Y., Takahashi, K., Enomoto, M., Tatsuno, T., *Food Cosmet. Toxicol.* (1972) **10,** 193.
237. Joffe, A. Z., *Microb. Toxins* (1971) **7,** 139.
238. Schoental, R., Joffe, A. Z., *J. Pathol.* (1974) **112,** 37.
239. Forgacs, J., Carll, W. T., *Adv. Vet. Sci.* (1962) **7,** 273.
239a. Schoental, R., *Int. J. Environ. Stud.* (1975) **8,** 171.
240. Kraybill, H. F., Shimkin, M. B., *Adv. Cancer Res.* (1964) **8,** 191.
241. G. N. Wogan, Ed., "Mycotoxins in Foodstuffs," M.I.T., Cambridge, 1965.
242. Wogan, G. N., *Bacteriol. Rev.* (1966) **30,** 460.
243. Schoental, R., *Ann. Rev. Pharmacol.* (1967) **7,** 343.
244. Goldblatt, L. A., "Aflatoxin, Scientific Background, Control, and Implications," Academic, New York and London, 1969.
245. Detroy, R. W., Lillehoj, E. B., Ciegler, A., *Microb. Toxins* (1971) **6,** 13.
246. Büchi, G., Rae, I. D., in "Aflatoxin, Scientific Background, Control, and Implications," L. A. Goldblatt, Ed., p. 55, Academic, New York and London, 1969.
247. Stubblefield, R. D., Shotwell, O. L., Shannon, G. M., Weisleder, D., Rohwedder, W. K., *J. Agr. Food Chem.* (1970) **18,** 391.
248. Detroy, R. W., Hesseltine, C. W., *Can. J. Biochem.* (1970) **48,** 830.
249. Dalezios, J., Wogan, G. N., Weinreb, S. M., *Science* (1971) **171,** 584.
250. Masri, M. S., Haddon, W. F., Loudin, R. E., Hsieh, D. P. H., *J. Agr. Food Chem.* (1974) **22,** 512.

251. Roberts, J. C., Sheppard, A. H., Knight, J. A., Roffey, P., *J. Chem. Soc.* (1968) 22.
252. Büchi, G., Weinreb, M., *J. Am. Chem. Soc.* (1971) **93**, 746.
253. Büchi, G., Spitzner, D., Paglialunga, S., Wogan, G. N., *Life Sci.* (1973) **13**, 1143.
254. Biollaz, M., Büchi, G., Milne, G., *J. Am. Chem. Soc.* (1970) **92**, 1035.
255. Elsworthy, G. C., Holker, J. S. E., McKeown, J. M., Robinson, J. B., Mulheirn, L. J., *Chem. Commun.* (1970) 1069.
256. Heathcote, J. G., Dutton, M. F., Hibbert, J. R., *Chem. Ind.* (1973) 1027.
257. Maggon, K. K., Venkitasubramanian, T. A., *Experientia* (1973) **29**, 1210.
258. Heathcote, J. G., Dutton, M. F., *Tetrahedron* (1969) **25**, 1497.
259. Krogh, P., Hald, B., Hasselager, E., Madsen, A., Mortensen, H. P., Larsen, A. E., Campbell, A. D., *Pure Appl. Chem.* (1973) **35**, 275.
260. Hanssen, E., Jung, M., *Pure Appl. Chem.* (1973) **35**, 239.
261. Hsieh, D. P. H., *J. Agr. Food Chem.* (1973) **21**, 468.
262. Patterson, D. S. P., *Food Cosmet. Toxicol.* (1973) **11**, 287.
263. Lijinsky, W., Butler, W. H., *Proc. Soc. Exp. Biol. Med.* (1966) **123**, 151.
264. Lancaster, M. C., *Cancer Res.* (1968) **28**, 2288.
265. Wales, J. H., Sinnhuber, R. O., *J. Natl. Cancer Inst.* (1972) **48**, 1529.
266. Gopalan, C., Tulpule, P. G., Krishnamurthi, D., *Food Cosmet. Toxicol.* (1972) **10**, 519.
267. Adamson, R. H., Correa, P., Dalgard, D. W., *J. Natl. Cancer Inst.* (1973) **50**, 549.
268. Epstein, S. M., Bartus, B., Farber, E., *Cancer Res.* (1969) **29**, 1045.
269. Butler, W. H., Greenblatt, M., Lijinsky, W., *Cancer Res.* (1969) **29**, 2206.
270. Butler, W. H., Barnes, J. M., *Nature* (1966) **209**, 90.
271. Newberne, P. M., Rogers, A. E., *J. Natl. Cancer Inst.* (1973) **50**, 439.
272. Vesselinovitch, S. D., Mihailovich, N., Wogan, G. N., Lombard, L. S., Rao, K. V. N., *Cancer Res.* (1972) **32**, 2289.
273. Grice, H. C., Moodie, C. A., Smith, D. C., *Cancer Res.* (1973) **33**, 262.
274. Walbeck, W. van, Scott, P. M., Tatcher, F. S., *Can. J. Microbiol.* (1968) **14**, 131.
275. Serck-Hanssen, A., *Arch. Environ. Health* (1970) **20**, 729.
276. Amla, I., Kamala, C. S., Gopalakrishna, G. S., Jayaraj, A. P., Sreenivasamurthy, V., Parpia, H. A. B., *Am. J. Clin. Nutr.* (1971) **24**, 609.
277. Shank, R. C., Bhamarapravati, N., Gordon, J. E., Wogan, G. N., *Food Cosmet. Toxicol.* (1972) **10**, 171.
278. Alpert, M. E., Hutt, M. S. R., Wogan, G. N., Davidson, C. S., *Cancer* (1971) **28**, 253.
279. Peers, F. G., Linsell, C. A., *Br. J. Cancer* (1973) **27**, 473.
280. Reddy, J. K., Svoboda, D., *Arch. Pathol.* (1972) **93**, 55.
281. Newberne, P. M., Rogers, A. E., *Plant Foods for Man* (1973) **1**, 23.
282. Sun Shib-Chien, Wei Ru-Dong, Schaeffer, B. T., *Lab. Invest.* (1971) **24**, 368.
283. Madhavan, T. V., Gopalan, C., *Arch. Pathol.* (1965) **85**, 133.
284. Sinnhuber, R. O., Lee, D. J., Wales, J. H., Ayres, J. L., *J. Natl. Cancer Inst.* (1968) **41**, 1293.
285. Hamilton, P. B., Tung, Hsi-Tang, Harris, J. R., Gainer, J. H., Donaldson, W. E., *Poult. Sci.* (1972) **51**, 165.
286. Rogers, A. E., Newberne, P. M., *Nature* (1971) **229**, 62.
287. Reddy, G. S., Tilak, T. B. G., Krishnamurthi, D., *Food Cosmet. Toxicol.* (1973) **11**, 467.
288. McLean, A. E. M., Marshall, A., *Br. J. Exp. Pathol.* (1971) **52**, 322.
289. Sinnhuber, R. O., Lee, D. J., Wales, J. H., Landers, M. K., Keyl, A. C., *Fed. Proc.* (1970) **29**, 568.
290. Pong, R. S., Wogan, G. N., *J. Natl. Cancer Inst.* (1971) **47**, 585.
291. Wogan, G. N., Paglialunga, S., *Food Cosmet. Toxicol.* (1974) **12**, 381.

292. Wogan, G. N., Edwards, G. S., Newberne, P. M., *Cancer Res.* (1971) **31,** 1936.
293. Ayres, J. L., Lee, D. J., Wales, J. H., Sinnhuber, R. O., *J. Natl. Cancer Inst.* (1971) **46,** 561.
294. Cheung, K. K., Sim, G. A., *Nature* (1964) **201,** 1185.
295. Van Soest, T. C., Peerdeman, A. F., *Acta Crystallogr.* (1970) **26B,** 1940, 1947, and 1956.
296. Masri, M. S., Lundin, R. E., Page, J. R., Garcia, V. C., *Nature* (1967) **215,** 753.
297. Portman, R. S., Plowman, K. M., Campbell, T. C., *Biochem. Biophys. Res. Commun.* (1968) **33,** 711.
298. Roebuck, B. D., Wogan, G. N., *Proc. Am. Assoc. Cancer Res.* (1974) **15,** 68, Abstr. 269.
299. Steyn, M., Pitout, M. J., Purchase, I. F. H., *Br. J. Cancer* (1971) **25,** 291.
300. Akao, M., Kuroda, K., Wogan, G. N., *Life Sci.* (1971) **10,** 495.
301. Neal, G. E., *Biochem. Pharmacol.* (1972) **21,** 3023.
302. Schoental, R., *Nature* (1970) **227,** 401.
303. Scaife, J. F., *FEBS Lett.* (1971) **12,** 143.
304. Garner, R. C., Miller, E. C., Miller, J. A., *Cancer Res.* (1972) **32,** 2058.
305. Swenson, D. H., Miller, J. A., Miller, E. C., *Biochem. Biophys. Res. Commun.* (1973) **53,** 1260.
306. Swenson, H., Miller, J. A., Miller, E. C., *Cancer Res.* (1975) **35,** 3811.
307. Heathcote, J. G., Hibbert, J. R., *Br. J. Cancer* (1974) **29,** 470.
308. Garner, R. C., Wright, C. M., *Br. J. Cancer* (1973) **28,** 544.
309. Tazima, Y., *Mutat. Res.* (1974) **26,** 225.
310. Friedman, L., Yim, L., Verrett, M. J., *Toxicol. Appl. Pharmacol.* (1972) **23,** 385.
311. Heathcote, J. G., Hibbert, J. R., *Biochem. Soc. Trans.* (1974) **2,** 301.
312. Bassett, C., Buchanan, M., Gallagher, R. T., Hodges, B., *Chem. Ind.* (1970) 1659.
313. Bullock, E., Roberts, J. C., Underwood, J. G., *J. Chem. Soc.* (1962) 4179.
314. Holzapfel, C. W., Purchase, I. F. H., Steyn, P. S., Gouws, L., *S. Afr. Med. J.* (1966) **40,** 1100.
315. Dickens, F., Jones, H. E. H., Waynforth, H. B., *Br. J. Cancer* (1966) **20,** 134.
316. Purchase, I. F. H., van der Watt, J. J., *Food Cosmet. Toxicol.* (1970) **8,** 289.
317. Purchase, I. F. H., van der Watt, J. J., *Toxicol. Appl. Pharmacol.* (1973) **26,** 274.
318. Van der Watt, J. J., "Sterigmatocystin," in "Mycotoxins," I. F. H. Purchase, Ed., Elsevier, Amsterdam, 1973.
319. Thiel, P. G., Steyn, M., *Biochem. Pharmacol.* (1973) **22,** 3267.
320. Burkhardt, H. J., Forgacs, J., *Tetrahedron* (1968) **24,** 717.
321. Rodricks, J. V., Henery-Logan, K. R., Campbell, A. D., Stoloff, L., Verrett, M. J., *Nature* (1968) **217,** 668.
322. Rance, M. J., Roberts, J. C., *J. Chem. Soc.* (1971) (C) 1247.
323. Holker, J. S. E., Kagal, S. A., *Chem. Commun.* (1968) 1574.
324. Bullock, E., Kirkaldy, D., Roberts, J. C., Underwood, J. G., *J. Chem. Soc.* (1963) 829.
325. Hamasaki, T., Hatsuna, Y., Terashima, N., Renbutsu, M., *Agr. Biol. Chem., Tokyo* (1965) **29,** 166 (Chem. Abstr. **62,** 16659).
326. *Ibid.,* 696 (Chem. Abstr. **63,** 10228).
327. Oxford, A. E., Raistrick, H., Simonart, P., *Biochem. J.* (1939) **33,** 240.
328. Grove, J. F., *Q. Rev. Chem. Soc. (London)* (1963) **17,** 1.
329. Grove, J. F., Ismay, D., MacMillan, J., Mulholland, T. P. C., Rogers, M. A. T., *Chem. Ind.* (1951) 219.
330. *WHO Chron.* (1966) **20,** 310.
331. Williams, D. I., Marten, R. H., Sarkany, I., *Lancet* (1958) **ii,** 1212.
332. Blank, H., *Am. J. Med.* (1965) **39,** 831.

333. Hurst, W. E., Paget, G. E., *Br. J. Dermatol.* (1963) **75,** 105.
334. De Matteis, F., Donnelly, A. J., Runge, W. J., *Cancer Res.* (1966) **26,** 721.
335. Epstein, S. S., Andrea, J., Joshi, S., Mantel, N., *Cancer Res.* (1967) **27,** 1900.
336. Paget, G. E., Walpole, A. L., *Nature* (1958) **182,** 1320.
337. Barich, L. L., Schwarz, J., Barich, D., *Cancer Res.* (1962) **22,** 53.
338. Boothroyd, B., Napier, E. J., Somerfield, G. A., *Biochem. J.* (1961) **80,** 34.
339. Bod, P., Szarka, E., Gyimesi, J., Horvath, Gy., Vajna-Mehesfalvi, Z., Horvath, I., *J. Antibiot.* (1973) **26,** 101.
340. Barnes, M. J., Boothroyd, B., *Biochem. J.* (1961) **78,** 41.
341. Harris, P. A., Riegelman, S., *J. Pharmacol. Sci.* (1969) **58,** 93.
342. Symchowicz, S., Wong, K. K., *Biochem. Pharmacol.* (1966) **15,** 1595.
343. *Ibid.*, 1601.
344. Lin, C., Chang, R., Magat, J., Symchowicz, S., *J. Pharm. Pharmacol.* (1972) **24,** 911.
345. Lin, C. C., Magat, J., Chang, R., McGlotten, J., Symchowicz, S., *J. Pharmacol. Exp. Ther.* (1973) **187,** 415.
346. Tomomatsu, S., Kitamura, J., *Chem. Pharm. Bull., Tokyo* (1960) **8,** 755.
347. Fisher, J. F., Mallette, M. F., *J. Gen. Physiol.* (1961) **45,** 1.
348. Farber, E., *Adv. Cancer Res.* (1963) **7,** 383.
349. Sternberg, S. S., Philips, F. S., Cronin, A. P., *Cancer Res.* (1972) **32,** 1029.
350. Maienhofer, P., *J. Am. Chem. Soc.* (1970) **92,** 3771.
351. Svoboda, D., Reddy, J., Harris, C., *Cancer Res.* (1970) **30,** 2271.
352. Herr, R. R., Jahnke, H. K., Argoudelis, A. D., *J. Am. Chem. Soc.* (1967) **89,** 4808.
353. Vavra, J. J., De Boer, C., Dietz, A., Hanka, L. J., Sokolski, W. T., *Antibiot. Ann.* (1959-60) **7,** 230.
354. Lewis, C., Barbiers, A. R., *Antibiot. Ann.* (1959-60) **7,** 247.
355. Rakieten, N., Rakieten, M. L., Nadkarni, M. V., *Cancer Chemother. Rept.* (1963) **29,** 91.
356. Rerup, C. C., *Pharmacol. Rev.* (1970) **22,** 484.
357. Gichner, T., Veleminsky, J., Krepinsky, J., *Mol. Gen. Genet.* (1968) **102,** 184.
358. Kolbye, S. McC., Legator, M. S., *Mutat. Res.* (1968) **6,** 387.
359. Evans, J. S., Gerritsen, G. C., Mann, K. M., Owen, S. P., *Cancer Chemother. Rep.* (1965) **48,** 1.
360. Murray-Lyon, I. M., Eddleston, A. L. W. F., Williams, R., Brown, M., Hogbin, B. M., Bennett, A., Edwards, J. C., Taylor, K. W., *Lancet* (1968) **ii,** 895.
361. Feldman, J. M., Quickel, K. E., Marecek, R. L., *Southern Med. J.* (1972) **65,** 1325.
362. Arison, R. N., Feudale, E. L., *Nature* (1967) **214,** 1254.
363. Rakieten, N., Gordon, B. S., Cooney, D. A., Davis, R. D., Schein, P. S., *Cancer Chemother. Rep.* (1968) **52,** 563.
364. Sibay, T. M., Hoyes, J. A., *Lancet* (1969) **ii,** 912.
365. Berman, L. D., Hayes, J. A., Sibay, T. M., *J. Natl. Cancer Inst.* (1973) **51,** 1287.
366. Mauer, S. M., Lee, C. S., Najarian, J. S., Brown, D. M., *Cancer Res.* (1974) **34,** 158.
367. Rakieten, N., Gordon, B. S., Beaty, A., Cooney, D. A., Davis, R. D., Schein, P. S., *Proc. Soc. Exp. Biol. Med.* (1971) **137,** 280.
368. Rosenkranz, H. S., Carr, H. S., *Cancer Res.* (1970) **30,** 112.
369. Gunnarsson, R., Berne, C., Hellerström, C., *Biochem. J.* (1974) **140,** 487.
370. Melmed, R. N., Benitez, C. J., Holt, S. J., *J. Cell. Sci.* (1973) **13,** 297.
371. Schein, P. S., Cooney, D. A., Vernon, M. L., *Cancer Res.* (1967) **27,** 2324.
372. Schein, P. S., Loftus, S., *Cancer Res.* (1968) **28,** 1501.
373. Schein, P. S., Cooney, D. A., McMenamin, M. G., Anderson, T., *Biochem. Pharmacol.* (1973) **22,** 2625.
374. Haskell, T. H., Ryder, A., Bartz, Q. R., *Antibiot. Chemother.* (1954) **4,** 141.

375. Ehrlich, J., Anderson, L. E., Coffey, G. L., Feldman, W. H., Fisher, M. W., Hillegas, A. B., Karlson, A. G., Knudsen, M. P., Weston, J. K., Youmans, A. S., Youmans, G. P., *Antibiot. Chemother.* (1954) **4**, 338.
376. Stevens, C. L., Gillis, B. T., French, J. C., Haskell, T. H., *J. Am. Chem. Soc.* (1958) **80**, 6088.
377. Ohkuma, K., Nakamura, G., Yamashita, S., *J. Antibiot. (Japan)* (1957) Ser. A. **10**, 224.
378. Schoental, R., *Nature* (1969) **221**, 765.
379. Schoental, R., *Gann Monograph* (1969) **8**, 289.
380. Schoental, R., "Toxicity and carcinogenic action in rats of elaiomycin, a metabolite of *Streptomyces hepaticus*," in "Toxins of Animal and Plant Origin," A. de Vries, E. Kochva, Eds., Gordon and Breach, London (1972) **2**, 781.
381. Schoental, R., Joffe, A. Z., Yagen, B., *Br. J. Cancer* (1978) in press

13

The Bracken Carcinogen

I. A. Evans, Department of Biochemistry and Soil Science,
University College of North Wales, Bangor, Wales, U.K.

SO COSMOPOLITAN A PLANT as the bracken fern needs little introduction, covering as it does millions of acres of the earth's land surface. Latitude does not inhibit its growth since it ranges from the Arctic Circle in Norway to the mid-tropics. With a preference for light acid soils, it is found in a variety of habitats from sea level up to 2000 ft in the British Isles but going much higher under continental conditions. Its own height can vary from 1 to 12 or 13 ft. The spread and persistence are attributable to the creeping underground rhizome. Its family, the *Polypodiaceae,* dates back to middle Mesozoic times, about 150 million years ago. Although Culpeper recommended its use as an abortant in 1652 (*1*), it was not until 1893 that its lethal properties were scientifically recognized (*2, 3, 4*). The earlier general literature on bracken was reviewed by Braid (*5*).

A great variety of research during this century showed that bracken assembles molecules with marked biological activity. These include an antheridiogen (*6, 7*), ecdysone and 20-hydroxyecdysone (*8*), and a phytotoxic agent which inhibits the growth of other plant seedlings (*9*). W. C. Evans *et al.* demonstrated the presence of the enzyme thiaminase, which was the first of its kind to be found in the plant kingdom (*10, 11, 12, 13*).

The enzyme, which is much more concentrated in the rhizome than the frond, can produce the typical nervous lesions of avitaminosis B_1 and can lead to death in simple-stomached animals if not treated in time—for example "bracken staggers" in the horse and related lesions in the pigeon, rat, pig, and sheep (*14–20*). The thiaminase belongs to Type 1 and requires a cofactor, such as an aromatic amine or sulfur containing amino acid, to inactivate thiamine (Figure 1). Currently, W. C. Evans extended this study successfully to include the production of experimental cerebro-cortical necrosis in lambs and sheep.

However, it is unlikely that the increased mortality of cattle, which accompanied the severe drought of 1893 in the British Isles, was caused by any of the above factors, although it was demonstrably produced by the bracken eaten in place of the missing fodder. The syndrome was quite dramatic. It was characterized by generalized hemorrhage, anorexia, extensive intestinal damage, and ulceration. In some cases, there was massive blood loss, severe pyrexia of 107–109°F, and death within a few weeks or months. This was termed "cattle bracken poisoning," and although it was realized that bovines were particularly susceptible, Boddie (*21*) made it clear that the true nature of the condition was not understood. There were ardent protagonists for the two contending theories of patent toxicity or hemorrhagic septicemia.

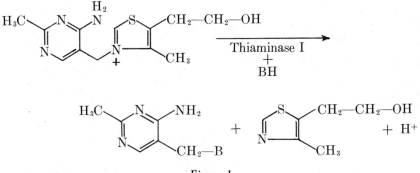

Figure 1.

Investigation of Biological Effects

Field case postmortems gave hints of low levels of leucocytes and platelets, but Shearer (*22*), recording erythrocytes, had not dealt with these parameters of myeloid origin. The fundamental lesions, destruction of the bone marrow leading to acute leukopenia and thrombocytopenia, together with severe terminal damage to the intestinal mucosa, were demonstrated by Evans, Evans and Hughes, (*23, 24*). Other changes in the circulation were recorded. Erythrocytes which have a much longer comparative life span take more time to demonstrate the aplastic nature of the hematogenous bone marrow, unless there is massive hemorrhage. Many of these findings were confirmed by Naftalin and Cushnie (*25, 26*), Guilhon and Julon (*27*), and Guilhon *et al.* (*28*). Essentially, the chemical in bracken causing this syndrome is acting in a mitotoxic manner. Since bone marrow and the intestinal mucosa are two indispensable sites of continuous cell division in the body, curtailment of their activity can lead to severe and frequently irreversible damage.

Unfortunately, in this day and age it is well known that radiation can produce the same syndrome as the one described above, and reports of the effect of radiation in bovines confirm the essential similarity of the two conditions (*29, 30, 31*). Attention was drawn to this possible radiomimetic nature of the cattle bracken toxin (*32, 33*). In the succeeding years much of the bracken research in Bangor concentrated on exploring the biological effects that bracken toxin and radiation have in common, according to the following simplified system (Table I).

A review of the results of this work (*34, 35*), undertaken by many workers and collaborators, shows that most of the features in the table have been reproduced by bracken or active extracts of the plant, and like radiation, the response depends on dose, administration, age, species, strain, individual, and tissue type. The experimental animals used in various sectors of the work included both immature and adult cattle, sheep, pigs, rats, mice, guinea pigs, quail, monkeys, hamsters, rabbits, and drosophila, with fish a very recent addition (33, 36–45).

Table I. The Radiation Syndrome

Category 1, Central Nervous Death (Hours)	Category 2, Gastrointestinal Death (Days)	Category 3, Bone Marrow Death (Weeks)	Category 4, Cancer Death (Years)
convulsions	destruction of GI mucosa	delayed bone marrow aplasia	a) local, e.g. bone, skin
immediate death	bone marrow aplasia	hemorrhages	b) whole body, e.g. gastrointestinal, lung, mammary
	electrolyte loss systemic toxemia	delayed gastro-intestinal syndrome	(species and strain dependent)
		histamine and heparin release	induction of mutations
		capillary fragility humoral changes including lipids	sterility

Decreasing dosage of radiation.

⎯⎯⎯⎯⎯⎯⎯⎯⎯⎯⎯⎯⎯⎯⎯⎯⎯⎯⎯⎯⎯⎯⎯⎯⎯⎯⎯⎯⎯⎯⎯⎯⎯⎯⎯⎯→

The typical form of cattle bracken poisoning belongs to Category 3 in the table and is accompanied by marked systemic inflammatory changes which occur quite independently from bacteremia and include humoral changes (proteins, lipids, lipases, mucopolysaccharides, histamine, and related amines) together with striking tissue invasions and wide fluctuations in numbers of the cells concerned with immunological reactions, particularly of the tissue-bound type. These findings led us to investigate the therapeutic potential of corticosteroids with marked success in both experimental and field cases (46).

The earliest evidence for the presence of a carcinogen in bracken was reported by Rosenberger and Heeschen (47), who described hematuria and changes of a polypus nature in the urinary bladder mucosa of five cattle fed bracken for long periods. Indirect evidence came from Georgiev et al. (48) who worked with an extract of urine of cattle fed hay from hematuria districts. This extract produced hemangioma-like lesions in the bladders of dogs and papilloma-type excrescences on mouse skin. Chronic enzoötic bovine hematuria has a wide distribution and was well characterized in different parts of the world although the etiology was unknown. Pamukcu (49) drew attention to the similar geographical distribution of the condition and bracken. He also suggested and worked on the possibility of a viral causative agent (*50*). There was, however, no conclusive evidence for either theory, and bracken could not be ruled out (*51*).

Since the carcinogenicity of bracken could only be firmly established by testing sufficient numbers of experimental animals, it was expedient to use rats and mice. In 1964 we started feeding them with pellets of one-third by weight dried, milled, June bracken fronds. This was maintained for nine weeks with the rats and five weeks with the mice. Between seven months and one year from the start of feeding, all 40 of the bracken rats had succumbed to multiple adenocarcinoma of the intestinal mucosa, predominantly in the ileal region. The tumors varied from early growths to the most malignant forms, often with very large diverticuli and frequent intussusceptions whereas nothing was found in the 40 control rats (*38*). The mice survived longer, but although they did not develop the ileal tumours, they had significantly high numbers of pulmonary adenomas, an average of 16 per mouse in 26 mice compared with 0.57 for 46 control mice (*39*). Subsequent experiments using both whole bracken and extracts, confirmed these results, extended the range of mouse tumors to include leukemias and gastric cancers, and demonstrated an age dependence in rats, the young animal being vulnerable (*34, 35, 43*). In mice single administrations of extract sometimes produced tumors, even squamous carcinoma of the stomach.

Other small experimental animals were tried, and we found the carcinogen to be strongly active in birds. Japanese quail died from adenocarcinoma, predominantly in the two ceca, which became increasingly hemorrhagic, and also in the colon and distal ileum. After 10 months, the incidence was 80% in the 34 bracken quail and 0% in the controls (*41*). Guinea pigs were especially interesting since they reproduced almost exactly the condition described for the chronic enzootic bovine hematuria. In this experiment, 13 animals had fresh bracken fronds offered to them in addition to their normal diet for 11 weeks, and it was terminated after 30 months by which time most of the animals had been sacrificed when in poor condition. The majority developed intermittent hematuria, and in all there was epithelial hyperplasia of the urinary bladder, advancing through papillomatous changes to papillary carcinoma and adenocarcinoma. Infilrating carcinoma and transitional cell carcinomas were frequent, sometimes with glandular or squamous metaplasia. One animal died with adenocarcinoma of the jejunum after 23 months. The control guinea pigs were all normal. With very limited numbers of animals, we have produced hematuria in rabbits and metastatic adenocarcinoma of the colon in a sheep and of the cecum and distal ileum in a hamster.

In 1965, Rosenberger (*52*) published further evidence obtained from nine experimental cows which he had fed both fresh and hay bracken. All developed chronic cystic hematuria 10½ to 15 months after feeding began, together with the same gross lesions of the vesical mucosa as obtained in the so-called spontaneous chronic field condition of cattle. Also in 1965, Sofrenovic *et al.* (*53*) described essentially similar results with five cattle fed long-term bracken. With the exception of one animal, they all developed vesicular hematuria together with the characteristic hemangiomas and papillomatous tumors. Later, Pamukcu *et al.* (*54, 55*) produced experimental bovine enzootic hematuria in 10 out of 18 cattle fed varying amounts of bracken over a mean period of 550 days. The majority of bladder neoplasms were papillomas and hemangiomas, and in some animals carcinomas were found as a late development. Survey studies by Döbereiner *et al.* (*56, 57*) associated bracken with enzootic hematuria in Brazil and also a slower developing epidermoid carcinoma of the upper digestive tract of cattle. Currently, Jarrett and co-workers are studying cases of esophageal cancer among Scottish cattle and are investigating the possibility of a combined action in which bracken acts as a derepressor for integrated DNA virus.

Our production of malignancies in rats and mice has since been confirmed by other workers. They fed the bracken for much longer periods of time than we had done, in some cases over a year, and reported the development of papillomas and carcinomas of the urinary bladder of rats in addition to the intestinal adenocarcinomas (*55, 58, 59*). Pamukcu *et al.* also report that the incidence of bladder tumors in rats can be increased by thiamine supplementation (*60, 61*) and decreased by chronic phenothiazine administration (*62*). They found that after adding bracken to the diet of mice on alternate weeks for 60 weeks, all those surviving had developed lymphatic leukemia and 15% had pulmonary tumors (*63*). In our experience, with a more restrained dosage, the incidence of mouse leukemias was lower and more varied.

The work of Hirono *et al.* (*59, 64*) in Japan is of particular interest since it is primarily in this country that direct human consumption of bracken occurs. It is eaten as salad and garnishing or cooked in a variety of ways. Unfortunately it is collected before the fronds have uncurled, in the fiddlehead or crozier stage, when there is a maximum content of toxin. Using rats as an assay, he reports that cooking the bracken in plain water only removes the carcinogen to some extent, but if an alkali such as wood ash or sodium bicarbonate is added, then only weak carcinogen activity is retained. This agrees completely with our findings that the acute toxicity and carcinogenicity are greatly reduced or destroyed under alkaline conditions and can be maintained best at acid pH. Hirono's work on the relative distribution of carcinogenic activity in the different parts of the bracken plant is of equal interest. As evidenced by the severity of rat intestinal tumors, the order of increasing activity goes from stalk to young frond to rhizome (*65*). If compared with our reports on the toxicity of bracken rhizomes in cattle (*36*), this lends additional weight to the common identiy of the carcinogen and the acute toxic factor. Two transplantable tumor lines, an adenocarcinoma and a sarcoma, were successfully established by the Japanese workers.

Sheep are more resistant to hemorrhagic bracken poisoning than cattle, but field cases have been described (*66, 67*), and it can be produced experimentally (*34, 68, 69*). Intestinal tumors in sheep occur in areas where bracken could be incriminated (*70, 71*), and McCrea described (*72*) the high incidence of both intestinal and jaw tumors in North Yorkshire Moor sheep observed after his long surveys of individual farms. Another disease of Yorkshire hill flocks which has been recognized by farmers for at least 50 years as "bright blindness" which is characterized by stenosis of the blood vessels and progressive retinal atrophy. This condition has been studied by Watson and Barnett, and they have produced it experimentally by feeding whole bracken (*73, 74, 75, 76, 77*).

Chemical Studies

The chemical isolation of the radiomimetic component has been bedeviled by two major factors—the nature of the assay system and the apparent instability of the toxin with progressive purification. In an effort to obviate the difficulties of long waits and expensive animals, various small scale biological assays have been tried and abandoned because of insufficient specificity.

Evans *et al.* (*78*) in 1958 first extracted the toxin into hot ethanol from dried milled bracken. Although they found it was also soluble from the fresh frond in hot acidulated water (*79*), the ethanol method has remained the initial step, allowing work all the year round. Widdop and I. A. Evans (*35, 39, 41*) used two further solvent extractions with heptane and acid ether pH 3 to show that both the cattle toxin and the carcinogen were insoluble in the first and only marginally soluble in the second. However, this greatly facilitated the purification of the plant extract. Further efforts with alkaline and continuous ether extraction led to activity loss.

Working with quail, Barber showed that bracken induced sterility in the male. He also demonstrated the production of dominant lethal mutations in both drosophila (orally) and male mice (intraperitoneal injection) (*34, 41, 42*). This mutagenicity test was used by Leach and Barber to reach a further stage of purification after charcoal had been introduced for the removal of lipids, etc. and a partition obtained with ethyl acetate. The ethyl acetate supernatant fraction was positive for the mutagenic factor, carcinogenic activity, and acute toxicity in mice. Following column and thin layer chromatography, the main constituent of the obtained fraction was given the preliminary molecular formula of $C_7H_8O_4$ (*43, 80*). In addition to producing dominant lethals in mice, the fraction later gave positive results when subjected to a microbiological mutation test (*81*). Further work on the chemistry of this compound by W. C. Evans and Osman corrected the formula to $C_7H_{10}O_5$, and the full analysis conclusively proved that it was shikimic acid, 3,4,5-trihydroxy-1-cyclohexene-1-carboxylic acid.

Since shikimic acid is common in plants, being on the biosynthetic pathway of aromatic ring compounds, and appears at first sight to be a harmless molecule, it was thought that the carcinogen would be found among the minor constituents of the fraction. Much time and effort was expended in this direction without positive results. Fortunately, some mice were given single administrations of commercially produced shikimic acid of tested purity and, against expectation, 9 of these 14 animals subsequently developed precancerous and cancerous lesions involving the glandular gastric mucosa and also malignant leukemias. None of 57 control mice treated in a similar manner with a varity of inert compounds and killed after comparable intervals of time produced any neoplasms. This demonstrated that the tumors were not the spontaneous ones of old age. When the mouse mutagen test was tried on the pure shikimic acid, it produced a high rate of dominant lethals when injected intraperitoneally and had marked activity even when given by stomach tube (82).

In light of these results we are currently extending the work on shikimic acid to include rats and other animals and a variety of administrative procedures. If these early results are confirmed, bracken may have led to the recognition of an environmental carcinogen much more ubiquitous than the weed itself.

We now have clear evidence from some of our previous experiments that the acute bovine bone marrow toxin and a strong carcinogen are both present in another and different bracken fraction which does not contain shikimic acid. In this case, single administrations (intraperitoneal and oral) can produce malignant squamous carcinoma of the mouse forestomach as well as the glandular gastric tumors, indicating a more powerful carcinogen. We are waiting for the long-term results to show which of these carcinogens is responsible for the rat and quail intestinal tumors. Meanwhile the fraction is being subjected to a full chemical investigation.

The findings of the Madison workers generally agree with our own. They fractionated the urine from cows fed on bracken and then used the urinary bladder implantation technique in mice. The acidic fraction of an ethyl acetate extraction produced bladder carcinomas in 5 out of 15 mice (83). Comparing the excretion of tryptophan metabolites in the urine of Turkish cows with and without bladder tumors they found that only acetylkynurenine was significantly higher in the former group (84). In similar studies Döbereiner et al. failed to find any consistent difference over 13 months (85). Starting with the whole plant, Pamukcu et al. confirmed that the carcinogenic activity can be extracted into methanol but is not significantly ether soluble (86).

Possible Human Hazards

This appraisal of bracken carcinogenicity would be incomplete without considering the possible human hazard by pathways, other than the direct consumption already mentioned, which might operate in all parts of the world where there are extensive bracken lands. The contamination of milk and dairy products and/or the water supply are the most likely possibilities. (One suspects that the brewing of bracken beer in Siberia and Norway may be somewhat limited (87), and we have concentrated attention on the first of these (88, 89, 90). Such enquiries are further prompted by the unexplained but very marked regional prevalence of some forms of human cancer such as that of the lips, mouth, esophagus, and stomach in Wales compared with the rest of the United Kingdom. It applies to both sexes, and farmers are particularly vulnerable. Japan shares top place in the world list for stomach cancer, and in this country also there is a marked regional distribution. If the contamination of cow's milk is relevant, then the greatest dangers in this respect would be in areas of marginal farming and free range practices, which have been characteristic of Welsh farming, and one is forcefully reminded that buttermilk (milk after lactic acid fermentation and fat removal) was until recently a staple item of diet of the poorer sections of the community.

Our first experiments with cows and mice showed that the toxin and a carcinogen could definitely pass the maternal barrier. Although there were records of placental passage in bovines (*32*), our most recent results with bovines and mice indicate that secretion *via* milk takes precedence over placental transference. With rats, however, there does not appear to be any maternal transference. When they are fed the milk of bracken-fed cows *ad libitum* for prolonged periods, no ileal tumors occur. When mice are fed the milk from bracken-fed cows daily—both as whole milk and processed into cream, sugar and salts, and protein—the incidence of the different kinds of tumors, particularly the leukemias, increases above control levels. In one of these experiments the rare, malignant, osteogenic sarcoma developed in two mice after a relatively short latent period. One animal was receiving the whole milk and the other the separated lipid fraction (*91*).

Our findings to date emphasize the importance of the neonatal period, especially during the early period of suckling. It is of special interest that mice so treated have produced gastric tumors, including squamous cell papilloma in non-glandular areas and carcinoma in the pyloric stomach. Mouse experiments in which we administered single sublethal doses orally and parenterally directly to the young animal produced gastric tumors as well as other varieties (*91*). Many other workers have emphasized the vulnerability of the neonatal period to some carcinogens, and there are cases in which it may be even confined to the first postpartural day (*92, 93, 94, 95*). These have reference to animal experiments, but Higginson, in a historical perspective on cancer incidence and migrant studies (96) drew two main conclusions:

"1. Migrant studies have to date confirmed that most cancers are not hereditary in origin and thus promoted general acceptance of the fact that 80–90% of human cancers are environmental and theoretically preventable. This has helped us to maintain a much more hopeful attitude to prevention.

2. They have shown that the cancerous process may be initiated very early in life and be irreversible."

With the thought of prevention in mind, we set up the nearest approach possible to a human experiment. We have been feeding eight Macaque monkeys with bracken extracts and in parallel have been giving eight baby monkeys the milk from our bracken-fed cows. The results so far show that, like other simple-stomached animals, this nonhuman primate does not have an acute reaction to bracken toxin at a dose level which would be lethal in bovines. Nevertheless, the fact that they are physiologically susceptible was demonstrated by the marked fluctuations discernible in bone marrow activity (*97*). Whatever the final outcome of this experiment, we hope that it may have some consequence for the human situation.

Literature Cited

1. Culpeper, N., "The English Physician, or an astrologo-physical discourse of the vulgar Herbs of this nation," London, 1652.

2. Storrer, D. N., *J. Comp. Pathol.* (1893) **6**, 276.
3. Penberthy, J., *J. Comp. Pathol.* (1893) **6**, 266.
4. Almond, N., *J. Comp. Pathol.* (1894) **7**, 165.
5. Braid, K. W., "Bracken: A Review of the Literature," Commonwealth Agricultural Bureau of Pasture and Field Crops No. **3**, 1959.
6. Döpp, W., *Ber. Deut. Bot. Ges.* (1950) **63**, 139.
7. Pringle, R. B., Näf, U., Braun, A. C., *Nature* (1960) **186**, 1066.
8. Kaplanis, J. N., Thompson, M. J., Robbins, W. E., Bryce, B. M., *Science* (1967) **157**, 1436.
9. Gliessman, R., Muller, C. H., *Madrōno* (1972) **21**, 299.
10. Evans, W. C., Jones, N. R., *Biochem. J.* (1952) **50**, 28.
11. Evans, W. C., Jones, N. R., Evans, R. A., *Biochem. J.* (1950) **47**, 12.
12. Thomas, A. J., Evans, I. A., Evans, W. C., *Biochem. J.* (1957) **65**, 5.
13. Watkin, J. E., Thomas, A. J., Evans, W. C., *Biochem. J.* (1953) **54**, 30.
14. Weswig, P. H., Freed, A. M, Haag, J. R., *J. Biol. Chem.* (1946) **165**, 737.
15. Evans, W. C., Evans, E. T. R., *Brit. Vet. J.* (1949) **105**, 175.
16. Thomas, B., Walker, H. F., *J. Soc. Chem. Ind.* (1949) **68**, 6.
17. Hadwen, S., Bruce, E. A., *Vet. J.* (1933) **89**, 120.
18. Evans, E. T. R., Evans, W. C., Roberts, H. E., *Brit. Vet. J.* (1951) **107**, 364, 399.
19. Evans, I. A., Humphreys, D. J., Goulden, L., Thomas, A. J., Evans, W. C., *J. Comp. Pathol.* (1963) **73**, 229.
20. Evans, W. C., Widdop, B., Harding, J. D. J., *Vet. Rec.* (1972) **90**, 471.
21. Boddie, G. F., *Vet. Rec.* (1947) **59**, 470.
22. Shearer, G. D., *J. Comp. Pathol.* (1945) **55**, 301.
23. Evans, E. T. R., Evans, W. C., Hughes, L. E., *Vet. Rec.* (1951) **63**, 444.
24. Evans, W. C., Evans, E. T. R., Hughes, L. E., *Brit. Vet. J.* (1954) **110**, 295, 365, 426.
25. Naftalin, J. M., Cushnie, G. H., *Vet. Rec.* (1951) **63**, 332.
26. Naftalin, J. M., Cushnie, G. H., *J. Comp. Pathol. Ther.* (1954) **64**, 54.
27. Guilhon, J., Julou, L., *Bull. Acad. Vét. Fr.* (1949) **22**, 407.
28. Guilhon, J., Oloy, J., Queinnec, G., *Bull. Acad. Vét. Fr.* (1955) **28**, 457.
29. Schultze, M. O., Perman, V., Mizuno, M. S., Bates, F. W., Sautter, J. H., Isbin, H. S., Lokeno, M. K., *Radiat. Res.* (1959) **11**, 399.
30. Brown, D. G., *J. Amer. Vet. Med. Ass.* (1962) **140**, 1051.
31. Brown, D. G., Thomas, R. E., Jones, L. J., Cross, F. H., Sasmore, D. P., *Radiat. Res.* (1961) **15**, 675.
32. Evans, I. A., Thomas, A. J., Evans, W. C., Edwards, C. M., *Brit. Vet. J.* (1958) **114**, 253.
33. Heath, G. B. S., Wood, B., *J. Comp. Pathol.* (1958) **68**, 201.
34. Evans, I. A., *Cancer Res.* (1968) **28**, 2252.
35. Evans, I. A., *Oncology 1970: Proc. Int. Cancer Congress 10th* (1972) **5**, 178.
36. Evans, W. C., Evans, I. A., Axford, R. F. E., Threlfall, G., Humphreys, D. J., Thomas, A. J., *Vet. Rec.* (1961) **35**, 852.
37. Evans, I. A., Howell, R. M. *Nature* (Lond) (1962) **194**, 584.
38. Evans, I. A., Mason, J., *Nature* (Lond.) (1965) **208**, 913.
39. Evans, I. A., Widdop, B., *British Empire Cancer Campaign for Research, Annual Report,* p. 377, 1966.
40. Howell, R. M., Evans, I. A., *J. Comp. Pathol.* (1967) **77**, 177.
41. Evans, I. A., Widdop, B., Barber, G. D., *British Empire Cancer Campaign for Research, Annual Report,* p. 411, 1967.
42. Evans, I. A., Barber, G. D., Jones, R. S., Leach, H., *British Empire Cancer Campaign for Research, Annual Report,* p. 416, 1968.
43. *Ibid.,* p. 446, 1969.
44. Naftalin, J. M., Cushnie, G. H., *J. Comp. Pathol.* (1956) **66**, 354.
45. Evans, I. A., Evans, W. C., Thomas, A. J., Threlfall, G., Humphreys, D. J., *Proc. Int. Congr. of Biochem. 5th* (1961) **10**, Section 16.

46. Widdop, B., Evans, I. A., unpublished data.
47. Rosenberger, von G., Heeschen, W., *Deut. Tierärztl. Wochschr.* (1960) **67**, 201.
48. Georgiev, R. A., Vrigasov, A., Antonov, S., Dimitrov, A., *Wien Tierärztl. Monatsschr.* (1963) **50**, 589.
49. Pamukcu, A. M., *Ann. N.Y. Acad. Sci.* (1963) **108**, 938.
50. Olson, C., Pamukcu, A. M., Brobst, D. F., *Cancer Res.* (1965) **25**, 840.
51. Donigiewicz, K., Kostuch, R., *Medycyny Weterynaryjnej* (1963) **5**, 237.
52. Rosenberger, von G., *Wien Tierärztl. Monatschr.* (1965) **52**, 415.
53. Sofrenovic, von Dj, Stamatovic, S., Bratanovic, U., *Deut. Tierärztl. Wochschr.* (1965) **72**, 409.
54. Pamukcu, A. M., Göksoy, S. K., Price, J. M., *Cancer Res.* (1967) **27**, 917.
55. Price, J. M., Pamukcu, A. M., *Cancer Res.* (1968) **28**, 2247.
56. Döbereiner, J. C., Tokarnia, C. H., Canella, C. F. C., *Pesq. Agropec., Brasil.* (1967) **2**, 329, 489.
57. Tokarnia, C. H., Döbereiner, J., Canella, C. F. C., *Pesq. Agropec., Brasil.* (1969) **4**, 209.
58. Pamukcu, A. M., Price, J. M., *J. Nat. Cancer Inst.* (1969) **43**, 275.
59. Hirono, I., Shibuya, C., Fushimi, K., Haga, M., *J. Nat. Cancer Inst.*, (1970) **45**, 179.
60. Pamukcu, A. M., Price, J. M., Bryan, G. T., *Proc. Amer. Ass. Cancer Res.* (1971) **12**, 7.
61. Pamukcu, A. M., Yalciner, S., Price, J. M., Bryan, G. T., *Cancer Res.* (1970) **30**, 2671.
62. Pamukcu, A. M., Wattenberg, I. W., Price, J. M., Bryan, G. T., *J. Nat. Cancer Inst.* (1971) **47**, 155.
63. Pamukcu, A. M., Ertürk, E., Price, J. M., Bryan, G. T., *Cancer Res.* (1972) **32**, 1442.
64. Hirono, I., Shibuya, C., Shimizu, M., Fushimi, K., *J. Nat. Cancer Inst.* (1972) **48**, 1245.
65. Hirono, I., Fushimi, K., Mori, H., Miwa, T., Haga, M., *J. Nat. Cancer Inst.* (1973) **50**, 1367.
66. Parker, W. H., McCrea, C. T., *Vet Record* (1965) **77**, 861.
67. Gardiner, M. R., Department of Agriculture, South Perth, Western Australia, personal communication.
68. Moon, F. E., Raafat, M. A., *J. Comp. Pathol.* (1951) **61**, 88.
69. Moon, F. E., McKeand, J. M., *Brit. Vet. J.* (1953) **109**, 321.
70. Dodd, D. C., *New Zealand Vet. J.* (1960) **8**, 109.
71. McDonald, J. W., Leaver, D. D., *Aust. Vet. J.* (1965) **41**, 269.
72. McCrea, C. T., personal communication.
73. Watson, W. A., Barlow, R. M., Barnett, K. C., *Vet. Rec.* (1965) **77**, 1060.
74. Barnett, K. C., Watson, W. A., *Veterinarian* (1968) **5**, 17.
75. Barnett, K. C., Watson, W. A., *Res. Vet. Sci.* (1970) **11**, 289.
76. Watson, W. A., Terlecki, S., Patterson, D. S. P., Sweasey, D., Herbert, C. M., Done, J. T., *Brit. Vet. J.* (1972) **128**, 457.
77. Watson, W. A., Barnett, K. C., Terlecki, S., *Vet. Rec.* (1972) **91**, 665.
78. Evans, W. C., Evans, I. A., Thomas, A. J., Watkin, J. E., Chamberlain, A. G., *Brit. Vet. J.* (1958) **114**, 180.
79. Evans, W. C., Evans, I. A., Chamberlain, A. G., Thomas, A. J., *Brit. Vet. J.* (1959) **115**, 1.
80. Leach, H., Barber, G. D., Evans, I. A., Evans, W. C., *Biochem. J.* (1971) **124**, 13.
81. Roberts, I. M., Shaw, D. S., Evans, W. C., *Biochem. J.* (1971) **124**, 13.
82. Evans, I. A., Osman, M. A., *Nature* (1974) **250**, 348.
83. Pamukcu, A. M., Olson, C., Price, J. M., *Cancer Res.* (1966) **26**, 1745.
84. Pamukcu, A. M., Brown, R. R., Price, J. M., *Cancer Res.* (1959) **19**, 321.

85. Döbereiner, J., Olson, C., Brown, R. R., Price, J. M., Yess, N., *Pesq. Agropec. Brasil.* (1966) **1**, 189.
86. Pamukcu, A. M., Price, J. M., Bryan, G. T., *Cancer Res.* (1970) **30**, 902.
87. Harrington, H. D., *Edible Native Plants of the Rocky Mountains*, pp. 122-125, University of New Mexico, 1967.
88. Evans, I. A., Widdop, B., Jones, R. S., Barber, G. D., Leach, H., Jones, D. L., Mainwaring-Burton, R., *Biochem. J.* (1971) **124**, 28.
89. Evans, I. A., Widdop, B., Jones, R. S., Barber, G. D., Leach, H., Jones, D. L., Mainwaring-Burton, R., Evans, W. C., *Proc. Int. Bladder Cancer Conf., Leeds*, 1971.
90. Evans, I. A., Jones, R. S., Mainwaring-Burton, R., *Nature* (1972) **237**, 107.
91. Jones, R. S., Evans, I. A., unpublished data.
92. Spatz, M., *Proc. Soc. Exp. Biol. Med.* (1968) **128**, 1005.
93. Hirono, I., *Fed. Proc.* (1972) **31**, 1493.
94. Toth, B., *Cancer Res.* (1968) **28**, 727.
95. Doll, R., Harold Dorn Memorial Lecture, *Oncology 1970: Proc. Int. Cancer Cong. 10th* (1972) **5**, 1.
96. Higginson, J., *Oncology 1970: Proc. Int. Cancer Congr. 10th* (1972) **5**, 300.
97. Evans, I. A., Mainwaring-Burton, R., Allport, B. R., Grey, N., *Medical Primatol.* (1972) **3**, 241.

14

Carcinogens in Food

P. Grasso and C. O'Hare, The British Industrial Biological Research
Association, Woodmansterne Road, Carshalton, Surrey, England

CHEMICAL CARCINOGENS COMPRISE organic compounds of many different types
and a few inorganic substances, and these can cause tumors in a wide range of
mammalian species including man. Pott (*1*) made the earliest observations
on man and first perceived an etiological relationship between the scrotal
cancer of chimney sweeps and the soot to which they were occupationally exposed. This observation was amply confirmed, and work in the 1930's by
Cook *et al.* (*2*) demonstrated that the responsible agents in soot were a family
of polycylic aromatic hydrocarbons (*see* Chapter 5).

Other chemicals have been firmly associated with the development of
cancer in man. For example, vesical cancer is caused by 2-naphthylamine
(*3*), lung cancer by mustard gas (*4*), hepatic cancer by vinyl chloride (*5*),
and vaginal cancer by diethylstilbestrol (*6*). All these chemicals were carcinogenic when administered to rodents, although the organ affected was not always
the same as in man. Mustard gas and vinyl chloride affected the same organ as
in man, but diethylstilbestrol induced mammary adenocarcinoma in the
mouse (*7*) instead of vaginal tumors, and 2-naphthylamine produced hepatic
tumors in the mouse (*8*). In the dog, 2-naphthylamine produced the same
type of tumor as it did in man (*9*).

Experiences of this sort have led to the generally accepted view that
laboratory animals could serve as a good indication of human carcinogenic
hazard, and animal results have served as the basis on which judgments are
made about the suitability of chemicals for addition to food.

Species Response

Apart from the compounds that have been shown to be carcinogenic in
man, there are numerous others that induced cancer when tested in animals
by various routes (*10*). An interesting feature of these results is the fact that
the carcinogens do not necessarily have the same activity in all species. In
fact, it is common in some circles to speak of a "species barrier," meaning a

resistance on the part of some animal species to tumor induction by certain carcinogens. This resistance may be total, as in the case of the guinea pig which resists tumor induction by the potent carcinogen 2-fluorenylacetamide (FAA, AAF) (11), or partial, as exemplified by the induction of hepatic nodular lesions of a questionable neoplastic nature in the mouse by doses of aflatoxin which are powerfully carcinogenic in the rat. This resistance almost certainly involves the manner in which the compound is metabolized. Thus, it is known that FAA is converted first to the N-hydroxy compound and then to the sulfate ester in the rat, and experiments have shown that this ester behaves as the ultimate carcinogen (12) (Chapter 16). In the guinea pig N-hydroxylation does not occur, so that the carcinogenic intermediate is not formed, and no hepatocarcinogenic effect ensues. The difference in the carcinogenic effect of aflatoxin between rat and mouse could possibly be explained on a similar basis (13). Differences of a less well defined nature may occur between strains within the same species and between the sexes, and young and old of the same strain.

Genetic Factors

Recent observations point to other factors which might also powerfully influence the carcinogenicity of a particular compound in mammals. Studies of a few human diseases with a proclivity toward cancer development indicated that these diseases are genetically transmitted and furthermore, the inherited defect involves a defective DNA repair mechanism. Thus Cleaver (14) demonstrated that the DNA from the epidermis of patients with xeroderma pigmentosum is defective in excision repair of dimers following uv damage and postulated that this defect may be the underlying cause of the susceptibility of these patients to skin carcinoma on exposure to uv light or to sunlight. A similar defect seems to be one of the main features of the DNA in patients with Fanconi's anaemia, a group in which a high incidence of spontaneous neoplasia occurs (15). In view of these observations, it is of interest that carcinogens appear not only to induce DNA damage but also to interfere with DNA repair. This type of lesion has been described in hepatic DNA following the administration of single doses of the hepatocarcinogens, N-nitrosodimethylamine, N-nitrosodiethylamine, N-nitrosomorpholine, N-nitrosopiperidine, and FAA to rats (16). There are some interesting exceptions. For example, aflatoxin damages hepatic DNA in the rat but does not seem to interfere with DNA repair (16).

Observations of this sort have a profound bearing on attempts to extrapolate from one animal species to another. Differences in metabolism usually indicate differences in enzyme pathways which in turn reflect genetic differences. Such differences between species may mean that compounds with a high carcinogenic risk in some species present little or no risk to others, as the examples of aflatoxin and FAA cited previously indicate. Obviously a better knowledge of these genetic differences with their implications in terms of carcinogenic risk would be a great asset in assisting in that important but hazardous step known to toxicologists as "extrapolation from animal data to man." Genetic differences seem also to be responsible for individual susceptibility within a particular species. The human examples cited above illustrate this. A better knowledge of these genetic differences may enable the identification of susceptible groups so that steps may be taken for their appropriate protection. At present, however, these considerations are of theoretical interest only and must await a more complete understanding of the biology of cancer before they are put into practice.

For the moment we can only follow the advice given by earlier authors (*17*) and assume that a substance which is carcinogenic for one species is strongly suspected to present the same type of hazard for other species, including man. As a result methods other than those using metabolic or genetic differences have to be used to assess this hazard.

The Statistical Approach

In general the recognition of a connection between the induction of a particular type of cancer in man and a particular chemical was made from observations of workers exposed under industrial conditions or, in the case of diethylstilbestrol, from the administration of high therapeutic doses. Under these conditions exposure tends to be fairly intensive, and there is a good chance that it may be identified. In other situations—and this applies particularly to food—the concentrations of the chemical carcinogens to which man is exposed are very low indeed. At present, much thought is being given to the relative hazards of these low levels and how they could be assessed. Certainly, no firm association has been established between any human cancer and the low levels of carcinogens which are found in food, but this may only reflect the imperfect state of the epidemiological investigations presently available. Consideration of current views on the mode of action of chemical carcinogens does not allow the hazard from these low levels to be ignored, especially since these exposures may occur throughout the lifetime of most of the general population.

At the molecular level carcinogens, either directly or/after metabolic transformation, interact with specific sites in the cell, resulting in changes which effectively transform the cell so that it is no longer controllable by homeostatic forces. The extent to which these interactions have to proceed to transform the cell is not known, so some workers (*18*) have drawn attention to the fact that the ultimate in chemical carcinogenesis is an interaction between one molecule of carcinogen and one molecule of target cell, implying that even at such levels the effects of carcinogens may not be disregarded. Against this view is the fact that not all animals in a group treated with appropriately high doses of carcinogens develop cancer, and in the human situation of high level industrial exposure only a proportion of workmen develop tumors. It thus appears that if in high risk situations a proportion of those exposed do not develop cancer, this proportion becomes increasingly greater as the concentration of the carcinogen becomes smaller, and in theory one could postulate a dose at which this risk is negligible.

Several attempts have been made to find an acceptable way of computing this "safe" dose. Mantel and Bryan (*17*) approached the problem from the epidemiological standpoint and considered that the virtually safe dose is one which would cause no more than one tumor in 100 million people. Experimentally, this sort of dose level has been extremely difficult to establish since it is virtually impossible to assess the carcinogenic effect of carcinogens at the low levels in which they are found in food, because of the large numbers of experimental animals that are required for this purpose. As a consequence there has been a tendency to develop mathematical models which are used to extrapolate the value of this safe dose from results obtained at dose levels which yield an unequivocally carcinogenic response.

Basically these methods depend on the numbers of tumors induced in animal groups of practicable size and rely on observations by several authors indicating that the number of tumors induced is related to the dose administered. This dose–response relationship has been expressed as a mathematical formula by Druckrey (19) in his studies on the pharmacological approach to carcinogenesis. Recently the members of an FDA panel on carcinogenesis attempted to extrapolate in realistic terms from the results of a "typical" dose–response study using high doses of a given chemical carcinogen and limited numbers of animals to the dose at which the tumor incidence would be one in 100 million. They found that the value of this dose varied according to the type of mathematical treatment selected for the extrapolation. This variation was so great that they concluded that extrapolation from the observable range to a safe dose has many of the perplexities and imponderables of extrapolation from animal to man, and it would be imprudent to place excessive reliance on mathematical sleight of hand, particularly when the dose–response curves used are largely empirical descriptions, lacking any theoretical, physical, or chemical basis (20).

Perhaps because of these difficulties other approaches have been proposed. These depend on the time of appearance of tumors in relation to the age of the animal or to the time interval after the first administration of the carcinogen (latent period). It is assumed that a certain proportion of the animals develop tumors naturally towards the end of their life span. This incidence, as well as the time of appearance, depend of course on the nature and type of the tumor. Carcinogens not only increase this incidence but also cause tumors to appear much earlier than would normally be expected. By appropriate mathematical treatment the age-related tumor incidence at a particular age of the animal can be computed.

An approach of this sort was suggested recently by Jones and Grendon (21) to assess the hazard presented by low levels of carcinogens in our environment. This approach seeks to establish the relationship of dose to time of appearance of cancer. By examining data of cancer incidence obtained from the survivors of the atomic bomb radiation at Hiroshima and Nagasaki, the latent period for the appearance of cancer was found to be inversely related to the cube root of the dose. This relationship also held when applied to the radiation-induced bone sarcoma incidence in workers in luminous paint factories. By application of this relationship expressed by the formula $T = t$ $(D_o/D)^{1/n}$ where $n = 3$, t = latent period for the carcinogenic dose D_o, D_o = applied dose, and D = the dose of the same carcinogen for which it is desired to calculate the latent period, T) it was possible to show that any tumors expected from exposure to natural levels of radiation would arise beyond the maximum expected life span of man. Hence it was possible to compute a virtually "safe" level of radiation.

This reasoning has been applied to chemical carcinogenicity studies with some degree of success. The recent concern about the safety of the small amounts of diethylstilbestrol likely to be present in beef from cattle treated with this hormone to improve feed conversion provides an interesting example. During the 1950's diethylstilbestrol was given in large doses (approximately 1.5 mg/day) to humans throughout pregnancy to avert the threat of an abortion. It came to light recently that a high incidence of vaginal adenocarcinoma developed in young girls whose mothers had this intensive hormone therapy during pregnancy. Approximately 58 cases of vaginal adenocarcinoma have been reported so far, many of them in women born in 1951–1955. If one assumes on the basis of the figures published by Heinonen (22), that 1% of all pregnant women received diethylstilbestrol, it can be calculated by the method of Jones and Grendon (21) that the maximum overall risk from diethylstilbestrol in beef, assuming it is present at the lowest detectable concentration of 2 ppb, is approximately 3×10^8 or, using the current birth rate in the U.S., about one birth every eight years. But this omits the fact that not all the diet is beef and that the figures on which the calculations were based are biased heavily to obtain the most pessimistic estimate. Jones and Grendon (21) calculate that a more realistic estimate of risk is one affected birth in ten million years.

Such reasoning and calculations were applied to three experimental situations: the calculation of risk tumor incidence in experimental animals from low doses of nitrosamines, urethane, and polycyclic aromatic hydrocarbons of the order found in the human environment and particularly in food or beverages. In all three situations tumor induction by these small doses would require a time period equivalent to ten or more times the average life span of the test species. If one assumes that man is as sensitive as the most sensitive species (which, fortunately in these particular instances, is the rat or mouse), then any tumors that these carcinogens are likely to cause from their presence in food or drink would appear at a time period corresponding to 10–20 times the human lifespan. The report of the FDA on carcinogenesis (20) and the paper of Jones and Grendon (21) discuss this important topic more fully.

Both nitrosamines and polycyclic aromatic hydrocarbons are found at low levels in food intended for human consumption and, in this chapter, the type of food in which they are found and the factors that are responsible for their presence are outlined. Attention has also been directed to other carcinogens which have been reported in food. Because of the extensive literature that has grown around this topic, it has only been possible to present a brief account of these, leaving considerations of the biochemistry and molecular biology of these compounds and other aspects which are not strictly related to food to the authors of other chapters.

Polycyclic Aromatic Hydrocarbons

This group of chemicals contains some of the most potent carcinogens known to man. Originally discovered in coal tar and shale oil (2), polycyclic aromatic hydrocarbons (PAHs) are now known to occur in various natural and cooked foods and in soil and water. A number of PAH compounds have been identified analytically, but for the majority data are either lacking or attempts to demonstrate carcinogenic activity have failed. Five of the compounds give a consistent carcinogenic response in experimental animals. The best known of these is benzo[a]pyrene (BP). The other four are dibenz[a,h] anthracene, benz[a]anthracene, benzo[b]fluoranthene, and benzo[k]fluoranthene (23). These occur either in raw or cooked foods in a range of concentrations. Table I gives levels likely to be found under average conditions. Some high figures have also been included to indicate the maximum PAH content probable.

Table I. Polycyclic Aromatic Hydrocarbons in Foods

Foodstuff	Benzo[a]-pyrene (ppb)	Benz[a]-anthracene (ppb)	Literature Cited
Fresh vegetables[a]	2.85–24.5	0.3–43.6	24, 25
Vegetable oils	0.4–1.4	0.8–1.1	27, 189, 190
Coconut oil	43.7	98.0	28, 29, 191
Margarine	0.4–0.5	1.4–3.0	192
Mayonnaise	0.4	2.2	192
Coffee	0.3–1.3	1.3–3.0	193, 194
Tea	3.9	2.9–4.6	193
Grain[a]	0.19–4.13	0.40–6.85	32, 195, 196
Oysters and mussels	1.5–9.0	—	197, 198
Smoked ham	3.2	2.8	26, 45, 199
Smoked fish[b]	0.83	1.9	40, 45, 199, 200
Smoked bonito	37	189	201
Cooked sausage	12.5–18.8	17.5–26.2	199, 202, 203
Singed meat	35–99	28–79	204
Broiled meat	0.17–0.63	0.2–0.4	44, 200, 205
Charcoal-broiled steak[a]	8.0	4.5	44, 205
Broiled mackerel	0.9	2.9	51
Barbecued beef	3.3	13.2	199
Barbecued ribs	10.5	3.6	44

[a] Dibenz[a,h]anthracene has been detected in charcoal-broiled meat (0.2 ppb), grain (0.1–0.61 ppb), and fresh vegetables (0.04–1.71 ppb).
[b] A number of Russian studies (206, 208) reported higher levels, up to 8.5 ppb of benzo[a]pyrene in smoked fish.

From Botanical Sources. PAHs have been demonstrated in a variety of raw edible green vegetables. Grimmer and Hildebrandt (24) identified 13 PAHs in lettuce, tomatoes, leeks, cabbage, and spinach from various parts of Germany. The latter two vegetables were especially rich in both carcinogenic (dibenz[a,h]anthracene, BP) and noncarcinogenic types. The presence of PAHs in edible green vegetables was confirmed by Gräf and Diehl (25) who also demonstrated their presence in the leaves of various trees.

Edible products manufactured from plants may also contain carcinogenic PAHs. They have been detected in refined vegetable oils derived from soybean, cottonseed, corn, olive, and peanut. The highest concentration of BP (1.5 ppb) was found in soybean oil and the highest total PAH concentration in peanut oil (*26*). Howard *et al.* (*27*) thought that the PAHs may have been transferred to the oil from solvents used in the refining process, but detailed analyses showed that this was unlikely. In a further study, Grimmer and Hildebrant (*28, 29*) analyzed some unrefined edible oils and fats for 13 PAH compounds. Crude coconut oil contained over 1 ppm phenanthrene, 129–402 ppb of other noncarcinogenic PAHs, 44 ppb BP, and smaller amounts of other carcinogenic PAHs while sunflower seed and palm kernal oils had the highest BP content. The widespread presence of PAHs in vegetable oils helps to explain the presense of these compounds in margine and mayonnaise.

Three sources of PAHs in plants have been postulated—endogenous synthesis, atmospheric pollution, and contamination from soil. Gräf and Diehl (*25*) showed that the PAH content increased up to fivefold in leaves during yellowing and in starchy bulbs and seeds soon after germination. Contamination from the environment or the soil to this extent was thought unlikely, and they suggested that biosynthesis of PAHs within the plants could account for this increase. Endogenous synthesis of PAHs could also account for some of the observations of Grimmer and Hildebrandt (*24*). These authors found that the degree of vegetable contamination appeared to depend on the surface area and on the exposure time before sale. Careful washing of the plant removed only one tenth of the PAH content, suggesting that environmental or soil contamination accounts for only a small proportion of the PAHs present.

Lower forms of plant life may also synthesize PAHs thus contributing to the total environmental content. Borneff and Fischer (*30*) identified at least 7 PAHs, among which was BP, in phytoplankton taken from the Bodensee in Germany. BP was found at a level of 2 ppm in the dried phytoplankton. PAHs have also been found in algae at levels much higher than environmental levels and in places remote from possible sources of PAH pollution, indicating synthesis within the plants. The synthesis of PAHs by phytoplankton is important since the compounds may enter the food chain which ends up in man, thus adding to the PAH burden. The synthesis of PAHs by the algal plants is interesting since it may contribute to the presence of PAHs in water and soil (*31*).

The data of Tilgner (*32*) suggest, however, that in certain areas atmospheric pollution may be an important source of crop contamination by PAH. Thus the PAH content of grain freshly harvested from fields close to heavily industrialized districts was about 10 times higher than that of grain grown far from industrial areas. Perhaps the PAH content of flour reported by various authors may have been from such sources, although in some instances drying by oil-fired burners might be a contributory factor (*33*). The soil itself may also contribute its small quota of PAHs.

The contribution of the soil to crop contamination by PAH is intriguing. Soil hydrocarbons were the subject of an intensive study by Blumer (*34*). The carcinogenic benzo[*a*]pyrene and the probably inactive benzo[*e*]pyrene were found in all samples of Swiss soil analyzed up to a level of 21 ppm. In samples of Connecticut and Massachusetts soils, the levels were in the region of 40–1300 μg/kg. PAHs were also found in Germany in soil from places far removed from industrial areas or human habitation. In some of the latter areas the PAHs were present in a concentration of 100–200 ppm. The presence of PAHs in these remote areas is difficult to explain on the basis of atmospheric pollution from industrial plants or others sources. The observations quoted in prevoius paragraphs suggest that PAHs in soil may be largely a residue from decaying vegetation. Their significance is not fully understood, but it would appear unlikely that they contribute to the PAH content of edible plants to any meaningful extent, although they may account for part of the PAH content of drinking water.

Decaying vegetation is not of course the only source of BP and other PAHs in water. Rain and storm water wash away PAHs together with other industrial pollutants into rivers and lakes. Eventually some of this finds its way into the sea. Extensive investigations established the content of PAHs, especially the carcinogenic ones, in water. Surface waters, chiefly lakes, rivers, and the sea, contain an average of 0.025–0.100 μg PAHs/l. Higher concentrations up to 1.0 μg/l. are found in heavily polluted rivers like the Rhine (35). The PAH concentration of the seabed is understandably quite high (up to 1,500 μg/kg dry sand or mud) close to the shores of industrialized countries like France, but a small amount of BP was also found off the west coast of Greenland, which is virtually unpopulated and far from any shipping lanes. In contrast, there seems to be little difference in the PAH content of samples of phytoplankton and other similar marine species taken from these two sources (36, 37).

Ground and drinking water contain less PAHs than the sea. The average range found in a number of samples taken from various countries in Europe is 0.001–0.010 μg/l. (35). Despite the sources of contamination mentioned, the PAH content of drinking water need not necessarily be high since it can be reduced by suitable filtration or chemical treatment (38). The maximum recommended concentration of PAHs in drinking water in terms of six specific compounds, which include the three carcinogens BP, benzo[b]fluoranthene and indeno [1,2,3-cd]pyrene, is 0.2 μg/l. (39).

The contribution of PAHs to human intake from water and other natural sources is much less than that resulting from some forms of cooking. A number of authors have shown that smoked fish and bacon contain small amounts of polynuclear hydrocarbons (40, 41, 42) while the early studies of Lijinsky and Shubik (43, 44) demonstrated the presence of these compounds, including the carcinogenic BP, in broiled meat. Barbecued pork, cured ham, and smoked whiting were found by Howard and Fazio (45) to contain 4.5, 3.2, and 6.9 ppb of BP, respectively. Charcoal-broiled meats contained even higher concentrations of BP—10.5 ppb in barbecued ribs and 50 ppb in some T-bone steaks.

In Cooked Food. The conditions leading to the formation of PAHs on cooking were studied in detail by Lijinsky and Ross (46). The higher the fat content, the greater was the amount of BP and other PAHs found after broiling. Thus a hamburger with a high fat content contained about 43 ppb of total PAHs, the BP content being 2.6 ppb. The lean variety contained 2.8 ppb PAH but no BP. Other cooking conditions also had a considerable influence on the PAH content. Thus cooking close to the flame led to a high content of PAH while slow cooking away from the heat source considerably diminished their concentration. Equally successful in this respect was the separation of dripping fat from the flame.

Separating the meat from the source of heat meant a lower cooking temperature at which only the simpler PAHs—pyrene and fluoranthrene—were formed. The authors concluded that to minimize carcinogen production, "the method of cooking should be such as to avoid contact of the food with cooking flames, to cook for a longer period at lower temperatures and to use meat with a minimum of fat." These conclusions are supported by the recent work of Rhee and Bratzler (47) who showed that wrapping meat in cellulose sheets prior to smoking can reduce the BP concentration in the final product from 11–12 to 4.5 ppb. A BP reduction of this order can also be achieved by discarding the fat released during the cooking of smoked bacon.

Lijinsky and Ross (46) recognized that their recommendations may alter considerably the flavor of the cooked meat but found it difficult to make suggestions in order to preserve it. They were more successful in preserving the flavor of smoked foods while reducing the PAH content considerably (48). They did this by developing "liquid smokes" produced by water absorption of wood smoke from which tarry droplets have been removed by filtration. This liquid smoke imparts the same flavor as the traditional methods. White (49) analyzed the BP content of several liquid smokes and of their tarry filtrates. He found no BP in the seven kinds of liquid smokes examined, but the tarry filtrates contained up to 3800 ppb of BP. The liquid smokes did, however, contain 1.7 ppb of 4-methyl BP, a substance which is a less potent carcinogen than BP.

Other sources of pollution with PAHs originate in industrial processes or other human activities. These may contaminate food exposed for sale in open markets but the amount contributed to the total PAH content is negligible. It would thus appear that there are two principal sources of PAH carcinogens— endogenous synthesis within a variety of plants and the traditional methods of cooking, namely smoking fish and meat and broiling meat. The latter source seems to be largely preventable by the use of "liquid smokes" and by avoiding fat pyrolysis. There are no means available at the moment to reduce the synthesis of polycyclic aromatic hydrocarbon carcinogens in vegetables.

The significance of these low levels of PAH carcinogens in food is difficult to assess. Undoubtedly, they are among the most potent carcinogens known, and every effort should be made to reduce their concentration in food. There are no clear indications, however, that they cause human cancer. Thus despite their fairly widespread distribution in the vegetable kingdom there is no indication that vegetarians have a higher cancer incidence than the rest of the population. Attempts to link the high incidence of stomach cancer in Japan and in some parts of Iceland with PAH carcinogens in food are not convincing (50, 51), and there are suggestions now that other articles of diet may be involved, for example bracken or asbestos in Japan. Furthermore, there are indications that low levels of BP, probably one of the most potent of the PAHs found in food, do not produce tumors in experimental animals. The repeated application of 1.25 μg of BP in acetone to the skin of mice for 68 weeks failed to produce tumors (52) while administration of BP in the diet to mice at 10 ppm or less also had no effect (53). Although one cannot accept these data without some reservations, they indicate that the hazard from PAHs in food may not be as great as might be expected on a first appraisal of the problem.

Nitrosamines

Considerable attention is currently being given to the presence of nitrosamines in food. Nitrosamines as a group, however, have been of interest to toxicologists and cancer research workers for several years (Chapter 11). In 1954 Barnes and Magee (54) reported three cases of jaundice with advanced cirrhosis of the liver suspected to have been caused by industrial exposure to N-nitrosodimethylamine (dimethylnitrosamine; DMN). They investigated the the toxicological properties of this nitrosamine in the rat and found it to be both a potent hepatotoxin and hepatocarcinogen (55, 56). A great number of nitrosamines homologous with DMN have been synthesized in the intervening years, and most of these are carcinogenic to laboratory animals. Cyclic nitrosamines and nitrosamides have been investigated as well in several species and, with few exceptions, the compounds were found to be carcinogenic (57, 58, 59).

In Fish. Food toxicologists were not interested in nitrosamines for several years. This seemed logical since the carcinogenic activity of these compounds was so well known that it was inconceivable that anyone would think of using them in any process which involved their contact with food. However, an epidemic of food poisoning in sheep which took place in Norway in 1962 (60) stimulated considerable interest in the possibility of a carcinogenic hazard to man from this group of compounds. The epidemic was traced to the consumption of nitrite-treated fish meal. Pathological examination of the stricken sheep revealed advanced hepatotoxic changes, and it was assumed that death was caused by hepatic failure (61). The economic loss caused to farmers attracted the attention of research workers who demonstrated the presence of DMN (62). The apparently spontaneous formation of DMN in nitrite-treated fish raised the possibility that a similar state of affairs might well occur in meat and other articles of diet treated with nitrates or nitrites.

Ender and his colleagues (63) paid attention to the factors that control the formation of nitrosamine in fish. The concentration of nitrite present and the temperature at which the fish was kept were found to be important in determining the amount of DMN present. In experiments carried out at 130°C for 2-hr periods, increasing the amount of nitrite 18-fold led to a 30-fold increase in the DMN level. At temperatures below 50°C this same increase in the amount of nitrite led to only a 13-fold increase in DMN. Since exposure to the higher temperature must have accelerated the protein degradation, the concentration of secondary amines in the food is clearly as important as that of the nitrite determining the amount of DMN formed. Presumably this is why fish that had been refrigerated yielded no more DMN than fresh fish on the addition of nitrite and heating at 130°C for 2 hr.

In one way or another cooking involves the application of heat, often at temperatures considerably higher than 130°C. This led Sen *et al.* (*64*) to investigate nitrosamine formation in cooked fish. They found that DMN, *N*-nitrosodiethylamine (DEN), and *N*-nitrosodi-*n*-propylamine could be detected in six varieties of fish after treating with up to 200 ppm nitrite and heating to 110°C for 60–70 min. No nitrosamines were detected in unheated specimens. The amount of nitrosamines found varied from 8 μg to less than 0.5 μg/100 g. The authors attributed the variation in the yield of carcinogens to the variable amount of secondary and tertiary amines in fish.

Compared with the studies on nitrosamine formation in fish, little has been published on nitrosamine formation in other foodstuffs. Ender's figures (*65*) (*see* Table II) indicate that nitrite-preserved meat contains small amounts

Table II. Volatile Nitrosamines in Some Types of Human Food

| Food | Nitrosamine[a] (ppb) | | | | | Literature Cited |
	Unspecified	DMN	PYR	DEN	PIP	
Herring meal	30–100 ppm	ND	ND	ND	ND	61
Kippers	40	ND	ND	ND	ND	65
Haddock	15	ND	ND	ND	ND	65
Sausage	0.8–2.4	ND	ND	ND	ND	65
Bacon	0.6–6.5	ND	ND	ND	ND	65
Ham	5.7	ND	ND	ND	ND	65
Mushrooms	1.4–30	ND	ND	ND	ND	65
Cheese	0–0.05 ppm	ND	ND	ND	ND	67
Fried bacon						
back pale Danish		0–4	0–4	ND	ND	69
back, pale		1–4	16–40	ND	ND	69
back smoked, Danish		<1	ND	<1	ND	69
back rashers, Danish smoked		ND	ND	ND	<1	69
Cod (salted, fresh or fried)		0–9	ND	ND	ND	69
Hake (fresh or fried)		0–9	ND	ND	ND	69
Haddock		0–9	ND	ND	ND	69
Luncheon meat		1–4	ND	ND	ND	69
Pork (Danish)		1–4	1–4	ND	ND	69
Salami (Hungarian)		1–4	ND	ND	ND	69

[a] DMN, *N*-nitrosodimethylamine; PYR, *N*-nitrosopyrrolidine; DEN, *N*-nitrosodiethylamine; PIP, *N*-nitrosopipendine; ND, not detected.

(0.5–5.0 ppb) of nitrosamines. Hedler and Marquardt (*66*) claimed to have isolated DMN from samples of wheat flour, grain, and plant in Germany as well as from milk and cheese. Earlier, Kroller (*67*) claimed to have found nitrosamines in cheese, a not-unexpected finding since cheese is in general rich in secondary amines, and some types of cheese are preserved with nitrate. Other sources may be responsible for the contamination of milk with nitrite.

Recent studies indicate that the amounts of nitrosames found may be greater than these figures suggest. Wasserman *et al.* (*86*) reported the presence of DMN from 3–48 μg/kg in frankfurters while Crosby *et al.* (*69*) reported levels of 0–40 μg/kg in fried bacon, 0–9 μg/kg in fish, and 0–4 μg/kg in cheeses. In addition to DMN these authors also found nitroso-pyrrolidine in the same range of concentrations and traces of DEN and nitrosopiperidine. These levels may not tell the whole story since, apart from inherent difficulties in quantitative analysis of these small concentrations, in-vestigations have been limited to volatile nitrosamines. A search for the nonvolatile compounds may tell a different story.

An interesting facet of investigations of nitrosamines in food is the frequent observation that no nitrosamines are detected. For example, Crosby *et al.* (*69*) failed to detect nitrosamines in gammon and other types of bacon, in kippers, herring, skate, mackerel, and plaice, in a number of salami and cheese samples, in smoked Westphalian ham, and in Irish bacon. The reasons for these negative results are not clear. The nitrosamine content may vary within wide limits and where negative results are recorded nitrosamines prob-ably are present below the detection level. The development of more sensitive analysis methods may show that a much wider variety of foodstuffs are con-taminated with nitrosamines than is presently thought. The variability in nitrosamine content emphasizes the importance of directing attention to the factors responsible for their formation in food.

Natural Occurrence. In the previous sections attention was directed to the formation of nitrosamines in those foods to which nitrate or nitrite is added intentionally as a preservative. The discovery of naturally occurring nitrosamines in mushrooms is probably as important as their discovery in nitrate and nitrite-treated fish meal. Formation of nitrosamines in this edible plant, presumably from endogenous nitrates, suggests that other plants with a high nitrate content, such as spinach, may also contain small but measurable amounts of these potent carcinogens.

An interesting observation in the Bantu tribe revealed the unexpected nature of the circumstances that might lead to the formation of nitrosamines in plant and their possible hazard. A high incidence of esophageal cancer was observed in certain circumscribed areas of the Transkei, and a search was made for possible carcinogenic effect of some article in the diet. During these investigations it was noted that the areas of high esophageal cancer coincided with areas of molybdenum deficiency in the leaves of important food plants such as pumpkins, beans, and maize. Molybdenum deficiency in these plants leads to a disturbance of nitrogen metabolism and the accumulation of nitrates in the food plants. This led Du Plessis *et al.* (*70*) to think of the possibility of nitrosamine formation under conditions of molybdenum deficiency. They selected for study the fruit of a plant, *Solanum incanum,* whose juice is used in the areas of high cancer incidence to curdle milk. An ethanolic extract of this fruit contained a nitrosamine fraction from which DMN was isolated. Commenting on this finding, Schoental (*71*) observed that *S. incanum* is widely used in parts of Central and East Africa as a herbal remedy and might be an important cause of liver cancer. Its etiological role in esophageal cancer is thought by this author to be of doubtful importance since DMN does not produce esophageal cancer experimentally.

Although experimental data are not available, some attention has been paid to the possible effect of cooking on nitrite-preserved meat. Lijinsky and Epstein (72) pointed out that during the cooking of meat, free amino acids (such as proline, arginine, and hydroxyproline) and secondary amines (such as pyrrolidine and piperidine) may be produced. The latter readily interact with nitrite to form the corresponding nitroso compounds. Since both nitrosopyrrolidine and nitrosopiperidine are hepatocarcinogenic to the rat (57), the speculation of Lijinsky and Epstein (72) is of great practical interest. Of much greater importance, however, are the claims outlined earlier that DMN and DEN are present in our food, since both these compounds are potent carcinogens to the rat. Thus DMN is reported to have produced hepatic tumors when fed to rats at 2 ppm and DEN to have induced tumors in the same organ when given in drinking water at 0.075 mg/kg (73, 73a). Despite intensive experimental investigations, however, it is difficult to assess the hazard to man from the small doses of carcinogens present in our environment, and until further experimental evidence is available no firm opinion can be given.

Formation *in Vivo*. So far we have limited our observation to the formation of nitrosamines in food before it is eaten. There is some experimental evidence and a good deal of speculation that interaction between nitrite and secondary amines may take place after ingestion. The principal site of their formation is thought to be the gastrointestinal tract. The conditions leading to nitrosamine formation differ according to the anatomical site. Thus in the stomach it is thought that the prevailing acidic conditions promote the chemical reaction leading to the formation of nitrosamines (74). Incubation of secondary amines with nitrite in the presence of gastric juice from a number of species has produced the corresponding N-nitroso compound (58, 75). The yield of nitrosamine was optimum in the pH range 1–3 and was much greater with weakly basic than with strongly basic secondary amines (76, 77).

Human and rabbit gastric juice, because of its low pH, was more effective in promoting this reaction than that of the rat. Perhaps because of the relatively high pH (4–5) of its stomach contents, the early experiments attempting to induce liver tumors in the rat by the feeding of sodium nitrite and diethylamine were unsuccessful (78). Later experiments with the feeding of nitrite and morpholine or N-methylbenzylamine produced malignant tumors in the liver or esophagus in rats, presumably from the corresponding nitroso compound (79).

In other parts of the gastrointestinal tract nitrosation of secondary amines is promoted by other agencies, principally bacterial action or chemical catalysis. *In vitro* coliform organisms of the type that inhabit the intestines of most mammals can nitrosate amines at pH values higher than the ones at which the reaction will occur spontaneously (76) while a hitherto unsuspected group of intestinal bacteria, including *clostridia, bacteroides*, and *lactobacilli*, effect this reaction at neutral pH (80).

These *in vitro* observations were recently confirmed *in vivo*. Alam, Saporoschetz, and Epstein (*81*) recovered nitrosopiperidine from the stomach or isolated loops of small intestine in rats after introducing piperidine and nitrate or nitrite. Earlier Sander and Seif (*82*) demonstrated the presence of the noncarcinogenic *N*-nitrosodiphenylamine in the gastric juice from human subjects who were previously given sodium nitrate and diphenylamine. The latter experiment is important in that it provides direct evidence of nitrate reduction to nitrite *in vivo*, probably by bacterial action.

Nitrosamine formation in the intestine may be assisted by chemical catalysts as well as by bacteria. Boyland *et al.* (*83*) demonstrated *in vitro* that both sodium iodide and sodium thiocyanate (1 mM conc. at pH 2) are effective catalysts of this reaction with nitrite concentrations as low as 0.1 mM. Sodium thiocyanate is a normal constituent of human saliva (0.06 mM) and was thought by the author to contribute to the synthesis of nitrosamines *in vivo*.

It is difficult however to assess this experimental evidence in relation to hazard to man. Undoubtedly, synthesis in the stomach is a possibility and in fact there is experimental evidence to support it. It is likely that if nitrosamine synthesis takes place here, it occurs either by virtue of the acidic pH or as a result of bacterial action. However, the concentrations of the precursors used in these model experiments are considerably higher than those normally met with in practice (*84*). One suspects that the test conditions are at or near the optimal ones for nitrosamine formation. It would be important to know to what extent, if at all, synthesis of nitrosamines occur at nitrate/nitrite concentrations usually taken in our food. Experimental results quoted earlier show conclusively that nitrosamine formation depends on the concentration of both the nitrate and the secondary amine present. Mirvish (*85*) showed from kinetic studies *in vitro* that the yield of nitrosamines under optimal conditions is directly proportional to the dimethylamine concentration and to the square of the concentration of nitrite. If the concentration of nitrite is low the nitrosamine formation rate may be very slow or indeed absent. Thus the minimum effective concentration of nitrite essential for nitrosamine formation by bacteria was found to be 12 mM (*80*). It may well be that for nitrosamine formation by direct or catalytic action some minimum effective concentration of both nitrite and secondary amine is required.

There are also other considerations to be taken into account. The human small intestine is virtually free of organisms so that any contribution from this source must be minimal. On the other hand, enzymatic degradation of protein proceeds here rapidly so substantial amounts of secondary amines might be present. The extent to which these are nitrosated would depend on the amount of nitrate/nitrite present, taking into account the possibility of its rapid absorption (*84*) and on the residence time of the secondary amines in the gut lumen. Since this is expected to be very short (*86*), the conditions for nitrosamine formation in the small intestine might not be quite optimal. In the colon and cecum the large numbers of coliform organisms present might be considered a potential source for nitrosamine formation. It is not certain, however, whether the nitrite or secondary amines are present in sufficient concentration to bring about nitrosamine synthesis. Thus, although from experimental evidence nitrosamine synthesis in the gut might be regarded a serious threat to health, there are grounds for doubting the validity of this conclusion, and a final judgment can not be reached until further work under more realistic conditions is carried out.

Plant Sources

Over the past few years, many often quite unrelated botanical species were identified as containing fractions which, when fed to laboratory animals, resulted in tumor formation. The overall hazard to man has to be evaluated in the light of this evidence. Whether the plant, and in particular the portion containing the carcinogen, is eaten occasionally or frequently by man and in what amounts is clearly the first and major consideration (Table III). Secondly, the possibility that the carcinogen may be removed by food processing methods has to be considered. In the long run appropriate epidemiological studies are needed, the results of which, in conjunction with experimental data and a knowledge of dietary habits, will considerably assist in evaluating human hazard.

Cycasin (Chapter 11), the toxic component of the cycad nut, is a good example of a carcinogen which is easily removed from food. The crude flour, prepared from unwashed nuts, induced malignant tumors in the liver and kidneys of rats when fed as 2% of the diet (*87*). Subsequent work has shown that the responsible carcinogenic agent is the glycoside beta-D-glucosyloxy-azoxymethane (*88*). In order to exercise its effect, the glycoside must be converted into methylazoxymethanol by the intestinal bacteria (*89*). Methylazoxymethanol is a potent carcinogen and induces a high incidence of tumors in rats after only one dose (*90*). Careful crushing and washing of the nuts during their preparation results in a flour free from the carcinogen. Indeed, rats have been maintained on diets containing up to 10% of commerical cycad flour without any evidence of a carcinogenic response (*91*). This conclusion is also verified by the limited epidemiological data available. As far as can be seen, the incidence of tumors, at least in the areas of Guam where some 95% of the population regularly eat cycad flour, is not significantly higher than one would expect (*92*). Nevertheless, further epidemiological data in Guam and the relevant areas of Japan would obviously be very useful in confirming this observation.

The pyrrolizidine alkaloids (Chapter 12), on the other hand, may present a real hazard to man, especially in the areas of the West Indies and Africa where they can be detected in bush teas and herbal remedies. They are found in many species of *Senecio, Crotalaria,* and *Heliotropium,* although the actual quantities involved and the type of alkaloid found vary widely (*93*). There can be little doubt that the alkaloids based on 1-hydroxymethyl-1,2-dehydropyr-rolizine can induce malignant liver tumors in laboratory animals (*94, 95*). Furthermore, liver lesions occur in the young of female rats fed pyrrolizidine alkaloids during pregnancy (*96, 97*), suggesting that the African practice of giving *Senecio*-based herbal remedies to pregnant women may be particularly dangerous (*98*). Opinion varies as to the mode of action of the pyrrolizidine

Table III.

Carcinogen	Food	Geographical Area
	Synthesis by Plants	
Pyrrolizidine alkaloids	bush teas and herbal remedies	Africa
Cycasin	cycad nuts and cycad flour	Guam, Japan
Thiourea	found in species of *Laburnum*	—
(Unidentified)	bracken	Japan, U.S., New Zealand
	Synthesis by Fungi	
Aflatoxin	total diet	Thailand
	peanuts	Uganda
	peanuts	Thailand
	peanut products	Taiwan
	peanut products	Thailand
	rice	Taiwan
	cassava	Uganda
	cereals	Thailand
	cereals	U.S.
	wine	Germany
	cottonseed meal	Universal
Luteoskyrin	rice	Japan
Sterigmatocystin	cereals and legumes	South Africa
	wheat and flour	universal

alkaloids (*95*), but whatever the results of this controversy, it will be necessary still to assess the actual hazard of the pyrrolizidine alkaloids. This is complicated by the fact that other carcinogens, *e.g.*, aflatoxin, are present in areas where these herbal remedies and bush teas are used (*98, 99, 100*).

Other natural products have been claimed to possess a carcinogenic potential. Safrole, for instance, the active ingredient of oil of sassafras, is a weak liver carcinogen to the rat (*101*). Although it is not now used as a flavoring for soft drinks, it is present in small quantities in cinnamon, nutmeg, and mace (*102*). Other methylenedioxyphenyls such as those present in sesame oil and myristicin occur in food.

Bracken (Chapter 13) is quite widely eaten as a delicacy in the United States, New Zealand, and Japan (*103*). The earliest feeding studies in which intestinal or bladder tumors were detected in the treated animals involved the incorporation of large quantities of bracken into the diet. With rats this was often 30–50% (*104, 105*), and with cattle a daily consumption of a half to one kilogram was not uncommon (*106, 107*). More recently it has been shown that many species are sensitive to the carcinogenic action of bracken and that the quantities involved may not be as large as was thought at first, at least with respect to the mouse (*108, 109*). Furthermore, the possibility remains that the carcinogen may be passed on to man in dairy products originating from cattle grazed on bracken. Transfer of the carcinogen to the offspring *via* the

Carcinogens in Food

Concentration	Literature Cited

Synthesis by Plants

usually $<0.1\%$; normal range $0.01–0.6\%$	*93, 209, 210*
usually $<1\%$; unusually as high as 2.2% (not found in commercial cycad flour)	*211, 212*
probably very low in human food	*100*
not known	*109*

Synthesis by Fungi

up to 1072 ng/kg/day intake	*135, 137, 138*
10 ppm	*213*
7–9 ppm	*135, 137, 138*
0.02–0.73 ppm	*214*
up to 6.5 ppm	*135, 137, 138*
0.2 ppm	*214*
1.7 ppm	*133*
0.4 ppm	*135, 137, 138*
2–19 ppb	*215*
$< 1 \mu g/1$	*216*
0.5 ppm	*217*
(work in progress)	*141*
(work in progress)	*144*
$< 0.10–0.15\%$	*218*

milk certainly occurs in mice (*110*). However, as the actual carcinogen has yet to be isolated, it is even more difficult to assess the potential hazard to man in this instance than with other carcinogens.

A survey of the genus *laburnum* shows that several species contain the well-known antithyroid compound, thiourea (*100*). Liver tumors (*111*), thyroid adenomas (*112*), and malignant tumors of the eyelid and ear duct (*113*) have all been induced in rats fed thiourea in their diet. Fortunately, these particular *laburnum* species are not known to be constituents of man's daily diet, although the related antithyroid compounds 1-5-vinyl-2-thioox-azolidone occurs in turnips, kale, cabbage, and rapeseed (*114*). Similarly, the liver tumors reported in rats fed very large quantities of red peppers and chillies (*115*) are not thought to have any great significance to man because of the grossly subnormal diet fed to the experimental animals (*116*). The overall hazard from either of these sources must be very low.

Several other foods or foodstuffs have been suggested as potential carcinogens as a result of epidemiological studies. It is realized that the results of such studies necessarily have to be interpreted with care. A correlation is not indicative of either a direct or indirect connection. Nevertheless, a wide range of food products have been linked with cancer in the past. Coffee consumption for instance has been correlated with pancreatic, ovarian, and prostatic cancer and with leukemia in one study (*117*) and with stomach cancer by another

(*118*). Similarly, spirit drinking has been suggested as a factor in the development of esophageal cancer in France (*119*). Others have claimed that diets containing sorghum or its tannins may well predispose to stomach cancer (*120*) or that saturated fats may increase the probability of fatal carcinomas (*121*). Further data on the latter claim (*122*) have shown that the correlation is almost certainly false. If the epidemiological factors influencing tumor production are as varied as some studies have shown (*123, 124*) it also seems likely that the list of correlations outlined above is not quite as simple as some workers would have us believe.

Fungal Sources

Microbial spoilage of food and the disease states associated with it have been recognized for many centuries. However, it has only recenly been realized that some microbial contaminants, especially fungi, could produce toxic and carcinogenic metabolites. The discovery of aflatoxin has stimulated work in the whole field of fungal contaminants with the result that many species are now seen to present a significant carcinogenic hazard both to farm animals and to man himself. While the individual toxins are now well known, there is still very little information on their combined effects, especially to those subsisting on nutritionally deficient diets. The incidence of liver tumors is high in many areas of the world where nutritional standards are low and where food is extremely prone to microbial attack, either from poor hygiene or from adverse climatic conditions. It will be many years before an overall evaluation of the hazard proffered by even common fungal contaminants can be made.

Aflatoxin is the most widely studied agent of the group. It is one of the most potent hepatocarcinogens known to man (Chapter 12). As little as 0.2 μg/day of aflatoxin B_1 is carcinogenic to the rat (*125*), and chronic feeding studies indicate that other species are equally susceptible, albeit at slightly higher levels of aflatoxin in the diet (*126*). Furthermore, a single dose as small as 0.5 mg of aflatoxin B_1 will induce a tumor incidence of 50% in rats over a subsequent period of 26 months (*127*). Nevertheless, some species have been sufficiently studied for a tentative tolerance limit to be set for aflatoxin contamination. Cattle for instance seem resistant if there is less than 0.66 ppm of aflatoxin in the diet (*128*). Similarly pigs are unaffected by levels of less than 0.4 ppm (*129*). In addition, although there is greater individual variation, it should also be possible to set safe levels of aflatoxin contamination for chickens, turkeys, and ducklings provided that the aflatoxin can be accurately determined and that sufficient allowance is made for these known variations (*130*).

There are four generally recognized aflatoxins, B_1, B_2, G_1, and G_2. Although they are generally associated with *Aspergillus flavus,* many other *Aspergillus* species and also members of the *Penicillium* and *Rhizopus* genera can also produce the carcinogens. This means that a range of both animal and human foodstuffs and not just the major source, peanuts, can become contaminated with aflatoxin (Table III). There is clearly therefore the possibility of a real hazard to man since the first criterion, the presence of the carcinogen in the diet, has been established. Not only can this arise directly but it could also result from the presence of aflatoxin M_1 and M_2 in the milk and cheese from cows fed aflatoxin-contaminated meal. These metabolites occur in the urine and milk of aflatoxin-treated animals and cause lesions in the duckling identical to those of aflatoxin B_1 (*131*). Aflatoxins M_1 and M_2 will have to be detected in milk and cheese on the open market, however, before this can be seen as a real hazard.

If aflatoxin occurs in the human diet, assuming that the human is affected like the rat, what evidence is there that it is a significant etiological factor in liver cancer? First of all, the incidence of this disease is high in the areas of the world where the climatic conditions are favorable for aflatoxin production, for example, in Uganda, South Africa, Nigeria, French East Africa, French West Africa, the East Indies, and Eastern Asia (*132*). While this could be caused by a number of other factors, the presence of aflatoxin in the food of these people does suggest that it may be at least one of the more important of these factors. It is of course very difficult to show specifically that aflatoxin has been the primary cause of a given liver lesion, although in one recent case (*133*) the author was very confident that contaminated cassava had caused the death of a young boy in Uganda. Histological examination of his liver showed centrilobular degeneration and necrosis very similar to that observed in a group of monkeys that consumed a comparable amount of aflatoxin (*134*).

A very recent study (*135, 136, 137, 138*) showed that aflatoxin contamination of food is extremely common in Southeast Asia and particularly in Thailand. Three two-day surveys over a period of one year in 144 randomly selected households showed that in some areas of Thailand 73–81 ng of aflatoxin/kg/day are ingested by most of the families. In some individual cases, intakes as high as 1972 ng/kg/day were recorded, and some children were found to consume as 163 μg/kg/day at the height of the peanut harvest. This is 20–30% of the intake required to induce 100% tumors in rats. On the other hand, peanuts and peanut meal represent one of the few high protein foods available to these people. Bearing this in mind, various authorities such as the Protein Advisory Group of FAO/WHO (*139*) have proposed, as an interim measure, that 30 μg/kg should be the upper limit of aflatoxin contamination which can be tolerated in human food. Even at this level, however, the intake of aflatoxin in affluent countries is considerably less than this figure would suggest since only a fraction of the total food intake is made up of components likely to contain aflatoxin.

Luteoskyrin, a metabolite of a number of *Penicillium* species, is another potent carcinogen found on contaminated food, in this case usually rice. The incorporation of the so-called "yellowed rice" into the diets of rats at a level of 5% produced hepatomas (*140*); the purified toxin is equally potent (*141*). Once again, liver cancer is common in the parts of the world where rice provides the staple diet but without detailed epidemiological studies it is impossible to assess the significance of luteoskyrin as a possible causative agent. On the other hand, a metabolite of *Aspergillus versicolor*, is thought to be closely connected with the high incidence of liver tumors in the Bantu tribe of South Africa. The hepatocellular carcinomas found in rats especially males fed diets containing as little as 10 ppm sterigmatocystin (*142*) suggest that it is of the same order of potency as aflatoxin to the rat and that the appearance of the tumors is very similar to those found in man in South Africa. Clearly sterigmatocystin may be as important a carcinogen in terms of its actual hazard to man as the more carcinogenic affatoxin (143). It is to be hoped that the recently published analytical method for detecting sterigmatocystin (144) will soon be put to use to quantitate the sterigmatocystin in the Bantu diet.

The case against patulin, penicillic acid, and the lactones, epoxides, and peroxides, closely related to them, is not as strong. It is well known that both patulin and penicillic acid are formed on cereal grains contaminated with *Penicillium* and *Aspergillus* species and that man therefore may be exposed to these compounds in his diet. A substantial list of structurally related fungal metabolites has also been drawn up (145), although their presence in food is not as well documented. More importantly, however, the validity of the methods used to demonstrate the carcinogenicity of penicillic acid, lactones, epoxides, and peroxides—that is repeated subcutaneous injections into rats (146, 147, 148)—has been put into serious doubt (149).

Finally, there are some fungi which produce metabolic products that, while themselves not recognized as carcinogens, are closely related to other chemicals which do possess these properties (145). Aromatic amines, alkyl nitroso compounds, and hydroxamates are the most commonly quoted sources of these potential carcinogens (150). Until the organisms producing them are found in human food and the metabolites identified in man's daily diet, they should not be allowed to overshadow the fungal toxins which are understood more fully and which do present a practical hazard to many thousands of people.

Metals

A number of the metals present in trace amounts in our food have produced tumors in experimental animals. Selenium produced hepatomas when fed to rats in the organic form or as the selenide at a level of 5–10 mg/kg (151). Lead induced renal tumors in rats when given parenterally as lead phosphate or orally as lead acetate (152, 153, 154), and cadmium produced testicular tumors in rats, in addition to local sarcomas, when injected subcutaneously (155, 156). The daily intake of these compounds is difficult to assess accurately because they occur in a variety of foodstuffs and in drinking water. It is estimated that the daily intake of selenium, based on the data of Smith and Westfall (157), is less than 1 mg., of lead is about 300 μg (158), and of cadmium is 100–300 μg (159).

There is some doubt regarding the validity of the carcinogenic hazard of these metals to man despite tumor production in animals. Selenium is an important trace element. The amounts taken daily are just about sufficient to satisfy our daily needs, and under these conditions it is unlikely that cell damage of any sort would occur. As regards lead, the significance to man of the kidney tumors produced in rats is very much in doubt since no increased susceptibility to malignancy has been reported in cases of chronic lead poisoning. In the case of cadmium, claims for carcinogenicity rest on the questionable value of the induction of local sarcomas and the equally questionable

Leydig cell tumors of the testis. Cadmium induces a severe irreversible testicular atrophy (*160, 161*), a condition which, according to Hinman and Smith (*162*), leads not infrequently to the development of these types of tumor in the rat when produced in other ways.

Arsenic in the pentavalent form also occurs naturally in a variety of foods and in drinking water. The daily intake is estimated to be about 100–800 μg from food and 10 μg from water (*163, 164*). Arsenic in this form is thought to be metabolically inert and is rapidly and almost quantitatively eliminated in the excreta (*165, 166*). Traces of trivalent arsenicals are also present in food and are derived mainly from trivalent organoarsenicals used as pesticides and herbicides (*163*). Organoarsenicals are also used as feed additives to poultry and livestock, as chemotherapeutic agents or to improve feed conversion. The majority of arsenicals used for this purpose however are the less toxic pentavalent organic compounds. The maximum allowable concentration of arsenic in food in the UK is 1 ppm (*167*). Arsenic, both in the inorganic and organic form, has been administered to rats and mice orally in a number of experiments without producing a carcinogenic response (*163, 168, 169*). Repeated application of an aqueous solution of sodium arsenate twice weekly to mouse skin for 60 weeks failed to elicit any skin tumors (*168*). In addition, Boutwell (*170*) has shown that arsenic is neither a tumor promoter nor initiator. Despite this negative evidence from animal experiments there is some epidemiological evidence that arsenic is connected with cancr produc- ton in man. Some workers claim to have found an increased incidence in workers occupationally exposed to arsenic, for example, chromate miners and those who spray crops with organoarsenicals (*171, 172, 173*). Recently Dob- son and Pinto (*174*) showed that chronic arsenical poisoning from a con- taminated source of drinking water in Taiwan was associated with a high incidence of skin tumors. The levels here were of the order of 0.8–2.5 ppm in the drinking water. Compared with the expected levels of intake in Great Britain, they are very high, and on the observations of Dobson and Pinto (*174*) it is questionable whether a cancer hazard exists from arsenic in the absence of clinical signs of chronic poisoning.

Food Additives and Frying Oils

Apart from the known carcinogens mentioned in this review there are other compounds suspected of carcinogenic activity present in food. Such com- pounds as sugar and salt, food colors, and other additives have been sus- pected by some authorities to possess carcinogenic activity either directly or through a contaminant because of the induction of local sarcoma in rats and mice by long-term repeated injection in the same subcutaneous site. As men- tioned earlier, this type of test is totally unreliable as an index of carcino- genicity potential so that a positive result cannot be taken as evidence of carcinogenicity (*148, 175*). Equally unreliable in this respect is the evidence produced for the carcinogenicity of propylene glycol and Citrus Red 2. These compounds produced bladder tumors in rodents on oral administration at high doses. These tumors were, however, accompanied by the formation of calcium oxalate stones, an event which precludes a conclusion of a carcinogenic effect

(176). Coumarin, a lactone widely found in edible plants such as strawberries, blackcurrents, apricots, and cherries has also been suspect because of the production of hepatic nodules on feeding to rats at very high concentrations only (5000 ppm). Low concentrations (1000 ppm) were without effect. In this instance the nature of the pathological lesion is in doubt (177, 178).

In addition to these groups of compounds, there is a large series of hydroxy-, epoxy-, and peroxy compounds and lactones (179, 180) that are formed in oils during frying and which in some quarters are suspected of carcinogenic activity because of their known reactive nature with biological macromolecules (181). Despite extensive feeding studies, these oils have not been shown to increase the tumor incidence in experimental animals (182). Furthermore, the extensive studies carried out by Van Duuren et al. (183) on model compounds of these chemical classes did not convincingly show that any of them were carcinogenic. It would thus seem that this type of traditional cooking does not constitute any carcinogenic hazard so that the British may enjoy the luxury of eating their fish and chips in tranquillity.

The sweetening agents saccharin and cyclamate have been under current scrutiny for possible carcinogenic activity. Concern about the safety of these agents arose after the publication by Price et al. (184) reporting the incidence of bladder carcinoma in rats fed a one-in-ten mixture of saccharin and cyclamate, to which cyclohexylamine, a bacterial metabolite of cyclamate had been added later in the experiment. For reasons unknown cyclamate was banned after the publication of these results both in the U.S. and in the U.K. This action followed so soon after the results became known that one suspects that cyclamate or one of its metabolites was incriminated as the causative agent of these tumors despite the fact that long-term feeding studies in rats and mice on both compounds proved negative (185, 186, 187). Recently, however, a number of studies revealed that saccharin fed at 5 and 7.5% (188) produced bladder tumors in rats indicating that possibly the carcinomas seen in the study by Price et al. could be caused by this compound. Interestingly, the saccharin that is claimed to have produced bladder tumors contains o-toluenesulfonamide as an impurity. Another type of saccharin, manufactured by a different process and not containing this impurity, has failed to induce tumors when fed at high levels to rats. At the time of writing this problem is being investigated further.

Conclusion

From the evidence available it would appear that carcinogens in food are derived from a number of unrelated sources. In edible plants the major sources of carcinogens are natural biosynthetic processes. These include synthesis by the plant itself or by fungi which infest the plant or its fruit or seed. By contrast carcinogens are formed in meat and fish as a result of traditional and time-honored methods of cooking or preservation. Environmental pollution contributes only a small fraction of these carcinogens.

The carcinogens found in plants or plant products are usually limited to fairly well defined geographical areas. Those found in meat and fish are less well defined geographically but there are substantial individual and racial differences in the intake of these carcinogens depending on the type of diet consumed and the cooking method.

The clear carcinogenic effect these compounds elicit in experimental animals is a cause for concern. The task of relating this evidence to human hazard is, however, a formidable one. Apart from inherent species differences in metabolism and sensitivity there are quantitative differences of several orders of magnitude between the amounts given to animals under experimental conditions and the amounts ingested by man in food. These difficulties are unlikely to be resolved until experimental methods are devised to assess the carcinogenic potency of low levels of carcinogens, until more attention is paid to metabolic pathways of carcinogens in different species, and until epidemiological studies are conducted on a more extensive scale than is being done at present.

Literature Cited

1. Pott, P., "Chirurgical observations," London, 1775.
2. Clayson, D. B., "Chemical Carcinogenesis," p. 135, J. & A. Churchill, London, 1962.
3. Case, R. A. M., Hosker, M. E., McDonald, D. B., Pearson, J. T., *Br. J. Ind. Med.* (1954) **11**, 75.
4. Wada, S., Miyanishi, M., Nishimoto, Y., Kambe, S., Miller, R. W., *Lancet* (1968) **i**, 1161.
5. Block, J. B., *J. Am. Med. Ass.* (1974) **229**, 53.
6. Herbst, A. L., Ulfelder, H., Poskanza, D. C., *N. Eng. J. Med.* (1971) **284**, 878.
7. Huseby, R. A., *Proc. Am. Ass. Cancer Res.* (1953) **1**, 25.
8. Bonser, G. M., Clayson, D. B., Jull, J. W., *Br. J. Cancer* (1956) **10**, 653.
9. Hueper, W. O., Wiley, F. H., Wolfe, H. D., *J. Ind. Hyg.* (1938) **20**, 46.
10. National Cancer Institute, "Survey of compounds which have been tested for carcinogenic activity," DHEW Publication No. (NIH) **73–453**, Public Health Service Publication No. **149**, 1970–71.
11. Miller, E. C., Miller, J. A., Enomoto, M., *Cancer Res.* (1964) **24**, 2018.
12. Miller, J. A., *Cancer Res.* (1970) **30**, 559.
13. Wogan, G. N., *Bacteriol. Rev.* (1966) **30**, 460.
14. Cleaver, J. E., *Nature* (1968) **218**, 652.
15. Poone, P. K., Parker, J. W., O'Brien, R. L., *Proc. Am. Ass. Cancer Res.* (1974) **15**, 19.
16. Keefe, D. A., Edwards, G. S., *Proc. Am. Ass. Cancer Res.* (1974) **15**, 19.
17. Mantel, N., Bryan, W. R., *J. Nat. Cancer Inst.* (1961) **27**, 455.
19. Druckrey, H., *Ciba Found. Sym. Carcinog. Mech. Action* (1959) 110.
19. Druckrey, H., *Ciba Found. Sym. Carcinog.—Mech. Action, 1959*, 110.
20. Food and Drug Administration Advisory Committee on Protocols for Safety Evaluation, *Toxicol. Appl. Pharmacol.* (1971) **20**, 419.
21. Jones, H. B., Grendon, A., *Food Cosmet. Toxicol.* (1975) **13**, 251.
22. Heinonen, O. P., *Cancer* (1973) **31**, 573.
23. Hoffman, D., Wynder, E. L., *Cancer* (1962) **15**, 93.
24. Grimmer, G., Hildebrandt, A., *Dt. Lebensmitt. Rundsch.* (1965) **61**, 237.
25. Gräf, W., Diehl, H., *Arch. Hyg. Bakteriol.* (1966) **150**, 49.
26. Howard, J. W., Teague, R. T., White, R. H., Fry, B. E., *J. Ass. Off. Anal. Chem.* (1966) **49**, 595.
27. Howard, J. W., Turicchi, E. W., White, R. H., Fazio, T., *J. Ass. Off. Anal. Chem.* (1966) **49**, 1236.

28. Grimmer, G., Hildebrandt, A., *Chem. Ind.* (1967) no. **47**, 2000.
29. Grimmer, G., Hildebrandt, A., *Arch. Hyg. Bakteriol.* (1968) **152**, 255.
30. Borneff, J., Fischer, R., *Arch. Hyg. (München)* (1962) **146**, 430.
31. Borneff, J., *Arch. Hyg. Berl.* (1964) **148**, 1.
32. Tilgner, D. J., *Food Manuf.* (1970) **45**, 47.
33. Rohrlich, M., Suckow, P., *Getreide Mehl.* (1970) **20**, 90.
34. Blumer, M., *Science N.Y.* (1961) **134**, 474.
35. Borneff, J., Kunte, H., *Arch. Hyg. Berl.* (1964) **148**, 585.
36. Bourcart, J., Lalou, C., Mallet, L., *C.R. Hebd. Séanc. Acad. Sci., Paris* (1961) **252**, 640.
37. Mallet, L., Perdriau, A., Perdriau, J., *Bull. Acad. Nat. Méd.* (1963) **147**, 320.
38. Andelman, J. B., Suess, M. J., *Bull. WHO* (1970) **43**, 479.
39. WHO Expert Committee on the Prevention of Cancer, *Tech. Rep. Ser. WHO* (1964) no. **276**.
40. Bailey, E. J., Dungal, N., *Br. J. Cancer* (1958) **12**, 348.
41. Dikin, P. P., *Vopr. Onkol.* (1965) **11**, 77.
42. Nugmanov, S. N., Gorelova, N. D., Dikin, P. P., *Vopr. Onkol.* (1961) **7**, 198.
43. Lijinsky, W., Shubik, P., *Toxicol. Appl. Pharmacol.* (1965) **7**, 337.
44. Lijinsky, W., Shubik, P., *Ind. Med. Surg.* (1965) **34**, 152.
45. Howard, J. W., Fazio, T., *J. Agric. Food Chem.* (1969) **17**, 527.
46. Lijinsky, W., Ross, A. E., *Food Cosmet. Toxicol.* (1967) **5**, 343.
47. Rhee, K. S., Bratzler, L. J., *J. Food Sci.* (1970) **35**, 146.
48. Lijinsky, W., Shubik, P., *Food Cosmet. Toxicol.* (1965) **3**, 145.
49. White, R. H., *J. Agric. Food Chem.* (1971) **19**, 43.
50. Dungal, N., Sigurjonsson, J., *Br. J. Cancer* (1967) **21**, 270.
51. Masuda, Y., Mori, K., Kuratsune, M., *Gann* (1966) **57**, 133.
52. Roe, F. J. C., *Acta Unio Int. Cancrum* (1963) **19**, 730.
53. Neal, J., Rigdon, R. H., *Tex. Rep. Biol. Med.* (1967) **25**, 553.
54. Barnes, J. M., Magee, P. N., *Br. J. Ind. Med.* (1954) **11**, 167.
55. Magee, P. N., *Biochem. J.* (1956) **64**, 676.
56. Magee, P. N., Barnes, J. M., *Br. J. Cancer* (1956) **10**, 114.
57. Druckrey, H., Preussmann, R., Ivankovic, S., Schmähl, D., *Z. Krebsforsch.* (1967) **69**, 103.
58. Magee, P. N., *Food Cosmet. Toxicol.* (1971) **9**, 207.
59. Magee, P. N., Barnes, J. M., *Adv. Cancer Res.* (1967) **10**, 163.
60. Böhler, *Nord. Veterinaermoede Beret., 9th* (1962) 774.
61. Sakshaug, J., Sögnen, E., Hansen, M. A., Koppang, N., *Nature* (1965) **206**, 1261.
62. Ender, F., Havre, G., Helgebostad, A., Koppang, N., Madsen, R., Čeh, L., *Naturwissenschaften* (1964) **51**, 637.
63. Ender, F., Havre, G. N., Madsen, R., Čeh, L., Helgebostad, A., *Z. Tierphysiol. Tierernähr. Futtermittelkd.* (1967) **22**, 133.
64. Sen, N. P., Smith, D. C., Schwinghamer, L., Howsam, B., *Can. Inst. Food Technol.* (1970) **3**, 66.
65. Ender, F., Čeh, L., *Food Cosmet. Toxicol.* (1968) **6**, 569.
66. Hedler, L., Marquardt, P., *Food Cosmet. Toxicol.* (1968) **6**, 341.
67. Kroller, E., *Dt. Lebensmitt. Rundsch.* (1967) **63**, 303.
68. Wasserman, A. E., Fiddler, W., Doerr, R. C., Osman, S. F., Dooley, C. J., *Food Cosmet. Toxicol.* (1972) **10**, 681.
69. Crosby, N. T., Foreman, J. K., Palframan, J. F., Sawyer, R., *Nature, London* (1972) **238**, 342.
70. Du Plessis, L. S., Nunn, J. R., Roach, W. A., *Nature, London* (1969) **222**, 1198.
71. Schoental, R., *Nature, London* (1969) **223**, 239.
72. Lijinsky, W., Epstein, S. S., *Nature, London* (1970) **225**, 21.
73. Terracini, B., Magee, P. N., Barnes, J. M., *Br. J. Cancer* (1967) **21**, 559.

73a. Druckrey, H., Potential Carcinogenic Hazard from Drugs, *U.I.C.C. Monogr.* (1959) **7**, 60.
74. Druckrey, H., Schildbach, A., Schmähl, D., Preussmann, R., Ivankovic, S., *Arzneimittel-Forsch.* (1963) **13**, 841.
75. Sen, N. P., Smith, D. C., Schwinghamer, L., *Food Cosmet. Toxicol.* (1969) **7**, 301.
76. Sander, J., *Hoppe-Seyler's Z. Physiol. Chem.* (1968) **349**, 429.
77. Sander, J., Schweinsberg, F., Manz, H. P., *Hoppe-Seyler's Z. Physiol. Chem.* (1968) **349**, 1691.
78. Druckrey, H., Steinhoff, D., Beuthner, H., Schneider, H., Klärner, P., *Arznei-mittel-Forsch.* (1963) **13**, 320.
79. Sander, J., Bürkle, G., *Z. Krebsforsch.* (1969) **73**, 54.
80. Hawksworth, G., Hill, M. J., *Biochem. J.* (1971) **122**, 28P.
81. Alam, B. S., Saporoschetz, I. B., Epstein, S. S., *Nature, London* (1971) **232**, 116, 199.
82. Sander, J., Seif, F., *Arzneimittel-Forsch.* (1969) **19**, 1091.
83. Boyland, E., Nice, E., Williams, K., *Food Cosmet. Toxicol.* (1971) **9**, 639.
84. Phillips, W. E. J., *Food Cosmet. Toxicol.* (1971) **9**, 219.
85. Mirvish, S. S., *J. Nat. Cancer Inst.* (1970) **44**, 633.
86. Fisher, R. B., *Br. Med. Bull.* (1967) **23**, 241.
87. Laqueur, G. L., Mickelsen, O., Whiting, M. G., Kurland, L. T., *J. Nat. Cancer Inst.* (1963) **31**, 919.
88. Spatz, Maria, Smith, D. W. E., McDaniel, E. G., Laqueur, G. L., *Proc. Soc. Exp. Biol. Med.* (1967) **124**, 691.
89. Spatz, M., *Ann. N.Y. Acad. Sci.* (1969) **163**, 848.
90. Hirono, L., Laqueur, G. L., Spatz, M., *J. Nat. Cancer Inst.* (1968) **40**, 1003.
91. Yang, M. G., Mickelsen, O., Campbell, M. E., Laqueur, G. L., Keresztesy, J. C., *J. Nutr.* (1966) **90**, 153.
92. Elizan, T. S., data presented to the 4th Conference on the Toxicity of Cycads, Bethesda, USA, April 1965, Marjorie G. Whiting, Ed., Public Health Service, U.S. Department of Health, Education, and Welfare.
93. Bull, L. B., Culvenor, C. C. J., Dick, A. T., "The Pyrrolizidine Alkaloids," North Holland, Amsterdam, 1968.
94. Schoental, R., *Cancer Res.* (1968) **28**, 2237.
95. McLean, Elizabeth K., *Pharmacol. Rev.* (1970) **22**, 429.
96. Schoental, R., *J. Pathol. Bacteriol.* (1959) **77**, 485.
97. Newberne, P. M., *Cancer Res.* (1968) **28**, 2327.
98. Williams, A. O., Schoental, R., *Trop. Geogr. Med.* (1970) **22**, 201.
99. Higginson, J., *Cancer Res.* (1963) **23**, 1624.
100. Miller, J. A., "Tumorigenic and carcinogenic natural Products," *Toxicants Occurring Nat. Food* (1966).
101. Long, E. L., Nelson, A. A., Fitzhugh, O. G., Hansen, W. H., *Arch. Pathol.* (1963) **75**, 595.
102. Kraybill, H. F., *Environ. Res.* (1969) **2**, 234.
103. Pamukcu, A. M., Yalciner, S., Price, J. M., Bryan, G. T., *Cancer Res.* (1970) **30**, 2671.
104. Evans, I. A., Mason, J., *Nature, London* (1965) **208**, 913.
105. Schacham, P., Philp, R. B., Gowdey, C. W., *Am. J. Vet. Res.* (1970) **31**, 191.
106. Price, J. M., Pamukcu, A. M., *Cancer Res.* (1968) **28**, 2247.
107. Pamukcu, A. M., Goksey, S. K., Price, J. M., *Cancer Res.* (1967) **27**, 917.
108. *New Scientist* (1970) **47**, 175.
109. Evans, I. A., paper presented to the 10th International Cancer Congress, Houston, 1970.
110. Evans, I. A., Barber, G. D., Jones, R. S., Leach, H., *Rep. Br. Emp. Cancer Campn.* (1968) **46**, 416.
111. Fitzhugh, O. G., Nelson, A. A., *Science, N.Y.* (1948) **108**, 626.

112. Purves, H. D., Griesbach, W. E., *Br. J. Exp. Pathol.* (1947) **28**, 46.
113. Rosin, A., Ungar, H., *Cancer Res.* (1957) **17**, 302.
114. Astwood, E. B., Greer, M. A., Ettlinger, M. G., *J. Biol. Chem.* (1949) **181**, 121.
115. Hoch-Ligeti, C., *Tex. Rep. Biol. Med.* (1952) **19**, 996.
116. Joint FAO/WHO Expert Committee on Food Additives, "Toxicological Evaluation of Some Extraction Solvents and Certain Other Substances," FAO Nutr. Mtg. Rep. Ser. no. **48A**, WHO/Food Add./70.39, 1970.
117. Stocks, P., *Br. J. Cancer* (1970) **24**, 215.
118. Cole, P., *Lancet* (1971) **i**, 1335.
119. Tuyns, A. J., *Int. J. Cancer* (1970) **5**, 152.
120. Morton, J. F., *Econ. Bot.* (1970) **24**, 217.
121. Pearce, M. L., Dayton, S., *Lancet* (1971) **i**, 464.
122. Ederer, F., Leren, P., Turpeinen, O., Frantz, I. D., Jr., *Lancet* (1971) **ii**, 203.
123. Shimkin, M. B., *Arch. Environ. Health* (1968) **16**, 503.
124. Martinex, I., *J. Nat. Cancer Inst.* (1969) **42**, 1069.
125. Wogan, G. N., Newberne, P. M., *Cancer Res.* (1967) **27**, 2370.
126. Butler, W. H., "Aflatoxin," L. A. Goldblatt, Ed., Academic, New York, London, Chapter VIII, 1969.
127. Carnaghan, R. B. A., *Br. J. Cancer* (1967) **21**, 811.
128. Horrocks, D., Burt, A. W. A., Thomas, D. C., Lancaster, M. C., *Anim. Prod.* (1965) **7**, 253.
129. Hintz, H. F., Booth, A. N., Cucullu, A. F., Gardner, H. K., Heitman, H., *Proc. Soc. Exp. Biol. Med.* (1967) **124**, 266.
130. Allcroft, R., "Aflatoxin," L. A. Goldblatt, Ed., Chapter IX, p. 250, Academic, New York, London, 1969.
131. Purchase, I. F. H., *Food Cosmet. Toxicol.* (1967) **5**, 339.
132. Stewart, H. L., "Primary Hepatoma," W. S. Burdette, Ed., p. 31, University of Utah, 1965.
133. Serek-Hanssen, A., *Arch. Environ. Health* (1970) **20**, 729.
134. Alpert, E., Serek-Hanssen, A., Rajagopolan, B., *Arch. Environ. Health* (1970) **20**, 723.
135. Shank, R. C., Wogan, G. N., Gibson, J. B., *Food Cosmet. Toxicol.* (1972) **10**, 51.
136. Shank, R. C., Bhamarapravati, N., Gordon, J. E., Wogan, G. N., *Food Cosmet. Toxicol.* (1972) **10**, 171.
137. Shank, R. C., Gordon, J. E., Wogan, G. N., Nondatsu, A., Subhamani, B., *Food Cosmet. Toxicol.* (1972) **10**, 71.
138. Shank, R. C., Wogan, G. N., Gibson, J. B., Nondatsu, A., *Food Cosmet. Toxicol.* (1972) **10**, 61.
139. Joint FAO/WHO Expert Committee on Nutrition, *FAO/WHO Protein Advisory Group Nutrition Document* **NU6**, October 31, 1966.
140. Kobayashi, Y., Urguchi, K., Sakai, F., Tatsuno, T., Tsukioka, M., Noguchi, Y., Tsunoda, H., Mijake, M., Saito, M., Enomoto, M., Shikata, T., Ishiko, T., *Proc. Jpn. Acad.* (1959) **35**, 501.
141. Uraguchi, K., Saito, M., Noguchi, Y., Takahashi, K., Enomoto, M., Tatsuno, T., *Food Cosmet. Toxicol.* (1972) **10**, 193.
142. Purchase, I. F. H., van der Watt, J. J., *Food Cosmet. Toxicol.* (1968) **6**, 555.
143. Holzapfel, C. W., Purchase, I. F. H., Steyn, P. S., Gorrins, L., *S. Afr. Med. J.* (1966) **40**, 1100.
144. Stack, M., Rodricks, J. V., *J. Ass. Off. Analyt. Chem.* (1971) **54**, 86.
145. Lillehoj, E. B., Ciegler, A., Detroy, R. W., "Fungal toxins," in "Essays in Toxicology," F. R. Blood, Ed., Academic, New York, London, 1970.
146. Dickens, F., Jones, H. E. H., *Br. J. Cancer* (1961) **15**, 85.
147. *Ibid.* (1963) **17**, 100.
148. Dickens, F., *Br. Med. Bull.* (1964) **20**, 96.
149. Grasso, P., Golberg, L., *Food Cosmet. Toxicol.* (1966) **4**, 297.

150. Miller, J. A., Miller, E. C., *Cancer Res.* (1965) **25,** 1292.
151. Nelson, A. A., Fitzhugh, O. G., Calvery, H. O., *Cancer Res.* (1943) **3,** 230.
152. Lollinger, H. U., *Virchows Arch.* (1953) **323,** 694.
153. Tönz, O., Z. *Ges. Exp. Med.* (1957) **128,** 361.
154. van Esch, G. J., van Genderen, H., Vink, H. H., *Br. J. Cancer* (1962) **16,** 289.
155. Kazantzis, G., *Nature, London* (1963) **198,** 1213.
156. Haddow, A., Dukes, C. E., Roe, F. J. C., Mitchley, B. C. V., Pugh, R. C. B., Cameron, K. M., *Rep. Br. Emp. Cancer Campn.* (1962) **40,** 34.
157. Smith, M. I., Westfall, B. B., *Public Health Rep., Washington* (1937) **52,** 1357.
158. Kehoe, R. A., *Arch. Environ. Health* (1961) **2,** 418.
159. *Food Cosmet. Toxicol.* (1972) **10,** 249.
160. Kar, A. B., Das, R. P., *Acta Biol. Med. Germ.* (1960) **5,** 153.
161. Meek, E. S., *Br. J. Exp. Pathol.* (1959) **40,** 503.
162. Hinman, F., Jr., Smith, G. I., *J. Urol.* (1960) **83,** 706.
163. Schroeder, H. A., Balassa, J. J., *J. Chronic Dis.* (1966) **19,** 85.
164. Somers, E., Smith, D. M., *Food Cosmet. Toxicol.* (1971) **9,** 185.
165. Overby, L. R., Frost, D. V., *Toxicol. Appl. Pharmacol.* (1962) **4,** 38.
166. Morgareidge, K., *J. Agr. Food Chem.* (1963) **11,** 377.
167. *Arsenic in Food Regulations, 1959,* Statutory Instrument 1959, No. **831,** HMSO, London.
168. Baroni, C., van Esch, F. J., Saffiotti, U., *Arch. Environ. Health* (1963) **7,** 668.
169. Oser, B. L., Morgareidge, K., Weinberg, M. S., Oser, M., *Toxicol. Appl. Pharmacol.* (1966) **9,** 528.
170. Boutwell, R. K., *J. Agr. Food Chem.* (1963) **11,** 381.
171. Currie, A. N., *Br. Med. Bull.* (1947) **4,** 402.
172. Neubauer, O., *Br. J. Cancer* (1947) **1,** 192.
173. Roth, F., *Virchows Arch.* (1958) **331,** 119.
174. Dobson, R. L., Pinto, J. S., "Advances in Biology of Skin," in "Carcinogenesis," W. Montagna, R. L. Dobson, Eds., Vol. **VII,** 1966.
175. Grasso, P., Gangolli, S. D., Golberg, L., Hooson, J., *Food Cosmet. Toxicol.* (1971) **9,** 463.
176. Grasso, P., *Chem. Brit.* (1970) **6,** 17.
177. Grasso, P., Lansdown, A. B. G., Kiss, I. S., Gaunt, I. F., Gangolli, S. D., *Food Cosmet. Toxicol.* (1969) **7,** 425.
178. Bär, F., Griepentrog, F., *Medizin Ernähr.* (1967) **8,** 244.
179. Raulin, J., *Ann. Nutr. Aliment.* (1967) **21,** 105.
180. Fioriti, J. A., Krampl, V., Sims, R. J., *J. Am. Oil Chem. Soc.* (1967) **44,** 534.
181. Zaldivar, R. S. D., *Nature, London* (1963) **199,** 1300.
182. O'Gara, R. W., Stewart, L., Brown, J., Hueper, W. C., *J. Nat. Cancer Inst.* (1969) **42,** 275.
183. Van Duuren, B. L., Langseth, L., Goldschmidt, B. M., Orris, L., *J. Nat. Cancer Inst.* (1967) **39,** 1217.
184. Price, J. M., Biava, C. G., Oser, B. L., Vogin, E. E., Steinfeld, J., Ley, H. L., *Science* (1970) **167,** 1131.
185. Roe, F. J. C., Levy, L. S., Carter, R. L., *Food Cosmet. Toxicol.* (1970) **8,** 135.
186. Brantom, P. G., Gaunt, I. F., Grasso, P., *Food Cosmet. Toxicol.* (1973) **11,** 735.
187. Schmähl, D. (1973), personal communication.
188. *Food Cosmet. Toxicol.* (1973) **11,** 1126.
189. Franke, C., Fritz, W., *Fette Seifen Anstrichm.* (1969) **71,** 23.
190. Borneff, J., Fábián, B., *Arch. Hyg. Bakteriol.* (1966) **150,** 485.
191. Bienorth, G., Rost, H. A., *Chem. Ind.* (1967) no. **47,** 2002.
192. Fritz, W., *Nahrung* (1968) **12,** 495.
193. Grimmer, G., Hildebrandt, A., *Dt. Lebensmitt. Rundsch.* (1966) **62,** 19.
194. Kuratsune, M., Hueper, W. C., *J. Nat. Cancer Inst.* (1960) **24,** 463.
195. Grimmer, G., Hildebrandt, A., *Z. Krebsforsch.* (1965) **67,** 272.

196. Fisher, N., Cooper, R. M., Bell, B. M., *Health Congr. R. Soc. Health, Pap. 78th* (1971) 7–10.
197. Mallet, L., *C.R. Hebd. Séances Acad. Sci., Paris* (1961) **253**, 168.
198. Cahnmann, H. J., Kuratsune, M., *Anal. Chem.* (1957) **29**, 1312.
199. Malonski, A. J., Greenfield, E. L., Barnes, C. J., Worthington, J. M., Joe, F. L., *J. Ass. Off. Anal. Chem.* (1968) **51**, 114.
200. Grimmer, G., Hildebrandt, A., *Z. Krebsforsch.* (1967) **69**, 223.
201. Masuda, Y., Kuratsune, M., *Gann* (1971) **62**, 27.
202. Fábián, B., *Arch. Hyg. Bakteriol.* (1968) **152**, 251.
203. Dikin, P. P., *Vopr. Pitan.* (1965) **24** (1), 31.
204. Thorsteinsson, T., Thordarson, G., *Cancer* (1968) **21**, 390.
205. Lijinsky, W., Shubik, P., *Science* (1964) **145**, 53.
206. Gorelova, N. D., Dikin, P. P., Gretskaya, O. P., Emshanova, A. V., *Vopr. Onkol.* (1965) **9** (8), 77.
207. Gretskaya, O. P., Yemshanova, A. V., Dikin, P. P., Gorelova, N. D., *Fish Ind. Moscow* (1962) **38**, 56.
208. Dikin, P. P., *Vopr. Onkol.* (1965) **11** (2), 77.
209. Mattocks, A. R., *Anal. Chem.* (1967) **39**, 443.
210. Kumari, S., Kapur, K. K., Atal, C. K., *Curr. Sci.* (1966) **35**, 546.
211. Palekar, R. S., Dastur, D. K., *Nature, London* (1965) **206**, 1363.
212. Dastur, D. K., Palekar, R. S., *Nature, London* (1966) **210**, 841.
213. Lopez, A., Crawford, M. A., *Lancet* (1967) **ii**, 1351.
214. Tung, T. C., Ling, K. H., *J. Vitaminol.* (1968) **14**, 48.
215. Shotwell, O. L., Hesseltine, C. W., Burmeister, H. R., Kowlek, W. F., Shannon, G. M., Hall, H. H., *Cereal Chem.* (1969) **46**, 454, 446.
216. Schuller, P. L., Ockhuizen, Th., Werringloen, J., Marquardt, P., *Arzneimittel-Forsch.* (1967) **17**, 888.
217. Loosmore, R. M., Allcroft, R., Tulton, E. A., Carnaghan, R. B. A., *Vet. Rec.* (1964) **76**, 64.
218. Fisher, J. F., Mallette, M. F., *J. Gen. Physiol.* (1961) **45**, 1.

Chapter

15

Asbestos Carcinogenesis

J. C. Wagner, Medical Research Council, Pneumoconiosis Unit,
Llandough Hospital, Penarth, Glamorgan, Wales

THE ASSOCIATION BETWEEN exposure to asbestos dust and the development of carcinomas of the lung and diffuse mesotheliomas of pleura and peritoneum has been studied intensively in recent years. There are several types of asbestos, and the materials have numerous uses. As a result of the epidemiological, pathological, physical, and chemical studies, a certain type of asbestos is more clearly implicated in tumor production than the others, and at present there is no evidence of risk to the general population.

In October 1972 a working group of experts met in Lyon under the auspices of the International Agency for Research on Cancer to assess the biological effects of asbestos. The working group consisted of clinicians, epidemiologists, pathologists, chemists, and physicists who had been studying the association between the various types of asbestos and cancer as part of an international study initiated at a meeting in New York in 1964 (1) following a New York Academy of Sciences Symposium on "The Biological Effects of Asbestos" (2). Recent evidence was presented and discussed. An advisory committee then reviewed and reported on the current knowledge of the roles of various types of asbestos as carcinogens. This report has clarified the situation in many respects, but numerous problems remain.

There are several types of asbestos. All are fibrous silicates and have similar properties. They are used mainly to produce fireproof insulation or to reinforce cement or plastics in building materials. Asbestos has hundreds of other uses and is essential in our industrial society. For example, the brakes of automobiles depend on the heat resistance of asbestos. The inhalation of asbestos dusts can lead to pulmonary fibrosis and carcinoma of the lung or to the development of diffuse mesotheliomas of the pleura and peritoneum. The problem has been to discover which type, or types, of asbestos are responsible for the development of the tumors. If a specific variety could be incriminated, then its use could be discouraged and that of the less harmful varieties recommended.

Asbestos—The Minerals

Three types of asbestos are important commercially: chrysotile (white), a magnesium silicate found mainly in serpentine, most aboundant and accounting for about 96% of the total; amosite (brown or grey); and crocidolite (blue), both amphiboles and occurring in banded ironstone. A small amount of anthophyllite is produced in Finland. Chrysotile is widely distributed, and the main mining areas are in Canada, Russia, Southern Africa, and Cyprus. Crocidolite is found in Cape Province and Transvaal in South Africa and until recently was produced in Western Australia; a deposit is also being developed in Bolivia. Amosite is mined in the Transvaal in South Africa.

The physical nature of the chrysotile fiber from different deposits varies considerably, as do the associated minerals found in the ore. However, after the fiber has been separated from the ore and processed in the mills, chrysotile fibers have a wavy coiled appearance. In contrast, the crocidolite and amosite fibers are much more rigid and straight. They are also more resistant to acids and alkalis. After 1900, crocidolite was in demand in the shipbuilding industry because chrysotile was not a good insulating material when exposed to seawater. Crocidolite is now used mainly to form a matrix in chrysotile asbestos cement products, pressure piping, and automobile battery boxes. Amosite binds well with plastics and is used in the manufacture of floor tiles and in decorative insulations to replace timber in passenger ships. The use of asbestos has increased tremendously in the last 20 years, and the annual consumption is now over four million tons.

Asbestos and the Asbestos Tumors

Asbestosis, the fibrosis of the lung caused by asbestos inhalation, was first detected at the turn of the century in France and Britain, but it was not until the early 1930's that it was shown to be a major occupational hazard in the asbestos textile industry (3). The first suggestion that there might be an association between asbestosis and bronchial carcinoma came from pathologists in Britain and the United States in 1935. This was reported in Britain by the Inspector of Factories, who reported that in 1947 (4) 15% of all death certificates for males which mentioned asbestosis attributed death to carcinoma of the lung. This excessive risk was confirmed in 1955 by Doll (5) who showed that those first employed before 1930 in scheduled occupations in an asbestos textile factory had a death rate from lung cancer 10 times greater than that of the general population. Later studies on the same population confirmed that the incidence of carcinoma dropped considerably with improved factory conditions. This suggested that carcinoma of the lung was associated with the incidence of severe pulmonary fibrosis caused by heavy asbestos exposure (6). In 1960, the situation was further complicated because exposure to asbestos dust was associated with the development of diffuse mesotheliomas of the pleura and peritoneum (7). This has several intriguing features.

1. These rare tumors were associated only with exposure to the crocidolite (blue) asbestos mined in the North West Cape Province and not to the chrysotile and amosite mining areas of Southern Africa or to the Transvaal crocidolite deposit adjoining the amosite area.

2. The association was with exposure to asbestos dust and not necessarily with the pulmonary fibrosis of asbestosis, and a number of the cases were environmental rather than occupational exposures.

3. The average latent period between initial exposure to asbestos dust and tumor development was over 40 years. This was the first indication that the different types of asbestos varied in their biological effects.

Crocidolite has been used in Britain since 1900, and by 1962 the Inspectorate of Factories had recorded 130 cancers of the lung in asbestos workers but no cases of mesothelioma (8). A search was therefore made in the departments of pathology and surgery, and cases were referred to a panel of pathologists formed to establish criteria for the diagnoses of these previously rare tumors (9, 10, 11).

By 1964 it was clear that mesotheliomas had occurred and were increasing in number (12, 13), but as most industrial asbestos workers had been exposed to more than one type of fiber, it was impossible to implicate a single type.

Epidemiological Investigations

To study the effect of exposure to one type of fiber, epidemiological studies were required in the mining areas. A comparison of the South African crocidolite mines with the chrysotile mines in Canada was needed. International coordination for this was possible through the working group of the International Union against Cancer (UICC), and a committee to implement these proposals was formed (1). Thus, it was possible to initiate international epidemiological surveys, develop a new radiological classification (14), organize international and national pathology panels, and prepare, characterize, and distribute reference samples of asbestos dust for experimental work (15).

The working party was reconvened in Lyon under the auspices of the International Agency for Research on Cancer (IARC), and results of the implementation of some of the 1964 recommendations were presented. The proceedings of this meeting were published as an IARC Scientific Report (16). Some of the more significant information is included in the following paragraphs.

A survey of Quebec asbestos miners was undertaken by epidemiologists of McGill University with support from the Quebec Asbestos Mining Association. They conducted a remarkably complete follow-up of about 12,000 workers which showed a slight excess of lung cancer in the most heavily exposed group. Despite the heavy general air pollution by chrysotile dust over many years, the crude death rates for lung cancer in the population of the two mining towns are less than the death rate for the province of Quebec (17). Only a few mesotheliomas were recorded in the mining population.

The situation was entirely different from that in the asbestos fields in the North West Cape.

In the United States, prospective mortality studies and social security records showed an excess risk of bronchial cancer in those working in an asbestos–textile factory just before World War II (18). New York insulation workers had death rates from lung cancer about seven times those expected (19). Mesotheliomas of the peritoneum were observed among those on the union books in 1942, but more recently employees show an increased incidence of pleural tumors. Carcinoma of the lung was particularly prevalent among heavy cigarette smokers, and the effect appeared to be multiplicative (20, 21, 22), but there was no correlation between cigarette smoking and the development of the mesotheliomas. Information about the type of asbestos used in the past by these workers is incomplete, but crocidolite, if used at all, was present in very small amounts compared with chrysotile and amosite.

The Soviet Union is second only to Canada in chrysotile production. At a meeting in Dresden in 1968, K. M. Kogan indicated an increased incidence of carcinoma of the lung in the asbestos area near Sverdlovsk. J. C. McDonald, who was in charge of the survey in Quebec, recently discussed results with Kogan, and they found that the situations in the Ural and Quebec asbestos fields are similar, with slight increase in carcinoma of the lung among heavily exposed workers and with no mesotheliomas. Similar results have been obtained in Finland among the anthophyllite miners (23).

In contrast, mesotheliomas have been reported from shipbuilding ports, particularly in dockyards in Britain, the U.S., Germany, and Holland. The whole situation was considered in Britain by a panel of authorities under the chairmanship of the Chief Medical Inspector of Factories. Their report, "Problems Arising from the Use of Asbestos" (24), concluded that there was sufficient evidence to suggest "other types of fiber should be substituted for crocidolite wherever possible." As a result, the law concerning the use of asbestos has been changed, and since 1970 the use of crocidolite has been subject to more rigorous standards than other types in Britain. It is disquieting to realize that, while the use of crocidolite has dropped rapidly during recent years in Britain, importation into the U.S., Western Germany, and Japan has steadily increased.

Experimental Studies

Possible reasons for the role of crocidolite in the production of mesotheliomas have been considered. In animal experiments the tumors can be produced easily after intrapleural inoculation of various types of asbestos (25). The suggestion was made that natural oils and waxes in the crocidolite (26) and contaminant oils from milling of all types of fiber (27) or from plastic storage bags (28) contributed to the tumors, but crocidolite from which oils had been removed gave very similar results to untreated fiber (25). This has been confirmed for the UICC standard reference samples by removing the oils from all samples and comparing them with untreated controls

(*29*). These findings indicate that neither the oils nor trace elements are responsible for the development of these mesotheliomas. Stanton and Wrench (*30*) showed that glass fibers could also induce mesotheliomas. Further studies by Wagner *et al.* (*31*) indicate that fine glass fibers produce mesotheliomas, but that coarser fibers more than 1 μm in diameter do not.

Dust Physics

Physicists have studied the aerodynamics of the different types of asbestos in relation to inhalation. To a first approximation, the rate of fall of an asbestos fiber depends on its diameter, not its length, so that when asbestos fibers are inhaled, deposition resulting from sedimentation is almost independent of length (*32*). This explains why long fibers (up to about 200 μm) can penetrate to the alveolar regions if they are thin enough (< 3 μm diameter). On the other hand, deposition by interception or wall collision, which is important in narrow airways, depends almost entirely on fiber length. Chrysotile fibers, which resemble stretched coils, are readily deposited by interception, especially at bifurcations, since the curvature increases the collision cross section area. Amphibole fibers, which are straight, are less readily deposited by interception, since they tend to turn into the direction of the streamlines in the airflow and thus have small collision cross sections. In an experiment in which rats were exposed by inhalation to dust clouds generated from the UICC reference samples, the retention of amphiboles was six times greater than for chrysotile (*33*). This ratio for the different types of fiber may be substantially higher in industry. Many chrysotile mining areas are characterized by dense clouds of dust, but a substantial proportion of particles are large flocks which settle quickly and are available for inhalation only during a short period. The small human risk of developing mesothelioma of the pleura from chrysotile may well arise from its curly nature which prevents most of it from reaching the pleura. Quantitative studies of the distribution of different types of fiber within the lungs after inhalation need further development.

By using the electron microscope for measurement, it was shown (*34*) that fibers of crocidolite mined in the North West Cape and Australia are much thinner and shorter than those of the crocidolite and amosite mined in the Transvaal and consequently have a much greater chance of reaching the pleura. This hypothesis could account for the high rate of pleural mesotheliomas in the North West Cape and only one case in the Transvaal (*35*).

Report of Advisory Committee

An Advisory Committee to the Director of the IARC reached the following conclusions on evidence available in the fall of 1972.

1. All major commercial types of asbestos have been associated with lung carcinoma. Since 1964 the evidence of a causal association has been increased by epidemiological studies showing exposure–response relationship for the incidence of lung carcinomas. The production of lung carcinomas in

certain animals by all types of asbestos supports this conclusion. The epidemiological evidence in man, however, shows that there are clear differences in risk with type of fiber and nature of exposure.

2. There is no evidence of an increased risk of lung carcinoma at low levels of exposure to asbestos, such as have been encountered by the general population in urban areas. The evidence of an exposure—response relationship based in part on past dust measurements and in part on the type of job within the industry suggests that an excess lung carcinoma risk is not detectable when the occupational exposure has been low. These low occupational exposures have almost certainly been much greater than that to the public from general air pollution.

3. Since 1964 the evidence relating past exposure to asbestos and mesotheliomas has been clarified. The evidence has been greatly strengthened by further prospective and retrospective mortality studies in many countries of populations exposed to asbestos. There is evidence that all commercial types of asbestos, except anthophyllite, may be responsible. Evidence for an important difference in risk in different occupations and with the type of asbestos has increased. The risk is greatest with crocidolite, less with amosite and apparently less with chrysotile. With amosite and chrysotile there appears to be a higher risk in manufacturing than in mining and milling. There is also evidence from population studies that a proportion of cases of mesothelioma have no known association with exposure to asbestos.

4. No evidence of an increased risk of mesothelial cancers at low levels of exposure to asbestos, such as have been encountered by the general population in urban areas, has been established. There is evidence of an association of mesothelial tumors with air pollution in the neighborhood of crocidolite mines and of factories using mixtures of asbestos fiber types. The evidence relates to conditions many years ago. There is evidence of no excess risk of mesotheliomas from asbestos air pollution which has existed in the neighborhood of chrysotile and amosite mines. There are reported differences on incidence of mesothelioma between urban and rural areas, the causes of which have not been established. There is no evidence of a risk to the general public at present.

5. Since 1964, information has been accumulated on the importance of other factors such as cigarette smoking, waxes, oils, and trace elements as contributory factors to the cancer risks. Cigarette smoking is an important factor enhancing the lung carcinoma risk in asbestos-exposed workers, in both men and women. Asbestos workers have specially strong grounds for giving up smoking to protect their health. No association has been demonstrated between cigarette smoking and mesotheliomas. Animal experiments designed thus far to test the importance of waxes and oils as contributory factors in the production of mesotheliomas have shown these contaminants are unlikely to be relevant. From animal experiments there are no good clues suggesting that trace elements are likely to be a major factor in the production of asbestos cancers.

6. Prospective surveys of occupational groups exposed to asbestos have in general shown a small excess risk of some other types of cancers (in addition to bronchial and mesothelial), especially those of the gastrointestinal tract and ovarian tumors. The excess of these tumors is relatively small compared with that for bronchial cancer.

7. In the present state of knowledge there is no evidence of an increased risk of cancer resulting from asbestos fibers present in water, beverages, food, or in the fluids used for the administration of drugs.

These statements, although generally acceptable, have received a certain amount of criticism, which on the whole has been more political than scientific. Scientific evidence produced since 1972 has tended to support the opinions expressed in the report. For example, Enterline and Henderson (*36*) have confirmed that the incidence of carcinoma of the lung and pulmonary fibrosis is greater in a cement factory using both crocidolite and chrysotile when compared with a factory using chrysotile alone. More evidence implicating crocidolite in the development of mesotheliomas has been reviewed by Wagner (*37*).

Conclusions

Carcinomas of the lung are associated with the moderate-to-severe fibrosis of asbestosis. It would seem that excessive exposure to all types of fiber could be responsible. There is evidence to support the contention that the incidence of carcinoma can be greatly reduced by good plant hygiene. Mesotheliomas may occur after only slight exposures, particularly to crocidolite. The use of this type of fiber should therefore be abandoned if not essential. The position of amosite is not yet clear, so that a high standard of dust control is required when it is used. The use of chrysotile may carry only a small risk when the dust control is at a level which is now practical and economic.

The evidence that fibrous particles if sufficiently fine, irrespective of chemical composition, may be responsible for the development of the pleural tumors may provide clues to the mechanism of tumor initiation at the cellular level. It is also important because it helps to judge the possible carcinogenicity of new fibrous materials, some of which are being produced as substitutes for asbestos.

Literature Cited

1. "Report and Recommendations of the Working Group on Asbestos and Cancer," *Ann. N.Y. Acad. Sci.* (1965) **132**, 706; *Br. J. Ind. Med.* (1965) **22**, 165.
2. Whipple, H. E., Ed., "Biological Effects of Asbestos," *Ann. N.Y. Acad. Sci.* (1965) **132**, Art. 1, 1-766.
3. Merewether, E. R. A., Price, C. W., "Report on Effects of Asbestos Dust on the Lung and Dust Suppression in the Asbestos Industry," HMSO, London, 1930.
4. Minister of Labour and National Service, "Annual Report of the Chief Inspector of Factories for the year 1947 (CMD. 7621)," HMSO, London, 1949.
5. Doll, R., *Br. J. Ind. Med.* (1955) **12**, 81.
6. Knox, J. F., Holmes, S., Doll, R., Hill, I. D., *Br. J. Ind. Med.* (1968) **25**, 293.
7. Wagner, J. C., Sleggs, C. A., Marchand, P., *Br. J. Ind. Med.* (1960) **17**, 260.
8. Buchanan, W. D., *Ann. N.Y. Acad. Sci.* (1965) **132**, 507.
9. Elmes, P. C., McCaughey, W. T. E., Wade, O. L., *Br. Med. J.* (1965) **1**, 350.
10. Hourihane, D. O'B., *Thorax* (1964) **19**, 268.

11. Owen, W. G., *Ann. N.Y. Acad. Sci.* (1965) **132,** 674.
12. Mancuso, T. F., Coulter, E. J., *Arch. Environ. Health* (1963) **6,** 210.
13. Gilson, J. C., *Trans. Soc. Occup. Med.* (1966) **16,** 62.
14. UICC Committee, *Chest* (1970) **58,** 57.
15. Timbrell, V., *Pneumoconiosis, Proc. Int. Conf., 3rd, 1969* (1970) 28.
16. Bogovski, P., Gilson, J. C., Timbrell, V., Wagner, J. C., Eds., "Biological effects of asbestos," *IARC Sci. Pub.* No. **8** (1973).
17. McDonald, J. C., McDonald, A. D., Gibbs, G. W., Siemiatycki, J., Rossiter, C. E., *Arch. Environ. Health* (1971) **22,** 677.
18. Mancuso, T. F., El-Attar, A. A., *J. Occup. Med.* (1967) **9,** 147.
19. Selikoff, I. J., Hammond, E. C., Churg, J., *Pneumoconiosis, Proc. Int. Conf., 3rd, 1969* (1970), 180.
20. Selikoff, I. J., Hammond, E. C., Churg, J., *J. Am. Med. Assoc.* (1968) **204,** 106.
21. Doll, R., *J.R. Statist. Soc. A.* (1971) **134,** 133.
22. Berry, G., Newhouse, M. L., Turok, M., *Lancet* (1972) **2,** 476.
23. Meurman, L. O., Kiviluoto, R., Hakama, M., *Br. J. Ind. Med.* (1974) **31,** 105.
24. Ministry of Labour, "Problems Arising from the Use of Asbestos," HMSO, London, 1967.
25. Wagner, J. C., Berry, G., *Br. J. Cancer* (1969) **23,** 567.
26. Harington, J. S., *Nature (Lond.)* (1962) **193,** 43.
27. Harington, J. S., Roe, F. J. C., *Ann. N.Y. Acad. Sci.* (1965) **132,** 439.
28. Commins, B. T., Gibbs, G. W., *Br. J. Cancer* (1969) **23,** 358.
29. Wagner, J. C., Berry, G., Timbrell, V., *Br. J. Cancer* (1973) **28,** 173.
30. Stanton, M. F., Wrench, C., *J. Natl. Cancer Inst.* (1972) **48,** 797.
31. Wagner, J. C., Berry, G., Skidmore, J. W., NIOSH Symposium on Occupational Exposure to Fibrous Glass, University of Maryland, June 1974, in press.
32. Timbrell, V., *Ann. N.Y. Acad. Sci.* (1965) **132,** 255.
33. Timbrell, V., Pooley, F., Wagner, J. C., *Pneumoconiosis, Proc. Int. Conf., 3rd, 1969* (1970), 120.
34. Timbrell, V., Griffiths, D. M., Pooley, F. D., *Nature (Lond.)* (1971) **232,** 55.
35. Harington, J. S., Gilson, J. C., Wagner, J. C., *Nature (Lond.)* (1971) **232,** 54.
36. Enterline, P. E., Henderson, V., *Arch. Environ. Health* (1973) **27,** 312.
37. Wagner, J. C., in Bucalossi, P., Veronesi, V., and Cascinelli, N., "Cancer epidemiology, environmental factors," *Excerpta Med. Int. Congr. Ser.* (1975) **351,** 323–326.

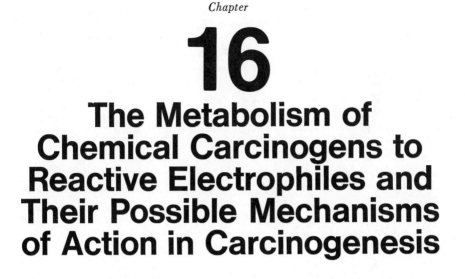

Chapter

16

The Metabolism of Chemical Carcinogens to Reactive Electrophiles and Their Possible Mechanisms of Action in Carcinogenesis

Elizabeth C. Miller and James A. Miller, McArdle Laboratory for Cancer Research, University of Wisconsin Medical Center, Madison Wis. 53706

CHEMICAL CARCINOGENS COMPRISE a diverse group of nonviral and nonradioactive organic and inorganic structures. These compounds generally have low molecular weights (less than 500 daltons) and various species and tissue specificities. A few of these agents are found in inanimate nature. Others are products of man's more or less routine activities and may enter his environment through industrial or nonindustrial activities or both. Most of the known carcinogenic chemicals are synthetic organic compounds, and some can be found in our environment. The fact that several chemical carcinogens have been found as metabolites of fungi or green plants has emphasized the need to monitor foods and other natural products for the possible presence of naturally occurring carcinogens and for other carcinogens which may have been introduced through production or handling. The large number and variety of chemical carcinogens and the wide distributions of some of these compounds emphasize the need for better means of assaying for the carcinogenic activities of chemicals, especially with respect to man, and for a better understanding of carcinogenic processes.

Accordingly, this review summarizes the current data and concepts of the active forms of chemical carcinogens and the reactions of these active forms with cellular constituents in the induction of neoplasia. While the principle of chemical carcinogen activation is now relatively well established, the molecular events involved in neoplasia induction are not yet defined for

737

any instance of carcinogenesis by chemicals, viruses, or radiations. Similarly, the molecular phenotype which is essential for the maintenance of any malignant state is not defined.

Definitions. In tumor induction chemical carcinogens must react, directly or indirectly, with critical informational macromolecules to produce alterations which lead to the seemingly irreversible changes in growth control characteristic of malignant transformations and which are perpetuated indefinitely in daughter cells. To provide more specific nomenclature for the following discussion, chemical carcinogens (*i.e.*, cancer-producing agents) are subdivided into several classes. Thus, we define a precarcinogen as a chemical which is administered to an animal or cell system to induce cancer, but which is not active in the form administered. Most chemical carcinogens are precarcinogens. An ultimate carcinogen is a chemical species which interacts with a critical cell constituent to induce cancer; it may be administered as such or it may be formed *in vivo*. A proximate carcinogen is a derivative of a precarcinogen and thus is a precursor of an ultimate carcinogen. In this discussion the word carcinogenesis is used in a general sense with little distinction between the induction of benign and malignant processes. This approach is justified in part by the fact that there seems to be no example of a chemical which, when adequately studied, induces only benign tumors.

Metabolic Activation of Chemical Carcinogens

General Aspects. Chemical carcinogens, like other chemicals, are subject to a variety of metabolic (usually enzymatic) reactions *in vivo*. If the carcinogen is not an ultimate carcinogen in the form administered, some of these reactions will be activation steps which produce proximate and ultimate carcinogenic derivatives. More than one ultimate carcinogenic derivative of a precarcinogen may be formed, and ultimate carcinogens may have no, one, or several proximate carcinogenic metabolites as precursors. The precarcinogen and its derivatives are usually also subject to deactivation reactions which lead to compounds with no carcinogenic activity or with less carcinogenic potential than the parent compound. The general situation is summarized in Figure 1. Thus, the carcinogenic activity of an administered compound is a function of both the potency of the ultimate carcinogen(s) which are formed and the relative proportions of the dose of administered compound which are funneled through the various activation and deactivation reactions. These considerations show that species, tissue, or other factors (hormonal, dietary, other agents, etc.) which affect the metabolic pathways of a precarcinogen or a proximate carcinogen may have profound effects on its carcinogenicity. Likewise, structural modifications of a carcinogen which affect its rate of metabolism by either activating or deactivating enzyme systems can be expected to modify the carcinogenic activity of the chemical.

A major generalization which has developed in the past few years is that the ultimate carcinogenic forms of chemical carcinogens are usually, if not always, electrophilic (*i.e.*, electron-deficient) reactants (*1, 2, 3*). This generalization is based in part on studies with carcinogenic alkylating agents. These compounds are electrophilic reagents per se and comprise a wide range of structures which have in common the ability to alkylate directly nucleophilic atoms in cellular macromolecules *in vitro* under physiological conditions (*see* Chapter 4). In those cases examined, the identities of the major alkylation products formed *in vivo* with those formed *in vitro* indicate that the reactions observed *in vitro* are appropriate models for the *in vivo* reactions (*4–11*). Some alkylating agents may, of course, be metabolized to

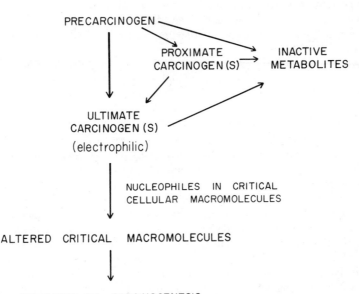

Figure 1. General pathways in the activation and deactivation of chemical carcinogens

forms with different alkylating activities. However, most chemical carcinogens are not reactive as such, but must be converted *in vivo* to electrophilic reactants, usually by enzymatic means. The electrophilic natures of the ultimate carcinogens derived from these precarcinogens were inferred from the structures of metabolic products, including the protein- and nucleic acid-bound derivatives, formed *in vivo* from a number of aromatic amines, amides, and nitro compounds as well as from various potential alkylating agents including the nitrosamines, nitrosamides, pyrrolizidine alkaloids, polycyclic aromatic hydrocarbons, and other compounds (*8, 9, 11–34*).

While proteins and nucleic acids contain several strongly nucleophilic (electron-rich) sites which are known or suspected to be targets of the chemical carcinogens *in vivo*, it seems unlikely that all the nucleophilic reaction sites are critical targets for carcinogenesis. Hence, exceptions to correlations suggested by earlier studies between the likelihood of tumor formation and the total amounts of protein- or nucleic acid-bound derivatives of certain carcinogens have developed (*34, 35, 36, 37, 38*). The critical reactions may involve only certain RNA's, certain proteins, certain portions of DNA, or combinations thereof, and it is possible that only a restricted group of reactions with one or more of these macromolecules is able to redirect a cell's activities toward malignancy.

In this review we consider some examples of the more extensively studied classes of chemical carcinogens with emphasis on the variety of electrophilic reactive forms which may arise in metabolism and which may be important in neoplasia induction. Several ultimate carcinogens may be derived from a single precarcinogen, and the amount and importance of each in a carcinogenic process may differ markedly, depending on the tissue, species, and other conditions.

Aromatic Amines, Amides, and Nitro Compounds. (*See* Chapter 8). *N*-Hydroxy metabolites were strongly implicated as proximate carcinogenic derivatives of aromatic amines and amides. Thus, in the rat and some other species, *N*-hydroxyamides and their conjugates were demonstrated to be metabolites of some aromatic amines and amides, including 2-fluorenamine, 2-fluorenylacetamide, 4-biphenylylacetamide, 4-stilbenylacetamide, and 2-phenanthrylacetamide (*3, 12*). Similarly, *N*-hydroxy-1- and 2-naphthylamine and *N*-hydroxy-4-biphenylamine or their conjugates are urinary metabolites of the corresponding amines in the dog (*39, 40, 41, 42*). Although the data on the metabolism of carcinogenic aromatic nitro compounds are less complete, they are also metabolized to hydroxylamines. The formation of 4-hydroxyaminoquinoline-1-oxide at the site of subcutaneous injection of 4-nitroquinoline-1-oxide was demonstrated in the rat (*43*). Evidence was also reported that certain carcinogenic nitrofuran derivatives were reduced to hydroxylamines by tissue preparations (*44, 45, 46, 47*). In a variety of studies *N*-hydroxy metabolites generally proved more carcinogenic than the parent compounds, especially at the administration sites; thus they are clearly proximate carcinogenic metabolites (*1, 2, 3, 41*).

Current concepts on the further metabolic activation of the aromatic *N*-hydroxyamines and *N*-hydroxyamides developed principally from studies on derivatives of 2-fluorenamine (*1, 2, 12*). *N*-Hydroxy-2-fluorenylacetamide is converted to its sulfuric acid ester in the rat liver (*48, 49, 50*), and this ester appears to be a major ultimate carcinogenic metabolite of *N*-hydroxy-2-fluorenylacetamide in this tissue. Under various conditions with two strains of rats and with other species, the hepatic sulfotransferase activity for *N*-hydroxy-2-fluorenylacetamide correlates well with hepatocarcinogenic activity (*48, 51*). Administration of *p*-hydroxyacetanilide or acetanilide to rats appears to deplete the sulfate available for esterification and thereby reduces the yield of the reactive sulfuric acid conjugate of *N*-hydroxy-2-fluorenylacetamide. The amounts of macromolecule-bound fluorene derivatives in the liver were reduced by administration of *p*-hydroxyacetanilide, and the hepatocarcinogenic activity of *N*-hydroxy-2-fluorenylacetamide was reduced by administration of acetanilide. Both inhibitions were largely overcome by the simultaneous administration of sodium sulfate (*52, 53*). The overall metabolism of 2-fluorenylacetamide in the male rat liver is outlined in Figure 2.

The enzymatic formation of the sulfuric acid ester of *N*-hydroxy-2-fluorenylacetamide by tissue preparations was assayed through the reaction of the ester with methionine to yield 1- and 3-methylmercapto-2-fluorenylacetamide or by reaction with nucleic acids to yield nucleic acid-bound fluorene residues. When the enzymatic formation of the sulfuric acid ester of other carcinogenic *N*-hydroxyarylamides was assayed in the rat liver system, lower levels of the methylmercaptoamides were obtained than with *N*-hydroxy-2-fluorenylacetamide as substrate (*48, 54*). Thus, these other *N*-hydroxyarylamides are either less readily esterified by the rat hepatic

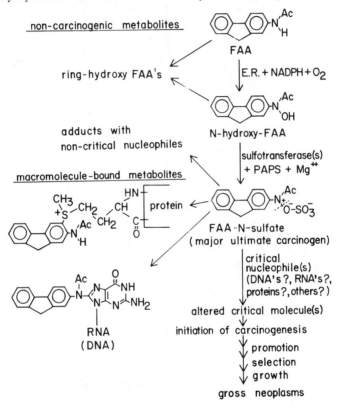

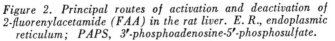

Figure 2. Principal routes of activation and deactivation of 2-fluorenylacetamide (FAA) in the rat liver. E. R., endoplasmic reticulum; PAPS, 3'-phosphoadenosine-5'-phosphosulfate.

sulfotransferase system, or the sulfuric acid esters are much less reactive, or, as seems likely, both of these explanations may be important. These data are consistent with the fact that 2-fluorenylacetamide and its *N*-hydroxy derivative are strong hepatocarcinogens in the rat whereas the other aromatic amides and, where tested, their *N*-hydroxy derivatives induced few liver tumors in the rat (*55–60*). Sulfotransferase activity toward 3-hydroxyxanthine and 3-hydroxyguanine was demonstrated in rat liver and rat fibroblasts *(61, 62)*. This finding is consistent with the observed hepatocarcinogenic and sarcomagenic activity of these *N*-hydroxy purines in the rat *(63)*.

Although the sulfuric acid ester is a major ultimate carcinogenic metabolite of *N*-hydroxy-2-fluorenylacetamide in the rat liver, other ultimate electrophilic derivatives are also probably involved in the carcinogenicity of this compound (Figure 3). No sulfotransferase activity for *N*-hydroxy-2-fluorenylacetamide was detected in the rat mammary gland, subcutaneous tissue, or sebaceous ear duct gland (Zymbal's gland) *(48, 64)*. Each of these tissues is a site in which *N*-hydroxy-2-fluorenylacetamide has strong carcinogenic activity. Furthermore, other metabolic reactions which convert

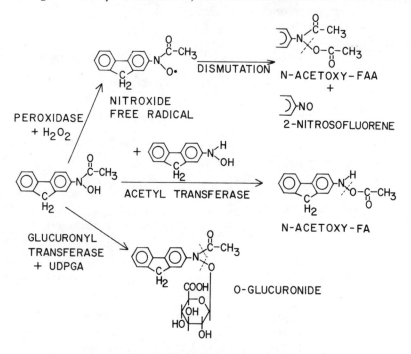

Figure 3. Pathways, in addition to sulfuric acid esterification, for the metabolism of N-hydroxy-2-fluorenylacetamide (N-HO-FAA) to electrophilic reactants in rat tissues. FA, 2-fluorenamine; UDPGA, uridine diphosphate glucuronic acid.

N-hydroxy-2-fluorenylacetamide to electrophilic reactants are known and are obvious reactions to examine as possible modes of *in vivo* activation, especially in extrahepatic tissues.

Phosphorylation of *N*-hydroxy-2-fluorenylacetamide appears to be, at most, a minor metabolic pathway for this carcinogen in rat liver *(48, 50 65, 66)*. The evidence for the reported phosphorylation of 4-hydroxyaminoquinoline-1-oxide by rat ascites hepatoma cells *(67)* was recently reinterpreted. More detailed studies now indicate that the reactive intermediate is an amino acid ester (primarily of serine) rather than a phosphoric acid ester *(68)*.

Two mechanisms were suggested for the formation of the acetic acid ester of N-hydroxy-2-fluorenylacetamide. The first is the nonenzymatic transfer of the acetyl group from S-acetyl coenzyme A. This reaction requires an alkaline pH, and no enzyme-catalyzed transfer from this coenzyme has been detected (*69*). A unique enzymatic means of generating the reactive ester, N-acetoxy-2-fluorenylacetamide, from N-hydroxy-2-fluorenylacetamide involves the one-electron oxidation of this hydroxamic acid by peroxidases and hydrogen peroxide (*70, 71, 72, 73*). The initial oxidation product, a free nitrooxide radical, readily dismutates to form N-acetoxy-2-fluorenylacetamide and 2-nitrosofluorene. Other N-hydroxyacetylaminoarenes behave in a similar manner (*73, 74*). Free radical formation was also reported from aromatic amines or amides, but the radicals have not been characterized (*75, 76*).

The glucuronide of N-hydroxy-2-fluorenylacetamide, a major metabolite of the carcinogen, reacts with nucleophilic centers at a very slow, but still measurable, rate (*77, 78*). The O-glucuronide of N-hydroxy-2-fluorenamine is a much more reactive electrophile than its acetylated derivative (*79*) and, if formed *in vivo*, could be an important reactive form. The urinary excretion of the O-glucuronide of N-hydroxy-4-biphenylamine by dogs dosed with 4-biphenylamine (*42*) makes the latter glucuronide an important candidate ultimate carcinogen for bladder tumor formation.

Esters of hydroxamic acids can act as acylating agents as well as arylamidating or arylating agents. Thus, considerable acetylation of guanosine occurs when it is incubated at neutrality with N-hydroxy-4-biphenylylacetamide or N-hydroxy-2-phenanthrylacetamide (*12*). The ε-amino-group of lysine in RNAse was acetylated when the enzyme was incubated with N-acetoxy-2-fluorenylacetamide (*80*). No evidence has been presented yet for the occurrence of these reactions *in vivo*.

N-Hydroxy-2-fluorenamine, an electrophilic reagent at acidic pH's, has little, if any, reactivity at neutrality (*77, 81*). Earlier reports on the apparent reactivity of this hydroxylamine on incubation with liver preparations now appear to be a consequence of N-acetoxy-2-fluorenamine formation (*65, 82, 83*). This very reactive ester is formed by the enzymatic transfer of the N-acetyl group of N-hydroxy-2-fluorenylacetamide to the oxygen of the hydroxylamine (*82, 83, 84*). This reaction is of further interest since strongly reactive acetic acid esters of several other carcinogenic aromatic hydroxylamines are formed by the same, or similar, enzyme systems and since a number of tissues catalyze the reaction (*82, 83, 84, 85*). While rat liver preparations use either 2-fluorenamine or 4-biphenylamine derivatives as substrates for this transacetylase system, the rat mammary gland system uses only the 4-biphenylamine derivatives (*85*). Since both N-hydroxy-2-fluorenylacetamide and N-hydroxy-4-biphenylylacetamide are carcinogenic for the rat mammary gland, no special role can be assigned the acetic acid esters of the hydroxylamines in mammary carcinoma induction (*56, 58, 86*). However, the observation emphasizes the probable importance of isozymic differences in determining the relative carcinogenic activities of related compounds in series of tissues.

The reactivities of the esters of the hydroxylamines and hydroxamic acids should not, however, obscure the possible importance of other metabolites in carcinogenesis. For instance, esters and the O-glucuronide of 2-amino-1-naphthol, a metabolite of 2-naphthylamine, arylate N-acetyl cysteine and glutathione at pH 7 to yield the corresponding S-(2-amino-1-naphthyl) derivatives (87). Further, the mutagenicity of the nitroso compounds related to a number of carcinogenic aromatic amines and amides, especially 2-nitrosofluorene, suggests the possible importance of this class of compounds in carcinogenesis (88); 2-nitrosofluorene is a moderately active carcinogen (89, 90, 91).

Polycyclic Aromatic Hydrocarbons. (*See* Chapter 5). Although first suggested over 20 years ago (92), the metabolic formation of epoxides of the polycyclic aromatic hydrocarbons, including several carcinogenic hydrocarbons, was clearly documented only in the past few years (31, 32, 33, 93, 94, 95). Epoxidation apparently occurs to some extent at most or all of the available sites on the aromatic rings (29, 30, 95, 96, 97, 98) (Figure 4), and the epoxides which were studied react nonenzymatically with nucleic acids and proteins (95, 97, 98, 99, 100, 101). However, until very recently the interest in epoxides as ultimate carcinogenic derivatives was focused on the K-region derivatives. The K-region epoxides of benz(*a*)anthracene, dibenz(*a,h*)anthracene, 3-methylcholanthrene, and benzo(*a*)pyrene are each more reactive in the induction of neoplastic transformations of mouse and hamster fibroblasts in culture than are the parent hydrocarbons or the corresponding phenols or dihydrodiols (102, 103, 104). On the other hand, the K-region epoxide of 7-methylbenz(*a*)anthracene had no more transforming activity than 7-methylbenz(*a*)anthracene. The 8,9-epoxide of 7-methylbenz(*a*)anthracene did not cause neoplastic transformation of hamster or mouse embryo fibroblasts under conditions where the 5,6-epoxide was active (103, 104).

However, comparison of the products formed on degradation of DNA incubated with the K-region epoxide of 7-methylbenz(*a*)anthracene with those formed on degradation of DNA from mouse embryo cells treated with 7-methylbenz(*a*)anthracene indicated that the K-region epoxide was not a precursor of the major DNA-bound derivatives formed by the cells (101). It now seems likely that the precursors of the DNA-bound hydrocarbon products formed *in vivo* are epoxides of dihydrodiols. Present data indicate that the epoxide groups are not in the K-region. Thus, the major product formed on degradation of DNA which was incubated with 8,9-dihydro-8,9-dihydroxybenz(*a*)anthracene-10,11-oxide showed the same chromatographic properties as the products formed on degradation of DNA from hamster embryo cells incubated with benz(*a*)anthracene (97). Recent results (98) likewise show that a degradation product from the DNA adduct formed from benzo(*a*)pyrene in cell systems co-chromatographed with a degradation product from DNA which was reacted with 7,8-dihydro-7,8-dihydroxybenzo-(*a*)pyrene in a fortified microsomal system.

The 6-oxobenzo(*a*)pyrene radical, which is formed on incubation of benzo(*a*)pyrene with skin or liver preparations was also suggested as a possible ultimate carcinogenic metabolite of this hydrocarbon (*105, 106*). This metabolite reacts readily with DNA at neutrality to yield covalently bound products (*107*), but so far it has shown only marginal carcinogenic activity (*105*). Radical cations which can be formed as intermediates in the one-electron oxidation of the hydrocarbons were also suggested as models for reactions which might take place metabolically (*106, 108, 109, 110, 111*).

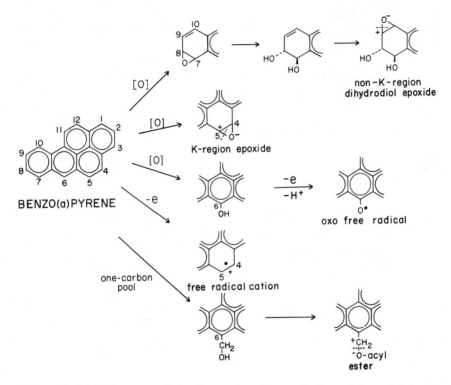

Figure 4. Multiple enzymatic pathways for the metabolism of benzo(a)pyrene to electrophilic reactants

Another suggested activation scheme is the metabolic oxidation of the methyl groups of 7-methylbenz(*a*)anthracene and 7,12-dimethylbenz(*a*)anthracene to hydroxymethyl derivatives (*112, 113*), although these hydroxymethyl derivatives usually showed less carcinogenic activity than the parent hydrocarbons (*114, 115, 116*). The corresponding benzylic bromide derivatives were studied as models for postulated metabolically formed esters of the hydroxymethyl compounds (*103, 104, 117*), and 7,12-bis(bromomethyl)benz(*a*)anthracene showed some carcinogenic activity (*117*). However, the lack of identity of the products formed on degradation of DNA treated with 7-bromomethylbenz(*a*)anthracene *in vitro* with those formed on degradation of the DNA isolated from cell cultures treated with 7-methylbenz(*a*)anthracene suggest that little or no cellular product was derived from an inter-

mediate hydroxymethyl derivative (*101*). 6-Hydroxymethylation of benzo-
(*a*)pyrene by rat liver preparations was reported (*118, 119*), but the significance of this reaction to benzo(*a*)pyrene carcinogenesis is not known.
Multiple pathways of benzo(*a*)pyrene metabolism to electrophilic reactants
that must be considered as possible ultimate carcinogens are shown in
Figure 4.

    Safrole. (*See* Chapter 12). Recent studies on the metabolism of the
naturally occurring carcinogen safrole (4-allyl-2-methylenedioxybenzene)
pointed to 1'-hydroxysafrole as a proximate carcinogenic metabolite (*120,
121*) (Figure 5). This metabolite is a considerably stronger hepatic carcinogen for the rat and mouse than the parent compound (*121*). 1'-Acetoxy-
safrole, a synthetic ester of 1'-hydroxysafrole with electrophilic reactivity
toward nucleophilic tissue constituents such as methionine and guanylic acid,

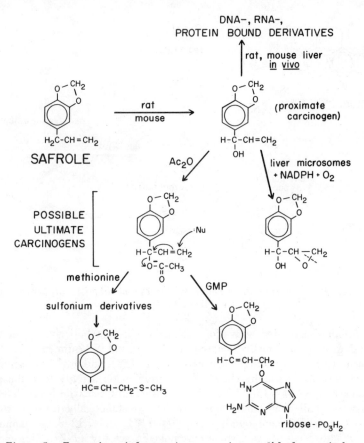

*Figure 5. Formation of the proximate carcinogen 1'-hydroxysafrole
from the naturally occurring precarcinogen safrole. Two possible
modes of further activation are shown, as well as the reactivity of
the model ester 1'-acetoxysafrole with methionine and 5'-guanylic
acid.*

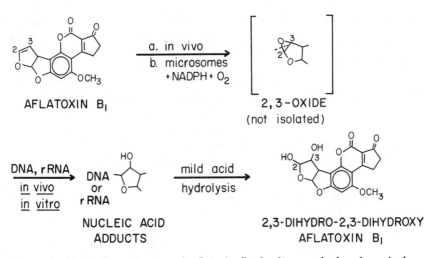

AFLATOXIN B₁

2,3-OXIDE
(not isolated)

NUCLEIC ACID
ADDUCTS

2,3-DIHYDRO-2,3-DIHYDROXY
AFLATOXIN B₁

Figure 6. Metabolic activation of aflatoxin B_1 by liver endoplasmic reticulum (E.R.) and the weak acid hydrolysis of nucleic acid adducts formed from the electrophilic intermediate

also has carcinogenic activity at administration sites (*120, 121*). However, the importance of esters of 1'-hydroxysafrole in the reactivity *in vivo* and carcinogenicity of 1'-hydroxysafrole is not clear. The detection of low levels of 3'-methylmercaptoisosafrole in the livers of rats and mice administered 1'-hydroxysafrole suggests that some esterification occurs (*122*). However, since the latter product accounts for only a small amount of the protein-bound tritium in the liver after administration of 1'-hydroxysafrole-2',3'-³H, other reactive metabolites are also apparently formed *in vivo*.

Other candidate ultimate carcinogenic derivatives of safrole include 1'-oxosafrole and the 2',3'-epoxides of safrole, 1'-hydroxysafrole, and 1'-oxosafrole (*122, 123, 124*). The latter epoxides show electrophilic reactivity, but are considerably less reactive than 1'-acetoxysafrole (*122*). 1'-Oxosafrole was not detected directly as a metabolite, but amine adducts of 1'-oxosafrole are excreted in trace amounts by animals administered safrole, 1'-hydroxysafrole, or 1'-oxosafrole (*124, 125, 126*). The reactivity of 1'-oxosafrole has not been adequately characterized, but its electrophilicity is apparent from its reaction with amines and by the formation of uncharacterized products on reaction with nucleosides and nucleotides (*122, 126*). 1'-Oxosafrole showed no carcinogenic activity while 1'-hydroxysafrole-2',3'-oxide initiated papilloma formation in mouse skin (*122*).

Aflatoxin B₁. (*See* Chapter 12). Several observations (*127*) suggest that the activity of this very potent hepatotoxic and hepatocarcinogenic mycotoxin depends on metabolic activation. Recent evidence indicates that the major metabolic precursor of the DNA- and RNA-bound derivatives in the livers of rodents administered aflatoxin B₁ is its 2,3-oxide (*127, 128, 129, 130, 131*) (Figure 6). The most convincing evidence comes from the finding that 2,3-dihydro-2,3-dihydroxyaflatoxin B₁ is released from the hepatic nucleic acids by weak acid hydrolysis (131). This dihydrodiol is also released from the nucleic acid-aflatoxin B_1 adducts formed by incubation of aflatoxin B_1 with NADPH-fortified rat or human liver microsomes and RNA or DNA (128, 131). The dihydrodiol is the product which would be expected on hydrolysis of the glycoside-like bond formed by reaction of aflatoxin B_1-2,3-oxide at carbon 2 with oxygen or nitrogen atoms in the nucleic acid.

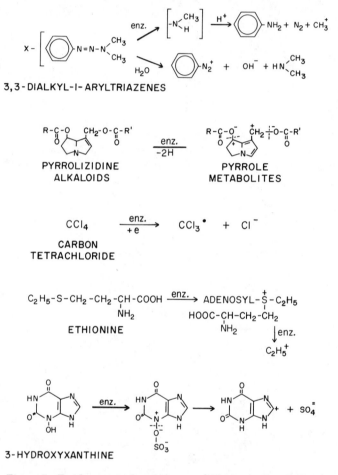

Figure 7. Further examples of the metabolic formation of reactive electrophiles from chemical carcinogens

The importance of the 2,3-double bond in the carcinogenicity of aflatoxin B_1 (132) suggests that the 2,3-oxide is also an ultimate carcinogenic metabolite of this mycotoxin.

The 2,3-oxide appears to be very labile and could not be isolated after presumed synthesis by chemical or enzymatic procedures. Aflatoxin B_1-2,3-dichloride, prepared as a possible model of the oxide, also is strongly electrophilic at carbon 2. This dichloride is more toxic and carcinogenic than aflatoxin B_1 for the skin of mice and subcutaneous tissue of rats (*133*).

Other Carcinogens. The relative abundance of strong nucleophilic sites and the dearth of electrophilic sites in components of informational macromolecules account for the electrophilic character of the majority of the agents that react readily with proteins and nucleic acids under physiologic conditions. These facts also account for the observation that the reactive forms of most, if not all, chemical carcinogens are strong electrophiles. Examples of electrophilic metabolites of a number of carcinogens other than those discussed above are presented in Figure 7. Most of the known chemical carcinogens produce alkylating and arylating species, but two carcinogenic acylating agents are known (*134, 135*). Additional carcinogenic acylating agents may be found.

6-Mercaptopurine is a possible exception to this generalization. It caused increased incidences of certain tumors of the hematopoietic system in rats and mice (*136*). Similarly, malignant transformations of hamster cells occurred after exposure to 1-β-D-arabinofuranosylcytosine, 5-fluorodeoxyuridine, or hydroxyurea (*137, 138*). It is not known whether or not the carcinogenic activities of these compounds are related to their effects on nucleic acid synthesis.

Molecular Targets of Ultimate Chemical Carcinogens

The covalent binding of certain chemical carcinogens to proteins in their target tissues was first recognized over 25 years ago (*139*). The reaction of some alkylating agents with tissue nucleic acids was first detected about 20 years ago (*140*). The covalent bindings of the more complex chemical carcinogens to RNA and DNA were first recognized nearly 15 years ago (*34, 141, 142, 143*). These studies provided the first data on the actions of chemical carcinogens on cells at a molecular level. The important message of these early studies was that chemical carcinogens can alter the structure of cellular nucleic acids and proteins. The exact consequences of any of these alterations in relation to the carcinogenic processes induced by these agents is still not known. However, the chemical natures of some of these interactions showed that they are the result of electrophilic attacks by carcinogen derivatives on nucleophilic centers in the proteins and nucleic acids.

Once formed, the electrophilic derivatives of the chemical carcinogens appear to react nonenzymatically with available nucleophiles in small molecules and in macromolecules (Table I). The nucleophilic sites which are substituted must depend on the formation site of the electrophile and the extent to which the stability, solubility, and charge of the electrophile permit its movement within the cell. The sites which are substituted must also be functions of the relative nucleophilicities of the various targets and the extents to which they are available for reaction. Thus, steric factors, charge distributions, and other factors which influence the approach of the electrophiles to the nucleophilic sites all play a role.

Ignorance of the molecular mechanisms by which chemical carcinogens induce neoplasia makes it difficult to understand the consequences of the reactions of chemical carcinogens with cellular molecules. Knowledge of the critical role of alterations in DNA bases in cellular mutagenesis makes it reasonable, in examining mutagenesis, to study only the effects of mutagenic agents on DNA. Since the critical target(s) for carcinogenesis are not defined, there is no similar guide in the study of chemical carcinogenesis. Because the hereditary nature of the neoplastic transformation appears to require that the critical alteration(s) responsible for transformation occur in one or more of the informational macromolecules of the cell, efforts were made to link the amounts and/or types of alterations of DNA's, RNA's, and proteins with the likelihood of the development of tumors under different conditions. In

Table I. Macromolecular Nucleophilic Targets of Chemical Carcinogens *in vivo*

	Sites Substituted	Reference[a]
Nucleic acids		
adenine	N-1, N-3, N-7	6, 9
cytosine	N-3	6, 9
guanine	N-3, N-7, O-6	6, 9
guanine	C-8	19
Proteins		
cysteine	S	153
histidine	N-1, N-3	144
methionine	S	13, 18
tyrosine	C-3	16

[a] The references are not inclusive; at least one well documented case is cited for each nucleophilic site.

many cases the attempted correlations concerned the total amounts of reaction products of a carcinogen covalently linked with the total DNA, RNA, or protein of a given tissue. While correlations were obtained within restricted carcinogen classes between binding to one or another of these classes of macromolecules and tumor incidences, exceptions were evident (*19, 20, 34–38, 145*). In almost every case these exceptions were situations in which the amounts of the macromolecule-bound derivatives were greater than were expected on the basis of the tumor incidences. This result would be expected if only a portion of the reactions of an ultimate carcinogen with the critical target were involved in the induction of neoplastic transformations. It would also be observed if reactions with only some species of a macromolecule were involved in the carcinogenic process.

Recent data suggest that characterization of specific reaction products may further elucidate the targets involved in carcinogenesis. Thus, studies with 2-fluorenylacetamide, 4-biphenylylacetamide, and their *N*-hydroxy derivatives indicated that the amounts of *N*-(guanosin-8-yl)-2-fluorenylacetamide or *N*-(guanosin-8-yl)-4-biphenylylacetamide residues in hepatic ribosomal RNA (rRNA) correlate more closely with the likelihood of liver tumor development than the amounts of the corresponding non-acetylated derivatives in rRNA, the amounts of these acetylated or non-acetylated derivatives in DNA, or the amounts of the 3-(guan-N^2-yl)-2-fluorenylacetamide in DNA (*19, 20, 25, 146, 147*). The mutagenic activities of several methylating and ethylating agents now appear to correlate much better with the extent of alkylation of the oxygen atom attached to C-6 of guanosine as compared with alkylation of the 7-nitrogen (*10, 148,* Chapter 4). Other differences were also noted in the relative proportions of various alkylation products on reaction of series of alkylating agents with nucleic acids (*6, 9,* Chapter 4). These and related studies should yield a firm basis from which to assess the effects of alkylation at various sites of the polymers on the functional capacities of nucleic acids.

Elucidation of the reactions essential to carcinogenesis also requires much more attention to the reactions of particular DNA's, RNA's, or proteins with the ultimate carcinogens. Aromatic amines and polycyclic hydrocarbons show some specificity with respect to the proteins of the target tissues to which they bind (*34, 149–162*). In the livers of rats administered ethionine the extent of ethylation of the transfer RNA's (*t*RNA's) is greater than that of rRNA (*163*). Administration of 2-fluorenylacetamide or its *N*-hydroxy derivative to rats likewise resulted in more extensive binding of fluorene residues to hepatic *t*RNA than to the *r*RNA (*146, 164, 165*). The administration of *N*-methyl-*N*-nitrosourea or *N*-nitrosodimethylamine (dimethylnitrosamine) to rats yielded several-fold greater substitution of hepatic mitochondrial DNA than of the nuclear DNA (*166, 167,* Chapter 11). These differences in the degree of reaction may reflect the relative proximities of different macromolecules to the formation sites of the electrophilic reagents or to differences in the half-lives of the substituted molecules and may or may not reflect the importance of the target molecule(s) in carcinogenesis. The differences in extent and type of binding to various macromolecules must be explored for their possible contributions to our knowledge of the initiation of carcinogenesis.

The above emphasis on covalently bound derivatives of chemical carcinogens arises from the fact that these relatively stable carcinogen-cell component interactions were the most obvious experimental findings that appeared to relate to carcinogenesis by these agents. Less stable covalent interactions, which may escape detection, may be important by causing alterations in cell macromolecules that persist after loss of the carcinogen residue (*168*). Similarly, important noncovalent binding may be evanescent and difficult to detect. Few studies of such interactions were made. In the case of the polycyclic aromatic hydrocarbons the physical binding of these compounds to polynucleotides did not correlate with carcinogenic activity (*169*). Likewise, only a few interactions of carcinogens with low molecular weight cellular components were noted. If such interactions are important in a carcinogenic process, it seems axiomatic that macromolecular informational molecules in the cell should ultimately be affected by the carcinogen—small molecule complex.

Mechanisms of Chemical Carcinogenesis

The molecular mechanisms by which chemicals (or other carcinogenic agents) cause the transformation of cells from a normal phenotype with responsiveness to growth-controlling factors to a tumor phenotype with a reduced or altered responsiveness to these factors have not been elucidated. In most cases the transformations appear to be essentially permanent and heritable in that tumor cells give rise to tumor cells. However, since these biological systems generally select for neoplastic cells through their greater capacity for multiplication than that of normal cells, the reversion to normal behavior of even large proportions of the cells in a tumor could be difficult to detect. Nevertheless, the relative permanence of the neoplastic state of many lines of tumor cells is supported by the high efficiencies with which some populations of malignant cells can be cloned indefinitely and still give rise to new colonies of similar cells in culture. On the other hand, some examples of the apparent reversibility of the neoplastic state were seen in the differentiation of teratoma cells (170) and the development of normal plants or parts thereof from plant tumor cell lines (171, but see critique in Ref. 172). Some apparent reversions of neoplastic animal cell lines yielded aneuploid cells with the phenotype, but not the genotype, of the parent cell (173, 174).

Genetic Mechanisms. For many years the lack of correspondence between the mutagenic and carcinogenic actions of chemicals argued against a mutagenic basis of carcinogenesis. However, as the proximate and ultimate carcinogenic forms of several precarcinogens were defined and these forms were tested for mutagenic activity, the correspondence between the mutagenic and carcinogenic activities of chemicals grew much stronger (175). As a first approximation the improved correspondence appears to argue that a causal relationship exists between these activities. However, closer inspection denies the necessity of this argument, and the relationship may be only a formal one. Thus, as discussed above, most, if not all, ultimate carcinogens are electrophilic reactants. Likewise, most ultimate mutagens (excluding hydroxylamine, bisulfite, and small groups of base analogs and simple intercalating frameshift mutagens) are electrophilic reactants (175). This formal correlation suggests that, with the exceptions noted above, most ultimate mutagens are ultimate carcinogens, and all ultimate carcinogens are ultimate mutagens, if they can reach the critical targets for each agent. However, this correlation does not specify the target for either type of agent or that the targets for mutagenesis and carcinogenesis are the same.

The genetic mechanism of carcinogenesis, e.g., the mutation of the nuclear DNA, was proposed in general terms (abnormal chromosome content) many years ago by Boveri (176) and has been debated ever since. In essence, this mechanism proposes that the basis of carcinogenesis is an alteration in the information coded in the nuclear DNA, either through base addition, base deletion, base alteration, or translocation of a portion of the genome. Newer observations in molecular biology expanded the scope of the mutational hypotheses. For instance, the finding of DNA in mitochondria and the observation that certain mutations in yeast (*e.g.*, petite mutants) can be a consequence of mutagenesis of mitochondrial DNA (*177*) raise the possibility that mutation of mitochondrial DNA could be involved in carcinogenesis (*178*). The greater degree of methylation of DNA in liver mitochondria as compared with that in liver nuclei from rats administered *N*-methyl-*N*-nitrosourea or *N*-nitrosodimethylamine lends credence to this suggestion (*166, 167*). Likewise, recent discoveries have highlighted the possible importance of mutagenesis of cellular RNA which might later be transcribed into DNA and then integrated into the nuclear DNA (protovirus hypothesis) (*179*). An assessment of the possible importance of this sequence of events in chemical carcinogenesis will depend in part on the development of information on the frequency with which RNA in eukaryotic cells is copied as DNA and integrated into the genomes of the cells.

Genetic mechanisms of chemical carcinogenesis are thought usually to depend on the chemical reaction or physical interaction of an ultimate carcinogen with a nucleic acid such that the genome of a line of daughter cells is different from that of the parent cell. However, other molecular mechanisms which have the same ultimate result would also be genetic in nature. The finding that strains of T4 phage which contain mutant DNA-directed polymerases have up to a 1000-fold greater incidences or much lower than normal incidences of spontaneous mutations than the wild-type phage (*180, 181*) has provided an interesting model of the extent to which alteration of a DNA polymerase can affect the genomes of progeny cells. The magnitude of the mutation frequency apparently depends on the relative exonuclease and polymerase activities of the enzyme since the exonuclease activity has a role in correcting the DNA as it is syntheiszed (*182*). It is evident that alteration by interaction with a chemical carcinogen of proteins such as DNA polymerase in a cell provides an opportunity for mutant (neoplastic) cells to form during replication (*183, 184*). This mechanism, like the direct alteration of one of the bases of the DNA (*185*), would require a round of replication to obtain a permanent, heritable lesion. Similarly, it was suggested that the mutant polymerases found in certain human leukemia cells may be important in the biological progression of these neoplasias (*186*).

Epigenetic Mechanisms. The quasi-permanence of the neoplastic state was used to support the assertion that neoplastic transformations are genetic changes. This argument meets a strong challenge, however, in the present-day interpretation of cell differentiation to yield the specialized tissues and organs of multicellular organisms. Thus, fertilized enucleated frog eggs bearing nuclei transplanted from differentiated frog cells or from renal tumors possess the genetic information which is needed for the development of swimming tadpoles (*187, 188, 189*). This finding, together with other information (*190*), generally interpreted as evidence that differentiation is a directed repression and derepression of the expression of genetic information rather than a directed mutation. A similar molecular mechanism for neoplasia induction would be consistent with the usual stability of the neoplastic state and the occasional cases of apparent reversion to at least a quasi-normal state (*170, 171*). This mechanism would include the differential repression and derepression of both apparently "normal" DNA genomes and other integrated information (*e.g.*, oncogenic viruses, oncogenes, bacterial genomes, etc.) which has accumulated through millions of cell generations. The greater susceptibility of cells previously infected with murine leukemia tumor virus to transformation by certain chemical carcinogens and the expression of certain RNA tumor virus antigens in chemically transformed cells suggest that oncogenic virus information may play a role in some chemically induced neoplastic transformations (*191, 192, 193*). However, the separation of concomitant effects from causally related conditions will require much more study.

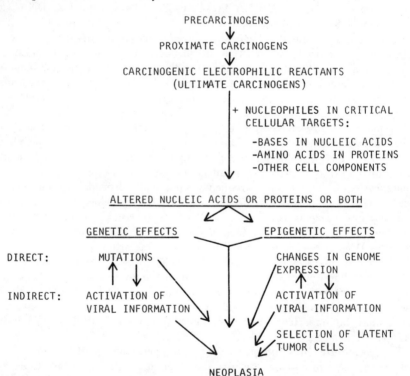

Figure 8. Metabolic activation of chemical carcinogens and possible mechanisms of action of these agents

From this point of view any change, exclusive of a genomic alteration, which can more or less permanently lessen the response of a cell and its descendants to growth controls within these cells or the host, or both, would provide an epigenetic mechanism for a neoplastic transformation. This type of alteration was exemplified by the Jacob–Monod circuitry in which the presence or absence of the appropriate repressor or derepressor can permit or prevent the expression of specific genomic information, including integrated tumor virus genomes, in a cell and its descendants (*194, 195*). The concept that differentiated cells differ with respect to the kinds of messenger RNA which are processed and transported from the nucleus to the cytoplasm (*196, 197*) suggests another site of epigenetic control, the mechanism of which is not known. Some differences of this type between tumor cells and their tissues of origin were reported (*198, 199, 200, 201*).

Throughout this review the term carcinogenesis has been used in the sense that the chemical initiates the conversion of normal cells to neoplastic cells. If one uses a wider definition in which carcinogenesis includes all of the processes leading to the appearance of a gross tumor, rather different epigenetic mechanisms can be envisioned. These are situations in which the prior presence of tumor cells is assumed, and the carcinogenic agent is assigned the role of adjusting conditions to favor the proliferation and survival of the tumor cell and its descendants (*202, 203, 204*). Thus, chemicals which reduce immunological surveillance by the host, which facilitate the development of an appropriate hormonal environment, or which otherwise promote the preferential growth of relatively quiescent tumor cells might be included in this class of agents. Since the effects of promoting agents (*see* Chapter 2), at least at early stages, are relatively reversible while those of initiating agents are essentially irreversible (*205, 206*, but *see also 207*), it is important that sufficient information be obtained to determine which chemicals are carcinogenic in the sense of initiating the neoplastic conversion and which facilitate the proliferation of more or less quiescent neoplastic cells. From a practical point reduction of exposure to promoting agents, even after prolonged exposure, could be important in reducing the risk of tumor development.

Figure 8 summarizes the known and possible steps involved in tumor induction on administration of chemical carcinogens. Each of the possible carcinogenesis mechanisms and their interplays, as discussed above, must be considered, and each may be predominant in specific cases.

Practical Applications

Whatever the mechanisms by which chemical carcinogens induce or facilitate the growth of neoplasms, it seems clear that the major route for controlling chemical carcinogenesis in man will be through controlling human exposures to these chemicals. In theory, at least, such control is relatively straightforward once an etiological agent is recognized. Thus, the chemical can then be removed from human contact by stopping its production or use, appropriate monitoring, education, and other devices. The major problem appears to be how best to identify the carcinogens in the environment and, particularly, how to decide whether or not they constitute risks for man.

The current knowledge on the ultimate forms of chemical carcinogens has two important roles in this problem. First, our increased knowledge of the metabolic alterations of administered chemicals and of the structures of ultimate chemical carcinogens permits much better deductions as to the metabolites which are likely to be formed *in vivo* and the probability that certain of them will be carcinogenic. Second, the knowledge that most, if not all, ultimate forms of chemical carcinogens and a major share of the ultimate forms of chemical mutagens are electrophilic reactants provides a logical basis for the preliminary screening of chemical carcinogens through their mutagenic activity. Mutagenicity assays are relatively inexpensive and rapid and are suited to screening large numbers of compounds. Their utility is greatly expanded by incorporation of the host-mediation principle (*208, 209*). Under these conditions animal tissues or extracts thereof are used to metabolize the test chemical, so that the assay tests the activity of both the administered chemical and any metabolites which are formed.

Short-term *in vitro* assays which use the malignant transformation of cells in cell or organ cultures as an endpoint also appear to be promising routine screens, since they combine the advantages of relative rapidity of assay with an endpoint which measures the induction of neoplasia (*210*). These cell transformation systems would be even more valuable in the form of host-mediated assays. The advantages of both the mutagenicity and transformation systems will be increased further as it becomes possible to use human cells as the test cells and various human tissues for the metabolic machinery. A combined *in vivo–in vitro* assay, in which the carcinogens are injected into pregnant mothers and the fetal tissues are analyzed for malignant potential *in vitro*, also showed promise (*211*).

While these tests can not yet supplant the whole animal life-span tests for assays of the carcinogenic activity of compounds seriously considered to pose risks for man, they can provide quicker interim information and should facilitate the ranking of the priorities of compounds to be assayed by the much more tedious and expensive *in vivo* carcinogenicity assays. Eventually such tests will probably take the place of the present life-span tests in rodents since the latter tests are not only cumbersome but will always be relatively inadequate and insensitive from both statistical and metabolic standpoints.

Literature Cited

1. Miller, J. A., *Cancer Res.* (1970) **30**, 559.
2. Miller, E. C., Miller, J. A., "Environment and Cancer," 24th Annual Symposium on Fundamental Cancer Research, p. 5, Williams and Wilkins, Baltimore, 1972.
3. Miller, J. A., Miller, E. C., "Physicochemical Mechanisms of Carcinogenesis," The Jerusalem Symposia on Quantum Chemistry and Biochemistry, E. D. Bergmann and B. Pullman, Eds., Vol. 1, p. 237, The Israel Academy of Sciences and Humanities, Jerusalem, 1969.
4. Ross, W. J. C., "Biological Alkylating Agents," Butterworth, London, 1962.
5. Lawley, P. D., *Progr. Nucleic Acid Res. Mol. Biol.* (1966) **5**, 89.
6. Lawley, P. D., Shah, S. A., *Biochem. J.* (1972) **128**, 117.
7. Preussmann, R., Druckrey, H., Ivankovic, S., Hodenberg, A.v., *Ann. N.Y. Acad. Sci.* (1969) **163**, 697.

8. Lawley, P. D., Brookes, P., Magee, P. N., Craddock, V. M., Swann, P. F., *Biochim. Biophys. Acta* (1968) **157,** 646.
9. O'Connor, P. J., Copps, M. J., Craig, A. W., Lawley, P. D., Shah, S. A., *Biochem. J.* (1972) **129,** 519.
10. Lawley, P. D., Thatcher, C. J., *Biochem. J.* (1970) **116,** 693.
11. Boutwell, R. K., Colburn, N. H., Muckerman, C. S., *Ann. N.Y. Acad. Sci.* (1969) **163,** 751.
12. Miller, J. A., Miller, E. C., *Progr. Exp. Tumor Res.* (1969) **11,** 273.
13. Scribner, J. D., Miller, J. A., Miller, E. C., *Biochem. Biophys. Res. Commun.* (1965) **20,** 560.
14. Poirier, L. A., Miller, J. A., Miller, E. C., Sato, K., *Cancer Res.* (1967) **27,** 1600.
15. Lin, J.-K., Miller, J. A., Miller, E. C., *Biochemistry* (1968) **7,** 1889.
16. *Ibid.,* **8,** 1573.
17. Kriek, E., Miller, J. A., Juhl, U., Miller, E. C., *Biochemistry* (1967) **6,** 177.
18. DeBaun, J. R., Miller, E. C., Miller, J. A., *Cancer Res.* (1970) **30,** 577.
19. Kriek, E., *Chem.-Biol. Interact.* (1969) **1,** 3.
20. *Ibid.* (1971) **3,** 19.
21. Lin, J.-K., Schmall, B., Sharpe, I. D., Miura, I., Miller, J. A., Miller, E. C., *Cancer Res.* (1975) **35,** 832.
22. Lin, J.-K., Miller, J. A., Miller, E. C., *Cancer Res.* (1975) **35,** 844.
23. Miller, E. C., Butler, B. W., Fletcher, T. L., Miller, J. A., *Cancer Res.* (1974) **34,** 2232.
24. Neumann, H.-G., Metzler, M., Töpner, W., *Abstracts, 2nd Meet. European Assoc. Cancer Res., Heidelberg* (Oct. 2-5, 1973) 159.
25. Kriek, E., *Biochim. Biophys. Acta* (1974) **355,** 177.
26. McLean, E. K., *Pharmacol. Rev.* (1970) **22,** 429.
27. Mattocks, A. R., *Nature (London)* (1968) **217,** 723.
28. Jago, M. V., Edgar, J. V., Smith, L. W., Culvenor, C. C. J. *Molec. Pharmacol.* (1970) **6,** 402.
29. Boyland, E., *Brit. Med. Bull.* (1964) **20,** 121.
30. Sims, P., *Biochem. J.* (1966) **98,** 215.
31. Selkirk, J. K., Huberman, E., Heidelberger, C., *Biochem. Biophys. Res. Commun.* (1971) **43,** 1010.
32. Grover, P. L., Hewer, A., Sims, P., *FEBS Lett.* (1971) **18,** 76.
33. Wang, I. Y., Rasmussen, R. E., Crocker, T. T., *Biochem. Biophys. Res. Commun.* (1972) **49,** 1142.
34. Miller, E. C., Miller, J. A., *Pharmacol. Rev.* (1966), **18,** 805.
35. DenEngelse, L., Bentvelzen, P. A. J., Emmelot, P., *Chem.-Biol. Interactions* (1970) **1,** 395.
36. Swann, P. F., Magee, P. N., *Biochem. J.* (1968) **110,** 39.
37. *Ibid.* (1971) **125,** 841.
38. Goshman, L. M., Heidelberger, C., *Cancer Res.* (1967) **27,** 1678.
39. Boyland, E., Manson, D., *Biochem. J.* (1966) **101,** 84.
40. Radomski, J. L., Brill, E., *Life Sciences* (1967) **6,** 2293.
41. Radomski, J. L., Brill, E., *Science* (1970), **167,** 992.
42. Radomski, J. L., Rey, A. A., Brill, E., *Cancer Res.* (1973) **33,** 1284.
43. Matsushima, T., Kobuna, I., Fukuoka, F., Sugimura, T., *Gann* (1968) **59,** 247.
44. Feller, D. R., Morita, M., Gillette, J. R., *Biochem. Pharmacol.* (1971) **20,** 203.
45. McCalla, D. R., Reuvers, A., Kaiser, C., *Biochem. Pharmacol.* (1971) **20,** 3532.
46. Lower, G. M., Jr., Bryan, G. T., *Proc. Amer. Ass. Cancer Res.* (1971) **12,** 3.
47. *Ibid.* (1972) **13,** 98.
48. DeBaun, J. R., Miller, E. C., Miller, J. A., *Cancer Res.* (1970) **30,** 577.

49. DeBaun, J. R., Rowley, J. Y., Miller, E. C., Miller, J. A., *Proc. Soc. Exp. Biol. Med.* (1968) **129**, 268.
50. King, C. M., Phillips, B., *Science* (1968) **159**, 1351.
51. Gutmann, H. R., Malejka-Giganti, D., Barry, E. J., Rydell, R. E., *Cancer Res.* (1972) **32**, 1554.
52. DeBaun, J. R., Smith, J. Y. R., Miller, E. C., Miller, J. A., *Science* (1970) **167**, 184.
53. Weisburger, J. H., Yamamoto, R. S., Williams, G. M., Grantham, P. H., Matsushima, T., Weisburger, E. K., *Cancer Res.* (1972) **32**, 491.
54. Zieve, F. J., Gutmann, H. R., *Cancer Res.* (1971) **31**, 471.
55. Clayson, D. B., "Chemical Carcinogenesis," Little, Brown, and Co., Boston, 1962.
56. Miller, E. C., Miller, J. A., Hartmann, H. A., *Cancer Res.* (1961) **21**, 815.
57. Miller, J. A., Sandin, R. B., Miller, E. C., Rusch, H. P., *Cancer Res.* (1955) **15**, 188.
58. Miller, J. A., Wyatt, C. S., Miller, J. A., Hartmann, H. A., *Cancer Res.* (1961) **21**, 1465.
59. Andersen, R. A., Enomoto, M., Miller, E. C., Miller, J. A., *Cancer Res.* (1964) **24**, 128.
60. Baldwin, R. W., Smith, W. R. D., *Brit. J. Cancer* (1965) **19**, 433.
61. Stöhrer, G., Corbin, E., Brown, G. B., *Cancer Res.* (1972) **32**, 637.
62. McDonald, J. J., Stöhrer, G., Brown, G. B., *Cancer Res.* (1973) **33**, 3319.
63. Sugiura, K., Teller, M. N., Parham, J. C., Brown, G. B., *Cancer Res.*, (1970) **30**, 184.
64. Irving, C. C., Janss, D. H., Russell, L. T., *Cancer Res.* (1971) **31**, 387.
65. King, C. M., Phillips, B., *J. Biol. Chem.* (1969) **244**, 6209.
66. Lotlikar, P. D., Wasserman, M. B., *Biochem. J.* (1970) **120**, 661.
67. Tada, M., Tada, M., *Biochim Biophys. Res. Commun.* (1972) **46**, 1025.
68. Tada, M., Tada, M., *Proc. Int. Cancer Cong. XIth* (1974) **3**, 339.
69. Lotlikar, P. D., Luha, L., *Biochem. J.* (1971) **124**, 69.
70. Bartsch, H., Traut, M., Hecker, E., *Biochim. Biophys. Acta.* (1971) **237**, 556.
71. Bartsch, H., Hecker, E., *Biochem. Biophys. Acta* (1971) **237**, 567.
72. King, C. M., Bednar, T. W., Linsmaier-Bednar, E. M., *Chem.-Biol. Interact.* (1973) **7**, 185.
73. Bartsch, H., Miller, J. A., Miller, E. C., *Biochim. Biophys. Acta* (1972) **273**, 40.
74. Forrester, A. R., Ogilvy, M. M., Thompson, R. H., *J. Chem. Soc.* (1970) 1081.
75. Wilk, M., Girke, W., "Physicochemical Mechanisms of Carcinogenesis," The Jerusalem Symposia on Quantum Chemistry and Biochemistry, E. D. Bergmann and B. Pullman, Eds., Vol. 1, p. 91. The Israel Academy of Sciences and Humanities, Jerusalem, 1969.
76. Stier, A., Reitz, I., Sackmann, E., *Naunyn-Schmiedeberg's Arch. Pharmacol.* (1972) **274**, 189.
77. Miller, E. C., Lotlikar, P. D., Miller, J. A., Butler, B. W., Irving, C. C., Hill, J. T., *Mol. Pharmacol.* (1968) **4**, 147.
78. Irving, C. C., Veazey, R. A., Hill, J. T., *Biochim. Biophys. Acta* (1969) **179**, 189.
79. Irving, C. C., Russell, L. T., *Biochemistry* (1970) **9**, 2471.
80. Barry, E. J., Gutmann, H. R., *J. Biol. Chem.* (1973) **248**, 2730.
81. Kriek, E., *Biochem. Biophys. Res. Commun.* (1965) **20**, 793.
82. Bartsch, H., Dworkin, M., Miller, J. A., Miller, E. C., *Biochim. Biophys. Acta* (1972) **286**, 272.
83. King, C. M., *Cancer Res.* (1974) **34**, 1503.
84. King, C. M., Olive, C. W., *Proc. Amer. Ass. Cancer Res.* (1974) **15**, 42.
85. Bartsch, H., Dworkin, C., Miller, J. A., Miller, E. C., *Biochim. Biophys. Acta* (1973) **304**, 42.

86. Miller, J. A., Enomoto, M., Miller, E. C., *Cancer Res.* (1962) **22**, 1381.
87. Manson, D., *Chem.-Biol. Interact.* (1972) **5**, 47.
88. Ames, B. N., Gurney, E. G., Miller, J. A., Bartsch, H., *Proc. Natl. Acad. Sci., U.S* (1972) **69**, 3128.
89. Miller, E. C., McKechnie, D., Poirier, M. M., Miller, J. A., *Proc. Soc. Exp. Biol. Med* (1965) **120**, 538.
90. Hecker, E., Traut, M., Hopp, M., *Z. Krebsforsch.* (1968) **71**, 81.
91. Gutmann, H. R., Leaf, D. S., Yost, Y., Rudell, R. E., Chen, C. C., *Cancer Res.* (1970) **30**, 1485.
92. Boyland, E., *Symp. Biochem. Soc.* (1950) **5**, **40**.
93. Jerina, D. M., Daly, J. W., Witkop, B., Zaltzman-Nirenberg, P., Udenfriend, S., *Biochemistry* (1970) **9**, 147.
94. Jerina, D. M., Daly, J. W., *Science* (1974) **185**, 573.
95. Sims, P., Grover, P. L., *Advan. Cancer Res.* (1974) **20**, 166.
96. Booth, J., Sims, P., *FEBS Lett.* (1974) **47**, 30.
97. Swaisland, A. J., Hewer, A., Pal, K., Keysell, G. R., Booth, J., Grover, P. L., Sims, P., *FEBS Letters* (1974) **47**, 34.
98. Sims, P., Grover, P. L., Swaisland, A., Pal, K., Hewer, A., *Nature* (1974) **252**, 326.
99. Grover, P. L., Sims, P., *Biochem. Pharmacol.* (1970) **19**, 2251.
100. *Ibid.* (1973) **22**, 661.
101. Baird, W. M., Dipple, A., Grover, P. L., Sims, P., Brookes, P., *Cancer Res.* (1973) **23**, 2386.
102. Grover, P. L., Sims, P., Huberman, E., Marquardt, H., Kuroki, T., Heidelberger, C., *Proc. Natl. Acad. Sci., U.S.A.* (1971) **68**, 1098.
103. Huberman, E., Kuroki, T., Marquardt, H., Selkirk, J. K., Heidelberger, C., Grover, P. L., Sims, P., *Cancer Res.* (1972) **32**, 1391.
104. Marquardt, H., Kuroki, T., Huberman, E., Selkirk, J. K., Heidelberger, C., Grover, P. L., Sims, P., *Cancer Res.* (1972) **32**, 716.
105. Nagata, C., Tagashira, Y., Kodama, M., "Chemical Carcinogenesis," P.O.P. Ts'o and J. A. DiPaolo, Eds., Part A, p. 87, Marcel Dekker, New York, 1974.
106. Ts'o, P.O.P., Caspary, W. J., Cohen, B. I., Leavitt, J. C., Lesko, S. A., Jr., Lorentzen, R. F., Schechtman, L. M., "Chemical Carcinogenesis," P. O. P. Ts'o and J. A. DiPaolo, Eds., Part A, p. 113, Marcel Dekker, New York, 1974.
107. Caspary, W., Lesko, S., Lorentzen, R., Ts'o, P., *Fed. Proc. Fed. Amer. Soc. Exp. Biol.* (1974) **33**, 1500.
108. Fried, J., Schumm, D. E., *J. Amer. Chem. Soc.* (1967) **89**, 5508.
109. Cavalieri, E., Calvin, M., *Proc. Natl. Acad. Sci., U.S.* (1971) **68**, 1251.
110. Cavalieri, E., *Proc. Amer. Ass. Cancer Res.* (1972) **13**, 125.
111. Johnson, M. D., Calvin, M., *Nature (London)* (1973) **241**, 271.
112. Boyland, E., Sims, P., *Biochem. J.* (1965) **95**, 780.
113. Jellinck, P. H., Smith, G., *Biochem. Pharmacol.* (1969) **18**, 679.
114. Boyland, E., Sims, P., *Int. J. Cancer* (1967) **2**, 500.
115. Flesher, J. W., Sydnor, K. L., *Cancer Res.* (1971) **31**, 1951.
116. Flaks, A., Hamilton, J. M., Clayson, D. B., Sims, P., *Int. J. Cancer* (1972) **10**, 548.
117. Dipple, A., Slade, T. A., *Eur. J. Cancer* (1970) **6**, 417.
118. Flesher, J. W., Sydnor, K. L., *Int. J. Cancer* (1973) **11**, 433.
119. Sloane, N. H., Davis, T. K., *Arch. Biochem. Biophys.* (1974) **163**, 46.
120. Borchert, P., Wislocki, P. G., Miller, J. A., Miller, E. C., *Cancer Res.* (1973) **33**, 575.
121. Borchert, P., Miller, J. A., Miller, E. C., Shires, T. K., *Cancer Res.* (1973) **33**, 590.
122. Wislocki, P. G., Ph.D. Thesis, University of Wisconsin, Madison, Wis., 1974.

123. Horning, M. G., Bell, L., Carman, M. J., Stillwell, W. G., *Abstracts, Soc. Toxicol. Ann. Meet. 13th, March 10-14, 1974,* 29, Washington, D. C.
124. Borchert, P., Ph.D. Thesis, University of Wisconsin, Madison, Wis., 1972.
125. Oswald, E. O., Fishbein, L., Corbett, B. J., Walker, M. P., *Biochim. Biophys. Acta* (1971) **230,** 237.
126. McKinney, J. D., Oswald, E., Fishbein, L., Walker, M. P., *Bull. Environ. Contam. Toxicol.* (1972) **7,** 305.
127. Garner, R. C., Miller, E. C., Miller, J. A., *Cancer Res.* (1972) **32,** 2058.
128. Swenson, D. H., Miller, J. A., Miller, E. C., *Biochem. Biophys. Res. Commun.* (1973) **53,** 1260.
129. Garner, R. C., *FEBS Letters* (1973) **36,** 261.
130. Gurtoo, J. L., Dave, C., *Res. Commun. Chem. Pathol. Pharmacol.* (1973) **5,** 635.
131. Swenson, D. H., Miller, E. C., Miller, J. A., *Biochem. Biophys. Res. Commun.* (1974) **60,** 1036.
132. Wogan, G. N., Edwards, G. S., Newberne, P. M., *Cancer Res.* (1971) **31,** 1936.
133. Swenson, D. H., Miller, J. A., Miller, E. C., *Proc. Amer. Ass. Cancer Res.* (1974) **15,** 43.
134. Dickens, F., Jones, H. E. H., *Br. J. Cancer* (1965) **19,** 392.
135. Van Duuren, B. L., Goldschmidt, B. M., Katz, C., Seidman, I., *J. Nat. Cancer Inst.* (1972) **48,** 1539.
136. Prejean, J. D., Griswold, D. P., Casey, A. E., Peckham, J. C., Weisburger, J. H., Weisburger, E. K., Wood, H. B., Jr., *Proc. Amer. Ass. Cancer Res.* (1972) **13,** 112.
138. Benedict, W. F., Jones, P. A., Baker, M. S., Bertram, J. S., *Abstracts, Int. Cancer Congr. XIth, Florence, Italy, Oct. 20-26, 1974* **3,** 421.
139. Miller, E. C., Miller, J. A., *Cancer Res.* (1947) **7,** 468.
140. Wheeler, G. P., Skipper, H. E., *Arch. Biochem. Biophys.* (1957) **72,** 465.
141. Marroquin, F., Farber, E., *Biochim. Biophys. Acta* (1962) **55,** 403.
142. Heidelberger, C., *J. Cell. Comp. Physiol. Suppl. 1* (1964) **64,** 129.
143. Brookes, P., Lawley, P. D., *Nature (London)* (1964) **202,** 781.
144. Craddock, V. M., *Biochem. J.* (1965) **94,** 323.
145. Miller, E. C., Miller, J. A., Sapp, R. W., Weber, G. M., *Cancer Res.* (1949) **9,** 336.
146. Irving, C. C., Veazey, R. A., *Cancer Res.* (1971) **31,** 19.
147. Kriek, E., *Cancer Res.* (1972) **32,** 2042.
148. Loveless, A., *Nature (London)* (1969) **223,** 206.
149. Sorof, S., Young, E. M., *Methods Cancer Res.,* **3,** 467, (1967).
150. Sorof, S., Young, E. M., McBride, R. A., Coffey, C. B., *Cancer Res.* (1970) **30,** 2029.
151. Sorof, S., Young, E. M., McBride, R. A., Coffey, C. B., Luongo, L., *Mol. Pharmacol.* (1969) **5,** 625.
152. Sani, B. P., Mott, D. M., Sorof, S., *Cancer Res.* (1974) **34,** 2476.
153. Ketterer, B., Christodoulides, L., *Chem.-Biol. Interact.* (1969) **1,** 173.
154. Litwack, G., Ketterer, B., Arias, I. M., *Nature* (1971) **234,** 466.
155. Ketterer, B., *Biochem. J.* (1971) **126,** 3P.
156. Singer, S., Litwack, G., *Cancer Res.* (1971) **31,** 1364.
157. Sugimoto, T., Terayama, H., *Chem.-Biol. Interact.* (1970) **2,** 391.
158. Sugimoto, T., Terayama, H., *Cancer Res.* (1971) **31,** 1478.
159. Barry, E. J., Ovechka, C. A., Gutmann, H. R., *J. Biol. Chem.* (1968) **243,** 51.
160. Tasseron, J. G., Diringer, H, Frohwirth, N., Mirvish, S. S., Heidelberger, C., *Biochemistry* (1970) **9,** 1636.
161. Kuroki, T., Heidelberger, C., *Biochemistry* (1972) **11,** 2116.
162. Albert, A. E., Warwick, G. P., *Chem.-Biol. Interact.* (1972) **5,** 61.
163. Farber, E., McConomy, J., Franzen, B., Marroquin, F., Stewart, G. A., Magee, P. N., *Cancer Res.* (1967) **27,** 1761.

164. Agarwal, M. K., Weinstein, I. B., *Biochemistry* (1970) **9**, 503.
165. Irving, C. C., Veazey, R. A., Williard, R. F., *Cancer Res.* (1967) **27**, 720.
166. Wunderlich, V., Schütt, M., Böttger, M., Graffi, A., *Biochem. J.* (1970) **118**, 99.
167. Wunderlich, V., Tetzlaff, I., Graffi, A., *Chem.-Biol. Interact.* (1972) **4**, 81.
168. King, C. M., Phillips, B., *Chem.-Biol. Interact.* (1970) **2**, 267.
169. Lesko, S. A., Jr., Smith, A., Ts'o, P. O. P., Umans, R. S., *Biochemistry* (1968) **7**, 434.
170. Pierce, G. B., *Fed. Proc. Fed. Amer. Soc. Exp. Biol.* (1970) **29**, 1248.
171. Braun, A. C., "Results and Problems in Cell Differentiation," (H. Ursprung, Ed.), Vol. 1, p. 128, Springer-Verlag, New York, 1968.
172. Melcher, G., "Mitteilungen aus der Max-Planck-Gesellschaft," Vol. 2, p. 72, Munich, 1971.
173. Bloch-Shtacher, N., Rabinowitz, Z., Sachs, L., *Int. J. Cancer* (1972) **9**, 632.
174. Nomura, S., Fischinger, P. J., Mattern, C. F. T., Peebles, P. T., Bassin, R. H., Friedman, G. P., *Virology* (1972) **50**, 51.
175. Miller, E. C., Miller, J. A., "Chemical Mutagens—Principles and Methods for Their Detection," A. Hollaender, Ed., Vol. 1, p. 83, Plenum Press, New York, 1971.
176. Boveri, T., "Zur Frage der Entstehung maligner Tumoren," Gustav Fischer, Jena, 1914.
177. Schwaier, R., Nashed, N., Zimmerman, F. K., *Mol. Gen. Genet.* (1968) **102**, 290.
178. Sager, R., "Cytoplasmic Genes and Organelles," pp. 105, 374, Academic, New York, 1972.
179. Temin, H. M., *J. Natl. Cancer Inst.* (1971) **46**, iii.
180. Speyer, J. F., Karam, J. D., Lenny, A. B., *Cold Spring Harb. Symp. Quant. Biol.*, 1966, **31**, 693.
181. Drake, J. W., Allen, E. F., *Cold Spring Harb. Symp. Quant. Biol.*, 1968, **33**, 339.
182. Muzyczks, N., Poland, R. L., Bessman, M. J., *J. Biol. Chem.* (1972) **247**, 7116.
183. Miller, J. A., Miller, E. C., *J. Natl. Cancer Inst.* (1971) **47**, vii.
184. Nelson, R. L., Mason, H. A., *J. Theor. Biol.* (1972) **37**, 197.
185. Borek, C., Sachs, L., *Proc. Natl. Acad. Sci., U.S.A.* (1967) **57**, 1522.
186. Loeb, L. A., Springgate, C. F., Battula, N., *Cancer Res.* (1974) **34**, 2311.
187. Gurdon, J. B., *Quarterly Rev. Biol.* (1963) **38**, 54.
188. Gurdon, J. B., "Current Topics in Developmental Biology," (Moscona, A. A., Monroy, A. Eds.), Vol. 1, p. 39, Academic Press, New York, 1970.
189. McKinnell, R. G., Deggins, B. A., Labat, D. D., *Science* (1969) **165**, 394.
190. "Results and Problems in Cell Differentiation," (H. Ursprung, Ed.), Vol. 1, Springer-Verlag, New York, 1968.
191. Price, P. J., Freeman, A. E., Lane, W. T., Huebner, R. J., *Nature New Biol.* (1971) **230**, 144.
192. Rhim, J. S., Cho, H. Y., Rabstein, L., Gordon, R. J., Bryan, R. J., Gardner, M. B., Huebner, R. J., *Nature* (1972) **239**, 103
193. Rhim, J. S., Vass, W., Cho, H. Y., Huebner, R. J., *Int. J. Cancer* (1971) **7**, 65.
194. Jacob, F., Monod, J., *Cold Spring Harb. Symp. Quant. Biol.* (1961) **26**, 193.
195. Pitot, H. C., Heidelberger, C., *Cancer Res.* (1963) **23**, 1964.
196. Church, R. B., McCarthy, B. J., *Proc. Nat. Acad. Sci., U.S.A.* (1967) **58**, 1548.
197. Church, R. B., McCarthy, B. J., *Biochim. Biophys. Acta* (1970) **199**, 103.
198. Drews, J., Brawerman, G., Morris, H. P., *Eur. J. Biochem.* (1968) **3**, 284.
199. Mendecki, J., Minc, B., Chorazy, M., *Biochem. Biophys. Res. Commun.* (1969) **36**, 494.

200. Shearer, R. W., Smuckler, E. A., *Cancer Res.* (1971) **31**, 2104.
201. *Ibid.*, **32**, 339.
202. Prehn, R. T., *Progr. Exp. Tumor Res.* (1971) **14**, 1.
203. Burnet, F. M., *Progr. Exp. Tumor Res.* (1970) **13**, 1.
204. Furth, J., *Harvey Lectures* (1969) **63**, 47.
205. Boutwell, R. K., *Progr. Exp. Tumor Res.* (1964) **4**, 207.
206. Boutwell, R. K., *CRC Critical Rev. Toxicol.* (1973) **2**, 418.
207. Roe, F. J., Carter, R. L., Mitchley, C. V., Peto, R., Hecker, E., *Int. J. Cancer* (1972) **9**, 264.
208. Legator, M. S., Malling, H. V., "Chemical Mutagens—Principles and Methods for Their Detection," (A. Hollaender, Ed.), Vol. 2, p. 569, Plenum, New York, 1971.
209. Ames, B. N., Durston, W. E., Yamasaki, E., Lee, F. D., *Proc. Nat. Acad. Sci., U.S.* (1973) **70**, 2281.
210. Heidelberger, C., *Advan. Cancer Res.* (1973) **18**, 317.
211. DiPaolo, J. A., Nelson, R. L., Donovan, P. J., *Nature (London)* (1972) **235**, 278.

Work supported by grants CA-07175 and CA-15785 of the National Institutes of Health, U.S. Public Health Service.

Index

Index

I

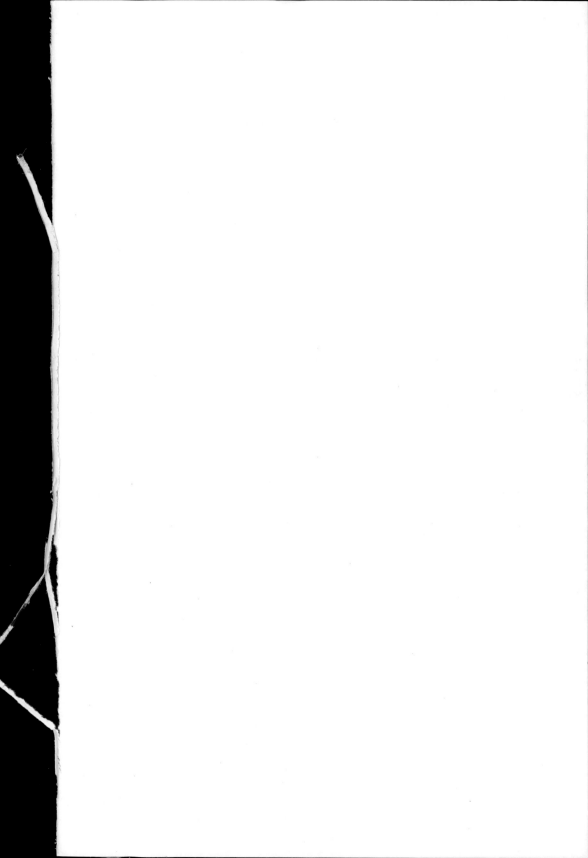